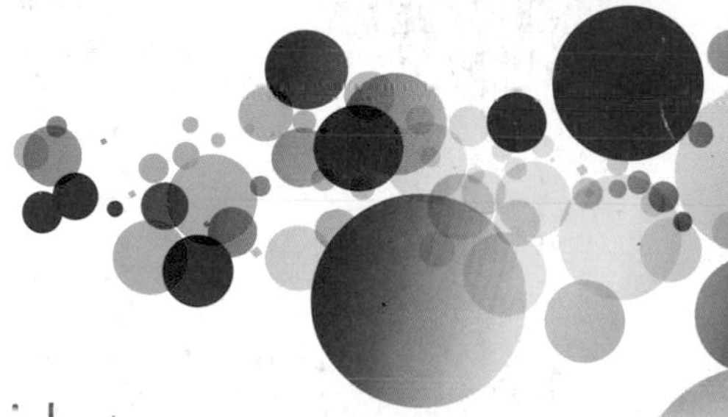

Mosby's Guide to

NURSING DIAGNOSIS

REVISED REPRINT WITH 2021-2023 NANDA-I® UPDATES

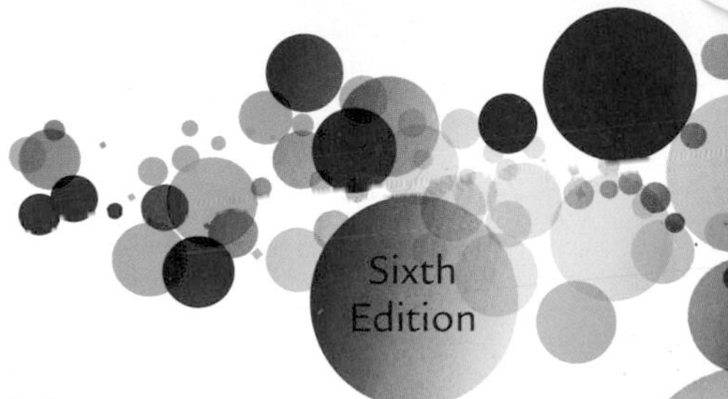

Mosby's Guide to

NURSING DIAGNOSIS

REVISED REPRINT WITH 2021-2023 NANDA-I® UPDATES

Gail B. Ladwig, MSN, RN

Betty J. Ackley, MSN, EdS, RN

Mary Beth Flynn Makic, PhD, RN, CCNS, FAAN, FNAP

Marina Reyna Martinez-Kratz, MS, RN, CNE

Melody Zanotti, BA, RN, LSW

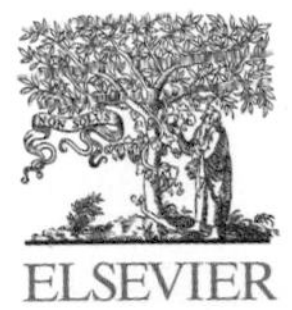
ELSEVIER

MOSBY'S GUIDE TO NURSING DIAGNOSIS, SIXTH EDITION
REVISED REPRINT WITH 2021-2023 NANDA-I® UPDATES ISBN: 978-0-323-87511-0

Senior Content Strategist: Sandra Clark
Senior Content Development Specialist: Jennifer Wade
Publishing Services Manager: Shereen Jameel
Project Manager: Rukmani Krishnan
Design Direction: Patrick Ferguson

Printed in Canada

Last digit is the print number: 9 8 7 6 5 4 3 2 1

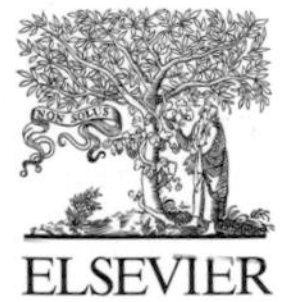

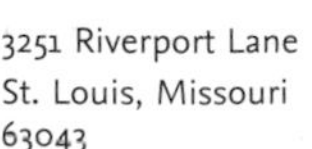

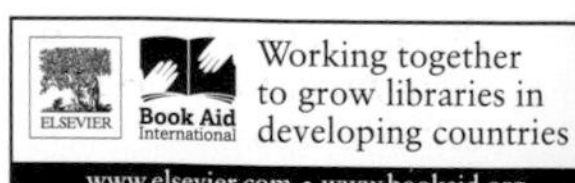

DEDICATION

In Loving Memory of Betty J. Ackley

Betty believed in dreams. This textbook was our dream. We set out to write the best nursing diagnosis textbook ever. Our book is now in 1400 nursing programs. I think her dream is realized. From a handout to students to an international publication. This is our 6th year of publication. Betty passed away in December 2014 at her home with her husband (Dale) and daughter (Dawn) present.

Thank you, dear friend Betty.

Betty saw a need and was able to help fill that need by working to complete this book and see it through to publication. She was very proud of each edition of this book. She always strived to make each edition as good as it could be.

Betty was a loving daughter, grandmother, mother, and wife. She cared about people and was always helping everyone to be their very best. This book will continue to be her way of giving to the profession she loved. Nursing gave a lot to Betty, and she returned the love of nursing by writing the most helpful book she could write.

Dale Ackley

Also Dedicated to

Jerry Ladwig, my wonderful husband, who, after 54 years, is still supportive and helpful—he has been "my right-hand man" in every revision of this book. Also, to my very special children, their spouses, and all of my grandchildren: Jerry, Kathy, Alexandra, Elizabeth, and Benjamin Ladwig; Christine, John, Sean, Ciara, and Bridget McMahon; Jennifer, Jim, Abby, Katelyn, Blake, and Connor Martin; Amy, Scott, Ford, and Vaughn Bertram—the greatest family anyone could ever hope for. A special thank you to my grandson Sean for his work on checking and incorporating the correct/new NANDA language for the diagnoses that I worked on.

Gail B. Ladwig

Thank you to my husband, Zlatko, and children, Alexander and Erik, whose unconditional love and support are ever present in my life. To my parents and sisters for always encouraging me to follow my passion. To Gail, for her incredible leadership and mentorship throughout the rigorous process of revising this essential text. And finally, to Betty, for her unwavering commitment to the profession of nursing through her roles as an expert teacher and prolific author. You are deeply missed but your spirit continues to inform nursing practice excellence.

Mary Beth Flynn Makic

To my best friend and the love of my life Kent Martinez-Kratz. To my children, Maxwell, Jesse and Sierra, whose love, inspiration and wit make my life complete. To my first fans, my parents and siblings. To Gail, for being the absolute best nursing professor, mentor, and comadre. And finally, to Betty's memory, for inspiring excellence in nursing education and practice.

Marina Martinez-Kratz

Thank you to my husband Marty for his infinite patience and encouragement in all my endeavors. To my amazing children, their spouses, and my grandchildren: Rachael, Frank, Corey, Zak, Dominic and Dylan, for their unconditional love and inspiration.

Thank you to my friend and mentor—Gail Ladwig—for offering me the opportunity to contribute to this incredible textbook. Your gifts of friendship, knowledge and positivity will stay with me forever. Your lifelong dedication and commitment to the field of nursing are truly inspiring.

Melody Zanotti

ACKNOWLEDGMENTS

The authors would like to thank the following individuals for their contributions to *Nursing Diagnosis Handbook: An Evidence-Based Guide to Planning Care*, Twelfth edition, by Betty J. Ackley, Gail B. Ladwig, Mary Beth Flynn Makic, Marina Martinez-Kratz, and Melody Zanotti, from which this book has been developed:

Michelle Acorn, DNP, NP PHC/Adult, BA, BScN/PHCNP, MN/ACNP, GNC(C), CGP

Keith Anderson, PhD, MSW

Amanda Andrews, BSc (Hons), MA

Kathaleen C. Bloom, PhD, CNM

Kathleen Patricia Buckheit, MPH, BSN, RN, CEN, COHN-S/CM, CCM, FAAOHN

Elyse Bueno, MS, ACCNS-AG, CCRN

Elizabeth Burkhart, PhD, RN, ANEF

Melodie Cannon, DNP, MSc/FNP, BHScN, RN(EC), NP-PHC, CEN, GNC(C)

Stacey Carroll, PhD, APRN-BC

Krystal Chamberlain, BSN, RN, CCRN

Nadia Charania, PhD, RN

Nichol Chesser, RN, CNM, DNP

JoAnn Coar, BSN, RN-BC, CWOCN, COS-C

Maureen F. Cooney, DNP, FNP-BC

Tara Cuccinelli, RN, MS, AGCNS-BC

Ruth Curchoe, RN, BSN, MSN, CIC

Mary Rose Day, DN, MA, PGDip PHN, BSc, Dip. Management (RCSI), RPHN, RM, RGN

Mary Alice DeWys, RN, BS, CIMI

Susan Dirkes, RN, MS, CCRN

Julianne E. Doubet, BSN, RN, EMT-B

Lorriane Duggan, MSN, ACNP-BC

Dawn Fairlie, PhD, NP

Arlene T. Farren, PhD, RN, AOCN, CTN-A, CNE

Judith Ann Floyd, PhD, RN, FNAP, FAAN

Katherine Foss, MSN, RN

Shari Froelich DNP, MSN, MSBA, ANP, BC, ACHPN, PMHNP, BC

Tracy P. George, DNP, APRN-BC, CNE

Susanne W. Gibbons PhD, C-ANP/GNP

Barbara Given, PhD, RN, FAAN

Sherry A. Greenberg, PhD, RN, GNP-BC

Marloes Harkema, BA

Dianne F. Hayward, RN, MSN, WHNP

Dina Hewett, PhD, RN, NEA-BC, CCRN-A

Patricia Hindin, PhD, CNM

Jackie Hogan, RD, CSO, LD

Paula D. Hopper MSN, RN, CNE

Wendie A. Howland, MN, RN-BC, CRRN, CCM, CNLCP, LNCC

Teri Hulett, RN, BSN, CIC, FAPIC

Olga F. Jarrín, PhD, RN

Rebecca Johnson, PhD, RN, FAAN, FNAP

Catherine Kleiner, PhD, MSN, BSN

Gail B. Ladwig, MSN, RN

Rosemary Koehl Lee, DNP, ARNP, ACNP-BC, CCNS, CCRN

Ellen MacKinnon, MS, RN, CNRN, AGCNS-BC

Mary Beth Flynn Makic, PhD, RN, CCNS, FAAN, FNAP

Marina Reyna Martinez-Kratz, MS, RN, CNE

Lauren McAlister, MSN, FNP, DNP Candidate

Marsha McKenzie, MA Ed, BSN, RN

Pauline McKinney Green, PhD, RN, CNE

Kimberly S. Meyer, PhD, ACNP-BC, CNRN

Annie Muller, DNP, APRN-BC

Morgan Nestingen, MSN, AGCNS, ONS

Katherina A. Nikzad-Terhune, PhD, MSW

Darcy O'Banion, RN, MS, ACCNS-AG

Mary E. Oesterle, MA, CCC-SLP

Wolter Paans, PhD
Margaret Padnos, RN, AB, BSN, MA
Kathleen Patusky, MA, PhD, RN, CNS
Kim Paxton, DNP, APRN, ANP-BC, LHIT-C
Sherry Pomeroy, PhD, RN
Ann Will Poteet, MS, RN, CNS, AGNP-C
Kerri Reid, MS, CNS, CCRN-K
Lori Rhudy, PhD, RN, CNRN, ACNS-BC
Shelley Sadler, BSN, MSN, APRN, WHNP-BC
Debra Siela, PhD, RN, CCNS, ACNS-BC, CCRN-K, CNE, RRT
Kimberly Silvey, MSN, RN, RAC-CT
Tammy Spencer, DNP, RN, CNE, AGCNS-BC, CCNS
Bernie St. Aubyn, BSc (hons), MSc
Elaine E. Steinke, PhD, APRN, CNS-BC, FAHA, FAAN
Denise Sullivan, MSN, ANP-BC
Cynthia DeLeon Thelen, MSN, BSN, RN
Rosemary Timmerman, DNP, APRN, CCNS, CCRN-CSC-CMC
Janelle Tipton, MSN, RN, AOCN
Stephanie Turrise, PhD, MSN, BSN
Carolien van der Velde
Anna van der Woude
Barbara Baele Vincensi, PhD, RN, FNP
Kerstin West-Wilson, BS, MS, BSN, RN, MS, IBCLC
Barbara Wheeler, RN, BN, MN, IBCLC
Suzanne White, MSN, RN, PHCNS, BC
Linda Williams, RN, MSN
Ruth A. Wittmann-Price, PhD, RN, CNS, CHSE, CNE, ANEF, FAAN
Melody Zanotti, BA, RN, LSW
Milou Zemering, BN

HOW TO USE *MOSBY'S GUIDE TO NURSING DIAGNOSIS*

Assess

Assess the client using the format provided by the clinical setting. Collect data including client's symptoms, clinical state, and known medical or psychiatric diagnoses.

Diagnosis

Use Section I, Guide to Nursing Diagnoses, and locate the client's symptoms, clinical state, medical or psychiatric diagnoses, and anticipated or prescribed diagnostic studies or surgical interventions (listed in alphabetical order). Note suggestions for appropriate nursing diagnoses.

Then use Section II, Guide to Planning Care, to evaluate each suggested nursing diagnosis and "related to" etiology statement. Section II is a listing of care plans according to NANDA-I, arranged alphabetically by diagnostic concept, for each nursing diagnosis referred to in Section I. Determine the appropriateness of each nursing diagnosis by comparing the Defining Characteristics and/or Risk Factors to the client data collected.

Determine Outcomes

Use Section II, Guide to Planning Care, to find appropriate outcomes for the client.

Plan Interventions

Use Section II, Guide to Planning Care, to find appropriate interventions for the client.

Give Nursing Care

Administer nursing care following the plan of care based on the interventions.

Evaluate Nursing Care

Evaluate nursing care administered using the Client Outcomes. If the outcomes were not met, and the nursing interventions were not effective, reassess the client and determine if the appropriate nursing diagnoses were made.

Document

Document all of the previous steps using the format provided in the clinical setting.

CONTENTS

SECTION I

Guide to Nursing Diagnoses

Section I is an alphabetical listing of client symptoms, client problems, medical diagnoses, psychosocial diagnoses, and clinical states. Each of these will have a list of possible nursing diagnoses. You may use this section to find suggestions for nursing diagnoses for your client.

- Assess the client using the format provided by the clinical setting.
- Locate the client's symptoms, problems, clinical state, diagnoses, surgeries, and diagnostic testing in the alphabetical listing contained in this section.
- Note suggestions given for appropriate nursing diagnoses.
- Evaluate the suggested nursing diagnoses to determine whether they are appropriate for the client and have information that was found in the assessment.
- Use Section II (which contains an alphabetized list of all NANDA-I approved nursing diagnoses) to validate this information and check the definition, related factors, and defining characteristics. Determine whether the nursing diagnosis you have selected is appropriate for the client.

A

A

ABDOMINAL DISTENTION

Constipation r/t decreased activity, decreased fluid intake, decreased fiber intake, pathological process

Dysfunctional Gastrointestinal motility r/t decreased perfusion of intestines, medication effect

Nausea r/t irritation of gastrointestinal tract

Imbalanced Nutrition: less than body requirements r/t nausea, vomiting

Acute Pain r/t retention of air, gastrointestinal secretions

Delayed Surgical recovery r/t retention of gas, secretions

ABDOMINAL HYSTERECTOMY

See Hysterectomy

ABDOMINAL PAIN

Dysfunctional Gastrointestinal motility r/t decreased perfusion, medication effect

Acute Pain r/t injury, pathological process

ABDOMINAL SURGERY

Constipation r/t decreased activity, decreased fluid intake, anesthesia, sopioids

Dysfunctional Gastrointestinal motility r/t medication or anesthesia effect, trauma from surgery

Imbalanced Nutrition: less than body requirements r/t high metabolic needs, decreased ability to ingest or digest food

Acute Pain r/t surgical procedure

Ineffective peripheral Tissue Perfusion r/t immobility, abdominal surgery

Risk for delayed Surgical recovery r/t extensive surgical procedure

Risk for Surgical Site Infection: Risk factor: invasive procedure

Readiness for enhanced Knowledge: expresses an interest in learning

See Surgery, Perioperative Care; Surgery, Postoperative Care; Surgery, Preoperative Care

ABDOMINAL TRAUMA

Disturbed Body Image r/t scarring, change in body function, need for temporary colostomy

Ineffective Breathing pattern r/t abdominal distention, pain

Deficient Fluid volume r/t hemorrhage, active fluid volume loss

Dysfunctional Gastrointestinal motility r/t decreased perfusion

Acute Pain r/t abdominal trauma

Risk for Bleeding: Risk factor: trauma and possible contusion/rupture of abdominal organs

Risk for Infection: Risk factor: possible perforation of abdominal structures

ABLATION, RADIOFREQUENCY CATHETER

Fear r/t invasive procedure

Risk for decreased Cardiac tissue perfusion: Risk factor: catheterization of heart

ABORTION, INDUCED

Compromised family Coping r/t unresolved feelings about decision

Acute Pain r/t surgical intervention

Chronic low Self-Esteem r/t feelings of guilt

Chronic Sorrow r/t loss of potential child

Risk for Bleeding: Risk factor: trauma from abortion

Risk for delayed Child Development: Risk factors: unplanned or unwanted pregnancy

Risk for Infection: Risk factors: open uterine blood vessels, dilated cervix

Risk for Post-Trauma syndrome: Risk factor: psychological trauma of abortion

Risk for Spiritual distress: Risk factor: perceived moral implications of decision

Readiness for enhanced Health literacy: expresses desire to enhance personal healthcare decisions

Readiness for enhanced Knowledge: expresses an interest in learning

ABORTION, SPONTANEOUS

Disturbed Body Image r/t perceived inability to carry pregnancy, produce child

Disabled family Coping r/t unresolved feelings about loss

Ineffective Coping r/t personal vulnerability

Interrupted Family processes r/t unmet expectations for pregnancy and childbirth

Fear r/t implications for future pregnancies

Acute Pain r/t uterine contractions, surgical intervention

Situational low Self-Esteem r/t feelings about loss of fetus

Chronic Sorrow r/t loss of potential child

Risk for Bleeding: Risk factor: trauma from abortion

Risk for Infection: Risk factors: septic or incomplete abortion of products of conception, open uterine blood vessels, dilated cervix

Risk for Post-Trauma syndrome: Risk factor: psychological trauma of abortion

Risk for Spiritual distress: Risk factor: loss of fetus

Readiness for enhanced Knowledge: expresses an interest in learning

ABRUPTIO PLACENTAE <36 WEEKS

Anxiety r/t unknown outcome, change in birth plans

Death Anxiety r/t unknown outcome, hemorrhage, or pain

Interrupted Family processes r/t unmet expectations for pregnancy and childbirth

Fear r/t threat to well-being of self and fetus

Impaired Gas exchange: placental r/t decreased uteroplacental area

Acute Pain r/t irritable uterus, hypertonic uterus

Impaired Tissue integrity: maternal r/t possible uterine rupture

Risk for Bleeding: Risk factor: separation of placenta from uterus causing bleeding

Risk for Infection: Risk factor: partial separation of placenta

Risk for disturbed Maternal–Fetal dyad: Risk factors: trauma of process, lack of energy of mother

Risk for Shock: Risk factor: separation of placenta from uterus

Readiness for enhanced Knowledge: expresses an interest in learning

ABSCESS FORMATION

Ineffective Protection r/t inadequate nutrition, abnormal blood profile, drug therapy, depressed immune function

Impaired Tissue integrity r/t altered circulation, nutritional deficit or excess

Readiness for enhanced Knowledge: expresses an interest in learning

ABUSE, CHILD

See Child Abuse

ABUSE, SPOUSE, PARENT, OR SIGNIFICANT OTHER

Anxiety r/t threat to self-concept, situational crisis of abuse

Caregiver Role Strain r/t chronic illness, self-care deficits, lack of respite care, extent of caregiving required

Impaired verbal Communication r/t psychological barriers of fear

Compromised family Coping r/t abusive patterns

Defensive Coping r/t low self-esteem

Dysfunctional Family processes r/t inadequate coping skills

A

Insomnia r/t psychological stress

Post-Trauma syndrome r/t history of abuse

Powerlessness r/t lifestyle of helplessness

Chronic low Self-Esteem r/t negative family interactions

Risk for impaired emancipated Decision-Making: Risk factor: inability to verbalize needs and wants

Risk for self-directed Violence: Risk factor: history of abuse

ACCESSORY MUSCLE USE (TO BREATHE)

Ineffective Breathing pattern (See **Breathing** pattern, ineffective, Section II)

See Asthma; Bronchitis; COPD (Chronic Obstructive Pulmonary Disease); Respiratory Infections, Acute Childhood (Croup, Epiglottis, Pertussis, Pneumonia, Respiratory Syncytial Virus)

ACCIDENT PRONE

Frail Elderly syndrome r/t history of falls

Acute Confusion r/t altered level of consciousness

Ineffective Coping r/t personal vulnerability, situational crises

Ineffective Impulse control (See **Impulse** control, ineffective, Section II)

Risk for Injury: Risk factor: history of accidents

ACHALASIA

Ineffective Coping r/t chronic disease

Acute Pain r/t stasis of food in esophagus

Impaired Swallowing r/t neuromuscular impairment

Risk for Aspiration: Risk factor: nocturnal regurgitation

ACID-BASE IMBALANCES

Risk for Electrolyte imbalance: Risk factors: renal dysfunction, diarrhea, treatment-related side effects (e.g., medications, drains)

ACIDOSIS, METABOLIC

Acute Confusion r/t acid-base imbalance, associated electrolyte imbalance

Impaired Memory r/t effect of metabolic acidosis on brain function

Imbalanced Nutrition: **less than body requirements** r/t inability to ingest, absorb nutrients

Risk for Electrolyte imbalance: Risk factor: effect of metabolic acidosis on renal function

Risk for Injury: Risk factors: disorientation, weakness, stupor

Risk for decreased Cardiac tissue perfusion: Risk factor: dysrhythmias from hyperkalemia

Risk for Shock: Risk factors: abnormal metabolic state, presence of acid state impairing function, decreased tissue perfusion

ACIDOSIS, RESPIRATORY

Decreased Activity tolerance r/t imbalance between oxygen supply and demand

Impaired Gas exchange r/t ventilation-perfusion imbalance

Impaired Memory r/t hypoxia

Risk for decreased Cardiac tissue perfusion: Risk factor: dysrhythmias associated with respiratory acidosis

ACNE

Disturbed Body Image r/t biophysical changes associated with skin disorder

Ineffective Health self-management r/t insufficient knowledge of therapeutic regimen

Impaired Skin integrity r/t hormonal changes (adolescence, menstrual cycle)

ACROMEGALY

Decreased Activity tolerance (See **Decreased** Activity tolerance, Section II)

Ineffective Airway clearance r/t airway obstruction by enlarged tongue

Disturbed Body Image r/t changes in body function and appearance

Impaired physical Mobility r/t joint pain

Risk for decreased Cardiac tissue perfusion: Risk factor: increased atherosclerosis from abnormal health status

Risk for unstable blood Glucose level: Risk factor: abnormal physical health status

Sexual dysfunction r/t changes in hormonal secretions

Risk for Overweight: Risk factor: energy expenditure less than energy intake

DECREASED ACTIVITY TOLERANCE, POTENTIAL TO DEVELOP

Decreased Activity tolerance (See **Decreased** Activity intolerance, Section II)

ACUTE ABDOMINAL PAIN

Deficient Fluid volume r/t air and fluids trapped in bowel, inability to drink

Acute Pain r/t pathological process

Risk for dysfunctional Gastrointestinal motility: Risk factor: ineffective gastrointestinal tissue perfusion

See Abdominal Pain

ACUTE ALCOHOL INTOXICATION

Ineffective Breathing pattern r/t depression of the respiratory center from excessive alcohol intake

Acute Confusion r/t central nervous system depression

Dysfunctional Family processes r/t abuse of alcohol

Risk for Aspiration: Risk factor: depressed reflexes with acute vomiting

Risk for Infection: Risk factor: impaired immune system from malnutrition associated with chronic excessive alcohol intake

Risk for Injury: Risk factor: chemical (alcohol)

ACUTE BACK PAIN

Anxiety r/t situational crisis, back injury

Constipation r/t decreased activity, effect of pain medication

Ineffective Coping r/t situational crisis, back injury

Impaired physical Mobility r/t pain

Acute Pain r/t back injury

Readiness for enhanced Knowledge: expresses an interest in learning

ACUTE CONFUSION

See Confusion, Acute

ACUTE CORONARY SYNDROME

Decreased Cardiac output r/t cardiac disorder

Risk for decreased Cardiac tissue perfusion (See **Cardiac** tissue perfusion, risk for decreased, Section II)

See Angina; Myocardial Infarction (MI)

ACUTE LYMPHOCYTIC LEUKEMIA (ALL)

See Cancer; Chemotherapy; Child with Chronic Condition; Leukemia

ACUTE RENAL FAILURE

See Renal Failure

ACUTE RESPIRATORY DISTRESS SYNDROME

See ARDS (Acute Respiratory Distress Syndrome)

ACUTE SUBSTANCE WITHDRAWAL SYNDROME

Anxiety r/t unknown outcome of withdrawal sequence, physiological effects

Imbalanced Energy Field r/t hyperactivity of energy flow

Impaired Comfort r/t restlessness and agitation

Acute Confusion r/t effects of substance withdrawal

Ineffective Coping r/t situational crisis, withdrawal

Labile Emotional Control r/t lack of control over the progression of withdrawal process

A

Fear r/t threat to well-being of self

Insomnia r/t physical and psychological effects of substance withdrawal

Imbalanced Nutrition: **less than body requirements** r/t nausea, anxiety

Powerlessness r/t loss of ability to control withdrawal process

Risk for acute Confusion: Risk factor: possible alteration in level of consciousness

Risk for Injury: Risk factor: alteration in sensory perceptual functioning

Risk for Suicidal Behavior: Risk factor: psychic pain

Risk for other-directed Violence: Risk factors: poor impulse control, hallucinations

Risk for self-directed Violence: Risk factors: poor impulse control, hallucinations

ADAMS–STOKES SYNDROME

See Dysrhythmia

ADDICTION

See Alcoholism; Substance Abuse

ADDISON'S DISEASE

Decreased Activity tolerance r/t weakness, fatigue

Disturbed Body Image r/t increased skin pigmentation

Deficient Fluid volume r/t failure of regulatory mechanisms

Imbalanced Nutrition: **less than body requirements** r/t chronic illness

Risk for Injury: Risk factor: weakness

Readiness for enhanced Knowledge: expresses an interest in learning

ADENOIDECTOMY

Acute Pain r/t surgical incision

Ineffective Airway clearance r/t hesitation or reluctance to cough as a result of pain, fear

Nausea r/t anesthesia effects, drainage from surgery

Acute Pain r/t surgical incision

Risk for Aspiration: Risk factors: postoperative drainage, impaired swallowing

Risk for Bleeding: Risk factor: surgical incision

Risk for deficient Fluid volume: Risk factors: decreased intake as a result of painful swallowing, effects of anesthesia

Risk for Dry Mouth: Risk factor: mouth breathing due to nasal congestion

Risk for imbalanced Nutrition: **less than body requirements**: Risk factor: reluctance to swallow

Readiness for enhanced Knowledge: expresses an interest in learning

ADHESIONS, LYSIS OF

See Abdominal Surgery

ADJUSTMENT DISORDER

Anxiety r/t inability to cope with psychosocial stressor

Labile Emotional Control r/t emotional disturbance

Risk-prone Health behavior r/t assault to self-esteem

Disturbed personal Identity r/t psychosocial stressor (specific to individual)

Situational low Self-Esteem r/t change in role function

Impaired Social interaction r/t absence of significant others or peers

ADJUSTMENT IMPAIRMENT

Risk-prone Health behavior (See **Health** behavior, risk-prone, Section II)

ADOLESCENT, PREGNANT

Anxiety r/t situational and maturational crisis, pregnancy

Disturbed Body Image r/t pregnancy superimposed on developing body

Decisional Conflict: **keeping child versus giving up child versus abortion** r/t lack of experience with decision-making, interference with decision-making, multiple or divergent sources of information, lack of support system

Disabled family Coping r/t highly ambivalent family relationships, chronically unresolved feelings of guilt, anger, despair

Ineffective Coping r/t situational and maturational crisis, personal vulnerability

Ineffective Denial r/t fear of consequences of pregnancy becoming known

Ineffective adolescent Eating dynamics r/t lack of knowledge of nutritional needs during pregnancy

Interrupted Family processes r/t unmet expectations for adolescent, situational crisis

Fear r/t labor and delivery

Deficient Knowledge r/t pregnancy, infant growth and development, parenting

Imbalanced Nutrition: less than body requirements r/t lack of knowledge of nutritional needs during pregnancy and as growing adolescent

Ineffective Role performance r/t pregnancy

Situational low Self-Esteem r/t feelings of shame and guilt about becoming or being pregnant

Impaired Social interaction r/t self-concept disturbance

Social Isolation r/t absence of supportive significant others

Risk for impaired Attachment: Risk factor: anxiety associated with the parent role

Risk for delayed Child Development: Risk factor: unplanned or unwanted pregnancy

Risk for urge urinary Incontinence: Risk factor: pressure on bladder by growing uterus

Risk for disturbed Maternal–Fetal dyad: Risk factors: immaturity, substance use

Risk for impaired Parenting: Risk factors: adolescent parent, unplanned or unwanted pregnancy, single parent

Readiness for enhanced Childbearing process: reports appropriate prenatal lifestyle

Readiness for enhanced Health literacy: expresses desire to enhance social support for health

Readiness for enhanced Knowledge: expresses an interest in learning

ADOPTION, GIVING CHILD UP FOR

Decisional Conflict r/t unclear personal values or beliefs, perceived threat to value system, support system deficit

Ineffective Coping r/t stress of loss of child

Interrupted Family processes r/t conflict within family regarding relinquishment of child

Insomnia r/t depression or trauma of relinquishment of child

Social isolation r/t making choice that goes against values of significant others

Chronic Sorrow r/t loss of relationship with child

Risk for Spiritual distress: Risk factor: perceived moral implications of decision

Readiness for enhanced Spiritual well-being: harmony with self-regarding final decision

ADRENOCORTICAL INSUFFICIENCY

Deficient Fluid volume r/t insufficient ability to reabsorb water

Ineffective Protection r/t inability to tolerate stress

Delayed Surgical recovery r/t inability to respond to stress

Risk for Shock: Risk factors: deficient fluid volume, decreased cortisol to initiate stress response to insult to body

See Addison's Disease; Shock, Hypovolemic

ADVANCE DIRECTIVES

Death Anxiety r/t planning for end-of-life health decisions

A

Decisional Conflict r/t unclear personal values or beliefs, perceived threat to value system, support system deficit

Readiness for enhanced Spiritual well-being: harmonious interconnectedness with self, others, higher power, God

AFFECTIVE DISORDERS

See Depression (Major Depressive Disorder); Dysthymic Disorder; Manic Disorder, Bipolar I; SAD (Seasonal Affective Disorder)

AGE-RELATED MACULAR DEGENERATION

See Macular Degeneration

AGGRESSIVE BEHAVIOR

Fear r/t real or imagined threat to own well-being

Risk for other-directed Violence (See **Violence**, other-directed, risk for, Section II)

AGING

Death Anxiety r/t fear of unknown, loss of self, impact on significant others

Impaired Dentition r/t ineffective oral hygiene

Risk for Frail Elderly syndrome: Risk factors: >70 years, decreased activity tolerance, impaired vision

Ineffective health maintenance behaviors r/t powerlessness

Hearing Loss r/t exposure to loud noises, aging

Disability-associated urinary Incontinence r/t impaired vision, impaired cognition, neuromuscular limitations, altered environmental factors

Impaired Resilience r/t aging, multiple losses

Sleep deprivation r/t aging-related sleep-stage shifts

Risk for Caregiver Role Strain: Risk factor: inability to handle increasing needs of significant other

Risk for Impaired emancipated Decision-Making: Risk factor: inability to process information regarding healthcare decisions

Risk for Injury: Risk factors: vision loss, hearing loss, decreased balance, decreased sensation in feet

Risk for Loneliness: Risk factors: inadequate support system, role transition, health alterations, depression, fatigue

Risk for Ineffective Thermoregulation: Risk factor: aging

Readiness for enhanced community Coping: providing social support and other resources identified as needed for elderly client

Readiness for enhanced family Coping: ability to gratify needs, address adaptive tasks

Readiness for enhanced Health Self-management: knowledge about medication, nutrition, exercise, coping strategies

Readiness for enhanced Knowledge: specify need to improve health

Readiness for enhanced Nutrition: need to improve health

Readiness for enhanced Relationship: demonstrates understanding of partner's insufficient function

Readiness for enhanced Sleep: need to improve sleep

Readiness for enhanced Spiritual well-being: one's experience of life's meaning, harmony with self, others, higher power, God, environment

AGITATION

Acute Confusion r/t side effects of medication, hypoxia, decreased cerebral perfusion, alcohol abuse or withdrawal, substance abuse or withdrawal, sensory deprivation or overload

Sleep deprivation r/t sustained inadequate sleep hygiene, sundown syndrome

AGORAPHOBIA

Anxiety r/t real or perceived threat to physical integrity

Ineffective Coping r/t inadequate support systems

Fear r/t leaving home, going out in public places

Impaired Social interaction r/t disturbance in self-concept

Social Isolation r/t altered thought process

AGRANULOCYTOSIS

Delayed Surgical recovery r/t abnormal blood profile

Risk for Infection: Risk factor: abnormal blood profile

Readiness for enhanced Knowledge: expresses an interest in learning

AIDS (ACQUIRED IMMUNODEFICIENCY SYNDROME)

Death Anxiety r/t fear of premature death

Disturbed Body Image r/t chronic contagious illness, cachexia

Caregiver Role Strain r/t unpredictable illness course, presence of situation stressors

Diarrhea r/t inflammatory bowel changes

Interrupted Family processes r/t distress about diagnosis of human immunodeficiency virus (HIV) infection

Fatigue r/t disease process, stress, decreased nutritional intake

Fear r/t powerlessness, threat to well-being

Hopelessness r/t deteriorating physical condition

Imbalanced Nutrition: less than body requirements r/t decreased ability to eat and absorb nutrients as a result of anorexia, nausea, diarrhea; oral candidiasis

Chronic Pain r/t tissue inflammation and destruction

Impaired Resilience r/t chronic illness

Situational low Self-Esteem r/t crisis of chronic contagious illness

Ineffective Sexuality pattern r/t possible transmission of disease

Social isolation r/t self-concept disturbance, therapeutic isolation

Chronic Sorrow r/t chronic illness

Spiritual distress r/t challenged beliefs or moral system

Risk for deficient Fluid volume: Risk factors: diarrhea, vomiting, fever, bleeding

Risk for Infection: Risk factor: inadequate immune system

Risk for Loneliness: Risk factor: social isolation

Risk for impaired Oral Mucous Membrane Integrity: Risk factor: immunological deficit

Risk for impaired Skin integrity: Risk factors: immunological deficit, diarrhea

Risk for Spiritual distress: Risk factor: physical illness

Readiness for enhanced Health literacy: expresses desire to enhance understanding of health information to make healthcare choices

Readiness for enhanced Knowledge: expresses an interest in learning

See AIDS, Child; Cancer; Pneumonia

AIDS, CHILD

Impaired Parenting r/t congenital acquisition of infection secondary to intravenous (IV) drug use, multiple sexual partners, history of contaminated blood transfusion

See AIDS (Acquired Immunodeficiency Syndrome); Child with Chronic Condition; Hospitalized Child; Terminally Ill Child, Adolescent; Terminally Ill Child, Infant/Toddler; Terminally Ill Child, Preschool Child; Terminally Ill Child, School-Age Child/Preadolescent; Terminally Ill Child/Death of Child, Parent

A

AIDS DEMENTIA

Chronic Confusion r/t viral invasion of nervous system

See Dementia

AIRWAY OBSTRUCTION/ SECRETIONS

Ineffective Airway clearance (See **Airway** clearance, ineffective, Section II)

ALCOHOL WITHDRAWAL

Anxiety r/t situational crisis, withdrawal

Acute Confusion r/t effects of alcohol withdrawal

Ineffective Coping r/t personal vulnerability

Dysfunctional Family processes r/t abuse of alcohol

Insomnia r/t effect of alcohol withdrawal, anxiety

Imbalanced Nutrition: less than body requirements r/t poor dietary habits

Chronic low Self-Esteem r/t repeated unmet expectations

Risk for deficient Fluid volume: Risk factors: excessive diaphoresis, agitation, decreased fluid intake

Risk for other-directed Violence: Risk factor: substance withdrawal

Risk for self-directed Violence: Risk factor: substance withdrawal

Readiness for enhanced Knowledge: expresses an interest in learning

ALCOHOLISM

Anxiety r/t loss of control

Risk-prone Health behavior r/t lack of motivation to change behaviors, addiction

Acute Confusion r/t alcohol abuse

Chronic Confusion r/t neurological effects of chronic alcohol intake

Defensive Coping r/t denial of reality of addiction

Disabled family Coping r/t codependency issues due to alcoholism

Ineffective Coping r/t use of alcohol to cope with life events

Labile Emotional Control r/t substance abuse

Ineffective Denial r/t refusal to acknowledge addiction

Dysfunctional Family processes r/t alcohol abuse

Ineffective Home Maintenance Behaviors r/t memory deficits, fatigue

Insomnia r/t irritability, nightmares, tremors

Impaired Memory r/t alcohol abuse

Self-Neglect r/t effects of alcohol abuse

Imbalanced Nutrition: less than body requirements r/t anorexia, inappropriate diet with increased carbohydrates

Powerlessness r/t alcohol addiction

Ineffective Protection r/t malnutrition, sleep deprivation

Chronic low Self-Esteem r/t failure at life events

Social isolation r/t unacceptable social behavior, values

Risk for Injury: Risk factor: alteration in sensory or perceptual function

Risk for Loneliness: Risk factor: unacceptable social behavior

Risk for other-directed Violence: Risk factors: reactions to substances used, impulsive behavior, disorientation, impaired judgment

Risk for self-directed Violence: Risk factors: reactions to substances used, impulsive behavior, disorientation, impaired judgment

ALCOHOLISM, DYSFUNCTIONAL FAMILY PROCESSES

Dysfunctional Family processes (See **Family** processes, dysfunctional, Section II)

ALKALOSIS

See Metabolic Alkalosis

ALL (ACUTE LYMPHOCYTIC LEUKEMIA)

See Cancer; Chemotherapy; Child with Chronic Condition; Leukemia

ALLERGIES

Latex Allergic reaction r/t hypersensitivity to natural rubber latex

Risk for Allergic reaction: Risk factors: chemical factors, dander, environmental substances, foods, insect stings, medications

Risk for Latex Allergic reaction: Risk factor: repeated exposure to products containing latex

Readiness for enhanced Knowledge: expresses an interest in learning

ALOPECIA

Disturbed Body Image r/t loss of hair, change in appearance

Readiness for enhanced Knowledge: expresses an interest in learning

ALS (AMYOTROPHIC LATERAL SCLEROSIS)

See Amyotrophic Lateral Sclerosis (ALS)

ALTERED MENTAL STATUS

See Confusion, Acute; Confusion, Chronic; Memory Deficit

ALZHEIMER'S DISEASE

Caregiver role strain r/t duration and extent of caregiving required

Chronic Confusion r/t loss of cognitive function

Compromised family Coping r/t interrupted family processes

Frail Elderly syndrome r/t alteration in cognitive functioning

Ineffective Home Maintenance Behaviors r/t impaired cognitive function, inadequate support systems

Hopelessness r/t deteriorating condition

Insomnia r/t neurological impairment, daytime naps

Impaired Memory r/t neurological disturbance

Impaired physical Mobility r/t severe neurological dysfunction

Self-Neglect r/t loss of cognitive function

Powerlessness r/t deteriorating condition

Self-Care deficit: specify r/t loss of cognitive function, psychological impairment

Social isolation r/t fear of disclosure of memory loss

Wandering r/t cognitive impairment, frustration, physiological state

Risk for chronic functional Constipation: Risk factor: impaired cognitive functioning

Risk for Injury: Risk factor: confusion

Risk for Loneliness: Risk factor: potential social isolation

Risk for Relocation stress syndrome: Risk factors: impaired psychosocial health, decreased health status

Risk for other-directed Violence: Risk factors: frustration, fear, anger, loss of cognitive function

Readiness for enhanced Knowledge: Caregiver: expresses an interest in learning

See Dementia

AMD (AGE-RELATED MACULAR DEGENERATION)

See Macular Degeneration

AMENORRHEA

Imbalanced Nutrition: less than body requirements r/t inadequate food intake

See Sexuality, Adolescent

AMI (ACUTE MYOCARDIAL INFARCTION)

See MI (Myocardial Infarction)

AMNESIA

Acute Confusion r/t alcohol abuse, delirium, dementia, drug abuse

A

Dysfunctional Family processes r/t alcohol abuse, inadequate coping skills

Impaired Memory r/t excessive environmental disturbance, neurological disturbance

Post-Trauma syndrome r/t history of abuse, catastrophic illness, disaster, accident

AMNIOCENTESIS

Anxiety r/t threat to self and fetus, unknown future

Decisional Conflict r/t choice of treatment pending results of test

Risk for Infection: Risk factor: invasive procedure

AMNIONITIS

See Chorioamnionitis

AMNIOTIC MEMBRANE RUPTURE

See Premature Rupture of Membranes

AMPUTATION

Disturbed Body Image r/t negative effects of amputation, response from others

Impaired physical Mobility r/t musculoskeletal impairment, limited movement

Acute Pain r/t surgery, phantom limb sensation

Chronic Pain r/t surgery, phantom limb sensation

Ineffective peripheral Tissue Perfusion r/t impaired arterial circulation

Impaired Skin integrity r/t poor healing, prosthesis rubbing

Risk for Bleeding: Risk factor: vulnerable surgical site

Risk for Impaired Tissue integrity: Risk factor: mechanical factors impacting site

Readiness for enhanced Knowledge: expresses an interest in learning

AMYOTROPHIC LATERAL SCLEROSIS (ALS)

Death Anxiety r/t impending progressive loss of function leading to death

Ineffective Breathing pattern r/t compromised muscles of respiration

Impaired verbal Communication r/t weakness of muscles of speech, deficient knowledge of ways to compensate and alternative communication devices

Decisional Conflict: **ventilator therapy** r/t unclear personal values or beliefs, lack of relevant information

Impaired Resilience r/t perceived vulnerability

Chronic Sorrow r/t chronic illness

Impaired Swallowing r/t weakness of muscles involved in swallowing

Impaired spontaneous Ventilation r/t weakness of muscles of respiration

Risk for Aspiration: Risk factor: impaired swallowing

Risk for Spiritual distress: Risk factor: chronic debilitating condition

See Neurological Disorders

ANAL FISTULA

See Hemorrhoidectomy

ANAPHYLACTIC SHOCK

Deficient Fluid volume r/t compromised regulatory mechanism

Ineffective Airway clearance r/t laryngeal edema, bronchospasm

Latex Allergic reaction r/t abnormal immune mechanism response

Impaired spontaneous Ventilation r/t acute airway obstruction from anaphylaxis process

ANAPHYLAXIS PREVENTION

Risk for Allergic reaction (See **Allergic reaction**, risk for, Section II)

ANASARCA

Excess Fluid volume r/t excessive fluid intake, cardiac/renal dysfunction, loss of plasma proteins

Risk for decreased Cardiac Output: Risk factor: imbalanced fluid volume

Risk for impaired Skin integrity: Risk factor: impaired circulation to skin from edema

ANEMIA

Anxiety r/t cause of disease

Impaired Comfort r/t feelings of always being cold from decreased hemoglobin and decreased metabolism

Fatigue r/t decreased oxygen supply to the body, increased cardiac workload

Impaired Memory r/t change in cognition from decreased oxygen supply to the body

Delayed Surgical recovery r/t decreased oxygen supply to body, increased cardiac workload

Risk for Bleeding (See **Bleeding**, risk for, Section II)

Risk for Injury: Risk factor: alteration in peripheral sensory perception

Readiness for enhanced Knowledge: expresses an interest in learning

ANEMIA, IN PREGNANCY

Anxiety r/t concerns about health of self and fetus

Fatigue r/t decreased oxygen supply to the body, increased cardiac workload

Risk for delayed Child Development: Risk factor: reduction in the oxygen-carrying capacity of blood

Risk for Infection: Risk factor: reduction in oxygen-carrying capacity of blood

Risk for disturbed Maternal–Fetal dyad: Risk factor: compromised oxygen transport

Readiness for enhanced Knowledge: expresses an interest in learning

ANEMIA, SICKLE CELL

See Anemia; Sickle Cell Anemia/Crisis

ANENCEPHALY

See Neural Tube Defects (Meningocele, myelomeningocele, Spina Bifida, Anencephaly)

ANEURYSM, ABDOMINAL AORTIC REPAIR SURGERY

Risk for deficient Fluid volume: Risk factor: hemorrhage r/t potential abnormal blood loss

Risk for Surgical Site Infection: Risk factor: invasive procedure

See Abdominal Surgery

ANEURYSM, CEREBRAL

See Craniectomy/Craniotomy; Subarachnoid Hemorrhage

ANGER

Anxiety r/t situational crisis

Defensive Coping r/t inability to acknowledge responsibility for actions and results of actions

Labile Emotional Control r/t stressors

Fear r/t environmental stressor, hospitalization

Risk-prone Health behavior r/t assault to self-esteem, disability requiring change in lifestyle, inadequate support system

Powerlessness r/t healthcare environment

Risk for compromised Human Dignity: Risk factors: inadequate participation in decision-making, perceived dehumanizing treatment, perceived humiliation, exposure of the body, cultural incongruity

Risk for Post-Trauma syndrome: Risk factor: inadequate social support

Risk for other-directed Violence: Risk factors: history of violence, rage reaction

A

Risk for self-directed Violence: Risk factors: history of violence, history of abuse, rage reaction

ANGINA

Decreased Activity tolerance r/t acute pain, dysrhythmias

Anxiety r/t situational crisis

Decreased Cardiac output r/t myocardial ischemia, medication effect, dysrhythmia

Ineffective Coping r/t personal vulnerability to situational crisis of new diagnosis, deteriorating health

Ineffective Denial r/t deficient knowledge of need to seek help with symptoms

Acute Pain r/t myocardial ischemia

Ineffective Sexuality pattern r/t disease process, medications, loss of libido

Readiness for enhanced Knowledge: expresses an interest in learning

See MI (Myocardial Infarction)

ANGIOCARDIOGRAPHY (CARDIAC CATHETERIZATION)

See Cardiac Catheterization

ANGIOPLASTY, CORONARY

Fear r/t possible outcome of interventional procedure

Ineffective peripheral Tissue Perfusion r/t vasospasm, hematoma formation

Risk for Bleeding: Risk factors: possible damage to coronary artery, hematoma formation

Risk for decreased Cardiac tissue perfusion: Risk factors: ventricular ischemia, dysrhythmias

Readiness for enhanced Knowledge: expresses an interest in learning

ANOMALY, FETAL/NEWBORN (PARENT DEALING WITH)

Anxiety r/t threat to role functioning, situational crisis

Decisional Conflict: interventions for fetus or newborn r/t lack of relevant information, spiritual distress, threat to value system

Disabled family Coping r/t chronically unresolved feelings about loss of perfect baby

Ineffective Coping r/t personal vulnerability in situational crisis

Interrupted Family processes r/t unmet expectations for perfect baby, lack of adequate support systems

Fear r/t real or imagined threat to baby, implications for future pregnancies, powerlessness

Hopelessness r/t long-term stress, deteriorating physical condition of child, lost spiritual belief

Deficient Knowledge r/t limited exposure to situation

Impaired Parenting r/t interruption of bonding process

Powerlessness r/t complication threatening fetus or newborn

Parental Role conflict r/t separation from newborn, intimidation with invasive or restrictive modalities, specialized care center policies

Situational low Self-Esteem r/t perceived inability to produce a perfect child

Social isolation r/t alterations in child's physical appearance, altered state of wellness

Chronic Sorrow r/t loss of ideal child, inadequate bereavement support

Spiritual distress r/t test of spiritual beliefs

Risk for impaired Attachment: Risk factor: ill infant unable to effectively initiate parental contact as result of altered behavioral organization

Risk for disorganized Infant behavior: Risk factor: congenital disorder

Risk for impaired Parenting: Risk factors: interruption of bonding process; unrealistic expectations for self, infant, or partner;

perceived threat to own emotional survival; severe stress; lack of knowledge

Risk for Spiritual distress: Risk factor: lack of normal child to raise and carry on family name

ANORECTAL ABSCESS

Disturbed Body Image r/t odor and drainage from rectal area

Acute Pain r/t inflammation of perirectal area

Risk for Constipation: Risk factor: fear of painful elimination

Readiness for enhanced Knowledge: expresses an interest in learning

ANOREXIA

Deficient Fluid volume r/t inability to drink

Imbalanced Nutrition: less than body requirements r/t loss of appetite, nausea, vomiting, laxative abuse

Delayed Surgical recovery r/t inadequate nutritional intake

Risk for delayed Surgical recovery: Risk factor: inadequate nutritional intake

ANOREXIA NERVOSA

Decreased Activity tolerance r/t fatigue, weakness

Disturbed Body Image r/t misconception of actual body appearance

Constipation r/t lack of adequate food, fiber, and fluid intake

Defensive Coping r/t psychological impairment, eating disorder

Disabled family Coping r/t highly ambivalent family relationships

Ineffective Denial r/t fear of consequences of therapy, possible weight gain

Diarrhea r/t laxative abuse

Interrupted Family processes r/t situational crisis

Ineffective adolescent Eating dynamics r/t food refusal

Ineffective family Health self-management r/t family conflict, excessive demands on family associated with complexity of condition and treatment

Imbalanced Nutrition: less than body requirements r/t inadequate food intake, excessive exercise

Chronic low Self-Esteem r/t repeated unmet expectations

Ineffective Sexuality pattern r/t loss of libido from malnutrition

Risk for Infection: Risk factor: malnutrition resulting in depressed immune system

Risk for Spiritual distress: Risk factor: low self-esteem

See Maturational Issues, Adolescent

ANOSMIA (SMELL, LOSS OF ABILITY TO)

Imbalanced Nutrition: less than body requirements r/t loss of appetite associated with loss of smell

ANTEPARTUM PERIOD

See Pregnancy, Normal; Prenatal Care, Normal

ANTERIOR REPAIR, ANTERIOR COLPORRHAPHY

Urinary Retention r/t edema of urinary structures

Risk for urge urinary Incontinence: Risk factor: trauma to bladder

Readiness for enhanced Knowledge: expresses an interest in learning

See Vaginal Hysterectomy

ANTICOAGULANT THERAPY

Risk for Bleeding: Risk factor: altered clotting function from anticoagulant

Risk for deficient Fluid volume: hemorrhage: Risk factor: altered clotting mechanism

Readiness for enhanced Knowledge: expresses an interest in learning

A

ANTISOCIAL PERSONALITY DISORDER

Defensive Coping r/t excessive use of projection

Ineffective Coping r/t frequently violating the norms and rules of society

Labile Emotional Control r/t psychiatric disorder

Hopelessness r/t abandonment

Impaired Social interaction r/t sociocultural conflict, chemical dependence, inability to form relationships

Spiritual distress r/t separation from religious or cultural ties

Ineffective Health self-management r/t excessive demands on family

Risk for Loneliness: Risk factor: inability to interact appropriately with others

Risk for impaired Parenting: Risk factors: inability to function as parent or guardian, emotional instability

Risk for Self-Mutilation: Risk factors: self-hatred, depersonalization

Risk for other-directed Violence: Risk factor: history of violence, altered thought patterns

ANURIA

See Renal Failure

ANXIETY

See **Anxiety**, Section II

ANXIETY DISORDER

Ineffective Activity planning r/t unrealistic perception of events

Anxiety r/t unmet security and safety needs

Death Anxiety r/t fears of unknown, powerlessness

Decisional Conflict r/t low self-esteem, fear of making a mistake

Defensive Coping r/t overwhelming feelings of dread

Disabled family Coping r/t ritualistic behavior, actions

Imbalanced Energy Field r/t feelings of restlessness and apprehension

Impaired Mood Regulation r/t functional impairment, impaired social functioning, alteration in sleep pattern

Ineffective Coping r/t inability to express feelings appropriately

Ineffective Denial r/t overwhelming feelings of hopelessness, fear, threat to self

Insomnia r/t psychological impairment, emotional instability

Labile Emotional Control r/t emotional instability

Powerlessness r/t lifestyle of helplessness

Self-Care deficit r/t ritualistic behavior, activities

Sleep deprivation r/t prolonged psychological discomfort

Risk for Spiritual distress: Risk factor: psychological distress

Readiness for enhanced Knowledge: expresses an interest in learning

AORTIC VALVULAR STENOSIS

See Congenital Heart Disease/Cardiac Anomalies

APHASIA

Anxiety r/t situational crisis of aphasia

Impaired verbal Communication r/t decrease in circulation to brain

Ineffective Coping r/t loss of speech

Ineffective health maintenance behaviors r/t deficient knowledge regarding information on aphasia and alternative communication techniques

APLASTIC ANEMIA

Decreased Activity tolerance r/t imbalance between oxygen supply and demand

Fear r/t ability to live with serious disease

Risk for Bleeding: Risk factor: inadequate clotting factors

Risk for Infection: Risk factor: inadequate immune function

Readiness for enhanced Knowledge: expresses an interest in learning

APNEA IN INFANCY

See Premature Infant (Child); Premature Infant (Parent); SIDS (Sudden Infant Death)

APNEUSTIC RESPIRATIONS

Ineffective Breathing pattern r/t perception or cognitive impairment, neurological impairment

APPENDECTOMY

Deficient Fluid volume r/t fluid restriction, hypermetabolic state, nausea, vomiting

Acute Pain r/t surgical incision

Delayed Surgical recovery r/t rupture of appendix

Risk for Infection: Risk factors: perforation or rupture of appendix, peritonitis

Risk for Surgical Site Infection: Risk factor: surgical incision

Readiness for enhanced Knowledge: expresses an interest in learning

See Hospitalized Child; Surgery, Postoperative Care

APPENDICITIS

Deficient Fluid volume r/t anorexia, nausea, vomiting

Acute Pain r/t inflammation

Risk for Infection: Risk factor: possible perforation of appendix

Readiness for enhanced Knowledge: expresses an interest in learning

APPREHENSION

Anxiety r/t threat to self-concept, threat to health status, situational crisis

Death Anxiety r/t apprehension over loss of self, consequences to significant others

ARDS (ACUTE RESPIRATORY DISTRESS SYNDROME)

Ineffective Airway clearance r/t excessive tracheobronchial secretions

Death Anxiety r/t seriousness of physical disease

Impaired Gas exchange r/t damage to alveolar capillary membrane, change in lung compliance

Impaired spontaneous Ventilation r/t damage to alveolar capillary membrane

See Ventilated Client, Mechanically

ARRHYTHMIA

See Dysrhythmia

ARTERIAL INSUFFICIENCY

Ineffective peripheral Tissue Perfusion r/t interruption of arterial flow

Delayed Surgical recovery r/t ineffective tissue perfusion

ARTHRITIS

Decreased activity tolerance r/t chronic pain, fatigue, weakness

Disturbed Body Image r/t ineffective coping with joint abnormalities

Impaired physical Mobility r/t joint impairment

Chronic Pain r/t progression of joint deterioration

Self-Care deficit: specify r/t pain with movement, damage to joints

Readiness for enhanced Knowledge: expresses an interest in learning

See JRA (Juvenile Rheumatoid Arthritis)

ARTHROCENTESIS

Acute Pain r/t invasive procedure

ARTHROPLASTY (TOTAL HIP REPLACEMENT)

See Total Joint Replacement (Total Hip/Total Knee/Shoulder); Surgery,

A

Perioperative Care; Surgery, Postoperative Care; Surgery, Preoperative Care

ARTHROSCOPY

Impaired physical Mobility r/t surgical trauma of knee

Readiness for enhanced Knowledge: expresses an interest in learning

ASCITES

Ineffective Breathing pattern r/t increased abdominal girth

Imbalanced Nutrition: less than body requirements r/t loss of appetite

Chronic Pain r/t altered body function

Readiness for enhanced Knowledge: expresses an interest in learning

See Ascites; Cancer; Cirrhosis

ASPERGER'S SYNDROME

Ineffective Relationship r/t poor communication skills, lack of empathy

See Autism

ASPHYXIA, BIRTH

Ineffective Breathing pattern r/t depression of breathing reflex secondary to anoxia

Ineffective Coping r/t uncertainty of child outcome

Fear (parental) r/t concern over safety of infant

Impaired Gas exchange r/t poor placental perfusion, lack of initiation of breathing by newborn

Impaired spontaneous Ventilation r/t brain injury

Risk for impaired Attachment: Risk factors: ill infant who is unable to initiate parental contact, hospitalization in critical care environment

Risk for delayed Child Development: Risk factor: lack of oxygen to brain

Risk for disorganized Infant behavior: Risk factor: lack of oxygen to brain

Risk for Injury: Risk factor: lack of oxygen to brain

Risk for ineffective Cerebral tissue perfusion: Risk factor: poor placental perfusion or cord compression resulting in lack of oxygen to brain

ASPIRATION, DANGER OF

Risk for Aspiration (See **Aspiration**, risk for, Section II)

ASSAULT VICTIM

Post-Trauma syndrome r/t assault

Rape-Trauma syndrome r/t rape

Impaired Resilience r/t frightening experience, post-trauma stress response

Risk for Post-Trauma syndrome: Risk factors: perception of event, inadequate social support, unsupportive environment, diminished ego strength, duration of event

Risk for Spiritual distress: Risk factors: physical, psychological stress

ASSAULTIVE CLIENT

Risk for Injury: Risk factors: confused thought process, impaired judgment

Risk for other-directed Violence: Risk factors: paranoid ideation, anger

ASTHMA

Decreased Activity tolerance r/t fatigue, energy shift to meet muscle needs for breathing to overcome airway obstruction

Ineffective Airway clearance r/t tracheobronchial narrowing, excessive secretions

Anxiety r/t inability to breathe effectively, fear of suffocation

Disturbed Body Image r/t decreased participation in physical activities

Ineffective Breathing pattern r/t anxiety

Ineffective Coping r/t personal vulnerability to situational crisis

Ineffective Health self-management (See **Health** management, ineffective, in Section II)

Ineffective Home Maintenance Behaviors r/t deficient knowledge regarding control of environmental triggers

Sleep deprivation r/t ineffective breathing pattern, cough

Readiness for enhanced Health self-management (See **Health** management, readiness for enhanced, in Section II)

Readiness for enhanced Knowledge: expresses an interest in learning

See Child with Chronic Condition; Hospitalized Child

ATAXIA

Anxiety r/t change in health status

Disturbed Body Image r/t staggering gait

Impaired physical Mobility r/t neuromuscular impairment

Risk for Adult Falls: Risk factors: gait alteration, instability

ATELECTASIS

Ineffective Breathing pattern r/t loss of functional lung tissue, depression of respiratory function or hypoventilation because of pain

Impaired Gas exchange r/t decreased alveolar-capillary surface

Anxiety r/t alteration in respiratory pattern

See Atelectasis

ATHEROSCLEROSIS

See MI (Myocardial Infarction); CVA (Cerebrovascular Accident); Peripheral Vascular Disease (PVD)

ATHLETE'S FOOT

Impaired Skin integrity r/t effects of fungal agent

Readiness for enhanced Knowledge: expresses an interest in learning

See Pruritus

ATN (ACUTE TUBULAR NECROSIS)

See Renal Failure

ATRIAL FIBRILLATION

See Dysrhythmia

ATRIAL SEPTAL DEFECT

See Congenital Heart Disease/Cardiac Anomalies

ATTENTION DEFICIT DISORDER

Risk-prone Health behavior r/t intense emotional state

Disabled family Coping r/t significant person with chronically unexpressed feelings of guilt, anxiety, hostility, and despair

Ineffective Impulse control r/t (See **Impulse** control, ineffective, Section II)

Chronic low Self-Esteem r/t difficulty in participating in expected activities, poor school performance

Social isolation r/t unacceptable social behavior

Risk for delayed Child Development: Risk factor: behavior disorders

Risk for Adult Falls: Risk factor: rapid non-thinking behavior

Risk for Loneliness: Risk factor: social isolation

Risk for impaired Parenting: Risk factor: lack of knowledge of factors contributing to child's behavior

Risk for Spiritual distress: Risk factor: poor relationships

AUTISM

Impaired verbal Communication r/t speech and language delays

Compromised family Coping r/t parental guilt over etiology of disease, inability to accept or adapt to child's condition, inability to help child and other family members seek treatment

B

Disturbed personal Identity r/t inability to distinguish between self and environment, inability to identify own body as separate from those of other people, inability to integrate concept of self

Self-Neglect r/t impaired socialization

Impaired Social interaction r/t communication barriers, inability to relate to others, failure to develop peer relationships

Risk for delayed Child Development: Risk factor: autism

Risk for Loneliness: Risk factor: difficulty developing relationships with other people

Risk for Self-Mutilation: Risk factor: autistic state

Risk for other-directed Violence: Risk factors: frequent destructive rages toward others secondary to extreme response to changes in routine, fear of harmless things

Risk for self-directed Violence: Risk factors: frequent destructive rages toward self, secondary to extreme response to changes in routine, fear of harmless things

See Child with Chronic Condition

AUTONOMIC DYSREFLEXIA

Autonomic Dysreflexia r/t bladder distention, bowel distention, noxious stimuli

Risk for Autonomic Dysreflexia: Risk factors: bladder distention, bowel distention, noxious stimuli

AUTONOMIC HYPERREFLEXIA

See Autonomic Dysreflexia

B

BABY CARE

Readiness for enhanced Childbearing process: demonstrates appropriate feeding and baby care techniques, along with attachment to infant and providing a safe environment

Anxiety r/t situational crisis, back injury

Ineffective Coping r/t situational crisis, back injury

Impaired physical Mobility r/t pain

Acute Pain r/t back injury

Chronic Pain r/t back injury

Risk for Constipation: Risk factors: decreased activity, side effect of pain medication

Risk for Disuse syndrome: Risk factor: severe pain

Readiness for enhanced Knowledge: expresses an interest in learning

BACTEREMIA

Risk for Infection: Risk factor: compromised immune system

Risk for Shock: Risk factor: development of systemic inflammatory response from presence of bacteria in bloodstream

See Infectious Processes

BALANCED ENERGY FIELD

Imbalanced Energy Field (See **Energy Field**, imbalanced, Section II)

BARREL CHEST

See Aging (if appropriate); COPD (Chronic Obstructive Pulmonary Disease)

BATHING/HYGIENE PROBLEMS

Impaired Mobility r/t chronic physically limiting condition

Self-Neglect (See **Self-Neglect**, Section II)

Bathing Self-Care deficit (See **Self-Care** deficit, bathing, Section II)

BATTERED CHILD SYNDROME

Dysfunctional Family processes r/t inadequate coping skills

Sleep deprivation r/t prolonged psychological discomfort

Chronic Sorrow r/t situational crises

Risk for Post-Trauma syndrome: Risk factors: physical abuse, incest, rape, molestation

Risk for Self-Mutilation: Risk factors: feelings of rejection, dysfunctional family

Risk for Suicidal Behavior: Risk factor: childhood abuse

See Child Abuse

BATTERED PERSON

See Abuse, Spouse, Parent, or Significant Other

BEDBUGS, INFESTATION

Ineffective Home Maintenance Behaviors r/t deficient knowledge regarding prevention of bedbug infestation

Impaired Skin integrity r/t bites of bedbugs

See Pruritus

BED MOBILITY, IMPAIRED

Impaired bed Mobility (See **Mobility**, bed, impaired, Section II)

BED REST, PROLONGED

Deficient Diversional activity engagement r/t prolonged bed rest

Impaired bed Mobility r/t neuromuscular impairment

Social isolation r/t prolonged bed rest

Risk for chronic functional Constipation: Risk factor: insufficient physical activity

Risk for Disuse syndrome: Risk factor: prolonged immobility

Risk for Frail Elderly syndrome: Risk factor: prolonged immobility

Risk for Loneliness: Risk factor: prolonged bed rest

Risk for Overweight: Risk factor: energy expenditure below energy intake

Risk for Adult Pressure Injury: Risk factor: prolonged immobility

BEDSORES

See Pressure Ulcer

BEDWETTING

Ineffective health maintenance behaviors r/t unachieved developmental level, neuromuscular immaturity, diseases of the urinary system

BELL'S PALSY

Disturbed Body Image r/t loss of motor control on one side of face

Imbalanced Nutrition: **less than body requirements** r/t difficulty with chewing

Acute Pain r/t inflammation of facial nerve

Risk for Injury (eye): Risk factors: decreased tears, decreased blinking of eye

Readiness for enhanced Knowledge: expresses an interest in learning

BENIGN PROSTATIC HYPERTROPHY

See BPH (Benign Prostatic Hypertrophy); Prostatic Hypertrophy

BEREAVEMENT

Insomnia r/t grief

Risk for maladaptive Grieving: Risk factor: emotional instability, lack of social support

Risk for Spiritual distress: Risk factor: death of a loved one

BILIARY ATRESIA

Anxiety r/t surgical intervention, possible liver transplantation

Impaired Comfort r/t inflammation of skin, itching

Imbalanced Nutrition: **less than body requirements** r/t decreased absorption of fat and fat-soluble vitamins, poor feeding

Risk for Bleeding: Risk factors: vitamin K deficiency, altered clotting mechanisms

Risk for ineffective Breathing pattern: Risk factors: enlarged liver, development of ascites

Risk for impaired Skin integrity: Risk factor: pruritus

See Child with Chronic Condition; Cirrhosis; Hospitalized Child; Terminally Ill: Child, Adolescent; Infant/Toddler; See Child with Chronic Condition; Cirrhosis; Hospitalized Child

BILIARY CALCULUS

See Cholelithiasis

BILIARY OBSTRUCTION

See Jaundice

BILIRUBIN ELEVATION IN NEONATE

See Hyperbilirubinemia, Neonatal

BIOPSY

Fear r/t outcome of biopsy

Readiness for enhanced Knowledge: expresses an interest in learning

BIOTERRORISM

Contamination r/t exposure to bioterrorism

Risk for Infection: Risk factor: exposure to harmful biological agent

Risk for Post-Trauma syndrome: Risk factor: perception of event of bioterrorism

BIPOLAR DISORDER I (MOST RECENT EPISODE, DEPRESSED OR MANIC)

Ineffective Activity planning r/t unrealistic perception of events

Fatigue r/t psychological demands

Risk-prone Health behavior r/t low state of optimism

Ineffective Health maintenance behaviors r/t lack of ability to make good judgments regarding ways to obtain help

Self-Care deficit: specify r/t depression, cognitive impairment

Chronic low Self-Esteem r/t repeated unmet expectations

Social isolation r/t ineffective coping

Risk for maladaptive Grieving: Risk factor: lack of previous resolution of former grieving response

Risk for Loneliness: Risk factors: stress, conflict

Risk for Spiritual distress: Risk factor: mental illness

Risk for Suicidal Behavior: Risk factors: psychiatric disorder, poor support system

See Depression (Major Depressive Disorder); Manic Disorder, Bipolar I

BIRTH ASPHYXIA

See Asphyxia, Birth

BIRTH CONTROL

See Contraceptive Method

BLADDER CANCER

Urinary Retention r/t clots obstructing urethra

See Cancer; TURP (Transurethral Resection of the Prostate)

BLADDER DISTENTION

Urinary Retention r/t high urethral pressure caused by weak detrusor, inhibition of reflex arc, blockage, strong sphincter

BLADDER TRAINING

Disturbed Body Image r/t difficulty maintaining control of urinary elimination

Disability-associated urinary Incontinence r/t altered environment; sensory, cognitive, mobility deficit

Stress urinary Incontinence r/t degenerative change in pelvic muscles and structural supports

Urge urinary Incontinence r/t decreased bladder capacity, increased urine concentration, overdistension of bladder

Readiness for enhanced Knowledge: expresses an interest in learning

BLADDER TRAINING, CHILD

See Toilet Training

BLEEDING TENDENCY

Risk for Bleeding (See **Bleeding**, risk for, Section II)

Risk for delayed Surgical recovery: Risk factor: bleeding tendency

BLEPHAROPLASTY

Disturbed Body Image r/t effects of surgery

Readiness for enhanced Knowledge: expresses an interest in learning

BLINDNESS

Interrupted Family processes r/t shift in health status of family member (change in visual acuity)

Ineffective Home Maintenance Behaviors r/t decreased vision

Ineffective Role performance r/t alteration in health status (change in visual acuity)

Self-Care deficit: **specify** r/t inability to see to be able to perform activities of daily living

Risk for delayed Child Development: Risk factor: vision impairment

Risk for Injury: Risk factor: sensory dysfunction

Readiness for enhanced Knowledge: expresses an interest in learning

BLOOD DISORDER

Ineffective Protection r/t abnormal blood profile

Risk for Bleeding: Risk factor: abnormal blood profile

See ITP (Idiopathic Thrombocytopenic Purpura); Hemophilia; Lacerations; Shock, Hypovolemic

BLOOD GLUCOSE CONTROL

Risk for unstable blood Glucose level (See **Glucose** level, blood, unstable, risk for, Section II)

BLOOD PRESSURE ALTERATION

See Hypotension; HTN (Hypertension)

See **Unstable Blood Pressure**, Risk for, Section II)

BLOOD TRANSFUSION

Anxiety r/t possibility of harm from transfusion

See Anemia

BODY DYSMORPHIC DISORDER

Anxiety r/t perceived defect of body

Disturbed Body Image r/t overinvolvement in physical appearance

Chronic low Self-Esteem r/t lack of self-valuing because of perceived body defects

Social isolation r/t distancing self from others because of perceived self-body defects

Risk for Suicidal Behavior: Risk factor: perceived defects of body affecting self-valuing and hopes

BODY IMAGE CHANGE

Disturbed Body Image (See **Body Image**, disturbed, Section II)

BODY TEMPERATURE, ALTERED

Ineffective Thermoregulation (See **Thermoregulation**, ineffective, Section II)

BONE MARROW BIOPSY

Fear r/t unknown outcome of results of biopsy

Acute Pain r/t bone marrow aspiration

Readiness for enhanced Knowledge: expresses an interest in learning

See Disease necessitating bone marrow biopsy (e.g., Leukemia)

BORDERLINE PERSONALITY DISORDER

Ineffective Activity planning r/t unrealistic perception of events

B

Anxiety r/t perceived threat to self-concept

Defensive Coping r/t difficulty with relationships, inability to accept blame for own behavior

Ineffective Coping r/t use of maladjusted defense mechanisms (e.g., projection, denial)

Powerlessness r/t lifestyle of helplessness

Social isolation r/t immature interests

Ineffective family Health self-management r/t manipulative behavior of client

Risk for Caregiver Role Strain: Risk factors: inability of care receiver to accept criticism, care receiver taking advantage of others to meet own needs or having unreasonable expectations

Risk for Self-Mutilation: Risk factors: ineffective coping, feelings of self-hatred

Risk for Spiritual distress: Risk factor: poor relationships associated with abnormal behaviors

Risk for self-directed Violence: Risk factors: feelings of need to punish self, manipulative behavior

BOREDOM

Decreased Diversional activity engagement r/t environmental lack of diversional activity

Impaired Mood regulation r/t emotional instability

Social isolation r/t altered state of wellness

BOTULISM

Deficient Fluid volume r/t profuse diarrhea

Readiness for enhanced Knowledge: expresses an interest in learning

BOWEL CONTINENCE, IMPAIRED

Impaired Bowel Continence r/t decreased awareness of need to defecate, loss of sphincter control, fecal impaction

Readiness for enhanced Knowledge: expresses an interest in learning

BOWEL OBSTRUCTION

Constipation r/t decreased motility, intestinal obstruction

Deficient Fluid volume r/t inadequate fluid volume intake, fluid loss in bowel

Imbalanced Nutrition: less than body requirements r/t nausea, vomiting

Acute Pain r/t pressure from distended abdomen

BOWEL RESECTION

See Abdominal Surgery

BOWEL SOUNDS, ABSENT OR DIMINISHED

Constipation r/t decreased or absent peristalsis

Deficient Fluid volume r/t inability to ingest fluids, loss of fluids in bowel

Delayed Surgical recovery r/t inability to obtain adequate nutritional status

Risk for dysfunctional Gastrointestinal motility (See **Gastrointestinal** motility, dysfunctional, risk for, Section II)

BOWEL SOUNDS, HYPERACTIVE

Diarrhea r/t increased gastrointestinal motility

BOWEL TRAINING

Impaired Bowel Continence r/t loss of control of rectal sphincter

Readiness for enhanced Knowledge: expresses an interest in learning

BOWEL TRAINING, CHILD

See Toilet Training

BPH (BENIGN PROSTATIC HYPERTROPHY)

Ineffective Health maintenance behaviors r/t deficient knowledge regarding self-care with prostatic hypertrophy

Insomnia r/t nocturia

Urinary Retention r/t obstruction of urethra

Risk for urge urinary Incontinence: Risk factors: detrusor muscle instability with impaired contractility, involuntary sphincter relaxation

Risk for Infection: Risk factors: urinary residual after voiding, bacterial invasion of bladder

Readiness for enhanced Knowledge: expresses an interest in learning

See Prostatic Hypertrophy

BRADYCARDIA

Decreased Cardiac output r/t slow heart rate supplying inadequate amount of blood for body function

Risk for ineffective Cerebral tissue perfusion: Risk factors: decreased cardiac output secondary to bradycardia, vagal response

Readiness for enhanced Knowledge: expresses an interest in learning

BRADYPNEA

Ineffective Breathing pattern r/t neuromuscular impairment, pain, musculoskeletal impairment, perception or cognitive impairment, anxiety, fatigue or decreased energy, effects of drugs

See Sleep apnea (See **Airway** clearance, ineffective, Section II)

BRAIN INJURY

See Intracranial Pressure, Increased

Risk for ineffective Thermoregulation: Risk factor: post-traumatic inflammation or infection

BRAIN SURGERY

See Craniectomy/Craniotomy

BRAIN TUMOR

Acute Confusion r/t pressure from tumor

Fear r/t threat to well-being

Acute Pain r/t pressure from tumor

Vision Loss r/t tumor growth compressing optic nerve and/or brain tissue

Risk for Injury: Risk factors: sensory-perceptual alterations, weakness

Risk for ineffective Thermoregulation: Risk factor: changes in metabolic activity of the brain

See Cancer; Chemotherapy; Child with Chronic Condition; Craniectomy/Craniotomy; Hospitalized Child; Radiation Therapy; Terminally Ill Child, Adolescent; Terminally Ill Child, Infant/Toddler; Terminally Ill Child, Preschool Child; Terminally Ill Child, School-Age Child/Preadolescent; Terminally Ill Child/Death of Child, Parent

BRAXTON HICKS CONTRACTIONS

Decreased activity tolerance r/t increased contractions with increased gestation

Anxiety r/t uncertainty about beginning labor

Fatigue r/t lack of sleep

Stress urinary Incontinence r/t increased pressure on bladder with contractions

Insomnia r/t contractions when lying down

Ineffective Sexuality pattern r/t fear of contractions associated with loss of infant

BREAST BIOPSY

Fear r/t potential for diagnosis of cancer

Risk for Spiritual distress: Risk factor: fear of diagnosis of cancer

Readiness for enhanced Knowledge: expresses an interest in learning

BREAST CANCER

Death Anxiety r/t diagnosis of cancer

Ineffective Coping r/t treatment, prognosis

Fear r/t diagnosis of cancer

Sexual dysfunction r/t loss of body part, partner's reaction to loss

B

Chronic Sorrow r/t diagnosis of cancer, loss of body integrity

Risk for Spiritual distress: Risk factor: fear of diagnosis of cancer

Readiness for enhanced Health literacy: expresses desire to enhance understanding of health information to make healthcare choices

Readiness for enhanced Knowledge: expresses an interest in learning

See Cancer; Chemotherapy; Mastectomy; Radiation Therapy

BREAST EXAMINATION, SELF

See SBE (Self-Breast Examination)

BREAST LUMPS

Fear r/t potential for diagnosis of cancer

Readiness for enhanced Knowledge: expresses an interest in learning

BREAST PUMPING

Risk for Infection: Risk factors: possible contaminated breast pump, incomplete emptying of breast

Risk for impaired Skin integrity: Risk factor: high suction

Readiness for enhanced Knowledge: expresses an interest in learning

BREASTFEEDING, EFFECTIVE

Readiness for enhanced Breastfeeding (See **Breastfeeding**, readiness for enhanced, Section II)

BREASTFEEDING, INEFFECTIVE

Ineffective Breastfeeding (See **Breastfeeding**, ineffective, Section II)

See Infant Feeding Pattern, Ineffective; Painful Breasts, Engorgement; Painful Breasts, Sore Nipples

BREASTFEEDING, INTERRUPTED

Interrupted Breastfeeding (See **Breastfeeding**, interrupted, Section II)

BREAST MILK PRODUCTION, INSUFFICIENT

Insufficient Breast Milk Production (See **Breast Milk Production**, insufficient, Section II)

BREATH SOUNDS, DECREASED OR ABSENT

See Atelectasis; Pneumothorax

BREATHING PATTERN ALTERATION

Ineffective Breathing pattern r/t neuromuscular impairment, pain, musculoskeletal impairment, perception or cognitive impairment, anxiety, decreased energy or fatigue

BREECH BIRTH

Fear: **maternal** r/t danger to infant, self

Impaired Gas exchange: **fetal** r/t compressed umbilical cord

Risk for Aspiration: **fetal**: Risk factor: birth of body before head

Risk for delayed Child Development: Risk factor: compressed umbilical cord

Risk for impaired Tissue integrity: **fetal**: Risk factor: difficult birth

Risk for impaired Tissue integrity: **maternal**: Risk factor: difficult birth

BRONCHITIS

Ineffective Airway clearance r/t excessive thickened mucus secretion

Readiness for enhanced Health self-management: wishes to stop smoking

Readiness for enhanced Knowledge: expresses an interest in learning

BRONCHOPULMONARY DYSPLASIA

Decreased activity tolerance r/t imbalance between oxygen supply and demand

Excess Fluid volume r/t sodium and water retention

Imbalanced Nutrition: less than body requirements r/t poor feeding, increased caloric needs as a result of increased work of breathing

See Child with Chronic Condition; Hospitalized Child; Respiratory Conditions of the Neonate

BRONCHOSCOPY

Risk for Aspiration: Risk factor: temporary loss of gag reflex

Risk for Injury: Risk factors: complication of pneumothorax, laryngeal edema, hemorrhage (if biopsy done)

BRUITS, CAROTID

Risk for ineffective Cerebral tissue perfusion: Risk factors: interruption of carotid blood flow to brain

BRYANT'S TRACTION

See Traction and Casts

BUCK'S TRACTION

See Traction and Casts

BUERGER'S DISEASE

See Peripheral Vascular Disease (PVD)

BULIMIA

Disturbed Body Image r/t misperception about actual appearance, body weight

Compromised family Coping r/t chronically unresolved feelings of guilt, anger, hostility

Defensive Coping r/t eating disorder

Diarrhea r/t laxative abuse

Fear r/t food ingestion, weight gain

Imbalanced Nutrition: less than body requirements r/t induced vomiting, excessive exercise, laxative abuse

Ineffective adolescent Eating dynamics r/t overeating, leading to purge

Powerlessness r/t urge to purge self after eating

Chronic low Self Esteem r/t lack of positive feedback

See Maturational Issues, Adolescent

BULLYING

Anxiety r/t specific or non-specific threat to self

Impaired Social Interaction r/t dysfunctional interactions with others

Fear r/t perceived threat to self

Risk for compromised Human Dignity: Risk factors: dehumanizing treatment, humiliation

Risk for other-directed violence: Risk factors: Social isolation, unresolved interpersonal conflicts

Risk for Powerlessness: Risk factor: ineffective coping strategies

Risk for impaired Resilience: Risk factor: insufficient familial and social support

Risk for Self-directed violence: Risk factors: unresolved interpersonal conflicts, social isolation

Risk for chronic low self-esteem: Risk factors: ineffective coping strategies, absence of sense of belonging, inadequate respect from others

BUNION

Readiness for enhanced Knowledge: expresses an interest in learning

BUNIONECTOMY

Impaired physical Mobility r/t sore foot

Impaired Walking r/t pain associated with surgery

Risk for Surgical Site Infection: Risk factors: surgical incision

Readiness for enhanced Knowledge: expresses an interest in learning

BURN RISK

Risk for Thermal injury (See **Thermal** injury, risk for, Section II)

BURNS

Anxiety r/t burn injury, treatments

Disturbed Body Image r/t altered physical appearance

Decreased Diversional activity engagement r/t long-term hospitalization

Fear r/t pain from treatments, possible permanent disfigurement

Deficient Fluid volume r/t loss of protective skin

Hypothermia r/t impaired skin integrity

Impaired physical Mobility r/t pain, musculoskeletal impairment, contracture formation

Imbalanced Nutrition: less than body requirements r/t increased metabolic needs, anorexia, protein and fluid loss

Acute Pain r/t burn injury, treatments

Chronic Pain r/t burn injury, treatments

Ineffective peripheral Tissue Perfusion r/t circumferential burns, impaired arterial/venous circulation

Post-Trauma syndrome r/t life-threatening event

Impaired Skin integrity r/t injury of skin

Delayed Surgical recovery r/t ineffective tissue perfusion

Risk for ineffective Airway clearance: Risk factors: potential tracheobronchial obstruction, edema

Risk for deficient Fluid volume: Risk factors: loss from skin surface, fluid shift

Risk for Infection: Risk factors: loss of intact skin, trauma, invasive sites

Risk for Peripheral Neurovascular dysfunction: Risk factor: eschar formation with circumferential burn

Risk for Post-Trauma syndrome: Risk factors: perception, duration of event that caused burns

Risk for ineffective Thermoregulation: Risk factor: disruption of skin integrity

Readiness for enhanced Knowledge: expresses an interest in learning

See Hospitalized Child; Safety, Childhood

BURSITIS

Impaired physical Mobility r/t inflammation in joint

Acute Pain r/t inflammation in joint

BYPASS GRAFT

See Coronary Artery Bypass Grafting (CABG)

CABG (CORONARY ARTERY BYPASS GRAFTING)

See Coronary Artery Bypass Grafting (CABG)

CACHEXIA

Frail Elderly syndrome r/t fatigue, feeding self-care deficit

Imbalanced Nutrition: less than body requirements r/t inability to ingest food because of physiological factors

Risk for Infection: Risk factor: inadequate nutrition

CALCIUM ALTERATION

See Hypercalcemia; Hypocalcemia

CANCER

Decreased activity tolerance r/t side effects of treatment, weakness from cancer

Death Anxiety r/t unresolved issues regarding dying

Disturbed Body Image r/t side effects of treatment, cachexia

Decisional Conflict r/t selection of treatment choices, continuation or discontinuation of treatment, "do not resuscitate" decision

Constipation r/t side effects of medication, altered nutrition, decreased activity

Compromised family Coping r/t prolonged disease or disability progression that exhausts supportive ability of significant others

Ineffective Coping r/t personal vulnerability in situational crisis, terminal illness

Ineffective Denial r/t maladaptive grieving process

Fear r/t serious threat to well-being

Ineffective Health maintenance behaviors r/t deficient knowledge regarding prescribed treatment

Hopelessness r/t loss of control, terminal illness

Insomnia r/t anxiety, pain

Impaired physical Mobility r/t weakness, neuromusculoskeletal impairment, pain

Imbalanced Nutrition: less than body requirements r/t loss of appetite, difficulty swallowing, side effects of chemotherapy, obstruction by tumor

Impaired Oral Mucous Membrane Integrity r/t chemotherapy, effects of radiation, oral pH changes, decreased oral secretions

Chronic Pain r/t metastatic cancer

Powerlessness r/t treatment, progression of disease

Ineffective Protection r/t cancer suppressing immune system

Ineffective Role performance r/t change in physical capacity, inability to resume prior role

Self-Care deficit: specify r/t pain, intolerance to activity, decreased strength

Impaired Skin integrity r/t immunological deficit, immobility

Social isolation r/t hospitalization, lifestyle changes

Chronic Sorrow r/t chronic illness of cancer

Spiritual distress r/t test of spiritual beliefs

Risk for Bleeding: Risk factor: bone marrow depression from chemotherapy

Risk for Disuse syndrome: Risk factors: immobility, fatigue

Risk for Infection: Risk factor: inadequate immune system

Risk for compromised Resilience: Risk factors: multiple stressors, pain, chronic illness

Risk for Spiritual distress: Risk factor: physical illness of cancer

Readiness for enhanced Knowledge: expresses an interest in learning

Readiness for enhanced Spiritual well-being: desire for harmony with self, others, higher power, God, when faced with serious illness

See Chemotherapy; Child with Chronic Condition; Hospitalized Child; Leukemia; Radiation Therapy; Terminally Ill Child, Adolescent; Terminally Ill Child, Infant/Toddler; Terminally Ill Child, Preschool Child; Terminally Ill Child, School-Age Child/Preadolescent; Terminally Ill Child/Death of Child, Parent

CANDIDIASIS, ORAL

Readiness for enhanced Knowledge: expresses an interest in learning

Impaired Oral Mucous Membrane Integrity r/t overgrowth of infectious agent, depressed immune function

Acute Pain r/t oral condition

CAPILLARY REFILL TIME, PROLONGED

Impaired Gas exchange r/t ventilation perfusion imbalance

Ineffective peripheral Tissue Perfusion r/t interruption of arterial flow

See Shock, Hypovolemic

CARBON MONOXIDE POISONING

See Smoke Inhalation

CARDIAC ARREST

Post-Trauma syndrome r/t experiencing serious life event

See Dysrhythmia; MI (Myocardial Infarction)

C

C

CARDIAC CATHETERIZATION

Fear r/t invasive procedure, uncertainty of outcome of procedure

Risk for Injury: hematoma: Risk factor: invasive procedure

Risk for decreased Cardiac tissue perfusion: Risk factors: ventricular ischemia, dysrhythmia

Risk for Peripheral Neurovascular dysfunction: Risk factor: vascular obstruction

Risk for Impaired Tissue integrity: Risk factor: invasive procedure

Readiness for enhanced Knowledge: expresses an interest in learning postprocedure care, treatment, and prevention of coronary artery disease

CARDIAC DISORDERS IN PREGNANCY

Decreased activity tolerance r/t cardiac pathophysiology, increased demand for cardiac output because of pregnancy, weakness, fatigue

Death Anxiety r/t potential danger of condition

Compromised family Coping r/t prolonged hospitalization or maternal incapacitation that exhausts supportive capacity of significant others

Ineffective Coping r/t personal vulnerability

Interrupted Family processes r/t hospitalization, maternal incapacitation, changes in roles

Fatigue r/t physiological, psychological, and emotional demands

Fear r/t potential maternal effects, potential poor fetal or maternal outcome

Powerlessness r/t illness-related regimen

Ineffective Role performance r/t changes in lifestyle, expectations from disease process with superimposed pregnancy

Situational low Self-Esteem r/t situational crisis, pregnancy

Social isolation r/t limitations of activity, bed rest or hospitalization, separation from family and friends

Risk for decreased Cardiac tissue perfusion: Risk factor: strain on compromised heart from work of pregnancy, delivery

Risk for delayed Child Development: Risk factor: poor maternal oxygenation

Risk for deficient Fluid volume: Risk factor: sudden changes in circulation after delivery of placenta

Risk for excess Fluid volume: Risk factors: compromised regulatory mechanism with increased afterload, preload, circulating blood volume

Risk for impaired Gas exchange: Risk factor: pulmonary edema

Risk for disturbed Maternal–Fetal dyad: Risk factor: compromised oxygen transport

Risk for compromised Resilience: Risk factors: multiple stressors, fear

Risk for Spiritual distress: Risk factor: fear of diagnosis for self and infant

Readiness for enhanced Knowledge: expresses an interest in learning

CARDIAC DYSRHYTHMIA

See Dysrhythmia

CARDIAC OUTPUT, DECREASED

Decreased Cardiac output r/t cardiac dysfunction

Decreased Cardiac output (See **Cardiac** output, decreased, Section II)

Oliguria r/t cardiac dysfunction

Risk for decreased Cardiac output (See **Cardiac** output, risk for decreased, Section II)

CARDIAC TAMPONADE

Decreased Cardiac output r/t fluid in pericardial sac

See Pericarditis

CARDIOGENIC SHOCK

See Shock, Cardiogenic

C

CAREGIVER ROLE STRAIN

Caregiver Role Strain (See **Caregiver Role Strain**, Section II)

Risk for compromised Resilience: Risk factor: stress of prolonged caregiving

CARIOUS TEETH

See Cavities in Teeth

CAROTID ENDARTERECTOMY

Fear r/t surgery in vital area

Risk for ineffective Airway clearance: Risk factor: hematoma compressing trachea

Risk for Bleeding: Risk factor: possible hematoma formation, trauma to region

Risk for ineffective Cerebral tissue perfusion: Risk factors: hemorrhage, clot formation

Readiness for enhanced Knowledge: expresses an interest in learning

CARPAL TUNNEL SYNDROME

Impaired physical Mobility r/t neuromuscular impairment

Chronic Pain r/t unrelieved pressure on median nerve

Self-Care deficit: bathing, dressing, feeding r/t pain

CARPOPEDAL SPASM

See Hypocalcemia

CASTS

Decreased Diversional activity engagement r/t physical limitations from cast

Impaired physical Mobility r/t limb immobilization

Self-Care deficit: bathing, dressing, feeding r/t presence of cast(s) on upper extremities

Self-Care deficit: toileting r/t presence of cast(s) on lower extremities

Impaired Walking r/t cast(s) on lower extremities, fracture of bones

Risk for Peripheral Neurovascular dysfunction: Risk factors: mechanical compression from cast, trauma from fracture

Risk for impaired Skin integrity: Risk factor: unrelieved pressure on skin from cast

Readiness for enhanced Knowledge: expresses an interest in learning

See Traction and Casts

CATARACT EXTRACTION

Anxiety r/t threat of permanent vision loss, surgical procedure

Risk for Injury: Risk factors: increased intraocular pressure, accommodation to new visual field

Readiness for enhanced Knowledge: expresses an interest in learning

CATATONIC SCHIZOPHRENIA

Impaired verbal Communication r/t cognitive impairment

Impaired Memory r/t cognitive impairment

Impaired physical Mobility r/t cognitive impairment, maintenance of rigid posture, inappropriate or bizarre postures

Imbalanced Nutrition: less than body requirements r/t decrease in outside stimulation, loss of perception of hunger, resistance to instructions to eat

Social isolation r/t inability to communicate, immobility

See Schizophrenia

CATHETERIZATION, URINARY

Risk for Infection: Risk factor: invasive procedure

Readiness for enhanced Knowledge: expresses an interest in learning

CAVITIES IN TEETH

Impaired Dentition r/t ineffective oral hygiene, barriers to self-care, economic barriers to professional care, nutritional deficits, dietary habits

C

CELIAC DISEASE

Diarrhea r/t malabsorption of food, immune effects of gluten on gastrointestinal system

Imbalanced Nutrition: less than body requirements r/t malabsorption caused by immune effects of gluten

Readiness for enhanced Knowledge: expresses an interest in learning

CELLULITIS

Acute Pain r/t inflammatory changes in tissues from infection

Impaired Tissue integrity r/t inflammatory process damaging skin and underlying tissue

Ineffective peripheral Tissue Perfusion r/t edema of extremities

Risk for Vascular Trauma: Risk factor: infusion of antibiotics

Readiness for enhanced Knowledge: expresses an interest in learning

CELLULITIS, PERIORBITAL

Acute Pain r/t edema and inflammation of skin/tissues

Impaired Skin integrity r/t inflammation or infection of skin, tissues

Vision Loss r/t decreased visual field secondary to edema of eyelids (*see care plan in Appendix*)

Readiness for enhanced Knowledge: expresses an interest in learning

See Hospitalized Child

CENTRAL LINE INSERTION

Risk for Infection: Risk factor: invasive procedure

Risk for Vascular Trauma (See **Vascular Trauma**, risk for, Section II)

Readiness for enhanced Knowledge: expresses an interest in learning

CEREBRAL ANEURYSM

See Craniectomy/Craniotomy; Intracranial Pressure, Increased; Subarachnoid Hemorrhage

CEREBRAL PALSY

Impaired verbal Communication r/t impaired ability to articulate or speak words because of facial muscle involvement

Decreased Diversional activity engagement r/t physical impairments, limitations on ability to participate in recreational activities

Impaired physical Mobility r/t spasticity, neuromuscular impairment or weakness

Imbalanced Nutrition: less than body requirements r/t spasticity, feeding or swallowing difficulties

Self-Care deficit: specify r/t neuromuscular impairments, sensory deficits

Impaired Social interaction r/t impaired communication skills, limited physical activity, perceived differences from peers

Chronic Sorrow r/t presence of chronic disability

Risk for Adult Falls: Risk factor: impaired physical mobility

Risk for Injury: Risk factors: muscle weakness, inability to control spasticity

Risk for impaired Parenting: Risk factor: caring for child with overwhelming needs resulting from chronic change in health status

Risk for Spiritual distress: Risk factor: psychological stress associated with chronic illness

See Child with Chronic Condition

CEREBRAL PERFUSION

Risk for ineffective Cerebral tissue perfusion (See **Cerebral** tissue perfusion, ineffective, risk for, Section II)

CEREBROVASCULAR ACCIDENT (CVA)

See CVA (Cerebrovascular Accident)

CERVICITIS

Ineffective Health maintenance behaviors r/t deficient knowledge regarding care and prevention of condition

Ineffective Sexuality pattern r/t abstinence during acute stage

Risk for Infection: Risk factors: spread of infection, recurrence of infection

CESAREAN DELIVERY

Disturbed Body Image r/t surgery, unmet expectations for childbirth

Interrupted Family processes r/t unmet expectations for childbirth

Fear r/t perceived threat to own well-being, outcome of birth

Impaired physical Mobility r/t pain

Acute Pain r/t surgical incision

Ineffective Role performance r/t unmet expectations for childbirth

Situational low Self-Esteem r/t inability to deliver child vaginally

Risk for Bleeding: Risk factor: surgery

Risk for imbalanced Fluid volume: Risk factors: loss of blood, fluid shifts

Risk for Surgical Site Infection: Risk factor: surgical incision

Risk for Urinary Retention: Risk factor: regional anesthesia

Readiness for enhanced Childbearing process: a pattern of preparing for, maintaining, and strengthening care of newborn

Readiness for enhanced Knowledge: expresses an interest in learning

CHEMICAL DEPENDENCE

See Alcoholism; Substance Abuse

CHEMOTHERAPY

Death Anxiety r/t chemotherapy not accomplishing desired results

Disturbed Body Image r/t loss of weight, loss of hair

Fatigue r/t disease process, anemia, drug effects

Nausea r/t effects of chemotherapy

Imbalanced Nutrition: less than body requirements r/t side effects of chemotherapy

Impaired Oral Mucous Membrane Integrity r/t effects of chemotherapy

Ineffective Protection r/t suppressed immune system, decreased platelets

Risk for Bleeding: Risk factors: tumor eroding blood vessel, stress effects on gastrointestinal system

Risk for Infection: Risk factor: immunosuppression

Risk for Vascular Trauma: Risk factor: infusion of irritating medications

Readiness for enhanced Knowledge: expresses an interest in learning

See Cancer

CHEST PAIN

Fear r/t potential threat of death

Acute Pain r/t myocardial injury, ischemia

Risk for decreased Cardiac tissue perfusion: Risk factor: ventricular ischemia

See Angina; MI (Myocardial Infarction)

CHEST TUBES

Ineffective Breathing pattern r/t asymmetrical lung expansion secondary to pain

Impaired Gas exchange r/t decreased functional lung tissue

Acute Pain r/t presence of chest tubes, injury

Risk for Injury: Risk factor: presence of invasive chest tube

CHEYNE-STOKES RESPIRATION

Ineffective Breathing pattern r/t critical illness

CHICKENPOX

See Communicable Diseases, Childhood

CHILD ABUSE

Interrupted Family processes r/t inadequate coping skills

Fear r/t threat of punishment for perceived wrongdoing

Insomnia r/t hypervigilance, fear

C

Imbalanced Nutrition: less than body requirements r/t inadequate caretaking

Acute Pain r/t physical injuries

Impaired Parenting r/t psychological impairment, physical or emotional abuse of parent, substance abuse, unrealistic expectations of child

Ineffective child Eating dynamics r/t hostile parental relationship

Post-Trauma syndrome r/t physical abuse, incest, rape, molestation

Chronic low Self-Esteem r/t lack of positive feedback, excessive negative feedback

Impaired Skin integrity r/t altered nutritional state, physical abuse

Social isolation: family imposed r/t fear of disclosure of family dysfunction and abuse

Risk for delayed Child Development: Risk factors: shaken baby syndrome, abuse

Risk for Poisoning: Risk factors: inadequate safeguards, lack of proper safety precautions

Risk for Suffocation: Risk factors: unattended child, unsafe environment

Risk for Physical Trauma: Risk factors: inadequate precautions, cognitive or emotional difficulties

CHILDBEARING PROBLEMS

Ineffective Childbearing process (See **Childbearing** process, ineffective, Section II)

Risk for ineffective Childbearing process: See **Childbearing** process, risk for ineffective, Section II)

CHILD NEGLECT

See Child Abuse; Failure to Thrive

CHILD WITH CHRONIC CONDITION

Decreased activity tolerance r/t fatigue associated with chronic illness

Compromised family Coping r/t prolonged overconcern for child; distortion of reality regarding child's health problem, including extreme denial about its existence or severity

Disabled family Coping r/t prolonged disease or disability progression that exhausts supportive capacity of significant others

Ineffective Coping: child r/t situational or maturational crises

Decisional Conflict r/t treatment options, conflicting values

Decreased Diversional activity engagement r/t immobility, monotonous environment, frequent or lengthy treatments, reluctance to participate, self-imposed social isolation

Interrupted Family processes r/t intermittent situational crisis of illness, disease, hospitalization

Ineffective Health maintenance behaviors r/t exhausting family resources (finances, physical energy, support systems)

Ineffective Home Maintenance Behaviors r/t overtaxed family members (e.g., exhausted, anxious)

Hopelessness: child r/t prolonged activity restriction, long-term stress, lack of involvement in or passively allowing care as a result of parental overprotection

Insomnia: child or parent r/t time-intensive treatments, exacerbation of condition, 24-hour care needs

Deficient Knowledge r/t knowledge or skill acquisition regarding health practices, acceptance of limitations, promotion of maximal potential of child, self-actualization of rest of family

Imbalanced Nutrition: less than body requirements r/t anorexia, fatigue from physical exertion

Risk for Overweight r/t effects of steroid medications on appetite

Chronic Pain r/t physical, biological, chemical, or psychological factors

Powerlessness: child r/t healthcare environment, illness-related regimen, lifestyle of learned helplessness

Parental Role conflict r/t separation from child as a result of chronic illness, home care of child with special needs, interruptions of family life resulting from home care regimen

Chronic low Self-Esteem r/t actual or perceived differences; peer acceptance; decreased ability to participate in physical, school, and social activities

Ineffective Sexuality pattern: parental r/t disrupted relationship with sexual partner

Impaired Social interaction r/t developmental lag or delay, perceived differences

Social Isolation: family r/t actual or perceived social stigmatization, complex care requirements

Chronic Sorrow r/t developmental stages and missed opportunities or milestones that bring comparisons with social or personal norms, unending caregiving as reminder of loss

Risk for delayed Child Development: Risk factor: chronic illness

Risk for Infection: Risk factor: debilitating physical condition

Risk for impaired Parenting: Risk factors: impaired or disrupted bonding, caring for child with perceived overwhelming care needs

Readiness for enhanced family Coping: impact of crisis on family values, priorities, goals, or relationships; changes in family choices to optimize wellness

CHILDBIRTH

Readiness for enhanced Childbearing process (See **Childbearing** process, readiness for enhanced, Section II)

See Labor, Normal; Postpartum, Normal Care

CHILDHOOD OBESITY

Obesity r/t disordered eating behaviors

Risk for Decreased activity tolerance: Risk factors: sedentary lifestyle, exertional discomfort

Risk for unstable Blood Glucose Level: Risk factor: excessive weight gain

Risk for Metabolic Syndrome: Risk factors: obesity, sedentary lifestyle

Readiness for Enhanced Knowledge: expresses desire to make healthier nutrition choices

CHILLS

Hyperthermia r/t infectious process

CHLAMYDIA INFECTION

See STD (Sexually Transmitted Disease)

CHLOASMA

Disturbed Body Image r/t change in skin color

CHOKING OR COUGHING WITH EATING

Impaired Swallowing r/t neuromuscular impairment

Risk for Aspiration: Risk factors: depressed cough and gag reflexes

CHOLECYSTECTOMY

Imbalanced Nutrition: less than body requirements r/t high metabolic needs, decreased ability to digest fatty foods

Acute Pain r/t trauma from surgery

Risk for deficient Fluid volume: Risk factors: restricted intake, nausea, vomiting

Risk for Surgical Site Infection: Risk factor: invasive procedure

Readiness for enhanced Knowledge: expresses an interest in learning

See Abdominal Surgery

CHOLELITHIASIS

Nausea r/t obstruction of bile

Imbalanced Nutrition: less than body requirements r/t anorexia, nausea, vomiting

Acute Pain r/t obstruction of bile flow, inflammation in gallbladder

Readiness for enhanced Knowledge: expresses an interest in learning

CHORIOAMNIONITIS

Anxiety r/t threat to self and infant

C

Hyperthermia r/t infectious process

Situational low Self-Esteem r/t guilt about threat to infant's health

Risk for Infection: Risk factors: infection transmission from mother to fetus; infection in fetal environment

CHRONIC CONFUSION

See Confusion, Chronic

CHRONIC FUNCTIONAL CONSTIPATION

(See **Constipation**, chronic functional, Section II)

(See **Constipation**, chronic functional, risk for, Section II)

CHRONIC LYMPHOCYTIC LEUKEMIA

See Cancer; Chemotherapy; Leukemia

CHRONIC OBSTRUCTIVE PULMONARY DISEASE (COPD)

See COPD (Chronic Obstructive Pulmonary Disease)

CHRONIC PAIN

See Pain Management, Chronic

CHRONIC RENAL FAILURE (CHRONIC RENAL DISEASE)

See Renal Failure

CHVOSTEK'S SIGN

See Hypocalcemia

CIRCUMCISION

Acute Pain r/t surgical intervention

Risk for Bleeding: Risk factor: surgical trauma

Risk for Infection: Risk factor: surgical wound

Readiness for enhanced Knowledge: parent: expresses an interest in learning

CIRRHOSIS

Chronic Confusion r/t chronic organic disorder with increased ammonia levels, substance abuse

Defensive Coping r/t inability to accept responsibility to stop substance abuse

Fatigue r/t malnutrition

Ineffective Health maintenance behaviors r/t deficient knowledge regarding correlation between lifestyle habits and disease process

Nausea r/t irritation to gastrointestinal system

Imbalanced Nutrition: less than body requirements r/t loss of appetite, nausea, vomiting

Chronic Pain r/t liver enlargement

Chronic low Self-Esteem r/t chronic illness

Chronic Sorrow r/t presence of chronic illness

Risk for Bleeding: Risk factors: impaired blood coagulation, bleeding from portal hypertension

Risk for Injury: Risk factors: substance intoxication, potential delirium tremens

Risk for impaired Oral Mucous Membrane Integrity: Risk factors: altered nutrition, inadequate oral care

Risk for impaired Skin integrity: Risk factors: altered nutritional state, altered metabolic state

CLEFT LIP/CLEFT PALATE

Ineffective Airway clearance r/t common feeding and breathing passage, postoperative laryngeal, incisional edema

Ineffective Breastfeeding r/t infant anomaly

Impaired verbal Communication r/t inadequate palate function, possible hearing loss from infected eustachian tubes

Fear: parental r/t special care needs, surgery

Ineffective infant Feeding dynamic r/t fear resulting in inadequate feeding

Ineffective infant suck-swallow response r/t cleft lip, cleft palate

Impaired physical Mobility r/t imposed restricted activity, use of elbow restraints

Impaired Oral Mucous Membrane Integrity r/t surgical correction

Acute Pain r/t surgical correction, elbow restraints

Impaired Skin integrity r/t incomplete joining of lip, palate ridges

Chronic Sorrow r/t birth of child with congenital defect

Risk for Aspiration: Risk factor: common feeding and breathing passage

Risk for disturbed Body Image: Risk factors: disfigurement, speech impediment

Risk for delayed Child Development: Risk factor: inadequate nutrition resulting from difficulty feeding

Risk for deficient Fluid volume: Risk factor: inability to take liquids in usual manner

Risk for Infection: Risk factors: invasive procedure, disruption of eustachian tube development, aspiration

Readiness for enhanced Knowledge: parent: expresses an interest in learning

CLOTTING DISORDER

Fear r/t threat to well-being

Risk for Bleeding: Risk factor: impaired clotting

Readiness for enhanced Knowledge: expresses an interest in learning

See Anticoagulant Therapy; DIC (Disseminated Intravascular Coagulation); Hemophilia

COCAINE BABY

See Neonatal Abstinence Syndrome

CODEPENDENCY

Caregiver Role Strain r/t codependency

Impaired verbal Communication r/t psychological barriers

Ineffective Coping r/t inadequate support systems

Decisional Conflict r/t support system deficit

Ineffective Denial r/t unmet self-needs

Powerlessness r/t lifestyle of helplessness

COLD, VIRAL

See Infectious Processes

COLECTOMY

Constipation r/t decreased activity, decreased fluid intake

Imbalanced Nutrition: less than body requirements r/t high metabolic needs, decreased ability to ingest or digest food

Acute Pain r/t recent surgery

Risk for Surgical Site Infection: Risk factor: invasive procedure

Readiness for enhanced Knowledge: expresses an interest in learning

See Abdominal Surgery

COLITIS

Diarrhea r/t inflammation in colon

Deficient Fluid volume r/t frequent stools

Acute Pain r/t inflammation in colon

Readiness for enhanced Knowledge: expresses an interest in learning

See Crohn's Disease; Inflammatory Bowel Disease (Child and Adult)

COLLAGEN DISEASE

See specific disease (e.g., Lupus erythematosus; JRA [juvenile rheumatoid arthritis]); Congenital Heart Disease/ Cardiac Anomalies

COLOSTOMY

Disturbed Body Image r/t presence of stoma, daily care of fecal material

Ineffective Sexuality pattern r/t altered body image, self-concept

Social isolation r/t anxiety about appearance of stoma and possible leakage of stool

C

Risk for Constipation: Risk factor: inappropriate diet

Risk for Diarrhea: Risk factor: inappropriate diet

Risk for impaired Skin integrity: Risk factor: irritation from bowel contents

Readiness for enhanced Knowledge: expresses an interest in learning

COLPORRHAPHY, ANTERIOR

See Vaginal Hysterectomy

COMA

Death Anxiety: **significant others** r/t unknown outcome of coma state

Interrupted Family processes r/t illness or disability of family member

Disability-associated urinary Incontinence r/t presence of comatose state

Self-Care deficit: r/t neuromuscular impairment

Ineffective family Health self-management r/t complexity of therapeutic regimen

Risk for Aspiration: Risk factors: impaired swallowing, loss of cough or gag reflex

Risk for Disuse syndrome: Risk factor: altered level of consciousness impairing mobility

Risk for Dry Mouth: Risk factor: inability to perform own oral care

Risk for Hypothermia: Risk factors: Inactivity, possible pharmaceutical agents, possible hypothalamic injury

Risk for Injury: Risk factor: potential seizure activity

Risk for corneal Injury: Risk factor: suppressed corneal reflex

Risk for urinary tract Injury: Risk factor: long-term use of urinary catheter

Risk for impaired Oral Mucous Membrane Integrity: Risk factors: dry mouth, inability to do own mouth care

Risk for Adult Pressure Injury: Risk factor: prolonged immobility

Risk for impaired Skin integrity: Risk factor: immobility

Risk for Spiritual distress: **significant others**: Risk factors: loss of ability to relate to loved one, unknown outcome of coma

Risk for impaired Tissue integrity: Risk factor: impaired physical mobility

See Head Injury; Subarachnoid Hemorrhage; Intracranial Pressure, Increased

COMFORT, LOSS OF

Impaired Comfort (See **Comfort**, impaired, Section II)

Readiness for enhanced Comfort (See **Comfort**, readiness for enhanced, Section II)

COMMUNICABLE DISEASES, CHILDHOOD (E.G., MEASLES, MUMPS, RUBELLA, CHICKENPOX, SCABIES, LICE, IMPETIGO)

Impaired Comfort r/t pruritus, inflammation or infection of skin, subdermal organisms

Decreased Diversional activity engagement r/t imposed isolation from peers, disruption in usual play activities, fatigue, decreased activity tolerance

Ineffective Health maintenance behaviors r/t nonadherence to appropriate immunization schedules, lack of prevention of transmission of infection

Acute Pain r/t impaired skin integrity, edema

Risk for Infection: **transmission to others**: Risk factor: contagious organisms

See Meningitis/Encephalitis; Respiratory Infections, Acute Childhood

COMMUNICATION

Readiness for enhanced Communication (See **Communication**, readiness for enhanced, Section II)

COMMUNICATION PROBLEMS

Impaired verbal Communication (See **Communication**, verbal, impaired, Section II)

COMMUNITY COPING

Ineffective community Coping (See **Coping**, community, ineffective, Section II)

Readiness for enhanced community Coping: community sense of power to manage stressors, social supports available, resources available for problem solving

COMMUNITY HEALTH PROBLEMS

Deficient community Health (See **Health**, deficient, community, Section II)

COMPANION ANIMAL

Anxiety r/t environmental and personal stressors

Impaired Comfort r/t insufficient environmental control

COMPARTMENT SYNDROME

Fear r/t possible loss of limb, damage to limb

Acute Pain r/t pressure in compromised body part

Ineffective peripheral Tissue Perfusion r/t increased pressure within compartment

COMPULSION

See OCD (Obsessive-Compulsive Disorder)

CONDUCTION DISORDERS (CARDIAC)

See Dysrhythmia

CONFUSION, ACUTE

Acute Confusion r/t older than 70 years of age with hospitalization, alcohol abuse, delirium, dementia, substance abuse

Frail Elderly syndrome r/t impaired memory

Risk for acute Confusion: Risk factor: alteration in level of consciousness

CONFUSION, CHRONIC

Chronic Confusion r/t dementia, Korsakoff's psychosis, multi-infarct dementia, cerebrovascular accident, head injury

Frail Elderly syndrome r/t impaired memory

Impaired Memory r/t fluid and electrolyte imbalance, neurological disturbances, excessive environmental disturbances, anemia, acute or chronic hypoxia, decreased cardiac output

Impaired Mood regulation r/t emotional instability

See Alzheimer's Disease; Dementia

CONGENITAL HEART DISEASE/ CARDIAC ANOMALIES

Decreased activity tolerance r/t fatigue, generalized weakness, lack of adequate oxygenation

Ineffective Breathing pattern r/t pulmonary vascular disease

Decreased Cardiac output r/t cardiac dysfunction

Excess Fluid volume r/t cardiac dysfunction, side effects of medication

Impaired Gas exchange r/t cardiac dysfunction, pulmonary congestion

Imbalanced Nutrition: less than body requirements r/t fatigue, generalized weakness, inability of infant to suck and feed, increased caloric requirements

Risk for delayed Child Development: Risk factor: inadequate oxygen and nutrients to tissues

Risk for deficient Fluid volume: Risk factor: side effects of diuretics

Risk for disorganized Infant behavior: Risk factor: invasive procedures

Risk for Poisoning: Risk factor: potential toxicity of cardiac medications

Risk for ineffective Thermoregulation: Risk factor: neonatal age

See Child with Chronic Condition; Hospitalized Child

CONGESTIVE HEART FAILURE (CHF)

See Heart Failure

CONJUNCTIVITIS

Acute Pain r/t inflammatory process

C

Vision Loss r/t change in visual acuity resulting from inflammation

C

CONSCIOUSNESS, ALTERED LEVEL OF

Acute Confusion r/t alcohol abuse, delirium, dementia, drug abuse, head injury

Chronic Confusion r/t multi-infarct dementia, Korsakoff's psychosis, head injury, cerebrovascular accident, neurological deficit

Disability-associated urinary Incontinence r/t neurological dysfunction

Impaired Memory r/t neurological disturbances

Self-Care deficit: **specify** r/t neuromuscular impairment

Risk for Aspiration: Risk factors: impaired swallowing, loss of cough or gag reflex

Risk for Disuse syndrome: Risk factor: impaired mobility resulting from altered level of consciousness

Risk for Dry Mouth: Risk factor: inability to perform own oral care

Risk for Adult Falls: Risk factor: diminished mental status

Risk for impaired Oral Mucous Membrane Integrity: Risk factors: dry mouth, interrupted oral care

Risk for ineffective Cerebral tissue perfusion: Risk factors: increased intracranial pressure, altered cerebral perfusion

Risk for impaired Skin integrity: Risk factor: immobility

See Coma; Head Injury; Subarachnoid Hemorrhage; Intracranial Pressure, Increased

CONSTIPATION

Constipation (See **Constipation**, Section II)

CONSTIPATION, CHRONIC FUNCTIONAL

Constipation (See **Constipation**, chronic functional, Section II)

CONSTIPATION, PERCEIVED

Perceived Constipation (See perceived **Constipation**, Section II)

CONSTIPATION, RISK FOR

Risk for Constipation (See **Constipation**, risk for, Section II)

Risk for chronic functional Constipation (See **Constipation**, chronic functional, risk for, Section II)

CONTAMINATION

Contamination (See **Contamination**, Section II)

Risk for Contamination (See **Contamination**, risk for, Section II)

CONTINENT ILEOSTOMY (KOCK POUCH)

Ineffective Coping r/t stress of disease, exacerbations caused by stress

Imbalanced Nutrition: **less than body requirements** r/t malabsorption from disease process

Risk for Injury: Risk factors: failure of valve, stomal cyanosis, intestinal obstruction

Readiness for enhanced Knowledge: expresses an interest in learning

See Abdominal Surgery; Crohn's Disease

CONTRACEPTIVE METHOD

Decisional Conflict: **method of contraception** r/t unclear personal values or beliefs, lack of experience or interference with decision-making, lack of relevant information, support system deficit

Ineffective Sexuality pattern r/t fear of pregnancy

Readiness for enhanced Health self-management: requesting information about available and appropriate birth control methods

CONVULSIONS

Anxiety r/t concern over controlling convulsions

Impaired Memory r/t neurological disturbance

Risk for Aspiration: Risk factor: impaired swallowing

Risk for delayed Child Development: Risk factor: seizures

Risk for Injury: Risk factor: seizure activity

Readiness for enhanced Knowledge: expresses an interest in learning

See Seizure Disorders, Adult; Seizure Disorders, Childhood

COPD (CHRONIC OBSTRUCTIVE PULMONARY DISEASE)

Decreased activity tolerance r/t imbalance between oxygen supply and demand

Ineffective Airway clearance r/t bronchoconstriction, increased mucus, ineffective cough, infection

Anxiety r/t breathlessness, change in health status

Death Anxiety r/t seriousness of medical condition, difficulty being able to "catch breath," feeling of suffocation

Interrupted Family processes r/t role changes

Impaired Gas exchange r/t ventilation-perfusion inequality

Ineffective Health self-management (See **Health** self-management, ineffective, Section II)

Imbalanced Nutrition: **less than body requirements** r/t decreased intake because of dyspnea, unpleasant taste in mouth left by medications, increased need for calories from work of breathing

Powerlessness r/t progressive nature of disease

Self-Care deficit: r/t fatigue from the increased work of breathing

Chronic low Self-Esteem r/t chronic illness

Sleep deprivation r/t breathing difficulties when lying down

Impaired Social interaction r/t social isolation because of oxygen use, decreased activity tolerance

Chronic Sorrow r/t presence of chronic illness

Risk for Infection: Risk factor: stasis of respiratory secretions

Readiness for enhanced Health self-management (See **Health** self-management, readiness for enhanced, Section II)

COPING

Readiness for enhanced Coping (See **Coping**, readiness for enhanced, Section II)

COPING PROBLEMS

Compromised family Coping (see **Coping**, compromised family, Section II)

Defensive Coping (See **Coping**, defensive, Section II)

Disabled family Coping (See **Coping**, disabled family, Section II)

Ineffective Coping (See **Coping**, ineffective, Section II)

Ineffective community Coping (see **Coping**, ineffective community, Section II)

CORNEAL INJURY

Risk for corneal Injury (See corneal **Injury**, risk for, Section II)

CORNEAL REFLEX, ABSENT

Risk for Injury: Risk factors: accidental corneal abrasion, drying of cornea

CORNEAL TRANSPLANT

Risk for Surgical Site Infection: Risk factors: invasive procedure, surgery

Readiness for enhanced Health self-management: describes need to rest and avoid strenuous activities during healing phase

C

CORONARY ARTERY BYPASS GRAFTING (CABG)

Decreased Cardiac output r/t dysrhythmia, depressed cardiac function, change in preload, contractility or afterload

Fear r/t outcome of surgical procedure

Deficient Fluid volume r/t intraoperative blood loss, use of diuretics in surgery

Acute Pain r/t traumatic surgery

Risk for Perioperative Positioning injury: Risk factors: hypothermia, extended supine position

Risk for Surgical Site Infection: Risk factor: surgical incision

Risk for Impaired Tissue integrity: Risk Factor: surgical procedure

Readiness for enhanced Knowledge: expresses an interest in learning

COSTOVERTEBRAL ANGLE TENDERNESS

See Kidney Stone; Pyelonephritis

COUGH, INEFFECTIVE

Ineffective Airway clearance r/t decreased energy, fatigue, normal aging changes

See Bronchitis; COPD (Chronic Obstructive Pulmonary Disease); Pulmonary Edema

CRACKLES IN LUNGS, COARSE

Ineffective Airway clearance r/t excessive secretions in airways, ineffective cough

See Heart Failure; Pneumonia; Pulmonary Edema

CRACKLES IN LUNGS, FINE

Ineffective Breathing pattern r/t fatigue, surgery, decreased energy

See Bronchitis or Pneumonia (if from pulmonary infection); Congestive Heart Failure (CHF) (if cardiac in origin); Infection, potential for

CRANIECTOMY/CRANIOTOMY

Frail Elderly syndrome r/t alteration in cognition

Fear r/t threat to well-being

Impaired Memory r/t neurological surgery

Acute Pain r/t recent brain surgery, increased intracranial pressure

Risk for ineffective Cerebral tissue perfusion: Risk factors: cerebral edema, increased intracranial pressure

Risk for Injury: Risk factor: potential confusion

See Coma (if relevant)

CREPITATION, SUBCUTANEOUS

See Pneumothorax

CRISIS

Anxiety r/t threat to or change in environment, health status, interaction patterns, situation, self-concept, or role functioning; threat of death of self or significant other

Death Anxiety r/t feelings of hopelessness associated with crisis

Compromised family Coping r/t situational or developmental crisis

Ineffective Coping r/t situational or maturational crisis

Fear r/t crisis situation

Impaired individual Resilience r/t onset of crisis

Situational low Self-Esteem r/t perception of inability to handle crisis

Stress overload (See **Stress** overload, Section II)

Risk for Spiritual distress: Risk factors: physical or psychological stress, natural disasters, situational losses, maturational losses

CROHN'S DISEASE

Anxiety r/t change in health status

Ineffective Coping r/t repeated episodes of diarrhea

Diarrhea r/t inflammatory process

Ineffective Health maintenance behaviors r/t deficient knowledge regarding management of disease

Imbalanced Nutrition: less than body requirements r/t diarrhea, altered ability to digest and absorb food

Acute Pain r/t increased peristalsis

Powerlessness r/t chronic disease

Risk for deficient Fluid volume: Risk factor: abnormal fluid loss with diarrhea

CROUP

See Respiratory Infections, Acute Childhood (Croup, Epiglottitis, Pertussis, Pneumonia, Respiratory)

CRYOSURGERY FOR RETINAL DETACHMENT

See Retinal Detachment

CUSHING'S SYNDROME

Decreased activity tolerance r/t fatigue, weakness

Disturbed Body Image r/t change in appearance from disease process

Excess Fluid volume r/t failure of regulatory mechanisms

Sexual dysfunction r/t loss of libido

Impaired Skin integrity r/t thin vulnerable skin from effects of increased cortisol

Risk for Infection: Risk factor: suppression of immune system caused by increased cortisol levels

Risk for Injury: Risk factors: decreased muscle strength, brittle bones

Readiness for enhanced Knowledge: expresses an interest in learning

CUTS (WOUNDS)

See Lacerations

CVA (CEREBROVASCULAR ACCIDENT)

Anxiety r/t situational crisis, change in physical or emotional condition

Disturbed Body Image r/t chronic illness, paralysis

Caregiver Role Strain r/t cognitive problems of care receiver, need for significant home care

Impaired verbal Communication r/t pressure damage, decreased circulation to brain in speech center informational sources

Chronic Confusion r/t neurological changes

Constipation r/t decreased activity

Ineffective Coping r/t disability

Interrupted Family processes r/t illness, disability of family member

Frail Elderly syndrome r/t alteration in cognitive functioning

Ineffective Home Maintenance Behaviors r/t neurological disease affecting ability to perform activities of daily living

Disability-associated urinary Incontinence r/t neurological dysfunction

Impaired Memory r/t neurological disturbances

Impaired physical Mobility r/t loss of balance and coordination

Unilateral Neglect r/t disturbed perception from neurological damage

Self-Care deficit: specify r/t decreased strength and endurance, paralysis

Impaired Social interaction r/t limited physical mobility, limited ability to communicate

Impaired Swallowing r/t neuromuscular dysfunction

Impaired Transfer Ability r/t limited physical mobility

Vision Loss r/t pressure damage to visual

C

C

centers in the brain (*see care plan in Appendix*)

Impaired Walking r/t loss of balance and coordination

Risk for Aspiration: Risk factors: impaired swallowing, loss of gag reflex

Risk for chronic functional Constipation: Risk factor: immobility

Risk for Disuse syndrome: Risk factor: paralysis

Risk for Adult Falls: Risk factor: paralysis, decreased balance

Risk for Injury: Risk factors: vision loss, decreased tissue perfusion with loss of sensation

Risk for ineffective Cerebral tissue perfusion: Risk factor: clot, emboli, or hemorrhage from cerebral vessel

Risk for impaired Skin integrity: Risk factor: immobility

Readiness for enhanced Knowledge: expresses an interest in learning

CYANOSIS, CENTRAL WITH CYANOSIS OF ORAL MUCOUS MEMBRANES

Impaired Gas exchange r/t alveolar-capillary membrane changes

CYANOSIS, PERIPHERAL WITH CYANOSIS OF NAIL BEDS

Ineffective peripheral Tissue Perfusion r/t interruption of arterial flow, severe vasoconstriction, cold temperatures

CYSTIC FIBROSIS

Decreased activity tolerance r/t imbalance between oxygen supply and demand

Ineffective Airway clearance r/t increased production of thick mucus

Anxiety r/t dyspnea, oxygen deprivation

Disturbed Body Image r/t changes in physical appearance, treatment of chronic lung disease (clubbing, barrel chest, home oxygen therapy)

Impaired Gas exchange r/t ventilation-perfusion imbalance

Ineffective Home Maintenance Behaviors r/t extensive daily treatment, medications necessary for health

Imbalanced Nutrition: less than body requirements r/t anorexia; decreased absorption of nutrients, fat; increased work of breathing

Chronic Sorrow r/t presence of chronic disease

Risk for Caregiver Role Strain: Risk factors: illness severity of care receiver, unpredictable course of illness

Risk for deficient Fluid volume: Risk factors: decreased fluid intake, increased work of breathing

Risk for Infection: Risk factors: thick, tenacious mucus; harboring of bacterial organisms; immunocompromised state

Risk for Spiritual distress: Risk factor: presence of chronic disease

See Child with Chronic Condition; Hospitalized Child; Terminally Ill Child, Adolescent; Terminally Ill Child, Infant/Toddler; Terminally Ill Child, Preschool Child; Terminally Ill Child, School-Age Child/Preadolescent; Terminally Ill Child/Death of Child, Parent

CYSTITIS

Acute Pain: dysuria r/t inflammatory process in bladder and urethra

Impaired Urinary elimination: frequency r/t urinary tract infection

Urge urinary Incontinence: Risk factor: infection in bladder

Readiness for enhanced Knowledge: expresses an interest in learning

CYSTOCELE

Stress urinary Incontinence r/t prolapsed bladder

Readiness for enhanced Knowledge: expresses an interest in learning

CYSTOSCOPY

Urinary Retention r/t edema in urethra obstructing flow of urine

Risk for Infection: Risk factor: invasive procedure

Readiness for enhanced Knowledge: expresses an interest in learning

DEAFNESS

Impaired verbal Communication r/t impaired hearing

Hearing Loss r/t alteration in sensory reception, transmission, integration

Risk for delayed Child Development: Risk factor: impaired hearing

Risk for Injury: Risk factor: alteration in sensory perception

DEATH

Risk for Sudden Infant Death (See **Sudden Infant Death**, risk for, Section II)

DEATH, ONCOMING

Death Anxiety r/t unresolved issues surrounding dying

Compromised family Coping r/t client's inability to provide support to family

Ineffective Coping r/t personal vulnerability

Fear r/t threat of death

Powerlessness r/t effects of illness, oncoming death

Social isolation r/t altered state of wellness

Spiritual distress r/t intense suffering

Readiness for enhanced Spiritual well-being: desire of client and family to be in harmony with each other and higher power, God

See Terminally Ill Child, Adolescent; Terminally Ill Child, Infant/Toddler; Terminally Ill Child, Preschool Child; Terminally Ill Child, School-Age Child/Preadolescent; Terminally Ill Child/Death of Child, Parent

DECISIONS, DIFFICULTY MAKING

Decisional Conflict r/t support system deficit, perceived threat to value system, multiple or divergent sources of information, lack of relevant information, unclear personal values or beliefs

Risk for impaired Emancipated Decision-Making: Risk factors: insufficient self-confidence in decision-making

Readiness for enhanced Decision-Making (See **Decision-Making**, readiness for enhanced, Section II)

DECUBITUS ULCER

See Pressure Ulcer

DEEP VEIN THROMBOSIS (DVT)

See DVT (Deep Vein Thrombosis); Venous Thromboembolism

DEFENSIVE BEHAVIOR

Defensive Coping r/t nonacceptance of blame, denial of problems or weakness

Ineffective Denial r/t inability to face situation realistically

DEHISCENCE, ABDOMINAL

Fear r/t threat of death, severe dysfunction

Acute Pain r/t stretching of abdominal wall

Impaired Skin integrity r/t altered circulation, malnutrition, opening in incision

Delayed Surgical recovery r/t altered circulation, malnutrition, opening in incision

Impaired Tissue integrity r/t exposure of abdominal contents to external environment

Risk for deficient Fluid volume: Risk factor: altered circulation associated with opening of wound and exposure of abdominal contents

Risk for Surgical Site Infection: Risk factors: loss of skin integrity, open surgical wound

DEHYDRATION

Deficient Fluid volume r/t active fluid volume loss

Impaired Oral Mucous Membrane Integrity r/t decreased salivation, fluid deficit

Risk for chronic functional Constipation: Risk factor: decreased fluid volume

D

Risk for Dry Mouth: Risk factor: decreased fluid volume

Risk for ineffective Thermoregulation: Risk factor: decreased fluid volume

Risk for Unstable Blood Pressure: Risk factor: hypotension caused by insufficient fluid volume

See Burns; Heat Stroke; Vomiting; Diarrhea

DELIRIUM

Acute Confusion r/t effects of medication, response to hospitalization, alcohol abuse, substance abuse, sensory deprivation or overload, infection, polypharmacy

Impaired Memory r/t delirium

Sleep deprivation r/t sustained inadequate sleep hygiene

Risk for Injury: Risk factor: altered level of consciousness

DELIRIUM TREMENS (DT)

See Alcohol Withdrawal

DELIVERY

See Labor, Normal

DELUSIONS

Impaired verbal Communication r/t psychological impairment, delusional thinking

Acute Confusion r/t alcohol abuse, delirium, dementia, substance abuse

Ineffective Coping r/t distortion and insecurity of life events

Fear r/t content of intrusive thoughts

Risk for other-directed Violence: Risk factor: delusional thinking

Risk for self-directed Violence: Risk factor: delusional thinking

DEMENTIA

Chronic Confusion r/t neurological dysfunction

Interrupted Family processes r/t disability of family member

Frail Elderly syndrome r/t alteration in cognitive functioning

Ineffective Home Maintenance Behaviors r/t inadequate support system, neurological dysfunction

Imbalanced Nutrition: less than body requirements r/t neurological impairment

Disability-associated urinary Incontinence r/t neurological dysfunction

Insomnia r/t neurological impairment, naps during the day

Impaired physical Mobility r/t alteration in cognitive function

Self-Neglect r/t cognitive impairment

Self-Care deficit: specify r/t psychological or neuromuscular impairment

Chronic Sorrow: Significant other r/t chronic long-standing disability, loss of mental function

Impaired Swallowing r/t neuromuscular changes associated with long-standing dementia

Risk for Caregiver Role Strain: Risk factors: number of caregiving tasks, duration of caregiving required

Risk for Chronic Functional Constipation: Risk factor: decreased fluid intake

Risk for Adult Falls: Risk factor: diminished mental status

Risk for Frail Elderly syndrome: Risk factors: cognitive impairment

Risk for Injury: Risk factors: confusion, decreased muscle coordination

Risk for impaired Skin integrity: Risk factors: altered nutritional status, immobility

DENIAL OF HEALTH STATUS

Ineffective Denial r/t lack of perception about the health status effects of illness

Ineffective Health self-management r/t denial of seriousness of health situation

DENTAL CARIES

Impaired Dentition r/t ineffective oral hygiene, barriers to self-care, economic barriers to professional care, nutritional deficits, dietary habits

Ineffective Health maintenance behaviors r/t lack of knowledge regarding prevention of dental disease

DEPRESSION (MAJOR DEPRESSIVE DISORDER)

Death Anxiety r/t feelings of lack of self-worth

Constipation r/t inactivity, decreased fluid intake

Fatigue r/t psychological demands

Ineffective Health maintenance behaviors r/t lack of ability to make good judgments regarding ways to obtain help

Hopelessness r/t feeling of abandonment, long-term stress

Impaired Mood Regulation r/t emotional instability

Insomnia r/t inactivity

Self-Neglect r/t depression, cognitive impairment

Powerlessness r/t pattern of helplessness

Chronic low Self-Esteem r/t repeated unmet expectations

Sexual dysfunction r/t loss of sexual desire

Social isolation r/t ineffective coping

Chronic Sorrow r/t unresolved grief

Risk for maladaptive Grieving: Risk factor: lack of previous resolution of former grieving response

Risk for Suicidal Behavior: Risk factor: grieving, hopelessness

DERMATITIS

Anxiety r/t situational crisis imposed by illness

Impaired Comfort r/t itching

Impaired Skin integrity r/t side effect of medication, allergic reaction

Readiness for enhanced Knowledge: expresses an interest in learning

See Itching

DESPONDENCY

Hopelessness r/t long-term stress

See Depression (Major Depressive Disorder)

DESTRUCTIVE BEHAVIOR TOWARD OTHERS

Risk-prone Health behavior r/t intense emotional state

Ineffective Coping r/t situational crises, maturational crises, disturbance in pattern of appraisal of threat

Risk for other-directed Violence (See **Violence**, other-directed, risk for, Section II)

DEVELOPMENTAL CONCERNS

Risk for delayed Child Development (See **Development**, delayed, risk for, Section II)

See Growth and Development Lag

DIABETES IN PREGNANCY

See Gestational Diabetes (Diabetes in Pregnancy)

DIABETES INSIPIDUS

Deficient Fluid volume r/t inability to conserve fluid

Ineffective Health maintenance behaviors r/t deficient knowledge regarding care of disease, importance of medications

DIABETES MELLITUS

Ineffective Health maintenance behaviors r/t complexity of therapeutic regimen

Ineffective Health self-management (See **Health** self-management, ineffective, Section II)

Imbalanced Nutrition: less than body requirements r/t inability to use glucose (type 1 [insulin-dependent] diabetes)

D

D

Risk for Overweight r/t excessive intake of nutrients (type 2 diabetes)

Ineffective peripheral Tissue perfusion r/t impaired arterial circulation

Powerlessness r/t perceived lack of personal control

Sexual dysfunction r/t neuropathy associated with disease

Vision Loss r/t ineffective tissue perfusion of retina

Risk for unstable blood Glucose level (See **Glucose** level, blood, unstable, risk for, Section II)

Risk for Infection: Risk factors: hyperglycemia, impaired healing, circulatory changes

Risk for Injury: Risk factors: hypoglycemia or hyperglycemia from failure to consume adequate calories, failure to take insulin

Risk for dysfunctional Gastrointestinal motility: Risk factor: complication of diabetes

Risk for Metabolic Syndrome: Risk factor: complication of diabetes

Risk for impaired Skin integrity: Risk factor: loss of pain perception in extremities

Risk for delayed Surgical recovery: Risk factor: impaired healing caused by circulatory changes

Readiness for enhanced Health literacy: expresses desire to enhance understanding of health information to make healthcare choices

Readiness for enhanced Health self-management (See **Health** self-management, readiness for enhanced, Section II)

Readiness for enhanced Knowledge: expresses an interest in learning

See Hyperglycemia; Hypoglycemia

DIABETES MELLITUS, JUVENILE (INSULIN-DEPENDENT DIABETES MELLITUS TYPE 1)

Risk-prone Health behavior r/t inadequate comprehension, inadequate social support, low self-efficacy, impaired adjustment attributable to adolescent maturational crises

Disturbed Body Image r/t imposed deviations from biophysical and psychosocial norm, perceived differences from peers

Impaired Comfort r/t insulin injections, peripheral blood glucose testing

Ineffective Health maintenance behaviors r/t (See **Health** maintenance behaviors, ineffective, Section II)

Imbalanced Nutrition: less than body requirements r/t inability of body to adequately metabolize and use glucose and nutrients, increased caloric needs of child to promote growth and physical activity participation with peers

Risk for Metabolic Syndrome: Risk factor: complication of diabetes

Readiness for enhanced Knowledge: expresses an interest in learning

See Diabetes Mellitus; Child with Chronic Condition; Hospitalized Child

DIABETIC COMA

Acute Confusion r/t hyperglycemia, presence of excessive metabolic acids

Deficient Fluid volume r/t hyperglycemia resulting in polyuria

Ineffective Health self-management r/t lack of understanding of preventive measures, adequate blood glucose control

Risk for unstable blood Glucose level (See **Glucose** level, blood, unstable, risk for, Section II)

Risk for Infection: Risk factors: hyperglycemia, changes in vascular system

See Diabetes Mellitus

DIABETIC KETOACIDOSIS

See Ketoacidosis, Diabetic

DIABETIC NEUROPATHY

See Neuropathy, Peripheral

DIABETIC RETINOPATHY

Ineffective Health maintenance behaviors r/t deficient knowledge regarding preserving vision with treatment if possible, use of low-vision aids

See Vision Impairment; Blindness

DIALYSIS

See Hemodialysis; Peritoneal Dialysis

DIAPHRAGMATIC HERNIA

See Hiatal Hernia

DIARRHEA

Diarrhea r/t infection, change in diet, gastrointestinal disorders, stress, medication effect, impaction

Deficient Fluid volume r/t excessive loss of fluids in liquid stools

Risk for Electrolyte imbalance: Risk factor: effect of loss of electrolytes from frequent stools

DIC (DISSEMINATED INTRAVASCULAR COAGULATION)

Fear r/t threat to well-being

Deficient Fluid volume: hemorrhage r/t depletion of clotting factors

Risk for Bleeding: Risk factors: microclotting within vascular system, depleted clotting factors

DIGITALIS TOXICITY

Decreased Cardiac output r/t drug toxicity affecting cardiac rhythm, rate

Ineffective Health self-management r/t deficient knowledge regarding action, appropriate method of administration of digitalis

DIGNITY, LOSS OF

Risk for compromised Human Dignity (See **Human Dignity**, compromised, risk for, Section II)

DILATION AND CURETTAGE (D&C)

Acute Pain r/t uterine contractions

Risk for Bleeding: Risk factor: surgical procedure

Risk for Surgical Site Infection: Risk factor: surgical procedure

Risk for ineffective Sexuality pattern: Risk factors: painful coitus, fear associated with surgery on genital area

Readiness for enhanced Knowledge: expresses an interest in learning

DIRTY BODY (FOR PROLONGED PERIOD)

Self-Neglect r/t mental illness, substance abuse, cognitive impairment

DISCHARGE PLANNING

Ineffective Home Maintenance Behaviors r/t family member's disease or injury interfering with home maintenance

Deficient Knowledge r/t lack of exposure to information for home care

Relocation stress syndrome: Risk factors: insufficient predeparture counseling, insufficient support system, unpredictability of experience

Readiness for enhanced Health literacy: expresses desire to enhance understanding of health information to make healthcare choices

Readiness for enhanced Knowledge: expresses an interest in learning

DISCOMFORTS OF PREGNANCY

Disturbed Body Image r/t pregnancy-induced body changes

Impaired Comfort r/t enlarged abdomen, swollen feet

Fatigue r/t hormonal, metabolic, body changes

Stress urinary Incontinence r/t enlarged uterus, fetal movement

D

Insomnia r/t psychological stress, fetal movement, muscular cramping, urinary frequency, shortness of breath

Nausea r/t hormone effect

Acute Pain: **headache** r/t hormonal changes of pregnancy

Acute Pain: **leg cramps** r/t nerve compression, calcium/phosphorus/potassium imbalance

Risk for Constipation: Risk factors: decreased intestinal motility, inadequate fiber in diet

Risk for Injury: Risk factors: faintness and/or syncope caused by vasomotor lability or postural hypotension, venous stasis in lower extremities

DISLOCATION OF JOINT

Acute Pain r/t dislocation of a joint

Self-Care deficit: r/t inability to use a joint

Risk for Injury: Risk factor: unstable joint

DISSECTING ANEURYSM

Fear r/t threat to well-being

See Abdominal Surgery; Aneurysm, Abdominal Aortic Repair Surgery

DISSEMINATED INTRAVASCULAR COAGULATION (DIC)

See DIC (Disseminated Intravascular Coagulation)

DISSOCIATIVE IDENTITY DISORDER (NOT OTHERWISE SPECIFIED)

Anxiety r/t psychosocial stress

Ineffective Coping r/t personal vulnerability in crisis of accurate self-perception

Disturbed personal Identity r/t inability to distinguish self—caused by multiple personality disorder, depersonalization, disturbance in memory

Impaired Memory r/t altered state of consciousness

See Multiple Personality Disorder (Dissociative Identity Disorder)

DISTRESS

Anxiety r/t situational crises, maturational crises

Death Anxiety r/t denial of one's own mortality or impending death

DISUSE SYNDROME, POTENTIAL TO DEVELOP

Risk for Disuse syndrome: Risk factors: paralysis, mechanical immobilization, prescribed immobilization, severe pain, altered level of consciousness

DIVERSIONAL ACTIVITY ENGAGEMENT, LACK OF

Decreased Diversional activity engagement r/t environmental lack of diversional activity as in frequent hospitalizations, lengthy treatments

DIVERTICULITIS

Constipation r/t dietary deficiency of fiber and roughage

Diarrhea r/t increased intestinal motility caused by inflammation

Deficient Knowledge r/t diet needed to control disease, medication regimen

Imbalanced Nutrition: **less than body requirements** r/t loss of appetite

Acute Pain r/t inflammation of bowel

Risk for deficient Fluid Volume: Risk factor: diarrhea

DIZZINESS

Decreased Cardiac output r/t alteration in heart rate and rhythm, altered stroke volume

Deficient Knowledge r/t actions to take to prevent or modify dizziness and prevent falls

Impaired physical Mobility r/t dizziness

Risk for Adult Falls: Risk factor: difficulty maintaining balance

Risk for ineffective Cerebral tissue perfusion: Risk factor: interruption of cerebral arterial blood flow

DOMESTIC VIOLENCE

Impaired verbal Communication r/t psychological barriers of fear

Compromised family Coping r/t abusive patterns

Defensive Coping r/t low self-esteem

Dysfunctional Family processes r/t inadequate coping skills

Fear r/t threat to self-concept, situational crisis of abuse

Insomnia r/t psychological stress

Post-Trauma syndrome r/t history of abuse

Powerlessness r/t lifestyle of helplessness

Situational low Self-Esteem r/t negative family interactions

Risk for compromised Resilience: Risk factor: effects of abuse

Risk for other-directed Violence: Risk factor: history of abuse

DOWN SYNDROME

See Child with Chronic Condition; Intellectual Disability

DRESS SELF (INABILITY TO)

Dressing Self-Care deficit r/t intolerance to activity, decreased strength and endurance, pain, discomfort, perceptual or cognitive impairment, neuromuscular impairment, musculoskeletal impairment, depression, severe anxiety

DRIBBLING OF URINE

Stress urinary Incontinence r/t degenerative changes in pelvic muscles and urinary structures

DROOLING

Impaired Swallowing r/t neuromuscular impairment, mechanical obstruction

Risk for Aspiration: Risk factor: impaired swallowing

DROPOUT FROM SCHOOL

Impaired individual Resilience (See **Resilience**, individual, impaired, Section II)

Anxiety r/t conflict about life goals

Ineffective Coping r/t inadequate resources

DRUG ABUSE

See Substance Abuse

DRUG WITHDRAWAL

See Acute Substance Withdrawal Syndrome

DRY EYE

Risk for dry Eye: Risk factors: (See dry **Eye**, risk for, Section II)

Risk for Corneal Injury: Risk factor: suppressed corneal reflex

Readiness for enhanced Knowledge: expresses an interest in learning

See Conjunctivitis; Keratoconjunctivitis Sicca (Dry Eye Syndrome)

DRY MOUTH

Risk for Dry Mouth: Risk factors: (See Dry Mouth, risk for, Section II)

Risk for impaired Oral Mucous Membrane Integrity: Risk factor: reduced quality or quantity of saliva caused by decreased fluid volume

DT (DELIRIUM TREMENS)

See Alcohol Withdrawal

DVT (DEEP VEIN THROMBOSIS)

Constipation r/t inactivity, bed rest

Impaired physical Mobility r/t pain in extremity

Acute Pain r/t vascular inflammation, edema

Ineffective peripheral Tissue perfusion r/t deficient knowledge of aggravating factors

Delayed Surgical recovery r/t impaired physical mobility

Readiness for enhanced Knowledge: expresses an interest in learning

Risk for ineffective Thermoregulation: Risk factor: inactivity

See Anticoagulant Therapy; Venous Thromboembolism, risk for *(See Section II)*

DYING CLIENT

See Terminally Ill Adult; Terminally Ill Adolescent; Terminally Ill Child, Infant/Toddler; Terminally Ill Child, Preschool Child; Terminally Ill Child, School-Age Child/Preadolescent; Terminally Ill Child/Death of Child, Parent

DYSFUNCTIONAL EATING PATTERN

Imbalanced Nutrition: less than body requirements r/t psychological factors

Risk for Overweight: Risk factor: psychological factors

See Anorexia Nervosa; Bulimia; Maturational Issues, Adolescent; Obesity

DYSFUNCTIONAL FAMILY UNIT

See Family Problems

DYSFUNCTIONAL VENTILATORY WEANING

Dysfunctional Ventilatory weaning response r/t physical, psychological, situational factors

DYSMENORRHEA

Nausea r/t prostaglandin effect

Acute Pain r/t cramping from hormonal effects

Readiness for enhanced Knowledge: expresses an interest in learning

DYSPAREUNIA

Sexual Dysfunction r/t lack of lubrication during intercourse, alteration in reproductive organ function

DYSPEPSIA

Anxiety r/t pressures of personal role

Acute Pain r/t gastrointestinal disease, consumption of irritating foods

Readiness for enhanced Knowledge: expresses an interest in learning

DYSPHAGIA

Impaired Swallowing r/t neuromuscular impairment

Risk for Aspiration: Risk factor: loss of gag or cough reflex

DYSPHASIA

Impaired verbal Communication r/t decrease in circulation to brain

Impaired social Interaction r/t difficulty in communicating

DYSPNEA

Decreased activity tolerance r/t imbalance between oxygen supply and demand

Ineffective Breathing pattern r/t compromised cardiac or pulmonary function, decreased lung expansion, neurological impairment affecting respiratory center, extreme anxiety

Fear r/t threat to state of well-being, potential death

Impaired Gas exchange r/t alveolar-capillary damage

Insomnia r/t difficulty breathing, positioning required for effective breathing

Sleep deprivation r/t ineffective breathing pattern

DYSRHYTHMIA

Decreased activity tolerance r/t decreased cardiac output

Decreased Cardiac output r/t alteration in heart rate, rhythm

Fear r/t threat of death, change in health status

Risk for ineffective Cerebral tissue perfusion: Risk factor: decreased blood supply to the brain from dysrhythmia

Readiness for enhanced Knowledge: expresses an interest in learning

DYSTHYMIC DISORDER

Ineffective Coping r/t impaired social interaction

Ineffective Health maintenance behaviors r/t inability to make good judgments regarding ways to obtain help

Insomnia r/t anxious thoughts

Chronic low Self-Esteem r/t repeated unmet expectations

Ineffective Sexuality pattern r/t loss of sexual desire

Social Isolation r/t ineffective coping

See Depression (Major Depressive Disorder)

DYSTOCIA

Anxiety r/t difficult labor, deficient knowledge regarding normal labor pattern

Ineffective Coping r/t situational crisis

Fatigue r/t prolonged labor

Acute Pain r/t difficult labor, medical interventions

Powerlessness r/t perceived inability to control outcome of labor

Risk for Bleeding: Risk factor: hemorrhage secondary to uterine atony

Risk for ineffective Cerebral tissue perfusion (fetal): Risk factor: difficult labor and birth

Risk for delayed Child Development (Infant): Risk factor: difficult labor and birth

Risk for Infection: Risk factor: prolonged rupture of membranes

Risk for impaired Tissue integrity (maternal and fetal): Risk factor: difficult labor

DYSURIA

Impaired Urinary elimination r/t infection/inflammation of the urinary tract

Risk for urge urinary Incontinence: Risk factor: detrusor hyperreflexia from infection in the urinary tract

Acute Pain r/t infection/inflammation of the urinary tract

E

EAR SURGERY

Acute Pain r/t edema in ears from surgery

Hearing Loss r/t invasive surgery of ears, dressings

Risk for delayed Child Development: Risk factor: hearing impairment

Risk for Adult Falls: Risk factor: dizziness from excessive stimuli to vestibular apparatus

Readiness for enhanced Knowledge: expresses an interest in learning

See Hospitalized Child

EARACHE

Acute Pain r/t trauma, edema, infection

Hearing Loss r/t altered sensory reception, transmission

EATING DYNAMICS, ADOLESCENT

Imbalanced Nutrition: less than body requirements r/t negative perception of one's body

Risk for Overweight: Risk factor: Media influence resulting in unhealthy choices, insufficient interest in physical activity

Readiness for enhanced Health Literacy: expresses desire to learn to make healthy food choices

EATING DYNAMICS, CHILD

Imbalanced Nutrition: less than body requirements r/t excessive of parental control over quantity and choices of foods

Risk for delayed Child Development: Risk factor: inadequate nutrition to meet metabolic needs for normal development

Risk for Overweight: Risk factors: unhealthy choices, frequent snacking, low physical activity

EATING DYNAMICS, INFANT

See Feeding Dynamics, Infant

ECLAMPSIA

Interrupted Family processes r/t unmet expectations for pregnancy and childbirth

Fear r/t threat of well-being to self and fetus

Risk for Aspiration: Risk factor: seizure activity

Risk for ineffective Cerebral tissue perfusion: fetal: Risk factor: uteroplacental insufficiency

Risk for delayed Child Development: Risk factor: uteroplacental insufficiency

Risk for excess Fluid volume: Risk factor: decreased urine output as a result of renal dysfunction

Risk for Unstable Blood Pressure: Risk factor: Hypertension caused by excess fluid volume

ECMO (EXTRACORPOREAL MEMBRANE OXYGENATOR)

Death Anxiety r/t emergency condition, hemorrhage

Decreased Cardiac output r/t altered contractility of the heart

Impaired Gas exchange (See **Gas** exchange, impaired, Section II)

See Respiratory Conditions of the Neonate

ECT (ELECTROCONVULSIVE THERAPY)

Decisional Conflict r/t lack of relevant information

Fear r/t real or imagined threat to well-being

Impaired Memory r/t effects of treatment

See Depression (Major Depressive Disorder)

ECTOPIC PREGNANCY

Death Anxiety r/t emergency condition, hemorrhage

Disturbed Body Image r/t negative feelings about body and reproductive functioning

Fear r/t threat to self, surgery, implications for future pregnancy

Acute Pain r/t stretching or rupture of implantation site

Ineffective Role performance r/t loss of pregnancy

Situational low Self-Esteem r/t loss of pregnancy, inability to carry pregnancy to term

Chronic Sorrow r/t loss of pregnancy, potential loss of fertility

Risk for Bleeding: Risk factor: possible rupture of implantation site, surgical trauma

Risk for ineffective Coping: Risk factor: loss of pregnancy

Risk for interrupted Family processes: Risk factor: situational crisis

Risk for Infection: Risk factors: traumatized tissue, surgical procedure

Risk for Spiritual distress: Risk factor: grief process

ECZEMA

Disturbed Body Image r/t change in appearance from inflamed skin

Impaired Comfort: pruritus r/t inflammation of skin

Impaired Skin integrity r/t side effect of medication, allergic reaction

Readiness for enhanced Knowledge: expresses an interest in learning

ED (ERECTILE DYSFUNCTION)

See Erectile Dysfunction (ED); Impotence

EDEMA

Excess Fluid volume r/t excessive fluid intake, cardiac dysfunction, renal dysfunction, loss of plasma proteins

Ineffective Health maintenance behaviors r/t deficient knowledge regarding treatment of edema

Risk for impaired Skin integrity: Risk factors: impaired circulation, fragility of skin

See Heart Failure; Renal Failure

ELDER ABUSE

See Abuse, Spouse, Parent, or Significant Other

ELDERLY

See Aging; Frail Elderly Syndrome

ELECTROCONVULSIVE THERAPY

See ECT (Electroconvulsive Therapy)

ELECTROLYTE IMBALANCE

Risk for Electrolyte imbalance (See **Electrolyte imbalance**, risk for, Section II)

Risk for Unstable Blood Pressure: Risk factor: fluid volume changes

EMACIATED PERSON

Frail Elderly syndrome r/t living alone, malnutrition, alteration in cognitive functioning

Imbalanced Nutrition: less than body requirements r/t inability to ingest food, digest food, absorb nutrients because of biological, psychological, economic factors

EMANCIPATED DECISION-MAKING, IMPAIRED

Risk for impaired emancipated Decision-Making: Risk factor: inability or unwillingness to verbalize needs and wants

Readiness for enhanced emancipated decision-making: expresses desire to enhance ability to understand available options

EMBOLECTOMY

Fear r/t threat of great bodily harm from embolus

Ineffective peripheral Tissue Perfusion r/t presence of embolus

Risk for Bleeding: Risk factors: postoperative complication, surgical area

See Surgery, Postoperative Care

EMBOLI

See Pulmonary Embolism (PE)

EMBOLISM IN LEG OR ARM

Ineffective peripheral Tissue Perfusion r/t arterial/venous obstruction from clot

See DVT (Deep Vein Thrombosis)

EMESIS

Nausea (See **Nausea**, Section II)

See Vomiting

EMOTIONAL PROBLEMS

See Coping Problems

EMPATHY

Readiness for enhanced community Coping: social supports, being available for problem solving

Readiness for enhanced family Coping: basic needs met, desire to move to higher level of health

Readiness for enhanced Spiritual Well-Being: desire to establish interconnectedness through spirituality

EMPHYSEMA

See COPD (Chronic Obstructive Pulmonary Disease)

EMPTINESS

Social isolation r/t inability to engage in satisfying personal relationships

Chronic Sorrow r/t unresolved grief

Spiritual distress r/t separation from religious or cultural ties

ENCEPHALITIS

See Meningitis/Encephalitis

E

ENDOCARDIAL CUSHION DEFECT

See Congenital Heart Disease/Cardiac Anomalies

ENDOCARDITIS

Decreased activity tolerance r/t reduced cardiac reserve, prescribed bed rest

Decreased Cardiac output r/t inflammation of lining of heart and change in structure of valve leaflets, increased myocardial workload

Risk for imbalanced Nutrition: less than body requirements: Risk factors: fever, hypermetabolic state associated with fever

Risk for ineffective Cerebral tissue perfusion: Risk factor: possible presence of emboli in cerebral circulation

Risk for ineffective peripheral Tissue perfusion: Risk factor: possible presence of emboli in peripheral circulation

Readiness for enhanced Knowledge: expresses an interest in learning

ENDOMETRIOSIS

Nausea r/t prostaglandin effect

Acute Pain r/t onset of menses with distention of endometrial tissue

Sexual dysfunction r/t painful intercourse

Readiness for enhanced Knowledge: expresses an interest in learning

ENDOMETRITIS

Anxiety r/t, fear of unknown

Ineffective Thermoregulation r/t infectious process

Acute Pain r/t infectious process in reproductive tract

Readiness for enhanced Knowledge: expresses an interest in learning

ENURESIS

Ineffective Health maintenance behaviors r/t unachieved developmental task, neuromuscular immaturity, diseases of urinary system

See Toilet Training

ENVIRONMENTAL INTERPRETATION PROBLEMS

See Confusion, Chronic

EPIDIDYMITIS

Anxiety r/t situational crisis, pain, threat to future fertility

Acute Pain r/t inflammation in scrotal sac

Ineffective Sexuality pattern r/t edema of epididymis and testes

Readiness for enhanced Knowledge: expresses an interest in learning

EPIGLOTTITIS

See Respiratory Infections, Acute Childhood (Croup, Epiglottitis, Pertussis, Pneumonia, Respiratory Syncytial Virus)

EPILEPSY

Anxiety r/t threat to role functioning

Ineffective Health self-management r/t deficient knowledge regarding seizure control

Impaired Memory r/t seizure activity

Risk for Aspiration: Risk factors: impaired swallowing, excessive secretions

Risk for delayed Child Development: Risk factor: seizure disorder

Risk for Injury: Risk factor: environmental factors during seizure

Readiness for enhanced Knowledge: expresses an interest in learning

See Seizure Disorders, Adult; Seizure Disorders, Childhood (Epilepsy, Febrile Seizures, Infantile Spasms)

EPISIOTOMY

Anxiety r/t fear of pain

Disturbed Body Image r/t fear of resuming sexual relations

Impaired physical Mobility r/t pain, swelling, tissue trauma

Acute Pain r/t tissue trauma

Sexual dysfunction r/t altered body structure, tissue trauma

Impaired Skin integrity r/t perineal incision

Risk for Infection: Risk factor: tissue trauma

EPISTAXIS

Fear r/t large amount of blood loss

Risk for deficient Fluid volume: Risk factor: excessive blood loss

EPSTEIN-BARR VIRUS

See Mononucleosis

ERECTILE DYSFUNCTION (ED)

Situational low Self-Esteem r/t physiological crisis, inability to practice usual sexual activity

Sexual dysfunction r/t altered body function

Readiness for enhanced Knowledge: information regarding treatment for erectile dysfunction

See Impotence

ESCHERICHIA COLI INFECTION

Fear r/t serious illness, unknown outcome

Deficient Knowledge r/t how to prevent disease; care of self with serious illness

See Gastroenteritis; Gastroenteritis, Child; Hospitalized Child

ESOPHAGEAL VARICES

Fear r/t threat of death from hematemesis

Risk for Bleeding: Risk factor: portal hypertension, distended variceal vessels that can easily rupture

See Cirrhosis

ESOPHAGITIS

Acute Pain r/t inflammation of esophagus

Readiness for enhanced Knowledge: expresses an interest in learning

EVISCERATION

See Dehiscence, Abdominal

EXHAUSTION

Impaired individual Resilience (See **Resilience**, individual, impaired, Section II)

Disturbed Sleep pattern (See **Sleep** pattern, disturbed, Section II)

EXPOSURE TO HOT OR COLD ENVIRONMENT

Hyperthermia r/t exposure to hot environment, abnormal reaction to anesthetics

Hypothermia r/t exposure to cold environment

Risk for ineffective Thermoregulation: Risk factors: extremes of environmental temperature, inappropriate clothing for environmental temperature

EXTERNAL FIXATION

Disturbed Body Image r/t trauma, change to affected part

Risk for Infection: Risk factor: presence of pins inserted into bone

See Fracture

EXTRACORPOREAL MEMBRANE OXYGENATOR (ECMO)

See ECMO (Extracorporeal Membrane Oxygenator)

EYE DISCOMFORT

Risk for dry Eye (See **Eye**, dry, risk for, Section II)

Risk for corneal Injury: Risk factors: exposure of the eyeball, blinking less than five times per minute

EYE SURGERY

Anxiety r/t possible loss of vision

Self-Care deficit: specify r/t impaired vision

Vision Loss r/t surgical procedure, eye pathology

Risk for Injury: Risk factor: impaired vision

Readiness for enhanced Knowledge: expresses an interest in learning

See Hospitalized Child

F

FAILURE TO THRIVE, CHILD

Disorganized Infant behavior (See **Infant** behavior, disorganized, Section II)

Ineffective Child Eating dynamics r/t lack of knowledge or resources regarding nutritional needs of child

Ineffective infant Feeding dynamics r/t lack of knowledge regarding nutritional needs of infant

Insomnia r/t inconsistency of caretaker; lack of quiet, consistent environment

Imbalanced Nutrition: less than body requirements r/t inadequate type or amounts of food for infant or child, inappropriate feeding techniques

Impaired Parenting r/t lack of parenting skills, inadequate role modeling

Chronic low Self-Esteem: parental r/t feelings of inadequacy, support system deficiencies, inadequate role model

Social isolation r/t limited support systems, self-imposed situation

Risk for impaired Attachment: Risk factor: inability of parents to meet infant's needs

Risk for delayed Child Development (See **Child Development,** delayed, risk for, Section II)

Readiness for enhanced Knowledge: parent expresses willingness to learn how to meet **infant/child nutritional needs**

FALLS, RISK FOR

Risk for Adult Falls (See **Adult Falls,** risk for, Section II)

FAMILY PROBLEMS

Compromised family Coping (See **Coping,** family, compromised, Section II)

Disabled family Coping (See **Coping,** family, disabled, Section II)

Interrupted Family Processes r/t situation transition and/or crises, developmental transition and/or crises

Ineffective family Health self-management (See family **Health** management, ineffective, Section II)

Readiness for enhanced family Coping: needs sufficiently gratified, adaptive tasks effectively addressed to enable goals of self-actualization to surface

FAMILY PROCESS

Dysfunctional Family processes (See **Family** processes, dysfunctional, Section II)

Interrupted Family processes (See **Family** processes, interrupted, Section II)

Readiness for enhanced Family processes (See **Family** processes, readiness for enhanced, Section II)

Readiness for enhanced Relationship (See **Relationship,** readiness for enhanced, Section II)

FATIGUE

Fatigue (See **Fatigue,** Section II)

FEAR

Death Anxiety r/t fear of death

Fear r/t identifiable physical or psychological threat to person

FEBRILE SEIZURES

See Seizure Disorders, Childhood (Epilepsy, Febrile Seizures, Infantile Spasms)

FECAL IMPACTION

See Impaction of Stool

(See **Constipation,** Section II)

(See **Constipation**, chronic functional, Section II)

FECAL INCONTINENCE

Impaired Bowel Continence r/t neurological impairment, gastrointestinal disorders, anorectal trauma, weakened perineal muscles

FEEDING DYNAMICS, INFANT

Risk for Caregiver Role Strain: Risk factor: fatigue leading to ineffective or insufficient feeding

Risk for Impaired Attachment: Risk factor: inability physically or psychologically to meet nutritional needs of newborn

Risk for Impaired Parenting: Risk factors: stress, sleep deprivation, insufficient knowledge, and/or social isolation

Readiness for enhanced Health literacy: expresses a desire to enhance knowledge of appropriate feeding dynamics for each developmental stage (See Ineffective **Feeding Dynamics**, Infant, Section II)

FEEDING PROBLEMS, NEWBORN

Ineffective Breastfeeding (See **Breastfeeding**, ineffective, Section II)

Insufficient Breast Milk Production (See **Breast Milk Production**, insufficient, Section II)

Disorganized Infant behavior r/t prematurity, immature neurological system

Ineffective infant Feeding dynamics r/t parental lack of knowledge of appropriate feeding methods for each stage of development

Ineffective infant suck-swallow response r/t prematurity, neurological impairment or delay, oral hypersensitivity, prolonged nothing-by-mouth status

Impaired Swallowing r/t prematurity

Risk for delayed Child Development: Risk factor: inadequate nutrition

Risk for deficient Fluid volume: Risk factor: inability to take in adequate amount of fluids

FEMALE GENITAL MUTILATION

Acute Pain r/t traumatic surgical procedure

Anxiety r/t situational crisis

Disturbed Body Image r/t scarring, changes in body function

Fear r/t threat to well-being

Powerlessness r/t absence of control of decision-making

Impaired Skin Integrity r/t traumatic surgical procedure

Impaired Tissue Integrity r/t wound, potential for infection

Risk for compromised Human Dignity: Risk factor: dehumanizing treatment

Risk for Infection: Risk factor: invasive procedure

Risk for Post-Trauma Syndrome: Risk factor: experiencing traumatic surgery

Risk for chronic low Self Esteem: Risk factor: cultural incongruence (See **Female Genital Mutilation**, Risk for, Section II)

FEMORAL POPLITEAL BYPASS

Anxiety r/t threat to or change in health status

Acute Pain r/t surgical trauma, edema in surgical area

Ineffective peripheral Tissue Perfusion r/t impaired arterial circulation

Risk for Bleeding: Risk factor: surgery on arteries

Risk for Surgical Site Infection: Risk factor: invasive procedure

FETAL ALCOHOL SYNDROME

See Neonatal Abstinence Syndrome

FETAL DISTRESS/ NONREASSURING FETAL HEART RATE PATTERN

Fear r/t threat to fetus

Ineffective peripheral Tissue Perfusion: fetal r/t interruption of umbilical cord blood flow

FEVER

Ineffective Thermoregulation r/t infectious process

FIBROCYSTIC BREAST DISEASE

See Breast Lumps

F

F

FILTHY HOME ENVIRONMENT

Ineffective Home Maintenance Behaviors (See **Home** maintenance behaviors, ineffective, Section II)

Self-Neglect r/t mental illness, substance abuse, cognitive impairment

FINANCIAL CRISIS IN THE HOME ENVIRONMENT

Ineffective Home Maintenance Behaviors r/t insufficient finances

FISTULECTOMY

See Hemorrhoidectomy

FLAIL CHEST

Ineffective Breathing pattern r/t chest trauma

Fear r/t difficulty breathing

Impaired Gas exchange r/t loss of effective lung function

Impaired spontaneous Ventilation r/t paradoxical respirations

FLASHBACKS

Post-Trauma syndrome r/t catastrophic event

FLAT AFFECT

Hopelessness r/t prolonged activity restriction creating isolation, failing or deteriorating physiological condition, long-term stress, abandonment, lost belief in transcendent values or higher power or God

Risk for Loneliness: Risk factors: social isolation, lack of interest in surroundings

See Depression (Major Depressive Disorder); Dysthymic Disorder

FLUID VOLUME DEFICIT

Deficient Fluid volume r/t active fluid loss, vomiting, diarrhea, failure of regulatory mechanisms

Risk for Shock: Risk factors: hypovolemia, sepsis, systemic inflammatory response syndrome (SIRS)

Risk for Unstable Blood Pressure: Risk factor: hypotension, excessive loss or insufficient intake of fluid

FLUID VOLUME EXCESS

Excess Fluid volume r/t compromised regulatory mechanism, excess sodium intake

Risk for Unstable Blood Pressure: Risk factor: hypertension, excessive intake or retention of fluid

FLUID VOLUME IMBALANCE, RISK FOR

Risk for imbalanced Fluid volume: Risk factor: major invasive surgeries

FOOD ALLERGIES

Diarrhea r/t immune effects of offending food on gastrointestinal system

Risk for Allergic reaction: Risk factor: specific foods

Readiness for enhanced Knowledge: expresses an interest in learning

See Anaphylactic Shock

FOODBORNE ILLNESS

Diarrhea r/t infectious material in gastrointestinal tract

Deficient Fluid volume r/t active fluid loss from vomiting and diarrhea

Deficient Knowledge r/t care of self with serious illness, prevention of further incidences of foodborne illness

Nausea r/t contamination irritating stomach

Risk for dysfunctional Gastrointestinal motility: Risk factor: contaminated food

See Gastroenteritis; Gastroenteritis, Child; Hospitalized Child; Escherichia coli Infection

FOOD INTOLERANCE

Risk for dysfunctional Gastrointestinal motility: Risk factor: food intolerance

FOREIGN BODY ASPIRATION

Ineffective Airway clearance r/t obstruction of airway

Ineffective Health maintenance behaviors r/t parental deficient knowledge regarding high-risk items

Risk for Suffocation: Risk factor: inhalation of small objects

See Safety, Childhood

FORMULA FEEDING OF INFANT

Risk for Constipation: **infant:** Risk factor: iron-fortified formula

Risk for Infection: **infant:** Risk factors: lack of passive maternal immunity, supine feeding position, contamination of formula

Readiness for enhanced Knowledge: expresses an interest in learning

FRACTURE

Decreased Diversional activity engagement r/t immobility

Impaired physical Mobility r/t limb immobilization

Acute Pain r/t muscle spasm, edema, trauma

Post-Trauma syndrome r/t catastrophic event

Impaired Walking r/t limb immobility

Risk for ineffective peripheral Tissue Perfusion: Risk factors: immobility, presence of cast

Risk for Peripheral Neurovascular dysfunction: Risk factors: mechanical compression, treatment of fracture

Risk for impaired Skin integrity: Risk factors: immobility, presence of cast

Readiness for enhanced Knowledge: expresses an interest in learning

FRACTURED HIP

See Hip Fracture

FRAIL ELDERLY SYNDROME

Decreased activity tolerance r/t sensory changes

Risk for Frail Elderly syndrome (see **Frail Elderly** syndrome, risk for, Section II)

Risk for Injury: Risk factors: impaired vision, impaired gait

Risk for Powerlessness: Risk factor: inability to maintain independence

FREQUENCY OF URINATION

Stress urinary Incontinence r/t degenerative change in pelvic muscles and structural support

Urge urinary Incontinence r/t decreased bladder capacity, irritation of bladder stretch receptors causing spasm, alcohol, caffeine, increased fluids, increased urine concentration, overdistended bladder

Impaired Urinary elimination r/t urinary tract infection

Urinary retention r/t high urethral pressure caused by weak detrusor, inhibition of reflex arc, strong sphincter, blockage

FRIENDSHIP

Readiness for enhanced Relationship: expresses desire to enhance communication between partners

FROSTBITE

Acute Pain r/t decreased circulation from prolonged exposure to cold

Ineffective peripheral Tissue Perfusion r/t damage to extremities from prolonged exposure to cold

Impaired Tissue integrity r/t freezing of skin and tissues

Risk for ineffective Thermoregulation: Risk factor: prolonged exposure to cold

See Hypothermia

FROTHY SPUTUM

See CHF (Congestive Heart Failure); Pulmonary Edema; Seizure Disorders, Adult; Seizure Disorders, Childhood (Epilepsy, Febrile Seizures, Infantile Spasms)

FUSION, LUMBAR

Anxiety r/t fear of surgical procedure, possible recurring problems

Impaired physical Mobility r/t limitations from surgical procedure, presence of brace

Acute Pain r/t discomfort at bone donor site, surgical operation

Risk for Injury: Risk factor: improper body mechanics

Risk for Perioperative Positioning injury: Risk factor: immobilization during surgery

Readiness for enhanced Knowledge: expresses an interest in learning

G

GAG REFLEX, DEPRESSED OR ABSENT

Impaired Swallowing r/t neuromuscular impairment

Risk for Aspiration: Risk factors: depressed cough or gag reflex

GALLOP RHYTHM

Decreased Cardiac output r/t decreased contractility of heart

GALLSTONES

See Cholelithiasis

GANG MEMBER

Impaired individual Resilience (See **Resilience,** individual, impaired, Section II)

GANGRENE

Fear r/t possible loss of extremity

Ineffective peripheral Tissue perfusion r/t obstruction of arterial flow

See Diabetes Mellitus; Peripheral Vascular Disease

GAS EXCHANGE, IMPAIRED

Impaired Gas exchange r/t ventilation-perfusion imbalance

GASTRIC ULCER

See GI Bleed (Gastrointestinal Bleeding); Ulcer, Peptic (Duodenal or Gastric)

GASTRITIS

Imbalanced Nutrition: less than body requirements r/t vomiting, inadequate intestinal absorption of nutrients, restricted dietary regimen

Acute Pain r/t inflammation of gastric mucosa

Risk for deficient Fluid volume: Risk factors: excessive loss from gastrointestinal tract from vomiting, decreased intake

GASTROENTERITIS

Diarrhea r/t infectious process involving intestinal tract

Deficient Fluid volume r/t excessive loss from gastrointestinal tract from diarrhea, vomiting

Nausea r/t irritation to gastrointestinal system

Imbalanced Nutrition: less than body requirements r/t vomiting, inadequate intestinal absorption of nutrients, restricted dietary intake

Acute Pain r/t increased peristalsis causing cramping

Risk for Electrolyte imbalance: Risk factor: loss of gastrointestinal fluids high in electrolytes

Readiness for enhanced Knowledge: expresses an interest in learning

See Gastroenteritis, Child

GASTROENTERITIS, CHILD

Impaired Skin integrity: diaper rash r/t acidic excretions on perineal tissues

Readiness for enhanced Knowledge: expresses an interest in learning

Acute Pain r/t increased peristalsis causing cramping

See Gastroenteritis; Hospitalized Child

GASTROESOPHAGEAL REFLUX (GERD)

Ineffective Airway clearance r/t reflux of gastric contents into esophagus and tracheal or bronchial tree

Ineffective Health maintenance behaviors r/t deficient knowledge regarding anti-reflux regimen (e.g., positioning, change in diet)

Acute Pain r/t irritation of esophagus from gastric acids

Risk for Aspiration: Risk factor: entry of gastric contents in tracheal or bronchial tree

GASTROESOPHAGEAL REFLUX, CHILD

Ineffective Airway clearance r/t reflux of gastric contents into esophagus and tracheal or bronchial tree

Anxiety: parental r/t possible need for surgical intervention

Deficient Fluid volume r/t persistent vomiting

Imbalanced Nutrition: less than body requirements r/t poor feeding, vomiting

Risk for Aspiration: Risk factor: entry of gastric contents in tracheal or bronchial tree

Risk for impaired Parenting: Risk factors: disruption in bonding as a result of irritable or inconsolable infant; lack of sleep for parents

Readiness for enhanced Knowledge: expresses an interest in learning

See Child with Chronic Condition; Hospitalized Child

GASTROINTESTINAL BLEEDING (GI BLEED)

See GI Bleed (Gastrointestinal Bleeding)

GASTROINTESTINAL HEMORRHAGE

See GI Bleed (Gastrointestinal Bleeding)

GASTROINTESTINAL SURGERY

Risk for Injury: Risk factor: inadvertent insertion of nasogastric tube through gastric incision line

See Abdominal Surgery

GASTROSCHISIS/OMPHALOCELE

Ineffective Airway clearance r/t complications of anesthetic effects

Impaired Gas exchange r/t effects of anesthesia, subsequent atelectasis

Risk for deficient Fluid volume: Risk factors: inability to feed because of condition, subsequent electrolyte imbalance

Risk for Infection: Risk factor: disrupted skin integrity with exposure of abdominal contents

Risk for Injury: Risk factors: disrupted skin integrity, ineffective protection

GASTROSTOMY

Risk for impaired Skin integrity: Risk factor: presence of gastric contents on skin

See Tube Feeding

GENDER DYSPHORIA

Anxiety r/t conflict between physical (assigned) gender and gender they identify with

Decisional Conflict r/t uncertainty about choices regarding gender reassignment

Disturbed Body Image r/t alteration in self-perception, inability to identify with own body

Ineffective Denial r/t insufficient emotional support

Fear r/t victimization

Disturbed Personal Identity r/t gender confusion

Ineffective Sexuality Pattern r/t conflict surrounding gender identity

Risk for Compromised Human Dignity: Risk factor: cultural incongruence, humiliation

Readiness for enhanced Decision-making: expresses desire to enhance understanding of choices for decision-making

GENITAL HERPES

See Herpes Simplex II

GENITAL WARTS

See STD (Sexually Transmitted Disease)

GERD

See Gastroesophageal Reflux (GERD)

GESTATIONAL DIABETES (DIABETES IN PREGNANCY)

Anxiety r/t threat to self and/or fetus

Impaired Nutrition: less than body requirements r/t decreased insulin production and glucose uptake in cells

Risk for Overweight: fetal: r/t excessive glucose uptake

Impaired Nutrition: more than body requirements: fetal r/t excessive glucose uptake

Risk for delayed Child Development: fetal: Risk factor: endocrine disorder of mother

Risk for unstable blood Glucose: Risk factor: excessive intake of carbohydrates

Risk for disturbed Maternal–Fetal dyad: Risk factor: impaired glucose metabolism

Risk for impaired Tissue integrity: fetal: Risk factors: large infant, congenital defects, birth injury

Risk for impaired Tissue integrity: maternal: Risk factor: delivery of large infant

Readiness for enhanced Knowledge: expresses an interest in learning

See Diabetes Mellitus

GI BLEED (GASTROINTESTINAL BLEEDING)

Fatigue r/t loss of circulating blood volume, decreased ability to transport oxygen

Fear r/t threat to well-being, potential death

Deficient Fluid volume r/t gastrointestinal bleeding, hemorrhage

Imbalanced Nutrition: less than body requirements r/t nausea, vomiting

Acute Pain r/t irritated mucosa from acid secretion

Risk for ineffective Coping: Risk factors: personal vulnerability in crisis, bleeding, hospitalization

Readiness for enhanced Knowledge: expresses an interest in learning

GINGIVITIS

Impaired Oral Mucous Membrane Integrity r/t ineffective oral hygiene

GLAUCOMA

Deficient Knowledge r/t treatment and self-care for disease

See Vision Impairment

GLOMERULONEPHRITIS

Excess Fluid volume r/t renal impairment

Imbalanced Nutrition: less than body requirements r/t anorexia, restrictive diet

Acute Pain r/t edema of kidney

Readiness for enhanced Knowledge: expresses an interest in learning

GLUTEN ALLERGY

See Celiac Disease

GONORRHEA

Acute Pain r/t inflammation of reproductive organs

Risk for Infection: Risk factor: spread of organism throughout reproductive organs

Readiness for enhanced Knowledge: expresses an interest in learning

See STD (Sexually Transmitted Disease)

GOUT

Impaired physical Mobility r/t musculoskeletal impairment

Chronic Pain r/t inflammation of affected joint

Readiness for enhanced Knowledge: expresses an interest in learning

GRANDIOSITY

Defensive Coping r/t inaccurate perception of self and abilities

GRAND MAL SEIZURE

See Seizure Disorders, Adult; Seizure Disorders, Childhood (Epilepsy, Febrile Seizures, Infantile Spasms)

GRANDPARENTS RAISING GRANDCHILDREN

Anxiety r/t change in role status

Decisional Conflict r/t support system deficit

Parental Role conflict r/t change in parental role

Compromised family Coping r/t family role changes

Interrupted Family processes r/t family roles shift

Ineffective Role performance r/t role transition, aging

Ineffective family Health self-management r/t excessive demands on individual or family

Risk for impaired Parenting: Risk factor: role strain

Risk for Powerlessness: Risk factors: role strain, situational crisis, aging

Risk for Spiritual distress: Risk factor: life change

Readiness for enhanced Parenting: physical and emotional needs of children are met

GRAVES' DISEASE

See Hyperthyroidism

GRIEVING, COMPLICATED

Maladaptive Grieving r/t expected or sudden death of a significant other with whom there was a volatile relationship, emotional instability, lack of social support

Risk for maladaptive Grieving: Risk factors: death of a significant other with whom there was a volatile relationship, emotional instability, lack of social support

GROOM SELF (INABILITY TO)

Bathing Self-Care deficit (See **Self-Care** deficit, bathing, Section II)

Dressing Self-Care deficit (See **Self-Care** deficit, dressing, Section II)

GROWTH AND DEVELOPMENT LAG

See Failure to Thrive, Child

GUILLAIN-BARRÉ SYNDROME

Impaired Spontaneous Ventilation r/t weak respiratory muscles

Risk for Aspiration: Risk factor: ineffective cough; depressed gag reflex

See Neurologic Disorders

GUILT

Impaired individual Resilience (See **Resilience,** individual, impaired, Section II)

Situational low Self-Esteem r/t unmet expectations of self

G

Risk for maladaptive Grieving: Risk factors: actual loss of significant person, animal, prized material possession, change in life role

Risk for Post-Trauma syndrome: Risk factor: exaggerated sense of responsibility for traumatic event

Readiness for enhanced Spiritual well-being: desire to be in harmony with self, others, higher power or God

H

H

HAIR LOSS

Disturbed Body Image r/t psychological reaction to loss of hair

Imbalanced Nutrition: less than body requirements r/t inability to ingest food because of biological, psychological, economic factors

HALITOSIS

Impaired Dentition r/t ineffective oral hygiene

Impaired Oral Mucous Membrane Integrity r/t ineffective oral hygiene

HALLUCINATIONS

Anxiety r/t threat to self-concept

Acute Confusion r/t alcohol abuse, delirium, dementia, mental illness, substance abuse

Ineffective Coping r/t distortion and insecurity of life events

Risk for Self-Mutilation: Risk factor: command hallucinations

Risk for other-directed Violence: Risk factors: catatonic excitement, manic excitement, rage or panic reactions, response to violent internal stimuli

Risk for self-directed Violence: Risk factors: catatonic excitement, manic excitement, rage or panic reactions, response to violent internal stimuli

HEADACHE

Acute Pain r/t lack of knowledge of pain control techniques or methods to prevent headaches

Ineffective Health self-management r/t lack of knowledge, identification, elimination of aggravating factors

HEAD INJURY

Ineffective Breathing pattern r/t pressure damage to breathing center in brainstem

Acute Confusion r/t increased intracranial pressure

Risk for ineffective Cerebral tissue perfusion: Risk factors: effects of increased intracranial pressure, trauma to brain

See Neurologic Disorders

HEALTH BEHAVIOR, RISK-PRONE

Risk-prone Health behavior: Risk factors (See **Health** behavior, risk-prone, Section II)

HEALTH MAINTENANCE PROBLEMS

Ineffective Health maintenance behaviors (See **Health** maintenance behaviors, ineffective, Section II)

Ineffective Health self-management (See **Health** self-management, ineffective family, Section II)

HEALTH-SEEKING PERSON

Readiness for enhanced Health literacy (See **Health** literacy, readiness for enhanced, Section II)

Readiness for enhanced Health self-management (See **Health** self-management, readiness for enhanced, Section II)

HEARING IMPAIRMENT

Impaired verbal Communication r/t inability to hear own voice

Hearing Loss (See **Hearing Loss,** Section II)

Social isolation r/t difficulty with communication

HEART ATTACK

See MI (Myocardial Infarction)

HEART FAILURE

Decreased activity tolerance r/t weakness, fatigue, shortness of breath

Decreased Cardiac output r/t impaired cardiac function, increased preload, decreased contractility, increased afterload

Constipation r/t decreased activity tolerance

Fatigue r/t disease process with decreased cardiac output

Fear r/t threat to one's own well-being

Excess Fluid volume r/t impaired excretion of sodium and water

Impaired Gas exchange r/t excessive fluid in interstitial space of lungs

Powerlessness r/t illness-related regimen

Risk for Shock (cardiogenic): Risk factors: decreased contractility of heart, increased afterload

Readiness for enhanced Health self-management (See **Health** management, readiness for enhanced, Section II)

See Child with Chronic Condition; Congenital Heart Disease/Cardiac Anomalies; Hospitalized Child

HEART SURGERY

See Coronary Artery Bypass Grafting (CABG)

HEARTBURN

Nausea r/t gastrointestinal irritation

Acute Pain: **heartburn** r/t inflammation of stomach and esophagus

Risk for imbalanced Nutrition: **less than body requirements:** Risk factor: pain after eating

Readiness for enhanced Knowledge: expresses an interest in learning

See Gastroesophageal Reflux (GERD)

HEAT STROKE

Deficient Fluid volume r/t profuse diaphoresis from high environmental temperature

Hyperthermia r/t vigorous activity, high environmental temperature, inappropriate clothing

HEMATEMESIS

See GI Bleed (Gastrointestinal Bleeding)

HEMATURIA

See Kidney Stone; UTI (Urinary Tract Infection)

HEMIANOPIA

Anxiety r/t change in vision

Unilateral Neglect r/t effects of disturbed perceptual abilities

Risk for Injury: Risk factor: disturbed sensory perception

HEMIPLEGIA

Anxiety r/t change in health status

Disturbed Body Image r/t functional loss of one side of body

Impaired physical Mobility r/t loss of neurological control of involved extremities

Self-Care deficit: **specify:** r/t neuromuscular impairment

Impaired Sitting r/t partial paralysis

Impaired Standing r/t partial paralysis

Impaired Transfer ability r/t partial paralysis

Unilateral Neglect r/t effects of disturbed perceptual abilities

Impaired Walking r/t loss of neurological control of involved extremities

Risk for Adult Falls: Risk factor: impaired mobility

Risk for impaired Skin integrity: Risk factors: alteration in sensation, immobility; pressure over bony prominence

See CVA (Cerebrovascular Accident)

H

HEMODIALYSIS

Ineffective Coping r/t situational crisis

Interrupted Family processes r/t changes in role responsibilities as a result of therapy regimen

Excess Fluid volume r/t renal disease with minimal urine output

Powerlessness r/t treatment regimen

Risk for Caregiver Role Strain: Risk factor: complexity of care receiver treatment

Risk for Electrolyte imbalance: Risk factor: effect of metabolic state on renal function

Risk for deficient Fluid volume: Risk factor: excessive removal of fluid during dialysis

Risk for Infection: Risk factors: exposure to blood products, risk for developing hepatitis B or C, impaired immune system

Risk for Injury: Risk factors: clotting of blood access, abnormal surface for blood flow

Risk for impaired Tissue integrity: Risk factor: mechanical factor associated with fistula formation

Readiness for enhanced Knowledge: expresses an interest in learning

See Renal Failure; Renal Failure, Child with Chronic Condition

HEMODYNAMIC MONITORING

Risk for Infection: Risk factor: invasive procedure

Risk for Injury: Risk factors: inadvertent wedging of catheter, dislodgment of catheter, disconnection of catheter

Risk for impaired Tissue integrity: Risk factor: invasive procedure

See Shock, Cardiogenic; Shock, Hypovolemic; Shock, Septic

HEMOLYTIC UREMIC SYNDROME

Fatigue r/t decreased red blood cells

Fear r/t serious condition with unknown outcome

Deficient Fluid volume r/t vomiting, diarrhea

Nausea r/t effects of uremia

Risk for Injury: Risk factors: decreased platelet count, seizure activity

Risk for impaired Skin integrity: Risk factor: diarrhea

See Hospitalized Child; Renal Failure, Acute/Chronic, Child

HEMOPHILIA

Fear r/t high risk for AIDS infection from contaminated blood products

Impaired physical Mobility r/t pain from acute bleeds, imposed activity restrictions, joint pain

Acute Pain r/t bleeding into body tissues

Risk for Bleeding: Risk factors: deficient clotting factors, child's developmental level, age-appropriate play, inappropriate use of toys or sports equipment

Readiness for enhanced Knowledge: expresses an interest in learning

See Child with Chronic Condition; Hospitalized Child; Maturational Issues, Adolescent

HEMOPTYSIS

Fear r/t serious threat to well-being

Risk for ineffective Airway clearance: Risk factor: obstruction of airway with blood and mucus

Risk for deficient Fluid volume: Risk factor: excessive loss of blood

HEMORRHAGE

Fear r/t threat to well-being

Deficient Fluid volume r/t massive blood loss

See Hypovolemic Shock

HEMORRHOIDECTOMY

Anxiety r/t embarrassment, need for privacy

Constipation r/t fear of pain with defecation

Acute Pain r/t surgical procedure

Urinary Retention r/t pain, anesthetic effect

Risk for Bleeding: Risk factors: inadequate clotting, trauma from surgery

Readiness for enhanced Knowledge: expresses an interest in learning

HEMORRHOIDS

Impaired Comfort r/t itching in rectal area

Constipation r/t painful defecation, poor bowel habits

Impaired Sitting r/t pain and pressure

Readiness for enhanced Knowledge: expresses an interest in learning

HEMOTHORAX

Deficient Fluid volume r/t blood in pleural space

See Pneumothorax

HEPATITIS

Decreased activity tolerance r/t weakness or fatigue caused by infection

Decreased Diversional activity engagement r/t isolation

Fatigue r/t infectious process, altered body chemistry

Imbalanced Nutrition: less than body requirements r/t anorexia, impaired use of proteins and carbohydrates

Acute Pain r/t edema of liver, bile irritating skin

Social isolation r/t treatment-imposed isolation

Risk for deficient Fluid volume: Risk factor: excessive loss of fluids from vomiting and diarrhea

Readiness for enhanced Knowledge: expresses an interest in learning

HERNIA

See Hiatal Hernia; Inguinal Hernia Repair

HERNIATED DISK

See Low Back Pain

HERNIORRHAPHY

See Inguinal Hernia Repair

HERPES IN PREGNANCY

Fear r/t threat to fetus, impending surgery

Situational low Self-Esteem r/t threat to fetus as a result of disease process

Risk for Infection (infant): Risk factors: transplacental transfer during primary herpes, exposure to active herpes during birth process

See Herpes Simplex II

HERPES SIMPLEX I

Impaired Oral Mucous Membrane Integrity r/t inflammatory changes in mouth

HERPES SIMPLEX II

Ineffective Health maintenance behaviors r/t deficient knowledge regarding treatment, prevention, spread of disease

Acute Pain r/t active herpes lesion

Situational low Self-Esteem r/t expressions of shame or guilt

Sexual dysfunction r/t disease process

Impaired Tissue integrity r/t active herpes lesion

Impaired Urinary elimination r/t pain with urination

HERPES ZOSTER

See Shingles

HHNS (HYPEROSMOLAR HYPERGLYCEMIC NONKETOTIC SYNDROME)

See Hyperosmolar Hyperglycemic Nonketotic Syndrome (HHNS)

HIATAL HERNIA

Ineffective Health maintenance behaviors r/t deficient knowledge regarding care of disease

Nausea r/t effects of gastric contents in esophagus

Imbalanced Nutrition: less than body requirements r/t pain after eating

Acute Pain r/t gastroesophageal reflux

HIP FRACTURE

Acute Confusion r/t sensory overload, sensory deprivation, medication side effects, advanced age, pain

Constipation r/t immobility, opioids, anesthesia

Fear r/t outcome of treatment, future mobility, present helplessness

Impaired physical Mobility r/t surgical incision, temporary absence of weight bearing, pain when walking

Acute Pain r/t injury, surgical procedure, movement

Powerlessness r/t healthcare environment

Self-Care deficit: specify r/t musculoskeletal impairment

Impaired Transfer ability r/t immobilization of hip

Impaired Walking r/t temporary absence of weight bearing

Risk for Bleeding: Risk factors: postoperative complication, surgical blood loss

Risk for Surgical Site Infection: Risk factor: invasive procedure

Risk for Injury: Risk factors: activities such as greater than 90-degree flexion of hips that can result in dislodged prosthesis, unsteadiness when ambulating

Risk for Perioperative Positioning injury: Risk factors: immobilization, muscle weakness, emaciation

Risk for Peripheral Neurovascular dysfunction: Risk factors: trauma, vascular obstruction, fracture

Risk for impaired Skin integrity: Risk factor: immobility

HIP REPLACEMENT

See Total Joint Replacement (Total Hip/ Total Knee/Shoulder)

HIRSCHSPRUNG'S DISEASE

Constipation: bowel obstruction r/t inhibited peristalsis as a result of congenital absence of parasympathetic ganglion cells in distal colon

Imbalanced Nutrition: less than body requirements r/t anorexia, pain from distended colon

Acute Pain r/t distended colon, incisional postoperative pain

Impaired Skin integrity r/t stoma, potential skin care problems associated with stoma

Readiness for enhanced Knowledge: expresses an interest in learning

See Hospitalized Child

HIRSUTISM

Disturbed Body Image r/t excessive hair

HITTING BEHAVIOR

Acute Confusion r/t dementia, alcohol abuse, drug abuse, delirium

Risk for other-directed Violence (See **Violence,** other-directed, risk for, Section II)

HIV (HUMAN IMMUNODEFICIENCY VIRUS)

Fear r/t possible death

Ineffective Protection r/t depressed immune system

Readiness for enhanced Health literacy: expresses desire to enhance understanding of health information to make healthcare choices

See AIDS (Acquired Immunodeficiency Syndrome)

HODGKIN'S DISEASE

See Anemia; Cancer; Chemotherapy

HOME MAINTENANCE PROBLEMS

Ineffective Home Maintenance Behaviors (See **Home** maintenance behaviors, ineffective, Section II)

Self-Neglect r/t mental illness, substance abuse, cognitive impairment

Powerlessness r/t interpersonal interactions

Risk for Physical Trauma: Risk factor: being in high-crime neighborhood

HOMELESSNESS

Ineffective Home Maintenance Behaviors r/t impaired cognitive or emotional functioning, inadequate support system, insufficient finances

HOPE

Readiness for enhanced Hope (See **Hope,** readiness for enhanced, Section II)

HOPELESSNESS

Hopelessness (See **Hopelessness,** Section II)

HOSPITALIZED CHILD

Decreased activity tolerance r/t fatigue associated with acute illness

Anxiety: separation (child) r/t familiar surroundings and separation from family and friends

Compromised family Coping r/t possible prolonged hospitalization that exhausts supportive capacity of significant people

Ineffective Coping: parent r/t possible guilt regarding hospitalization of child, parental inadequacies

Decreased Diversional activity engagement r/t immobility, monotonous environment, frequent or lengthy treatments, reluctance to participate, therapeutic isolation, separation from peers

Interrupted Family processes r/t situational crisis of illness, disease, hospitalization

Fear r/t deficient knowledge or maturational level with fear of unknown, mutilation, painful procedures, surgery

Hopelessness: child r/t prolonged activity restriction, uncertain prognosis

Insomnia: child or parent r/t 24-hour care needs of hospitalization

Acute Pain r/t treatments, diagnostic or therapeutic procedures, disease process

Powerlessness: child r/t healthcare environment, illness-related regimen

Risk for impaired Attachment: Risk factor: separation

Risk for delayed Child Development: regression: Risk factors: disruption of normal routine, unfamiliar environment or caregivers, developmental vulnerability of young children

Risk for Injury: Risk factors: unfamiliar environment, developmental age, lack of parental knowledge regarding safety (e.g., side rails, intravenous (IV) site/pole)

Risk for imbalanced Nutrition: less than body requirements: Risk factors: anorexia, absence of familiar foods, cultural preferences

Readiness for enhanced family Coping: impact of crisis on family values, priorities, goals, relationships in family

See Child with Chronic Condition

HOSTILE BEHAVIOR

Risk for other-directed Violence: Risk factor: antisocial personality disorder

HTN (HYPERTENSION)

Ineffective Health self-management (See **Health** self-management, ineffective, Section II)

Readiness for enhanced Health self-management (See **Health** self-management, readiness for enhanced, Section II)

Risk for Overweight: Risk factor: lack of knowledge of relationship between diet and disease process

HUMAN ENERGY FIELD

Energy Field, Imbalanced (See **Imbalanced Energy Field**, Section II)

HUMILIATING EXPERIENCE

Risk for compromised Human Dignity (See **Human Dignity,** compromised, risk for, Section II)

H

HUNTINGTON'S DISEASE

Decisional Conflict r/t whether to have children

See Neurologic Disorders

HYDROCELE

Acute Pain r/t severely enlarged hydrocele

Ineffective Sexuality pattern r/t recent surgery on area of scrotum

H

HYDROCEPHALUS

Decisional Conflict r/t unclear or conflicting values regarding selection of treatment modality

Interrupted Family processes r/t situational crisis

Imbalanced Nutrition: **less than body requirements** r/t inadequate intake as a result of anorexia, nausea, vomiting, feeding difficulties

Risk for delayed Child Development: Risk factor: sequelae of increased intracranial pressure

Risk for Infection: Risk factor: sequelae of invasive procedure (shunt placement)

Risk for ineffective Cerebral tissue perfusion: Risk factors: interrupted flow, hypervolemia of cerebral ventricles

Risk for Adult Falls: Risk factors: acute illness, alteration in cognitive functioning

See Normal Pressure Hydrocephalus (NPH); Child with Chronic Condition; Hospitalized Child; Premature Infant (Child); Premature Infant (Parent)

HYGIENE, INABILITY TO PROVIDE OWN

Frail Elderly syndrome r/t living alone

Self-Neglect (See **Self-Neglect,** Section II)

Bathing Self-Care deficit (See **Self-Care** deficit, bathing, Section II)

HYPERACTIVE SYNDROME

Decisional Conflict r/t multiple or divergent sources of information regarding education, nutrition, medication regimens; willingness to change own food habits; limited resources

Parental Role conflict: **when siblings present** r/t increased attention toward hyperactive child

Compromised family Coping r/t unsuccessful strategies to control excessive activity, behaviors, frustration, anger

Ineffective Impulse control r/t disorder of development, environment that might cause frustration or irritation

Ineffective Role performance: **parent** r/t stressors associated with dealing with hyperactive child, perceived or projected blame for causes of child's behavior, unmet needs for support or care, lack of energy to provide for those needs

Chronic low Self-Esteem r/t inability to achieve socially acceptable behaviors; frustration; frequent reprimands, punishment, or scolding for uncontrolled activity and behaviors; mood fluctuations and restlessness; inability to succeed academically; lack of peer support

Impaired Social interaction r/t impulsive and overactive behaviors, concomitant emotional difficulties, distractibility and excitability

Risk for delayed Child Development: Risk factor: behavior disorders

Risk for impaired Parenting: Risk factor: disruptive or uncontrollable behaviors of child

Risk for other-directed Violence: **parent or child:** Risk factors: frustration with disruptive behavior, anger, unsuccessful relationships

HYPERBILIRUBINEMIA, NEONATAL

Anxiety: **parent** r/t threat to infant, unknown future

Parental Role conflict r/t interruption of family life because of care regimen

Neonatal Hyperbilirubinemia r/t abnormal breakdown of red blood cells following birth

Imbalanced Nutrition: less than body requirements (infant) r/t disinterest in feeding because of jaundice-related lethargy

Risk for Injury: infant: Risk factors: kernicterus, phototherapy lights

Risk for ineffective Thermoregulation: Risk factor: phototherapy

Readiness for enhanced Health self-management (parents): expresses desire to manage treatment: assessment of jaundice when infant is discharged from the hospital, when to call the physician, and possible preventive measures such as frequent breastfeeding (See **Neonatal Hyperbilirubinemia**, Risk for, Section II)

HYPERCALCEMIA

Decreased Cardiac output r/t bradydysrhythmia

Impaired physical Mobility r/t decreased muscle tone

Imbalanced Nutrition: less than body requirements r/t gastrointestinal manifestations of hypercalcemia (nausea, anorexia, ileus)

Risk for Disuse syndrome: Risk factor: comatose state impairing mobility

HYPERCAPNIA

Fear r/t difficulty breathing

Impaired Gas exchange r/t ventilation-perfusion imbalance, retention of carbon dioxide

See ARDS (Adult Respiratory Distress Syndrome); COPD (Chronic Obstructive Pulmonary Disorder); Sleep Apnea

HYPEREMESIS GRAVIDARUM

Anxiety r/t threat to self and infant, hospitalization

Deficient Fluid volume r/t excessive vomiting

Ineffective Home Maintenance Behaviors r/t chronic nausea, inability to function

Nausea r/t hormonal changes of pregnancy

Imbalanced Nutrition: less than body requirements r/t excessive vomiting

Powerlessness r/t healthcare regimen

Social isolation r/t hospitalization

Risk for Electrolyte imbalance: Risk factor: vomiting

HYPERGLYCEMIA

Ineffective Health self-management r/t complexity of therapeutic regimen, decisional conflicts, economic difficulties, unsupportive family, insufficient cues to action, deficient knowledge, mistrust, lack of acknowledgment of seriousness of condition

Risk for unstable blood Glucose level (See **Glucose** level, blood, unstable, risk for, Section II)

See Diabetes Mellitus

HYPERKALEMIA

Risk for Decreased activity tolerance: Risk factor: muscle weakness

Risk for decreased Cardiac tissue perfusion: Risk factor: abnormal electrolyte level affecting heart rate and rhythm

Risk for excess Fluid volume: Risk factor: untreated renal failure

HYPERNATREMIA

Risk for deficient Fluid volume: Risk factors: abnormal water loss, inadequate water intake

HYPEROSMOLAR HYPERGLYCEMIC NONKETOTIC SYNDROME (HHNS)

Acute Confusion r/t dehydration, electrolyte imbalance

Deficient Fluid volume r/t polyuria, hyperglycemia, inadequate fluid intake

Risk for Electrolyte imbalance: Risk factor: effect of metabolic state on kidney function

Risk for Injury: seizures: Risk factors: hyperosmolar state, electrolyte imbalance

See Diabetes Mellitus; Diabetes Mellitus, Juvenile (Insulin-Dependent Diabetes Mellitus Type 1)

H

HYPERPHOSPHATEMIA

Deficient Knowledge r/t dietary changes needed to control phosphate levels

See Renal Failure

HYPERSENSITIVITY TO SLIGHT CRITICISM

Defensive Coping r/t situational crisis, psychological impairment, substance abuse

H

HYPERTENSION (HTN)

See HTN (Hypertension)

Risk for decreased Cardiac output: Risk factors: decreased contractility and altered conductivity associated with myocardial damage

Risk for Unstable Blood Pressure: (See **Unstable Blood Pressure,** Risk for, Section II)

HYPERTHERMIA

Hyperthermia (See **Hyperthermia,** Section II)

HYPERTHYROIDISM

Anxiety r/t increased stimulation, loss of control

Diarrhea r/t increased gastric motility

Insomnia r/t anxiety, excessive sympathetic discharge

Imbalanced Nutrition: less than body requirements r/t increased metabolic rate, increased gastrointestinal activity

Risk for Injury: **eye damage:** Risk factor: protruding eyes without sufficient lubrication

Readiness for enhanced Knowledge: expresses an interest in learning

HYPERVENTILATION

Ineffective Breathing pattern r/t anxiety, acid-base imbalance

See Anxiety Disorder; Dyspnea; Heart Failure

HYPOCALCEMIA

Decreased activity tolerance r/t neuromuscular irritability

Ineffective Breathing pattern r/t laryngospasm

Imbalanced Nutrition: less than body requirements r/t effects of vitamin D deficiency, renal failure, malabsorption, laxative use

HYPOGLYCEMIA

Acute Confusion r/t insufficient blood glucose to brain

Ineffective Health self-management r/t deficient knowledge regarding disease process, self-care

Imbalanced Nutrition: **less than body requirements** r/t imbalance of glucose and insulin level

Risk for unstable blood Glucose level (See **Glucose** level, blood, unstable, risk for, Section II)

See Diabetes Mellitus; Diabetes Mellitus, Juvenile (IDDM Type 1)

HYPOKALEMIA

Decreased activity tolerance r/t muscle weakness

Risk for decreased Cardiac tissue perfusion: Risk factor: possible dysrhythmia from electrolyte imbalance

HYPOMAGNESEMIA

Imbalanced Nutrition: **less than body requirements** r/t deficient knowledge of nutrition, alcoholism

See Alcoholism

HYPOMANIA

Insomnia r/t psychological stimulus

See Manic Disorder, Bipolar I

HYPONATREMIA

Acute Confusion r/t electrolyte imbalance

Excess Fluid volume r/t excessive intake of hypotonic fluids

Risk for Injury: Risk factors: seizures, new onset of confusion

HYPOPLASTIC LEFT LUNG

See Congenital Heart Disease/Cardiac Anomalies

HYPOTENSION

Decreased Cardiac output r/t decreased preload, decreased contractility

Risk for deficient Fluid volume: Risk factor: excessive fluid loss

Risk for ineffective Cerebral tissue perfusion: Risk factors: hypovolemia, decreased contractility, decreased afterload

Risk for Shock (See **Shock,** risk for, Section II)

Risk for Unstable Blood Pressure (See **Unstable Blood Pressure,** Risk for, Section II)

See Dehydration; Heart Failure; MI (Myocardial Infarction)

HYPOTHERMIA

Hypothermia (See **Hypothermia,** Section II)

Risk for Hypothermia (see **Hypothermia,** risk for, Section II)

HYPOTHYROIDISM

Decreased activity tolerance r/t muscular stiffness, shortness of breath on exertion

Constipation r/t decreased gastric motility

Impaired Gas exchange r/t respiratory depression

Impaired Skin integrity r/t edema, dry or scaly skin

Risk for Overweight: Risk factor: decreased metabolic process

HYPOVOLEMIC SHOCK

See Shock, Hypovolemic

HYPOXIA

Acute Confusion r/t decreased oxygen supply to brain

Fear r/t breathlessness

Impaired Gas exchange r/t altered oxygen supply, inability to transport oxygen

Risk for Shock (See **Shock,** risk for, Section II)

HYSTERECTOMY

Constipation r/t opioids, anesthesia, bowel manipulation during surgery

Ineffective Coping r/t situational crisis of surgery

Acute Pain r/t surgical injury

Sexual dysfunction r/t disturbance in self-concept

Urinary retention r/t edema in area, anesthesia, opioids, pain

Risk for Bleeding: Risk factor: surgical procedure

Risk for Constipation: Risk factors: opioids, anesthesia, bowel manipulation during surgery

Risk for ineffective peripheral Tissue perfusion: Risk factor: deficient knowledge of aggravating factors

Risk for Surgical Site Infection: Risk factor: invasive procedure

Readiness for enhanced Knowledge: Expresses an interest in learning

See Surgery, Perioperative Care; Surgery, Preoperative Care; Surgery, Postoperative Care

I

IBS (IRRITABLE BOWEL SYNDROME)

Constipation r/t low-residue diet, stress

Diarrhea r/t increased motility of intestines associated with disease process, stress

Ineffective Health self-management r/t deficient knowledge, powerlessness

Chronic Pain r/t spasms, increased motility of bowel

Risk for Electrolyte imbalance: Risk factor: diarrhea

Readiness for enhanced Health self-management: expresses desire to manage illness and prevent onset of symptoms

ICD (IMPLANTABLE CARDIOVERTER/DEFIBRILLATOR)

Anxiety r/t possible dysrhythmia, threat of death

Decreased Cardiac output r/t possible dysrhythmia

Readiness for enhanced Knowledge: expresses an interest in learning

IDDM (INSULIN-DEPENDENT DIABETES)

See Diabetes Mellitus

IDENTITY DISTURBANCE/ PROBLEMS

Disturbed personal Identity r/t situational crisis, psychological impairment, chronic illness, pain

Risk for disturbed personal Identity (See **Identity**, personal, risk for disturbed in Section II)

IDIOPATHIC THROMBOCYTOPENIC PURPURA (ITP)

See ITP (Idiopathic Thrombocytopenic Purpura)

ILEAL CONDUIT

Disturbed Body Image r/t presence of stoma

Ineffective Health self-management r/t new skills required to care for appliance and self

Ineffective Sexuality pattern r/t altered body function and structure

Social isolation r/t alteration in physical appearance, fear of accidental spill of urine

Risk for Latex Allergic reaction: Risk factor: repeated exposures to latex associated with treatment and management of disease

Risk for impaired Skin integrity: Risk factor: difficulty obtaining tight seal of appliance

Readiness for enhanced Knowledge: expresses an interest in learning

ILEOSTOMY

Disturbed Body Image r/t presence of stoma

Diarrhea r/t dietary changes, alteration in intestinal motility

Deficient Knowledge r/t limited practice of stoma care, dietary modifications

Ineffective Sexuality pattern r/t altered body function and structure

Social isolation r/t alteration in physical appearance, fear of accidental spill of ostomy contents

Risk for impaired Skin integrity: Risk factors: difficulty obtaining tight seal of appliance, caustic drainage

Readiness for enhanced Knowledge: expresses an interest in learning

ILEUS

Deficient Fluid volume r/t loss of fluids from vomiting, fluids trapped in bowel

Dysfunctional Gastrointestinal motility r/t effects of surgery, decreased perfusion of intestines, medication effect, immobility

Nausea r/t gastrointestinal irritation

Acute Pain r/t pressure, abdominal distention

Readiness for enhanced Knowledge: expresses an interest in learning

IMMIGRATION TRANSITION, RISK FOR COMPLICATED

Anxiety r/t changes in safety and security needs

Fear r/t unfamiliar environment, separation from support system, possible language barrier

Impaired Social Interaction r/t possible communication or sociocultural barriers

Risk for Loneliness: Risk factor: separation from support system

Risk for Powerlessness: Risk factor: insufficient social support

Risk for Relocation Stress Syndrome: Risk factors: insufficient support system, social isolation, and potential communication barriers

Risk for Impaired Resilience: Risk factor: decreased ability to adapt to adverse or changing situations

Readiness for enhanced Coping: expresses desire to enhance social support

Readiness for enhanced Knowledge: expresses a desire to become familiar with resources within their environment

IMMOBILITY

Ineffective Breathing pattern r/t inability to deep breathe in supine position

Acute Confusion: **elderly** r/t sensory deprivation from immobility

Constipation r/t immobility

Risk for Frail Elderly syndrome: Risk factors: low physical activity, bed rest

Impaired physical Mobility r/t medically imposed bed rest

Ineffective peripheral Tissue Perfusion r/t interruption of venous flow

Powerlessness r/t forced immobility from healthcare environment

Impaired Walking r/t limited physical mobility, deconditioning of body

Risk for Disuse syndrome: Risk factor: immobilization

Risk for impaired Skin integrity: Risk factors: pressure over bony prominences, shearing forces when moved; pressure from devices

Risk for Impaired Tissue Integrity: Risk factors: mechanical factors from pressure over bony prominences, shearing forces when moved; pressure from devices

Risk for Overweight: Risk factor: energy expenditure less than energy intake

Readiness for enhanced Knowledge: expresses an interest in learning

IMMUNIZATION

See Readiness for enhanced **Health** literacy, Section II

See Readiness for enhanced **Health** management, Section II

IMMUNOSUPPRESSION

Risk for Infection: Risk factors: immunosuppression; exposure to disease outbreak

Impaired Social interaction r/t therapeutic isolation

IMPACTION OF STOOL

Constipation r/t decreased fluid intake, less than adequate amounts of fiber and bulk-forming foods in diet, medication effect, or immobility

IMPAIRED SITTING

Impaired physical Mobility r/t musculoskeletal, cognitive, or neuromuscular disorder

IMPAIRED STANDING

Decreased activity tolerance r/t insufficient physiological or psychological energy

Powerlessness r/t loss of function

IMPERFORATE ANUS

Anxiety r/t ability to care for newborn

Deficient Knowledge r/t home care for newborn

Impaired Skin integrity r/t pruritus

IMPETIGO

Impaired Skin integrity r/t infectious disease

Readiness for enhanced Knowledge: expresses an interest in learning

See Communicable Diseases, Childhood (e.g., Measles, Mumps, Rubella, Chickenpox, Scabies, Lice)

IMPLANTABLE CARDIOVERTER/ DEFIBRILLATOR (ICD)

See ICD (Implantable Cardioverter/ Defibrillator)

IMPOTENCE

Situational low Self-Esteem r/t physiological crisis, inability to practice usual sexual activity

Sexual dysfunction r/t altered body function

Readiness for enhanced Knowledge: treatment information for erectile dysfunction

See Erectile Dysfunction (ED)

IMPULSIVENESS

Ineffective Impulse control r/t (See **Impulse** control, ineffective in Section II)

INACTIVITY

Decreased activity tolerance r/t imbalance between oxygen supply and demand, sedentary lifestyle, weakness, immobility

Hopelessness r/t deteriorating physiological condition, long-term stress, social isolation

Impaired physical Mobility r/t intolerance to activity, decreased strength and endurance, depression, severe anxiety, musculoskeletal impairment, perceptual or cognitive impairment, neuromuscular impairment, pain, discomfort

Risk for Constipation: Risk factor: insufficient physical activity

INCOMPETENT CERVIX

See Premature Dilation of the Cervix (Incompetent Cervix)

INCONTINENCE OF STOOL

Disturbed Body Image r/t inability to control elimination of stool

Impaired Bowel Continence r/t decreased awareness of need to defecate, loss of sphincter control

Toileting Self-Care deficit r/t cognitive impairment, neuromuscular impairment, perceptual impairment, weakness

Situational low Self-Esteem r/t inability to control elimination of stool

Risk for impaired Skin integrity: Risk factor: presence of stool

INCONTINENCE OF URINE

Disability-associated urinary Incontinence r/t altered environment; sensory, cognitive, or mobility deficits

Stress urinary Incontinence (See **Incontinence,** urinary, stress, Section II)

Urge urinary Incontinence (See **Incontinence,** urinary, urge, Section II)

Toileting Self-Care deficit r/t cognitive impairment

Situational low Self-Esteem r/t inability to control passage of urine

Risk for impaired Skin integrity: Risk factor: presence of urine on perineal skin

INDIGESTION

Nausea r/t gastrointestinal irritation

Imbalanced Nutrition: less than body requirements r/t discomfort when eating

INDUCTION OF LABOR

Anxiety r/t medical interventions, powerlessness

Decisional Conflict r/t perceived threat to idealized birth

Ineffective Coping r/t situational crisis of medical intervention in birthing process

Acute Pain r/t contractions

Situational low Self-Esteem r/t inability to carry out normal labor

Risk for Injury: maternal and fetal: Risk factors: hypertonic uterus, potential prematurity of newborn

Readiness for enhanced Family processes: family support during induction of labor

INFANT APNEA

See Premature Infant (Child); Respiratory Conditions of the Neonate; Sudden Infant Death Syndrome (SIDS)

INFANT BEHAVIOR

Disorganized Infant behavior r/t pain, oral/motor problems, feeding intolerance, environmental overstimulation, lack of containment or boundaries, prematurity, invasive or painful procedures

Risk for disorganized Infant behavior: Risk factors: pain, oral/motor problems, environmental overstimulation, lack of containment or boundaries

Readiness for enhanced organized Infant behavior: stable physiologic measures, use of some self-regulatory measures

INFANT CARE

Readiness for enhanced Childbearing process: a pattern of preparing for, maintaining, and strengthening care of newborn infant

INFANT FEEDING PATTERN, INEFFECTIVE

Ineffective infant suck-swallow response r/t prematurity, neurological impairment or delay, oral hypersensitivity, prolonged nothing-by-mouth order

INFANT OF DIABETIC MOTHER

Decreased Cardiac output r/t cardiomegaly

Deficient Fluid volume r/t increased urinary excretion and osmotic diuresis

Imbalanced Nutrition: less than body requirements r/t hypotonia, lethargy, poor sucking, postnatal metabolic changes from hyperglycemia to hypoglycemia and hyperinsulinism

Risk for delayed Child Development: Risk factor: prolonged and severe postnatal hypoglycemia

Risk for impaired Gas exchange: Risk factors: increased incidence of cardiomegaly, prematurity

Risk for unstable blood Glucose level: Risk factor: metabolic change from hyperglycemia to hypoglycemia and hyperinsulinism

Risk for disturbed Maternal–Fetal dyad: Risk factor: impaired glucose metabolism

See Premature Infant (Child); Respiratory Conditions of the Neonate

INFANT OF SUBSTANCE-ABUSING MOTHER

See Neonatal Abstinence Syndrome

INFANTILE POLYARTERITIS

See Kawasaki Disease

INFECTION, POTENTIAL FOR

Risk for Infection (See **Infection,** risk for, Section II)

INFECTIOUS PROCESSES

Impaired Comfort r/t distressing symptoms

Diarrhea r/t gastrointestinal inflammation

Ineffective Health maintenance behaviors r/t knowledge deficit regarding transmission, symptoms, and treatment

Ineffective Health Self-Management r/t lack of knowledge regarding preventative immunizations

Ineffective Protection r/t inadequate nutrition, abnormal blood profiles, drug therapies, treatments

Impaired Social interaction r/t therapeutic isolation

Risk for Electrolyte Imbalance: Risk factors: vomiting, diarrhea

Risk for deficient Fluid Volume: Risk factors: vomiting, diarrhea, inadequate fluid intake

Risk for Infection: Risk factor: increased environmental exposure when in close proximity to infected persons

Risk for ineffective Thermoregulation: Risk factor: infectious process

Readiness for enhanced Knowledge: expresses desire for information regarding prevention and treatment

INFERTILITY

Ineffective Health self-management r/t deficient knowledge about infertility

Powerlessness r/t infertility

Chronic Sorrow r/t inability to conceive a child

Spiritual distress r/t inability to conceive a child

INFLAMMATORY BOWEL DISEASE (CHILD AND ADULT)

Ineffective Coping r/t repeated episodes of diarrhea

Diarrhea r/t effects of inflammatory changes of the bowel

Deficient Fluid volume r/t frequent and loose stools

Imbalanced Nutrition: less than body requirements r/t anorexia, decreased absorption of nutrients from gastrointestinal tract

Acute Pain r/t abdominal cramping and anal irritation

Impaired Skin integrity r/t frequent stools, development of anal fissures

Social isolation r/t diarrhea

See Child with Chronic Condition; Crohn's Disease; Hospitalized Child; Maturational Issues, Adolescent

INFLUENZA

See Infectious Processes

INGUINAL HERNIA REPAIR

Impaired physical Mobility r/t pain at surgical site and fear of causing hernia to rupture

Acute Pain r/t surgical procedure

Urinary retention r/t possible edema at surgical site

Risk for Surgical Site Infection: Risk factor: surgical procedure

INJURY

Risk for Adult Falls: Risk factors: orthostatic hypotension, impaired physical mobility, diminished mental status

Risk for Injury: Risk factor: environmental conditions interacting with client's adaptive and defensive resources

Risk for corneal Injury: Risk factors: blinking less than five times per minute, mechanical ventilation, pharmaceutical agent, prolonged hospitalization

Risk for Thermal injury: Risk factors: cognitive impairment, inadequate supervision, developmental level

Risk for urinary tract Injury: Risk factor: inflammation and/or infection from long-term use of urinary catheter

INSANITY

See Mental Illness; Psychosis

INSOMNIA

(See **Insomnia,** Section II)

INSULIN SHOCK

See Hypoglycemia

INTELLECTUAL DISABILITY

Impaired verbal Communication r/t developmental delay

Interrupted Family processes r/t crisis of diagnosis and situational transition

Deficient community Health r/t lack of programs to address developmental deficiencies

Ineffective Home Maintenance Behaviors r/t insufficient support systems

Self-Neglect r/t learning disability

Self-Care deficit: bathing, dressing, feeding, toileting r/t perceptual or cognitive impairment

Self-Mutilation r/t inability to express tension verbally

Social isolation r/t delay in accomplishing developmental tasks

Spiritual distress r/t chronic condition of child with special needs

Stress overload r/t intense, repeated stressor (chronic condition)

Impaired Swallowing r/t neuromuscular impairment

Risk for ineffective Activity planning r/t inability to process information

Risk for delayed Child Development: Risk factor: cognitive or perceptual impairment

Risk for impaired Religiosity: Risk factor: social isolation

Risk for Self-Mutilation: Risk factors: separation anxiety, depersonalization

Readiness for enhanced family Coping: adaptation and acceptance of child's condition and needs

See Child with Chronic Condition; Safety, Childhood

INTERMITTENT CLAUDICATION

Deficient Knowledge r/t lack of knowledge of cause and treatment of peripheral vascular diseases

Acute Pain r/t decreased circulation to extremities with activity

Ineffective peripheral Tissue Perfusion r/t interruption of arterial flow

Risk for Injury: Risk factor: tissue hypoxia

Readiness for enhanced Knowledge: prevention of pain and impaired circulation

See Peripheral Vascular Disease (PVD)

INTERNAL CARDIOVERTER/ DEFIBRILLATOR (ICD)

See ICD (Implantable Cardioverter/ Defibrillator)

INTERNAL FIXATION

Impaired Walking r/t repair of fracture

Risk for Infection: Risk factors: traumatized tissue, broken skin

See Fracture

INTERSTITIAL CYSTITIS

Acute Pain r/t inflammatory process

Impaired Urinary elimination r/t inflammation of bladder

Risk for Infection: Risk factor: suppressed inflammatory response

Readiness for enhanced Knowledge: expresses an interest in learning

INTERVERTEBRAL DISK EXCISION

See Laminectomy

INTESTINAL OBSTRUCTION

See Ileus; Bowel Obstruction

INTESTINAL PERFORATION

See Peritonitis

INTOXICATION

Anxiety r/t loss of control of actions

Acute Confusion r/t alcohol abuse

Ineffective Coping r/t use of mind-altering substances as a means of coping

Impaired Memory r/t effects of alcohol on mind

Risk for Aspiration: Risk factors: diminished mental status, vomiting

Risk for Adult Falls: Risk factor: diminished mental status

Risk for other-directed Violence: Risk factor: inability to control thoughts and actions

INTRAAORTIC BALLOON COUNTERPULSATION

Anxiety r/t device providing cardiovascular assistance

Decreased Cardiac output r/t heart dysfunction needing counterpulsation

Compromised family Coping r/t seriousness of significant other's medical condition

Impaired physical Mobility r/t restriction of movement because of mechanical device

Risk for Peripheral Neurovascular dysfunction: Risk factors: vascular obstruction of balloon catheter, thrombus formation, emboli, edema

Risk for Infection: Risk factor: invasive procedure

Risk for impaired Tissue integrity: Risk factor: invasive procedure

INTRACRANIAL PRESSURE, INCREASED

Ineffective Breathing pattern r/t pressure damage to breathing center in brainstem

Acute Confusion r/t increased intracranial pressure

Impaired Memory r/t neurological disturbance

Vision Loss r/t pressure damage to sensory centers in brain

Risk for ineffective Cerebral tissue perfusion: Risk factors: body position, cerebral vessel circulation deficits

See Head Injury; Subarachnoid Hemorrhage

INTRAUTERINE GROWTH RETARDATION

Anxiety: **maternal** r/t threat to fetus

Ineffective Coping: **maternal** r/t situational crisis, threat to fetus

Impaired Gas exchange r/t insufficient placental perfusion

Imbalanced Nutrition: **less than body requirements** r/t insufficient placenta

Situational low Self-Esteem: **maternal** r/t guilt about threat to fetus

Spiritual distress r/t unknown outcome of fetus

Risk for Powerlessness: Risk factor: unknown outcome of fetus

INTRAVENOUS THERAPY

Risk for Vascular Trauma: Risk factor: infusion of irritating chemicals

INTUBATION, ENDOTRACHEAL OR NASOGASTRIC

Disturbed Body Image r/t altered appearance with mechanical devices

Impaired verbal Communication r/t endotracheal tube

Imbalanced Nutrition: **less than body requirements** r/t inability to ingest food because of the presence of tubes

Impaired Oral Mucous Membrane r/t presence of tubes

Acute Pain r/t presence of tube

IODINE REACTION WITH DIAGNOSTIC TESTING

Risk for adverse reaction to iodinated Contrast Media (See reaction to iodinated **Contrast Media**, risk for adverse, Section II)

IRREGULAR PULSE

See Dysrhythmia

IRRITABLE BOWEL SYNDROME (IBS)

See IBS (Irritable Bowel Syndrome)

ISOLATION

Impaired individual Resilience (See **Resilience**, individual, impaired, Section II)

Social isolation (See **Social** isolation, Section II)

ITCHING

See Pruritus

ITP (IDIOPATHIC THROMBOCYTOPENIC PURPURA)

Decreased Diversional activity engagement r/t activity restrictions, safety precautions

Ineffective Protection r/t decreased platelet count

Risk for Bleeding: Risk factors: decreased platelet count, developmental level, age-appropriate play

See Hospitalized Child

J

JAUNDICE

Imbalanced Nutrition: less than body requirements r/t decreased appetite with liver disorder

Risk for Bleeding: Risk factor: impaired liver function

Risk for impaired Liver function: Risk factors: possible viral infection, medication effect

Risk for impaired Skin integrity: Risk factors: pruritus, itching

See Cirrhosis; Hepatitis

JAUNDICE, NEONATAL

See Hyperbilirubinemia, Neonatal

JAW PAIN AND HEART ATTACKS

See Angina; Chest Pain; MI (Myocardial Infarction)

JAW SURGERY

Deficient Knowledge r/t emergency care for wired jaws (e.g., cutting bands and wires), oral care

Imbalanced Nutrition: less than body requirements r/t jaws wired closed, difficulty eating

Acute Pain r/t surgical procedure

Impaired Swallowing r/t edema from surgery

Risk for Aspiration. Risk factor: wired jaws

JITTERY

Anxiety r/t unconscious conflict about essential values and goals, threat to or change in health status

Death Anxiety r/t unresolved issues relating to end of life

Risk for Post-Trauma syndrome: Risk factors: occupation, survivor's role in event, inadequate social support

JOCK ITCH

Ineffective Health self-management r/t prevention and treatment of disorder

Impaired Skin integrity r/t moisture and irritating or tight-fitting clothing

See Pruritus

JOINT DISLOCATION

See Dislocation of Joint

JOINT PAIN

See Arthritis; Bursitis; JRA (Juvenile Rheumatoid Arthritis); Osteoarthritis; Rheumatoid Arthritis (RA)

JOINT REPLACEMENT

Risk for Peripheral Neurovascular dysfunction: Risk factor: orthopedic surgery

Risk for impaired Tissue integrity: Risk factor: invasive procedure

See Total Joint Replacement (Total Hip/ Total Knee/Shoulder)

JRA (JUVENILE RHEUMATOID ARTHRITIS)

Impaired Comfort r/t altered health status

Fatigue r/t chronic inflammatory disease

Impaired physical Mobility r/t pain, restricted joint movement

Acute Pain r/t swollen or inflamed joints, restricted movement, physical therapy

Self-Care deficit: feeding, bathing, dressing, toileting r/t restricted joint movement, pain

Risk for compromised Human Dignity: Risk factors: perceived intrusion by clinicians, invasion of privacy

Risk for Injury: Risk factors: impaired physical mobility, splints, adaptive devices, increased bleeding potential from antiinflammatory medications

Risk for compromised Resilience: Risk factor: chronic condition

Risk for situational low Self-Esteem: Risk factor: disturbed body image

Risk for impaired Skin integrity: Risk factors: splints, adaptive devices

See Child with Chronic Condition; Hospitalized Child

KAPOSI'S SARCOMA

Risk for maladaptive Grieving: Risk factor: loss of social support

Risk for impaired Religiosity: Risk factors: illness/hospitalization, ineffective coping

Risk for impaired Resilience: Risk factor: serious illness

See AIDS (Acquired Immunodeficiency Syndrome)

KAWASAKI DISEASE

Anxiety: **parental** r/t progression of disease, complications of arthritis, and cardiac involvement

Impaired Comfort r/t altered health status

Hyperthermia r/t inflammatory disease process

Imbalanced Nutrition: **less than body requirements** r/t impaired oral mucous membrane integrity

Impaired Oral Mucous Membrane Integrity r/t inflamed mouth and pharynx; swollen lips that become dry, cracked, fissured

Acute Pain r/t enlarged lymph nodes; erythematous skin rash that progresses to desquamation, peeling, denuding of skin

Impaired Skin integrity r/t inflammatory skin changes

Risk for imbalanced Fluid volume: Risk factor: hypovolemia

Risk for decreased Cardiac tissue perfusion: Risk factor: cardiac involvement

Risk for Dry Mouth: Risk factor: decreased fluid intake

See Hospitalized Child

KELOIDS

Disturbed Body Image r/t presence of scar tissue at site of a healed skin injury

Readiness for enhanced Health self-management: desire to have information to manage condition

KERATOCONJUNCTIVITIS SICCA (DRY EYE SYNDROME)

Risk for dry Eye: Risk factors: aging, staring at a computer screen for long intervals

Risk for Infection: Risk factor: dry eyes that are more vulnerable to infection

Risk for corneal Injury: Risk factors: dry eye; exposure of the eyeball

See Conjunctivitis

KERATOPLASTY

See Corneal Transplant

KETOACIDOSIS, ALCOHOLIC

See Alcohol Withdrawal; Alcoholism

KETOACIDOSIS, DIABETIC

Deficient Fluid volume r/t excess excretion of urine, nausea, vomiting, increased respiration

Impaired Memory r/t fluid and electrolyte imbalance

Imbalanced Nutrition: less than body requirements r/t body's inability to use nutrients

Risk for unstable blood Glucose level: Risk factor: deficient knowledge of diabetes management (e.g., action plan)

Risk for Powerlessness: Risk factor: illness-related regimen

Risk for impaired Resilience: Risk factor: complications of disease

See Diabetes Mellitus

KEYHOLE HEART SURGERY

See MIDCAB (Minimally Invasive Direct Coronary Artery Bypass)

KIDNEY DISEASE SCREENING

Readiness for enhanced Health management: seeks information for screening

KIDNEY FAILURE

See Renal Failure

KIDNEY FAILURE ACUTE/ CHRONIC, CHILD

See Renal Failure, Acute/Chronic, Child

KIDNEY FAILURE, NONOLIGURIC

See Renal Failure, Nonoliguric

KIDNEY STONE

Acute Pain r/t obstruction from kidney calculi

Impaired Urinary elimination: urgency and frequency r/t anatomical obstruction, irritation caused by stone

Risk for Infection: Risk factor: obstruction of urinary tract with stasis of urine

Readiness for enhanced Knowledge: expresses an interest in learning about prevention of stones

KIDNEY TRANSPLANT

Ineffective Protection r/t immunosuppressive therapy

Readiness for enhanced Decision-making: expresses desire to enhance understanding of choices

Readiness for enhanced Family processes: adapting to life without dialysis

Readiness for enhanced Health self-management: desire to manage the treatment and prevention of complications after transplantation

Readiness for enhanced Spiritual well-being: heightened coping, living without dialysis

See Renal Failure, Kidney Transplantation, Donor; Kidney Transplantation, Recipient; Nephrectomy; Surgery, Perioperative Care; Surgery, Postoperative Care; Surgery, Preoperative Care

KIDNEY TRANSPLANTATION, DONOR

Impaired emancipated Decision-Making r/t harvesting of kidney from traumatized donor

Moral Distress r/t conflict among decision-makers, end-of-life decisions, time constraints for decision-making

Risk for Surgical Site Infection: Risk factor: surgical procedure

K

Readiness for enhanced Communication: expressing thoughts and feelings about situation

Readiness for enhanced family Coping: decision to allow organ donation

Readiness for enhanced emancipated Decision-Making: expresses desire to enhance understanding and meaning of choices

Readiness for enhanced Resilience: decision to donate organs

Readiness for enhanced Spirituality: inner peace resulting from allowance of organ donation

See Nephrectomy

K

KIDNEY TRANSPLANTATION, RECIPIENT

Anxiety r/t possible rejection, procedure

Ineffective Health maintenance behaviors r/t long-term home treatment after transplantation, diet, signs of rejection, use of medications

Deficient Knowledge r/t specific nutritional needs, possible paralytic ileus, fluid or sodium restrictions

Impaired Urinary elimination r/t possible impaired renal function

Risk for Bleeding: Risk factor: surgical procedure

Risk for Infection: Risk factor: use of immunosuppressive therapy to control rejection

Risk for Surgical Site Infection: Risk factor: surgical procedure

Risk for Shock: Risk factor: possible hypovolemia

Risk for Spiritual distress: Risk factor: obtaining transplanted kidney from someone's traumatic loss

Readiness for enhanced Spiritual well-being: acceptance of situation

KIDNEY TUMOR

See Wilms' Tumor

KISSING DISEASE

See Mononucleosis

KNEE REPLACEMENT

See Total Joint Replacement (Total Hip/Total Knee/Shoulder)

KNOWLEDGE

Readiness for enhanced Knowledge (See **Knowledge,** readiness for enhanced, Section II)

KNOWLEDGE, DEFICIENT

Ineffective Health maintenance behaviors r/t lack of or significant alteration in communication skills (written, verbal, and/or gestural)

Deficient Knowledge (See **Knowledge,** deficient, Section II)

Readiness for enhanced Knowledge (See **Knowledge,** readiness for enhanced, Section II)

KOCK POUCH

See Continent Ileostomy (Kock Pouch)

KORSAKOFF'S SYNDROME

Acute Confusion r/t alcohol abuse

Dysfunctional Family processes r/t alcoholism as possible cause of syndrome

Impaired Memory r/t neurological changes associated with excessive alcohol intake

Self-Neglect r/t cognitive impairment from chronic alcohol abuse

Risk for Adult Falls: Risk factor: cognitive impairment from chronic alcohol abuse

Risk for Injury: Risk factors: sensory dysfunction, lack of coordination when ambulating from chronic alcohol abuse

Risk for impaired Liver function: Risk factor: substance abuse (alcohol)

Risk for imbalanced Nutrition: less than body requirements: Risk factor: lack of adequate balanced intake from chronic alcohol abuse

L

LABOR, INDUCTION OF

See Induction of Labor

LABOR, NORMAL

Anxiety r/t fear of the unknown, situational crisis

Impaired Comfort r/t labor

Fatigue r/t childbirth

Deficient Knowledge r/t lack of preparation for labor

Labor Pain r/t uterine contractions, stretching of cervix and birth canal

Impaired Tissue Integrity r/t passage of infant through birth canal, episiotomy

Risk for ineffective Childbearing process (See **Childbearing** process, Section II)

Risk for Adult Falls: Risk factors: excessive loss or shift in intravascular fluid volume, orthostatic hypotension

Risk for deficient Fluid volume: Risk factor: excessive loss of blood

Risk for Infection: Risk factors: multiple vaginal examinations, tissue trauma, prolonged rupture of membranes

Risk for Injury: fetal: Risk factor: hypoxia

Risk for Post-Trauma syndrome: Risk factors: trauma or violence associated with labor pains, medical or surgical interventions, history of sexual abuse

Readiness for enhanced Childbearing process: responds appropriately, is proactive, bonds with infant, uses support systems

Readiness for enhanced family Coping: significant other provides support during labor

Readiness for enhanced Health self-management: prenatal care and childbirth education birth process

Readiness for enhanced Power: expresses readiness to enhance participation in choices regarding treatment during labor

LABOR PAIN

Labor Pain r/t uterine contractions, stretching of cervix and birth canal

LABYRINTHITIS

Ineffective Health self-management r/t delay in seeking treatment for respiratory and ear infections

Risk for Injury r/t dizziness

Readiness for enhanced Health self-management: management of episodes

See Ménière's Disease

LACERATIONS

Readiness for enhanced Health management: appropriate care of injury

Risk for Infection: Risk factor: broken skin

Risk for Physical Trauma: Risk factor: children playing with dangerous objects

LACTATION

See Breastfeeding, Ineffective; Breastfeeding, Interrupted

LACTIC ACIDOSIS

Decreased Cardiac output r/t altered heart rate/rhythm, preload, and contractility

Risk for Electrolyte imbalance: Risk factor: impaired regulatory mechanism

Risk for decreased Cardiac tissue perfusion: Risk factor: hypoxia

See Ketoacidosis, Diabetic

LACTOSE INTOLERANCE

Readiness for enhanced Knowledge: interest in identifying lactose intolerance, treatment, and substitutes for milk products

See Abdominal Distention; Diarrhea

LAMINECTOMY

Anxiety r/t change in health status, surgical procedure

Impaired Comfort r/t surgical procedure

Deficient Knowledge r/t appropriate postoperative and postdischarge activities

Impaired physical Mobility r/t neuromuscular impairment

Acute Pain r/t localized inflammation and edema

Urinary retention r/t competing sensory impulses, effects of opioids or anesthesia

Risk for Bleeding: Risk factor: surgery

Risk for Surgical Site Infection: Risk factor: invasive procedure, surgery

Risk for Perioperative Positioning injury: Risk factor: prone position

See Surgery, Perioperative Care; Surgery, Postoperative Care; Surgery, Preoperative Care

L

LANGUAGE IMPAIRMENT

See Speech Disorders

LAPAROSCOPIC LASER CHOLECYSTECTOMY

See Cholecystectomy; Laser Surgery

LAPAROSCOPY

Urge urinary Incontinence r/t pressure on the bladder from gas

Acute Pain: shoulder r/t gas irritating the diaphragm

LAPAROTOMY

See Abdominal Surgery

LARGE BOWEL RESECTION

See Abdominal Surgery

LARYNGECTOMY

Ineffective Airway clearance r/t surgical removal of glottis, decreased humidification

Death Anxiety r/t unknown results of surgery

Disturbed Body Image r/t change in body structure and function

Impaired Comfort r/t surgery

Impaired verbal Communication r/t removal of larynx

Interrupted Family processes r/t surgery, serious condition of family member, difficulty communicating

Ineffective Health self-management r/t deficient knowledge regarding self-care with laryngectomy

Imbalanced Nutrition: less than body requirements r/t absence of oral feeding, difficulty swallowing, increased need for fluids

Impaired Oral Mucous Membrane r/t absence of oral feeding

Chronic Sorrow r/t change in body image

Impaired Swallowing r/t edema, laryngectomy tube

Risk for Electrolyte imbalance: Risk factor: fluid imbalance

Risk for maladaptive Grieving: Risk factors: loss, major life event

Risk for compromised Human Dignity: Risk factor: inability to communicate

Risk for Surgical Site Infection: Risk factors: invasive procedure, surgery

Risk for Powerlessness: Risk factors: chronic illness, change in communication

Risk for impaired Resilience: Risk factor: change in health status

Risk for situational low Self-Esteem: Risk factor: disturbed body image

LASER SURGERY

Impaired Comfort r/t surgery

Constipation r/t laser intervention in vulval and perianal areas

Deficient Knowledge r/t preoperative and postoperative care associated with laser procedure

Acute Pain r/t heat from laser

Risk for Bleeding: Risk factor: surgery

Risk for Infection: Risk factor: delayed heating reaction of tissue exposed to laser

Risk for Injury: Risk factor: accidental exposure to laser beam

LASIK EYE SURGERY (LASER-ASSISTED IN SITU KERATOMILEUSIS)

Impaired Comfort r/t surgery

Decisional Conflict r/t decision to have surgery

Risk for Infection: Risk factor: invasive procedure/surgery

Readiness for enhanced Health self-management: surgical procedure preoperative and postoperative teaching and expectations

LATEX ALLERGIC REACTION

Latex Allergic reaction (See **Latex Allergic** reaction, Section II)

Risk for Latex Allergic reaction (See **Latex Allergic** reaction, risk for, Section II)

Readiness for enhanced Knowledge: prevention and treatment of exposure to latex products

LAXATIVE ABUSE

Perceived Constipation r/t health belief, faulty appraisal, impaired thought processes

LEAD POISONING

Contamination r/t flaking, peeling paint in presence of young children

Ineffective Home Maintenance Behaviors r/t presence of lead paint

Risk for delayed Child Development: Risk factor: lead poisoning

LEFT HEART CATHETERIZATION

See Cardiac Catheterization

LEGIONNAIRES' DISEASE

Contamination r/t contaminated water in air-conditioning systems

See Pneumonia

LENS IMPLANT

See Cataract Extraction; Vision Impairment

LETHARGY/LISTLESSNESS

Frail Elderly syndrome r/t alteration in cognitive function

Fatigue r/t decreased metabolic energy production

Insomnia r/t internal or external stressors

Risk for ineffective Cerebral tissue perfusion: Risk factor: carbon dioxide retention and/or lack of oxygen supply to brain

LEUKEMIA

Ineffective Protection r/t abnormal blood profile

Fatigue r/t abnormal blood profile and/or side effects of chemotherapy treatment

Risk for imbalanced Fluid volume: Risk factors: nausea, vomiting, bleeding, side effects of treatment

Risk for Infection: Risk factor: ineffective immune system

Risk for impaired Resilience: Risk factor: serious illness

See Cancer; Chemotherapy

LEUKOPENIA

Ineffective Protection r/t leukopenia

Risk for Infection: Risk factor: low white blood cell count

LEVEL OF CONSCIOUSNESS, DECREASED

See Confusion, Acute; Confusion, Chronic

LICE

Impaired Comfort r/t inflammation, pruritus

Readiness for enhanced Health self-management: preventing and treating infestation

Ineffective Home Maintenance Behaviors r/t close unsanitary, overcrowded conditions

Self-Neglect r/t lifestyle

See Communicable Diseases, Childhood (e.g., Measles, Mumps, Rubella, Chickenpox, Scabies, Lice)

LIFESTYLE, SEDENTARY

Sedentary lifestyle (See **Sedentary** lifestyle, Section II)

Risk for ineffective peripheral Tissue Perfusion: Risk factor: lack of movement

LIGHTHEADEDNESS

See Dizziness; Vertigo

LIMB REATTACHMENT PROCEDURES

Anxiety r/t unknown outcome of reattachment procedure, use and appearance of limb

Disturbed Body Image r/t unpredictability of function and appearance of reattached body part

Spiritual distress r/t anxiety about condition

Stress overload r/t multiple coexisting stressors, physical demands

Risk for Bleeding: Risk factor: severed vessels

Risk for Perioperative Positioning injury: Risk factor: immobilization

Risk for Peripheral Neurovascular dysfunction: Risk factors: trauma, orthopedic and neurovascular surgery, compression of nerves and blood vessels

Risk for Powerlessness: Risk factor: unknown outcome of procedure

Risk for impaired Religiosity: Risk factors: suffering, hospitalization

See Surgery, Postoperative Care

LIPOSUCTION

Disturbed Body Image r/t dissatisfaction with unwanted fat deposits in body

Risk for impaired Resilience: Risk factor: body image disturbance

Readiness for enhanced Decision-Making: expresses desire to make decision regarding liposuction

Readiness for enhanced Self-Concept: satisfaction with new body image

See Surgery, Perioperative Care; Surgery, Postoperative Care; Surgery, Preoperative Care

LITHOTRIPSY

Readiness for enhanced Health self-management: expresses desire for information related to procedure and aftercare and prevention of stones

See Kidney Stone

LIVER BIOPSY

Anxiety r/t procedure and results

Risk for deficient Fluid volume: Risk factor: hemorrhage from biopsy site

Risk for Infection: Risk factor: invasive procedure

Risk for Powerlessness: Risk factor: inability to control outcome of procedure

LIVER CANCER

Risk for Bleeding: Risk factor: liver dysfunction

Risk for Adult Falls: Risk factor: confusion associated with liver dysfunction

Risk for impaired Liver function: Risk factor: disease process

Risk for impaired Resilience: Risk factor: serious illness

See Cancer; Chemotherapy; Radiation Therapy

LIVER DISEASE

See Cirrhosis; Hepatitis

LIVER FUNCTION

Risk for impaired Liver function (See **Liver** function, impaired, risk for, Section II)

LIVER TRANSPLANT

Impaired Comfort r/t surgical pain

Decisional Conflict r/t acceptance of donor liver

Ineffective Protection r/t immunosuppressive therapy

Risk for impaired Liver function: Risk factors: possible rejection, infection

Readiness for enhanced Family processes: change in physical needs of family member

Readiness for enhanced Health self-management: desire to manage the treatment and prevention of complications after transplantation

Readiness for enhanced Spiritual well-being: heightened coping

See Surgery, Perioperative Care; Surgery, Postoperative Care; Surgery, Preoperative Care

LIVING WILL

Moral Distress r/t end-of-life decisions

Readiness for enhanced Decision-Making: expresses desire to enhance understanding of choices for decision-making

Readiness for enhanced Relationship: shares information with others

Readiness for enhanced Religiosity: request to meet with religious leaders or facilitators

Readiness for enhanced Resilience: uses effective communication

Readiness for enhanced Spiritual well-being: acceptance of and preparation for end of life

See Advance Directives

LOBECTOMY

See Thoracotomy

LONELINESS

Spiritual distress r/t loneliness, social alienation

Risk for Loneliness (See **Loneliness,** risk for, Section II)

Risk for impaired Religiosity: Risk factor: lack of social interaction

Readiness for enhanced Hope: expresses desire to enhance interconnectedness with others

Readiness for enhanced Relationship: expresses satisfaction with complementary relationship between partners

LOOSE STOOLS (BOWEL MOVEMENTS)

Diarrhea r/t increased gastric motility

Risk for dysfunctional Gastrointestinal motility (See **Gastrointestinal** motility, dysfunctional, risk for, Section II)

See Diarrhea

LOSS OF BLADDER CONTROL

See Incontinence of Urine

LOSS OF BOWEL CONTROL

See Incontinence of Stool

LOU GEHRIG'S DISEASE

See Amyotrophic Lateral Sclerosis (ALS)

LOW BACK PAIN

Impaired Comfort r/t back pain

Ineffective Health maintenance behaviors r/t deficient knowledge regarding self-care with back pain

Impaired physical Mobility r/t back pain

Chronic Pain r/t degenerative processes, musculotendinous strain, injury, inflammation, congenital deformities

Urinary Retention r/t possible spinal cord compression

Risk for Powerlessness: Risk factor: living with chronic pain

Readiness for enhanced Health self-management: expresses desire for information to manage pain

LOW BLOOD GLUCOSE

See Hypoglycemia

LOW BLOOD PRESSURE

See Hypotension

LOWER GI BLEEDING

See GI Bleed (Gastrointestinal Bleeding)

LUMBAR PUNCTURE

Anxiety r/t invasive procedure and unknown results

Deficient Knowledge r/t information about procedure

Acute Pain r/t possible loss of cerebrospinal fluid

Risk for ineffective Cerebral tissue perfusion: Risk factor: treatment-related side effects

Risk for Infection: Risk factor: invasive procedure

L

LUMPECTOMY

Decisional Conflict r/t treatment choices

Readiness for enhanced Knowledge: preoperative and postoperative care

Readiness for enhanced Spiritual well-being: hope of benign diagnosis

See Cancer

LUNG CANCER

See Cancer; Chemotherapy; Radiation Therapy; Thoracotomy

LUNG SURGERY

See Thoracotomy

LUPUS ERYTHEMATOSUS

Disturbed Body Image r/t change in skin, rash, lesions, ulcers, mottled erythema

Fatigue r/t increased metabolic requirements

Ineffective Health maintenance behaviors r/t deficient knowledge regarding medication, diet, activity

Acute Pain r/t inflammatory process

Powerlessness r/t unpredictability of course of disease

Impaired Religiosity r/t ineffective coping with disease

Chronic Sorrow r/t presence of chronic illness

Spiritual distress r/t chronicity of disease, unknown etiology

Risk for decreased Cardiac tissue perfusion: Risk factor: altered circulation

Risk for impaired Resilience: Risk factor: chronic disease

Risk for impaired Skin integrity: Risk factors: chronic inflammation, edema, altered circulation

LYME DISEASE

Impaired Comfort r/t inflammation

Fatigue r/t increased energy requirements

Deficient Knowledge r/t lack of information concerning disease, prevention, treatment

Acute Pain r/t inflammation of joints, urticaria, rash

Risk for decreased Cardiac output: Risk factor: dysrhythmia

Risk for Powerlessness: Risk factor: possible chronic condition

LYMPHEDEMA

Disturbed Body Image r/t change in appearance of body part with edema

Excess Fluid volume r/t compromised regulatory system; inflammation, obstruction, or removal of lymph glands

Deficient Knowledge r/t management of condition

Risk for Infection: Risk factors: abnormal lymphatic system allowing stasis of fluids with decreased resistance to infection

Risk for situational low Self-Esteem: Risk factor: disturbed body image

LYMPHOMA

See Cancer

M

MACULAR DEGENERATION

Ineffective Coping r/t visual loss

Compromised family Coping r/t deteriorating vision of family member

Risk-prone Health behavior r/t deteriorating vision while trying to maintain usual lifestyle

Hopelessness r/t deteriorating vision

Sedentary lifestyle r/t visual loss

Self-Neglect r/t change in vision

Social Isolation r/t inability to drive because of visual changes

Risk for Adult Falls: Risk factor: visual difficulties

Risk for Injury: Risk factor: inability to distinguish traffic lights and safety signs

Risk for Powerlessness: Risk factor: deteriorating vision

Risk for impaired Religiosity: Risk factor: possible lack of transportation to church

Risk for impaired Resilience: Risk factor: changing vision

Readiness for enhanced Health self-management: appropriate choices of daily activities for meeting the goals of a treatment program

MAGNETIC RESONANCE IMAGING (MRI)

See MRI (Magnetic Resonance Imaging)

MAJOR DEPRESSIVE DISORDER

See Depression (Major Depressive Disorder)

MALABSORPTION SYNDROME

Diarrhea r/t lactose intolerance, gluten sensitivity, resection of small bowel

Dysfunctional Gastrointestinal motility r/t disease state

Deficient Knowledge r/t lack of information about diet and nutrition

Imbalanced Nutrition: less than body requirements r/t inability of body to absorb nutrients because of physiological factors

Risk for Electrolyte imbalance: Risk factors: hypovolemia, hyponatremia, hypokalemia

Risk for imbalanced Fluid volume: Risk factors: diarrhea, hypovolemia

See Abdominal Distention

MALADAPTIVE BEHAVIOR

See Crisis; Post-Trauma Syndrome; Suicide Attempt

MALAISE

See Fatigue

MALARIA

Contamination r/t geographic area

Risk for Contamination: Risk factors: increased environmental exposure (not wearing protective clothing, not using insecticide or repellant on skin, clothing, and in room in areas in which infected mosquitoes are present); inadequate defense mechanisms (inappropriate use of prophylactic regimen)

Risk for impaired Liver function: Risk factor: complications of disease

Readiness for enhanced community Coping: uses resources available for problem solving

Readiness for enhanced Health self-management: expresses desire to enhance immunization status/vaccination status

Readiness for enhanced Resilience: immunization status

See Anemia

MALE INFERTILITY

See Erectile Dysfunction (ED); Infertility

MALIGNANCY

See Cancer

MALIGNANT HYPERTENSION (ARTERIOLAR NEPHROSCLEROSIS)

Decreased Cardiac output r/t altered afterload, altered contractility

Fatigue r/t disease state, increased blood pressure

Excess Fluid volume r/t decreased kidney function

Risk for ineffective Cerebral tissue perfusion: Risk factor: elevated blood pressure damaging cerebral vessels

Risk for acute Confusion: Risk factors: increased blood urea nitrogen or creatinine levels

Risk for imbalanced Fluid volume: Risk factors: hypertension, altered kidney function

Risk for Unstable Blood Pressure: Risk factor: damaged vessels due to disease process

Readiness for enhanced Health self-management: expresses desire to manage the illness, high blood pressure

MALIGNANT HYPERTHERMIA

Hyperthermia r/t anesthesia reaction associated with inherited condition

Readiness for enhanced Health management: knowledge of risk factors

MALNUTRITION

Insufficient Breast Milk Production r/t (See **Breast Milk,** insufficient production, Section II)

Frail Elderly syndrome r/t undetected malnutrition

Deficient Knowledge r/t misinformation about normal nutrition, social isolation, lack of food preparation facilities

Imbalanced Nutrition: less than body requirements r/t inability to ingest food, digest food, or absorb nutrients because of biological, psychological, or economic factors; institutionalization (i.e., lack of menu choices)

Ineffective Protection r/t inadequate nutrition

Ineffective Health self-management r/t inadequate nutrition

Self-Neglect r/t inadequate nutrition

Risk for Powerlessness: Risk factor: possible inability to provide adequate nutrition

MAMMOGRAPHY

Readiness for enhanced Health self-management: follows guidelines for screening

Readiness for enhanced Resilience: responsibility for self-care

MANIC DISORDER, BIPOLAR I

Anxiety r/t change in role function

Ineffective Coping r/t situational crisis

Ineffective Denial r/t fear of inability to control behavior

Interrupted Family processes r/t family member's illness

Risk-prone Health behavior r/t low self-efficacy

Ineffective Health self-management r/t unpredictability of client, excessive demands on family, chronic illness, social support deficit

Ineffective Home Maintenance Behaviors r/t altered psychological state, inability to concentrate

Disturbed personal Identity r/t manic state

Insomnia r/t constant anxious thoughts

Imbalanced Nutrition: less than body requirements r/t lack of time and motivation to eat, constant movement

Impaired individual Resilience r/t psychological disorder

Ineffective Role performance r/t impaired social interactions

Self-Neglect r/t manic state

Sleep deprivation r/t hyperagitated state

Risk for ineffective Activity planning r/t inability to process information

Risk for Caregiver Role Strain: Risk factor: unpredictability of condition

Risk for imbalanced Fluid volume: Risk factor: hypovolemia

Risk for Powerlessness: Risk factor: inability to control changes in mood

Risk for Spiritual distress: Risk factor: depression

Risk for Suicidal Behavior: Risk factor: bipolar disorder

Risk for self-directed Violence: Risk factors: hallucinations, delusions

Risk for other-directed Violence: Risk factor: pathologic intoxication

Readiness for enhanced Hope: expresses desire to enhance problem-solving goals

MANIPULATIVE BEHAVIOR

Defensive Coping r/t superior attitude toward others

Ineffective Coping r/t inappropriate use of defense mechanisms

Self-Mutilation r/t use of manipulation to obtain nurturing relationship with others

Self-Neglect r/t maintaining control

Impaired Social interaction r/t self-concept disturbance

Risk for Loneliness: Risk factor: inability to interact appropriately with others

Risk for situational low Self-Esteem: Risk factor: history of learned helplessness

Risk for Self-Mutilation: Risk factor: inability to cope with increased psychological or physiological tension in healthy manner

MARFAN SYNDROME

Decreased Cardiac output r/t dilation of the aortic root, dissection or rupture of the aorta

Risk for decreased Cardiac tissue perfusion: Risk factor: heart-related complications from Marfan syndrome

Readiness for enhanced Health self-management: describes reduction of risk factors

See Mitral Valve Prolapse; Scoliosis

MASTECTOMY

Disturbed Body Image r/t loss of sexually significant body part

Impaired Comfort r/t altered body image; difficult diagnosis

Death Anxiety r/t threat of mortality associated with breast cancer

Fatigue r/t increased metabolic requirements

Fear r/t change in body image, prognosis

Deficient Knowledge r/t self-care activities

Nausea r/t chemotherapy

Acute Pain r/t surgical procedure

Sexual dysfunction r/t change in body image, fear of loss of femininity

Chronic Sorrow r/t disturbed body image, unknown long-term health status

Spiritual distress r/t change in body image

Risk for Surgical Site Infection: Risk factors: surgical procedure, broken skin

Risk for impaired physical Mobility: Risk factors: nerve or muscle damage, pain

Risk for Post-Trauma syndrome: Risk factors: loss of body part, surgical wounds

Risk for Powerlessness: Risk factor: fear of unknown outcome of procedure

Risk for impaired Resilience: Risk factor: altered body image

See Cancer; Modified Radical Mastectomy; Surgery, Perioperative Care; Surgery, Postoperative Care; Surgery, Preoperative Care

MASTITIS

Anxiety r/t threat to self, concern over safety of milk for infant

Ineffective Breastfeeding r/t breast pain, conflicting advice from healthcare providers

Deficient Knowledge r/t antibiotic regimen, comfort measures

Acute Pain r/t infectious disease process, swelling of breast tissue

Ineffective Role performance r/t change in capacity to function in expected role

MATERNAL INFECTION

Ineffective Protection r/t invasive procedures, traumatized tissue

See Postpartum, Normal Care

MATURATIONAL ISSUES, ADOLESCENT

Ineffective Coping r/t maturational crises

Risk-prone Health behavior r/t inadequate comprehension, negative attitude toward healthcare

Interrupted Family processes r/t developmental crises of adolescence resulting from challenge of parental authority and values, situational crises from change in parental marital status

M

Deficient Knowledge: potential for enhanced health maintenance r/t information misinterpretation, lack of education regarding age-related factors

Impaired Social interaction r/t ineffective, unsuccessful, or dysfunctional interaction with peers

Social isolation r/t perceived alteration in physical appearance, social values not accepted by dominant peer group

Risk for Ineffective Activity planning: Risk factor: unrealistic perception of personal competencies

Risk for disturbed personal Identity: Risk factor: maturational issues

Risk for Injury: Risk factor: thrill-seeking behaviors

Risk for chronic low Self-Esteem: Risk factor: lack of sense of belonging in peer group

Risk for situational low Self-Esteem: Risk factor: developmental changes

Readiness for enhanced Communication: expressing willingness to communicate with parental figures

Readiness for enhanced Relationship: expresses desire to enhance communication with parental figures

See Sexuality, Adolescent; Substance Abuse (if relevant)

MAZE III PROCEDURE

See Dysrhythmia; Open Heart Surgery

MD (MUSCULAR DYSTROPHY)

See Muscular Dystrophy (MD)

MEASLES (RUBEOLA)

See Communicable Diseases, Childhood (e.g., Measles, Mumps, Rubella, Chickenpox, Scabies, Lice)

MECONIUM ASPIRATION

See Respiratory Conditions of the Neonate

MECONIUM DELAYED

Risk for neonatal hyperbilirubinemia: Risk factor: delayed meconium

MEDICAL MARIJUANA

Imbalanced Nutrition: less than body requirements r/t eating disorder, appetite loss, effects of chemotherapy

Chronic Pain Syndrome r/t persistence of pain as a result of physical injury or condition

Nausea r/t effects of chemotherapy

MELANOMA

Disturbed Body Image r/t altered pigmentation, surgical incision

Fear r/t threat to well-being

Ineffective Health maintenance behaviors r/t deficient knowledge regarding self-care and treatment of melanoma

Acute Pain r/t surgical incision

Chronic Sorrow r/t disturbed body image, unknown long-term health status

Readiness for enhanced Health self-management: describes reduction of risk factors; protection from sunlight's ultraviolet rays

See Cancer

MELENA

Fear r/t presence of blood in feces

Risk for imbalanced Fluid volume: Risk factor: hemorrhage

See GI Bleed (Gastrointestinal Bleeding)

MEMORY DEFICIT

Impaired Memory (See **Memory,** impaired, Section II)

MÉNIÈRE'S DISEASE

Risk for Injury: Risk factor: symptoms of disease

Readiness for enhanced Health self-management: expresses desire to manage illness

See Dizziness; Nausea; Vertigo

MENINGITIS/ENCEPHALITIS

Ineffective Airway clearance r/t seizure activity

Impaired Comfort r/t altered health status

Excess Fluid volume r/t increased intracranial pressure, syndrome of inappropriate secretion of antidiuretic hormone

Impaired Mobility r/t neuromuscular or central nervous system insult

Acute Pain r/t biological injury

Risk for Aspiration: Risk factor: seizure activity

Risk for acute Confusion: Risk factor: infection of brain

Risk for Adult Falls: Risk factors: neuromuscular dysfunction and confusion

Risk for Injury: Risk factor: seizure activity

Risk for impaired Resilience: Risk factor: illness

Risk for Shock: Risk factor: infectious process

Risk for ineffective Cerebral tissue perfusion: Risk factors: cerebral tissue edema and inflammation of meninges, increased intracranial pressure; infection

Risk for ineffective Thermoregulation: Risk factor: infectious process

See Hospitalized Child

MENINGOCELE

See Neural Tube Defects

MENOPAUSE

Impaired Comfort r/t symptoms associated with menopause

Insomnia r/t hormonal shifts

Impaired Memory r/t change in hormonal levels

Sexual dysfunction r/t menopausal changes

Ineffective Sexuality pattern r/t altered body structure, lack of lubrication, lack of knowledge of artificial lubrication

Ineffective Thermoregulation r/t changes in hormonal levels

Risk for urge urinary Incontinence: Risk factor: changes in hormonal levels affecting bladder function

Risk for Overweight: Risk factor: change in metabolic rate caused by fluctuating hormone levels

Risk for Powerlessness: Risk factor: changes associated with menopause

Risk for impaired Resilience: Risk factor: menopause

Risk for situational low Self-Esteem: Risk factors: developmental changes, menopause

Readiness for enhanced Health self-management: verbalized desire to manage menopause

Readiness for enhanced Self-Care: expresses satisfaction with body image

Readiness for enhanced Spiritual well-being: desire for harmony of mind, body, and spirit

MENORRHAGIA

Fear r/t loss of large amounts of blood

Risk for deficient Fluid volume: Risk factor: excessive loss of menstrual blood

MENTAL ILLNESS

Defensive Coping r/t psychological impairment, substance abuse

Ineffective Coping r/t situational crisis, coping with mental illness

Compromised family Coping r/t lack of available support from client

Disabled family Coping r/t chronically unexpressed feelings of guilt, anxiety, hostility, or despair

Ineffective Denial r/t refusal to acknowledge abuse problem, fear of the social stigma of disease

Risk-prone Health behavior r/t low self-efficacy

Disturbed personal Identity r/t psychoses

Ineffective Relationship r/t effects of mental illness in partner relationship

Chronic Sorrow r/t presence of mental illness

Stress overload r/t multiple coexisting stressors

Ineffective family Health self-management r/t chronicity of condition, unpredictability of client, unknown prognosis

Risk for Loneliness: Risk factor: social isolation

Risk for Powerlessness: Risk factor: lifestyle of helplessness

Risk for impaired Resilience: Risk factor: chronic illness

Risk for chronic low Self-Esteem: Risk factor: presence of mental illness/repeated negative reinforcement

METABOLIC ACIDOSIS

See Ketoacidosis, Alcoholic; Ketoacidosis, Diabetic

METABOLIC ALKALOSIS

Deficient Fluid volume r/t fluid volume loss, vomiting, gastric suctioning, failure of regulatory mechanisms

METABOLIC IMBALANCE SYNDROME

Ineffective Health Maintenance behaviors r/t deficient knowledge regarding basic health practice

Obesity r/t energy expenditure below energy intake

Risk for unstable Blood Glucose level: Risk factor: variations in serum glucose levels

METASTASIS

See Cancer

METHICILLIN-RESISTANT *STAPHYLOCOCCUS AUREUS* (MRSA)

See MRSA (Methicillin-Resistant Staphylococcus aureus)

MI (MYOCARDIAL INFARCTION)

Decreased activity tolerance r/t imbalance between oxygen supply and demand

Anxiety r/t threat of death, possible change in role status

Death Anxiety r/t seriousness of medical condition

Constipation r/t decreased peristalsis from decreased physical activity, medication effect, change in diet

Ineffective family Coping r/t spouse or significant other's fear of partner loss

Ineffective Denial r/t fear, deficient knowledge about heart disease

Interrupted Family processes r/t crisis, role change

Fear r/t threat to well-being

Ineffective Health maintenance behaviors r/t deficient knowledge regarding self-care and treatment

Acute Pain r/t myocardial tissue damage from inadequate blood supply

Situational low Self-Esteem r/t crisis of MI

Ineffective Sexuality pattern r/t fear of chest pain, possibility of heart damage

Risk for Powerlessness: Risk factor: acute illness

Risk for Shock: Risk factors: hypotension, myocardial dysfunction, hypoxia

Risk for Spiritual distress: Risk factor: physical illness

Risk for decreased Cardiac output: Risk factors: alteration in heart rate, rhythm, and contractility

Risk for decreased Cardiac tissue perfusion: Risk factors: coronary artery spasm, hypertension, hypotension, hypoxia

Readiness for enhanced Knowledge: expresses an interest in learning about condition

See Angioplasty, Coronary; Coronary Artery Bypass Grafting (CABG)

MIDCAB (MINIMALLY INVASIVE DIRECT CORONARY ARTERY BYPASS)

Risk for Bleeding: Risk factor: surgery

Readiness for enhanced Health self-management: preoperative and postoperative care associated with surgery

Risk for Surgical Site Infection: Risk factor: surgical procedure

See Angioplasty, Coronary; Coronary Artery Bypass Grafting (CABG)

MIDLIFE CRISIS

Ineffective Coping r/t inability to deal with changes associated with aging

Powerlessness r/t lack of control over life situation

Spiritual distress r/t questioning beliefs or value system

Risk for disturbed Personal Identity: Risk factor: alteration in social roles

Risk for chronic low Self-Esteem: Risk factor: ineffective coping with loss

Readiness for enhanced Relationship: meets goals for lifestyle change

Readiness for enhanced Spiritual well-being: desire to find purpose and meaning to life

MIGRAINE HEADACHE

Ineffective Health maintenance behaviors r/t deficient knowledge regarding prevention and treatment of headaches

Readiness for enhanced Health management: expresses desire to manage illness

Acute Pain: headache r/t vasodilation of cerebral and extracerebral vessels

Risk for impaired Resilience: Risk factors: chronic illness, disabling pain

MILITARY FAMILIES, PERSONNEL

Anxiety r/t apprehension and helplessness caused by uncertainty of family members' situation

Interrupted Family Processes r/t possible change in family roles, decrease in available emotional support

Relocation Stress Syndrome r/t unpredictability of experience, powerlessness, significant environmental change

MILK INTOLERANCE

See Lactose Intolerance

MINIMALLY INVASIVE DIRECT CORONARY BYPASS (MIDCAB)

See MIDCAB (Minimally Invasive Direct Coronary Artery Bypass)

MISCARRIAGE

See Pregnancy Loss

MITRAL STENOSIS

Decreased activity tolerance r/t imbalance between oxygen supply and demand

Anxiety r/t possible worsening of symptoms, decreased activity tolerance, fatigue

Decreased Cardiac output r/t incompetent heart valves, abnormal forward or backward blood flow, flow into a dilated chamber, flow through an abnormal passage between chambers

Fatigue r/t reduced cardiac output

Ineffective Health maintenance behaviors r/t deficient knowledge regarding self-care with disorder

Risk for decreased Cardiac tissue perfusion: Risk factor: incompetent heart valve

Risk for Infection: Risk factors: invasive procedure, risk for endocarditis

MITRAL VALVE PROLAPSE

Anxiety r/t symptoms of condition: palpitations, chest pain

Fatigue r/t abnormal catecholamine regulation, decreased intravascular volume

Fear r/t lack of knowledge about mitral valve prolapse, feelings of having heart attack

Ineffective Health maintenance behaviors r/t deficient knowledge regarding methods to relieve pain and treat dysrhythmia and shortness of breath, need for prophylactic antibiotics before invasive procedures

Acute Pain r/t mitral valve regurgitation

Risk for ineffective Cerebral tissue perfusion: Risk factor: postural hypotension

Risk for Infection: Risk factor: invasive procedures

Risk for Powerlessness: Risk factor: unpredictability of onset of symptoms

Readiness for enhanced Knowledge: expresses interest in learning about condition

MOBILITY, IMPAIRED BED

Impaired bed Mobility (See **Mobility**, bed, impaired, Section II)

MOBILITY, IMPAIRED PHYSICAL

Impaired physical Mobility (See **Mobility**, physical, impaired, Section II)

Risk for Adult Falls: Risk factor: impaired physical mobility

MOBILITY, IMPAIRED WHEELCHAIR

Impaired wheelchair Mobility (See **Mobility**, wheelchair, impaired, Section II)

MODIFIED RADICAL MASTECTOMY

Readiness for enhanced Communication: willingness to enhance communication

See Mastectomy

MONONUCLEOSIS

Decreased activity tolerance r/t generalized weakness

Impaired Comfort r/t sore throat, muscle aches

Fatigue r/t disease state, stress

Ineffective Health maintenance behaviors r/t deficient knowledge concerning transmission and treatment of disease

Acute Pain r/t enlargement of lymph nodes, oropharyngeal edema

Impaired Swallowing r/t enlargement of lymph nodes, oropharyngeal edema

Risk for Injury: Risk factor: possible rupture of spleen

Risk for Loneliness: Risk factor: social isolation

MOOD DISORDERS

Caregiver Role Strain r/t overwhelming needs of care receiver, unpredictability of mood alterations

Labile Emotional Control r/t (See Labile **Emotional Control**, Section II)

Risk-prone Health behavior r/t hopelessness, altered locus of control

Impaired Mood regulation r/t (See **Mood** regulation, impaired, Section II)

Self-Neglect r/t inability to care for self

Social isolation r/t alterations in mental status

Risk for situational low Self-Esteem: Risk factor: unpredictable changes in mood

Readiness for enhanced Communication: expresses feelings

See specific disorder: Depression (Major Depressive Disorder); Dysthymic Disorder; Hypomania; Manic Disorder, Bipolar I

MOON FACE

Disturbed Body Image r/t change in appearance from disease and medication(s)

Risk for situational low Self-Esteem: Risk factor: change in body image

See Cushing's Syndrome

MORAL/ETHICAL DILEMMAS

Impaired emancipated Decision-Making r/t questioning personal values and belief, which alter decision

Moral Distress r/t conflicting information guiding moral or ethical decision-making

Risk for Powerlessness: Risk factor: lack of knowledge to make a decision

Risk for Spiritual distress: Risk factor: moral or ethical crisis

Readiness for enhanced emancipated Decision-Making: expresses desire to enhance congruency of decisions with personal values and goals

Readiness for enhanced Religiosity: requests assistance in expanding religious options

Readiness for enhanced Resilience: vulnerable state

Readiness for enhanced Spiritual well-being: request for interaction with others regarding difficult decisions

MORNING SICKNESS

See Hyperemesis Gravidarum; Pregnancy, Normal

MOTION SICKNESS

See Labyrinthitis

MOTTLING OF PERIPHERAL SKIN

Ineffective peripheral Tissue Perfusion r/t interruption of arterial flow, decreased circulating blood volume

Risk for Shock: Risk factor: inadequate circulation to perfuse body

MOUTH LESIONS

See Mucous Membrane Integrity, Impaired Oral

MRI (MAGNETIC RESONANCE IMAGING)

Anxiety r/t fear of being in closed spaces

Readiness for enhanced Health management: describes reduction of risk factors associated with exam

Deficient Knowledge r/t unfamiliarity with information resources; exam information

Readiness for enhanced Knowledge: expresses interest in learning about exam

MRSA (METHICILLIN-RESISTANT *STAPHYLOCOCCUS AUREUS*)

Impaired Skin integrity r/t infection

Delayed Surgical recovery r/t infection

Ineffective Thermoregulation r/t severe infection stimulating immune system

Impaired Tissue integrity r/t wound, infection

Risk for Loneliness: Risk factor: physical isolation

Risk for impaired Resilience: Risk factor: illness

Risk for Shock: Risk factor: sepsis

MUCOCUTANEOUS LYMPH NODE SYNDROME

See Kawasaki Disease

MUCOUS MEMBRANE INTEGRITY, IMPAIRED ORAL

Impaired Oral Mucous Membrane Integrity (See **Oral Mucous Membrane Integrity**, impaired, Section II)

MULTI-INFARCT DEMENTIA

See Dementia

M

MULTIPLE GESTATIONS

Anxiety r/t uncertain outcome of pregnancy

Death Anxiety r/t maternal complications associated with multiple gestations

Insufficient Breast Milk Production r/t multiple births

Ineffective Childbearing process r/t unavailable support system

Fatigue r/t physiological demands of a multifetal pregnancy and/or care of more than one infant

Ineffective Home Maintenance Behaviors r/t fatigue

Stress urinary Incontinence r/t increased pelvic pressure

Insomnia r/t impairment of normal sleep pattern; parental responsibilities

Deficient Knowledge r/t caring for more than one infant

Neonatal Hyperbilirubinemia r/t feeding pattern not well established

Deficient Knowledge r/t caring for more than one infant

Imbalanced Nutrition: less than body requirements r/t physiological demands of a multifetal pregnancy

Stress overload r/t multiple coexisting stressors, family demands

Impaired Walking r/t increased uterine size

Risk for ineffective Breastfeeding: Risk factors: lack of support, physical demands of feeding more than one infant

Risk for delayed Child Development: fetus: Risk factor: multiple gestations

Risk for neonatal hyperbilirubinemia: Risk factors: abnormal weight loss, prematurity, feeding pattern not well-established

Readiness for enhanced Childbearing process: demonstrates appropriate care for infants and mother

Readiness for enhanced Family processes: family adapting to change with more than one infant

MULTIPLE PERSONALITY DISORDER (DISSOCIATIVE IDENTITY DISORDER)

Anxiety r/t loss of control of behavior and feelings

Disturbed Body Image r/t psychosocial changes

Defensive Coping r/t unresolved past traumatic events, severe anxiety

Ineffective Coping r/t history of abuse

Hopelessness r/t long-term stress

Disturbed personal Identity r/t severe child abuse

Chronic low Self-Esteem r/t rejection, failure

Risk for Self-Mutilation: Risk factor: need to act out to relieve stress

Readiness for enhanced Communication: willingness to discuss problems associated with condition

See Dissociative Identity Disorder (Not Otherwise Specified)

MULTIPLE SCLEROSIS (MS)

Ineffective Activity planning r/t unrealistic perception of personal competence

Ineffective Airway clearance r/t decreased energy or fatigue

Impaired physical Mobility r/t neuromuscular impairment

Self-Neglect r/t functional impairment

Powerlessness r/t progressive nature of disease

Self-Care deficit: specify r/t neuromuscular impairment

Sexual dysfunction r/t biopsychosocial alteration of sexuality

Chronic Sorrow r/t loss of physical ability

Spiritual distress r/t perceived hopelessness of diagnosis

Urinary Retention r/t inhibition of the reflex arc

Risk for Disuse syndrome: Risk factor: physical immobility

Risk for Injury: Risk factors: altered mobility, sensory dysfunction

Risk for imbalanced Nutrition: less than body requirements: Risk factors: impaired swallowing, depression

Risk for Powerlessness: Risk factor: chronic illness

Risk for impaired Religiosity: Risk factor: illness

Risk for Thermal Injury: Risk factor: neuromuscular impairment

Readiness for enhanced Health self-management: expresses a desire to manage condition

Readiness for enhanced Self-Care: expresses desire to enhance knowledge of strategies and responsibility for self-care

Readiness for enhanced Spiritual well-being: struggling with chronic debilitating condition

See Neurologic Disorders

MUMPS

See Communicable Diseases, Childhood (e.g., Measles, Mumps, Rubella, Chickenpox, Scabies, Lice)

MURMURS

Decreased Cardiac output r/t altered preload/afterload

Risk for decreased Cardiac tissue perfusion: Risk factor: incompetent valve

Risk for Fatigue: Risk factor: decreased cardiac output

MUSCULAR ATROPHY/WEAKNESS

Risk for Disuse syndrome: Risk factor: impaired physical mobility

Risk for Adult Falls: Risk factor: impaired physical mobility

MUSCULAR DYSTROPHY (MD)

Decreased activity tolerance r/t fatigue, muscle weakness

Ineffective Activity planning r/t unrealistic perception of personal competence

Ineffective Airway clearance r/t muscle weakness and decreased ability to cough

Constipation r/t immobility

Fatigue r/t increased energy requirements to perform activities of daily living

Impaired physical Mobility r/t muscle weakness and development of contractures

Imbalanced Nutrition: less than body requirements r/t impaired swallowing or chewing

Self-Care deficit: feeding, bathing, dressing, toileting r/t muscle weakness and fatigue

Self-Neglect r/t functional impairment

Impaired Transfer ability r/t muscle weakness

Impaired Swallowing r/t neuromuscular impairment

Impaired Walking r/t muscle weakness

Risk for Aspiration: Risk factor: impaired swallowing

Risk for decreased Cardiac tissue perfusion: Risk factor: hypoxia associated with cardiomyopathy

Risk for Disuse syndrome: Risk factor: complications of immobility

Risk for Adult Falls: Risk factor: muscle weakness

Risk for Infection: Risk factor: pooling of pulmonary secretions as a result of immobility and muscle weakness

Risk for Injury: Risk factors: muscle weakness and unsteady gait

Risk for Overweight: Risk factor: inactivity

Risk for Powerlessness: Risk factor: chronic condition

Risk for impaired Religiosity: Risk factor: illness

Risk for impaired Resilience: Risk factor: chronic illness

Risk for situational low Self-Esteem: Risk factor: presence of chronic condition

Readiness for enhanced Self-Concept: acceptance of strength and abilities

Risk for impaired Skin integrity: Risk factors: immobility, braces, or adaptive devices

M

See Child with Chronic Condition; Hospitalized Child

MVC (MOTOR VEHICLE CRASH)

See Fracture; Head Injury; Injury; Pneumothorax

MYASTHENIA GRAVIS

Ineffective Airway clearance r/t decreased ability to cough and swallow

Interrupted Family processes r/t crisis of dealing with diagnosis

Fatigue r/t paresthesia, aching muscles, weakness of muscles

Impaired physical Mobility r/t defective transmission of nerve impulses at the neuromuscular junction

Imbalanced Nutrition: less than body requirements r/t difficulty eating and swallowing

Impaired Swallowing r/t neuromuscular impairment

Risk for Caregiver Role Strain: Risk factors: severity of illness of client, overwhelming needs of client

Risk for impaired Religiosity: Risk factor: illness

Risk for impaired Resilience: Risk factor: new diagnosis of chronic, serious illness

Readiness for enhanced Spiritual well-being: heightened coping with serious illness

See Neurologic Disorders

MYCOPLASMA PNEUMONIA

See Pneumonia

MYELOCELE

See Neural Tube Defects

MYELOMENINGOCELE

See Neural Tube Defects

MYOCARDIAL INFARCTION (MI)

See MI (Myocardial Infarction)

MYOCARDITIS

Decreased activity tolerance r/t reduced cardiac reserve and prescribed bed rest

Decreased Cardiac output r/t altered preload/afterload

Deficient Knowledge r/t treatment of disease

Risk for decreased Cardiac tissue perfusion: Risk factors: hypoxia, hypovolemia, cardiac tamponade

Readiness for enhanced Knowledge: treatment of disease

See Heart Failure, if appropriate

MYRINGOTOMY

Fear r/t hospitalization, surgical procedure

Ineffective Health maintenance behaviors r/t deficient knowledge regarding care after surgery

Acute Pain r/t surgical procedure

Risk for Surgical Site Infection: Risk factor: invasive procedure

See Ear Surgery

MYXEDEMA

See Hypothyroidism

N

NARCISSISTIC PERSONALITY DISORDER

Defensive Coping r/t grandiose sense of self

Impaired emancipated Decision-Making r/t lack of realistic problem-solving skills

Interrupted Family processes r/t taking advantage of others to achieve own goals

Risk-prone Health behavior r/t low self-efficacy

Disturbed personal Identity r/t psychological impairment

Ineffective Relationship r/t lack of mutual support/respect between partners

Impaired individual Resilience r/t psychological disorders

Impaired Social interaction r/t self-concept disturbance

Risk for Loneliness: Risk factors: emotional deprivation, social isolation

NARCOLEPSY

Anxiety r/t fear of lack of control over falling asleep

Disturbed Sleep pattern r/t uncontrollable desire to sleep

Risk for Physical Trauma: Risk factor: falling asleep during potentially dangerous activity

Readiness for enhanced Sleep: expresses willingness to enhance sleep

NARCOTIC USE

See Opiod Use

NASOGASTRIC SUCTION

Impaired Oral Mucous Membrane Integrity r/t presence of nasogastric tube

Risk for Electrolyte imbalance: Risk factor: loss of gastrointestinal fluids that contain electrolytes

Risk for imbalanced Fluid volume: Risk factor: loss of gastrointestinal fluids without adequate replacement

Risk for dysfunctional Gastrointestinal motility: Risk factor: decreased intestinal motility

NAUSEA

Nausea (See **Nausea,** Section II)

NEAR-DROWNING

Ineffective Airway clearance r/t aspiration of fluid

Aspiration r/t aspiration of fluid into lungs

Fear: parental r/t possible death of child, possible permanent and debilitating sequelae

Impaired Gas exchange r/t laryngospasm, holding breath, aspiration, inflammation

Ineffective Health maintenance behaviors r/t parental deficient knowledge regarding safety measures appropriate for age

Hypothermia r/t central nervous system injury, prolonged submersion in cold water

Risk for delayed Child Development: Risk factors: hypoxemia, cerebral anoxia

Risk for maladaptive Grieving: Risk factors: potential death of child, unknown sequelae, guilt about accident

Risk for Infection: Risk factors: aspiration, invasive monitoring

Risk for ineffective Cerebral tissue perfusion: Risk factor: hypoxia

Readiness for enhanced Spiritual well-being: struggle with survival of life-threatening situation

See Child with Chronic Condition; Hospitalized Child; Safety, Childhood; Terminally Ill Child/Death of Child, Parent

NEARSIGHTEDNESS

Readiness for enhanced Health self-management: need for correction of myopia

NEARSIGHTEDNESS; CORNEAL SURGERY

See LASIK Eye Surgery (Laser-Assisted in Situ Keratomileusis)

NECK VEIN DISTENTION

Decreased Cardiac output r/t decreased contractility of heart resulting in increased preload

Excess Fluid volume r/t excess fluid intake, compromised regulatory mechanisms

See Congestive Heart Failure (CHF); Heart Failure

NECROSIS, KIDNEY TUBULAR; NECROSIS, ACUTE TUBULAR

See Renal Failure

NECROTIZING ENTEROCOLITIS

Ineffective Breathing pattern r/t abdominal distention, hypoxia

Diarrhea r/t infection

Deficient Fluid volume r/t vomiting, gastrointestinal bleeding

Neonatal Hyperbilirubinemia r/t feeding pattern not well established

Imbalanced Nutrition: less than body requirements r/t decreased ability to absorb nutrients, decreased perfusion to gastrointestinal tract

Risk for dysfunctional Gastrointestinal motility: Risk factor: infection

Risk for Infection: Risk factors: bacterial invasion of gastrointestinal tract, invasive procedures

See Hospitalized Child; Premature Infant (Child)

NEGATIVE FEELINGS ABOUT SELF

Chronic low Self-Esteem r/t long-standing negative self-evaluation

Self-Neglect r/t negative feelings

Readiness for enhanced Self-Concept: expresses willingness to enhance self-concept

NEGLECT, UNILATERAL

Unilateral Neglect (See **Unilateral Neglect**, Section II)

NEGLECTFUL CARE OF FAMILY MEMBER

Caregiver Role Strain r/t overwhelming care demands of family member, lack of social or financial support

Disabled family Coping r/t highly ambivalent family relationships, lack of respite care

Interrupted Family processes r/t situational transition or crisis

Deficient Knowledge r/t care needs

Impaired individual Resilience r/t vulnerability from neglect

Risk for compromised Human Dignity: Risk factor: inadequate participation in decision-making

NEONATAL ABSTINENCE SYNDROME

Ineffective Airway clearance r/t pooling of secretions from lack of adequate cough reflex, effects of viral or bacterial lower airway infection as a result of altered protective state

Interrupted Breastfeeding r/t use of drugs or alcohol by mother

Ineffective Childbearing process r/t inconsistent prenatal health visits, suboptimal maternal nutrition, substance abuse

Impaired Comfort r/t irritability and inability to relax

Diarrhea r/t effects of withdrawal, increased peristalsis from hyperirritability

Disorganized infant Behavior r/t exposure and/or withdrawal from toxic substances (alcohol or drugs), lack of attachment

Ineffective infant suck-swallow response r/t uncoordinated or ineffective sucking reflex

Imbalanced Nutrition: less than body requirements r/t feeding problems; uncoordinated or ineffective suck and swallow; effects of diarrhea, vomiting, or colic associated with maternal substance abuse

Impaired Parenting r/t impaired or absent attachment behaviors, inadequate support systems

Ineffective infant suck-swallow response r/t neurological delay

Disturbed Sleep Pattern r/t hyperirritability or hypersensitivity to environmental stimuli

Risk for impaired Attachment: Risk factor: (parent) substance misuse, inability to meet infant's needs

Risk for delayed Child Development: Risk factor: effects of prenatal substance abuse

Risk for Infection: skin, meningeal, respiratory: Risk factor: stress effects of withdrawal

Risk for Disturbed Maternal–fetal Dyad: Risk factor: substance abuse

Risk for Sudden Infant Death: Risk factor: prenatal illicit drug exposure

Risk for ineffective Thermoregulation: Risk factor: immature nervous system

See Anomaly, fetal/Newborn (Parent Dealing with); Cerebral Palsy; Child with Chronic Condition; Failure to Thrive; Hospitalized Child; Hyperactive Syndrome; Premature Infant/Child; Sudden Infant Death Syndrome (SIDS)

NEONATAL HYPERBILIRUBINEMIA

Neonatal Hyperbilirubinemia (See neonatal **Hyperbilirubinemia,** Section II)

NEONATE

Readiness for enhanced Childbearing process: appropriate care of newborn

See Newborn, Normal; Newborn, Postmature; Newborn, Small for Gestational Age (SGA)

NEOPLASM

Fear r/t possible malignancy

See Cancer

NEPHRECTOMY

Anxiety r/t surgical recovery, prognosis

Ineffective Breathing pattern r/t location of surgical incision

Constipation r/t lack of return of peristalsis

Acute Pain r/t incisional discomfort

Spiritual distress r/t chronic illness

Risk for Bleeding: Risk factor: surgery

Risk for imbalanced Fluid volume: Risk factors: vascular losses, decreased intake

Risk for Surgical Site Infection: Risk factors: surgical procedure

NEPHROSTOMY, PERCUTANEOUS

Acute Pain r/t invasive procedure

Impaired Urinary elimination r/t nephrostomy tube

Risk for Infection: Risk factor: invasive procedure

NEPHROTIC SYNDROME

Decreased activity tolerance r/t generalized edema

Disturbed Body Image r/t edematous appearance and side effects of steroid therapy

Excess Fluid volume r/t edema resulting from oncotic fluid shift caused by serum protein loss and kidney retention of salt and water

Imbalanced Nutrition: less than body requirements r/t anorexia, protein loss

Imbalanced Nutrition: more than body requirements r/t increased appetite attributable to steroid therapy

Social isolation r/t edematous appearance

Risk for Infection: Risk factor: altered immune mechanisms caused by disease and effects of steroids

Risk for impaired Skin integrity: Risk factor: edema

See Child with Chronic Condition; Hospitalized Child

NEURAL TUBE DEFECTS (MENINGOCELE, MYELOMENINGOCELE, SPINA BIFIDA, ANENCEPHALY)

Chronic functional Constipation r/t immobility or less than adequate mobility

Total urinary Incontinence r/t neurogenic impairment

Urge urinary Incontinence r/t neurogenic impairment

Impaired Mobility r/t neuromuscular impairment

Chronic low Self-Esteem r/t perceived differences, decreased ability to participate in physical and social activities at school

Impaired Skin integrity r/t incontinence

Risk for delayed Child Development: Risk factor: inadequate nutrition

Risk for Latex Allergic reaction: Risk factor: multiple exposures to latex products

Risk for imbalanced Nutrition: more than body requirements: Risk factors: diminished, limited, or impaired physical activity

Risk for Powerlessness: Risk factor: debilitating disease

Risk for impaired Skin integrity: lower extremities: Risk factor: decreased sensory perception

Readiness for enhanced family Coping: effective adaptive response by family members

Readiness for enhanced Family processes: family supports each other

See Child with Chronic Condition; Premature Infant (Child)

N

NEURALGIA

See Trigeminal Neuralgia

NEURITIS (PERIPHERAL NEUROPATHY)

Decreased activity tolerance r/t pain with movement

Ineffective Health maintenance behaviors r/t deficient knowledge regarding self-care with neuritis

Acute Pain r/t stimulation of affected nerve endings, inflammation of sensory nerves

See Neuropathy, Peripheral

NEUROGENIC BLADDER

Urinary Retention r/t interruption in the lateral spinal tracts

Risk for Latex Allergic reaction: Risk factor: repeated exposures to latex associated with possible repeated catheterizations

NEUROLOGIC DISORDERS

Ineffective Airway clearance r/t perceptual or cognitive impairment, decreased energy, fatigue

Acute Confusion r/t dementia, alcohol abuse, drug abuse, delirium

Ineffective Coping r/t disability requiring change in lifestyle

Interrupted Family processes r/t situational crisis, illness, or disability of family member

Ineffective Home Maintenance Behaviors r/t client's or family member's disease

Risk for corneal Injury: Risk factor: lack of spontaneous blink reflex

Impaired Memory r/t neurological disturbance

Impaired physical Mobility r/t neuromuscular impairment

Imbalanced Nutrition: less than body requirements r/t impaired swallowing, depression, difficulty feeding self

Powerlessness r/t progressive nature of disease

Self-Care deficit: specify r/t neuromuscular dysfunction

Sexual dysfunction r/t biopsychosocial alteration of sexuality

Social isolation r/t altered state of wellness

Impaired Swallowing r/t neuromuscular dysfunction

Risk for Disuse syndrome: Risk factors: physical immobility, neuromuscular dysfunction

Risk for Injury: Risk factors: altered mobility, sensory dysfunction, cognitive impairment

Risk for ineffective Cerebral tissue perfusion: Risk factor: cerebral disease/ injury

Risk for impaired Religiosity: Risk factor: life transition

Risk for impaired Skin integrity: Risk factors: altered sensation, altered mental status, paralysis

See specific condition: Alcohol Withdrawal; Amyotrophic Lateral Sclerosis (ALS); CVA (Cerebrovascular Accident); Delirium; Dementia; Guillain-Barré Syndrome; Head Injury; Huntington's

Disease; Spinal Cord Injury; Myasthenia Gravis, Muscular Dystrophy (MD); Parkinson's Disease

NEUROPATHY, PERIPHERAL

Chronic Pain r/t damage to nerves in the peripheral nervous system as a result of medication side effects, vitamin deficiency, or diabetes

Ineffective Thermoregulation r/t decreased ability to regulate body temperature

Risk for Injury: Risk factors: lack of muscle control, decreased sensation

Risk for impaired Skin integrity: Risk factor: poor perfusion

Risk for Thermal Injury r/t nerve damage

See Peripheral Vascular Disease (PVD)

NEUROSURGERY

See Craniectomy/Craniotomy

NEWBORN, NORMAL

Breastfeeding r/t normal oral structure and gestational age greater than 34 weeks

Ineffective Thermoregulation r/t immaturity of neuroendocrine system

Risk for Sudden Infant Death: Risk factors: lack of knowledge regarding infant sleeping in prone or side-lying position, prenatal or postnatal infant smoke exposure, infant overheating or overwrapping, loose articles in the sleep environment

Risk for Infection: Risk factors: open umbilical stump, immature immune system

Risk for Injury: Risk factors: immaturity, need for caretaking

Readiness for enhanced Childbearing process: appropriate care of newborn

Readiness for enhanced organized Infant behavior: demonstrates adaptive response to pain

Readiness for enhanced Parenting: providing emotional and physical needs of infant

NEWBORN, POSTMATURE

Hypothermia r/t depleted stores of subcutaneous fat

Impaired Skin integrity r/t cracked and peeling skin as a result of decreased vernix

Risk for ineffective Airway clearance: Risk factor: meconium aspiration

Risk for unstable blood Glucose level: Risk factor: depleted glycogen stores

NEWBORN, SMALL FOR GESTATIONAL AGE (SGA)

Neonatal Hyperbilirubinemia r/t neonate age and difficulty feeding

Imbalanced Nutrition: less than body requirements r/t history of placental insufficiency

Ineffective Thermoregulation r/t decreased brown fat, subcutaneous fat

Risk for delayed Child Development: Risk factor: history of placental insufficiency

Risk for Injury: Risk factors: hypoglycemia, perinatal asphyxia, meconium aspiration

Risk for Sudden Infant Death: Risk factor: low birth weight

NICOTINE ADDICTION

Risk-prone Health behavior r/t smoking

Ineffective Health maintenance behaviors r/t lack of ability to make a judgment about smoking cessation

Risk for impaired Skin integrity: Risk factor: poor tissue perfusion associated with nicotine

Powerlessness r/t perceived lack of control over ability to give up nicotine

Readiness for enhanced emancipated Decision-Making: expresses desire to enhance understanding and meaning of choices

Readiness for enhanced Health literacy: expresses desire to enhance understanding of health information to make healthcare choices

Readiness for enhanced Health self-management: expresses desire to learn measures to stop smoking

NIDDM (NON-INSULIN-DEPENDENT DIABETES MELLITUS)

Readiness for enhanced Health self-management: expresses desire for information on exercise and diet to manage diabetes

See Diabetes Mellitus

NIGHTMARES

Post-Trauma syndrome r/t disaster, war, epidemic, rape, assault, torture, catastrophic illness, or accident

NIPPLE SORENESS

Impaired Comfort r/t physical condition

See Painful Breasts, Sore Nipples; Sore Nipples, Breastfeeding

NOCTURIA

Urge urinary Incontinence r/t decreased bladder capacity, irritation of bladder stretch receptors causing spasm, alcohol, caffeine, increased fluids, increased urine concentration, overdistention of bladder

Impaired Urinary elimination r/t sensory motor impairment, urinary tract infection

Risk for Powerlessness: Risk factor: inability to control nighttime voiding

NOCTURNAL MYOCLONUS

See Restless Leg Syndrome; Stress

NOCTURNAL PAROXYSMAL DYSPNEA

See PND (Paroxysmal Nocturnal Dyspnea)

NON–INSULIN-DEPENDENT DIABETES MELLITUS (NIDDM)

See Diabetes Mellitus

NORMAL PRESSURE HYDROCEPHALUS (NPH)

Impaired verbal Communication r/t obstruction of flow of cerebrospinal fluid affecting speech

Acute Confusion r/t increased intracranial pressure caused by obstruction to flow of cerebrospinal fluid

Impaired Memory r/t neurological disturbance

Risk for ineffective Cerebral tissue perfusion: Risk factor: fluid pressing on the brain

Risk for Adult Falls: Risk factor: unsteady gait as a result of obstruction of cerebrospinal fluid

NSTEMI (NON-ST-ELEVATION MYOCARDIAL INFARCTION)

See MI (Myocardial Infarction)

NURSING

See Breastfeeding, Effective; Breastfeeding, Ineffective; Breastfeeding, Interrupted

NUTRITION

Readiness for enhanced Nutrition (See **Nutrition,** readiness for enhanced, Section II)

NUTRITION, IMBALANCED

Imbalanced Nutrition: less than body requirements (See **Nutrition: less than body requirements**, imbalanced, Section II)

Obesity (See **Obesity,** Section II)

Overweight (See **Overweight,** Section II)

Risk for Overweight (See **Overweight,** risk for, Section II)

OBESITY

Disturbed Body Image r/t eating disorder, excess weight

Risk-prone Health behavior: r/t negative attitude toward healthcare

Obesity (See **Obesity**, Section II)

Chronic low Self-Esteem r/t ineffective coping, overeating

Risk for Metabolic Syndrome: Risk factor: obesity

Risk for ineffective peripheral Tissue Perfusion: Risk factor: sedentary lifestyle

Readiness for enhanced Nutrition: expresses willingness to enhance nutrition

OBS (ORGANIC BRAIN SYNDROME)

See Organic Mental Disorders; Dementia

OBSESSIVE-COMPULSIVE DISORDER (OCD)

See OCD (Obsessive-Compulsive Disorder)

OBSTRUCTION, BOWEL

See Bowel Obstruction

OBSTRUCTIVE SLEEP APNEA

Insomnia r/t blocked airway

Obesity r/t excessive intake related to metabolic need

See PND (Paroxysmal Nocturnal Dyspnea)

OCD (OBSESSIVE-COMPULSIVE DISORDER)

Ineffective Activity planning r/t unrealistic perception of events

Anxiety r/t threat to self-concept, unmet needs

Impaired emancipated Decision-Making r/t inability to make a decision for fear of reprisal

Disabled family Coping r/t family process being disrupted by client's ritualistic activities

Ineffective Coping r/t expression of feelings in an unacceptable way, ritualistic behavior

Risk-prone Health behavior r/t inadequate comprehension associated with repetitive thoughts

Powerlessness r/t unrelenting repetitive thoughts to perform irrational activities

Impaired individual Resilience r/t psychological disorder

Risk for situational low Self-Esteem: Risk factor: inability to control repetitive thoughts and actions

OCCUPATIONAL INJURY

Fatigue r/t lack of sleep

Deficient Knowledge r/t inadequate training, improper use of equipment

Stress Overload r/t feelings of pressure

Risk for Occupational Injury (See **Risk for Occupational Injury**, Section II)

ODD (OPPOSITIONAL DEFIANT DISORDER)

Anxiety r/t feelings of anger and hostility toward authority figures

Ineffective Coping r/t lack of self-control or perceived lack of self-control

Disabled Family coping r/t feelings of anger, hostility; defiant behavior toward authority figures

Risk-prone Health behavior r/t multiple stressors associated with condition

Ineffective Impulse control r/t anger/compunction to engage in disruptive behaviors

Chronic or situational low Self-Esteem r/t poor self-control and disruptive behaviors

Impaired Social interaction r/t being touchy or easily annoyed, blaming others for own mistakes, constant trouble in school

Social isolation r/t unaccepted social behavior

Ineffective family Health self-management r/t difficulty in limit setting and managing oppositional behaviors

Risk for ineffective Activity planning: Risk factors: unrealistic perception of events, hedonism, insufficient social support

Risk for impaired Parenting: Risk factors: children's difficult behaviors and inability to set limits

Risk for Powerlessness: Risk factor: inability to deal with difficult behaviors

Risk for Spiritual distress: Risk factors: anxiety and stress in dealing with difficult behaviors

Risk for other-directed Violence: Risk factors: history of violence, threats of violence against others, history of antisocial behavior, history of indirect violence

OLDER ADULT

See Aging

OLIGURIA

Deficient Fluid volume r/t active fluid loss, failure of regulatory mechanism, inadequate intake

See Cardiac Output, Decreased; Renal Failure; Shock, Hypovolemic

O

OMPHALOCELE

See Gastroschisis/Omphalocele

OOPHORECTOMY

Risk for ineffective Sexuality pattern: Risk factor: altered body function

See Surgery, Perioperative Care; Surgery, Postoperative Care; Surgery, Preoperative Care

OPCAB (OFF-PUMP CORONARY ARTERY BYPASS)

See Angioplasty, Coronary; Coronary Artery Bypass Grafting (CABG)

OPEN HEART SURGERY

Risk for decreased Cardiac tissue perfusion: Risk factor: cardiac surgery

See Coronary Artery Bypass Grafting (CABG); Dysrhythmia

OPEN REDUCTION OF FRACTURE WITH INTERNAL FIXATION (FEMUR)

Anxiety r/t outcome of corrective procedure

Impaired physical Mobility r/t postoperative position, abduction of leg, avoidance of acute flexion

Powerlessness r/t loss of control, unanticipated change in lifestyle

Risk for Surgical Site Infection: Risk factor: surgical procedure

Risk for Perioperative Positioning injury: Risk factor: immobilization

Risk for peripheral neurovascular dysfunction: Risk factors: mechanical compression, orthopedic surgery, immobilization

See Surgery, Postoperative Care

OPIOID USE

Acute Pain r/t physical injury or surgical procedure

Chronic Pain syndrome r/t prolonged use of opioids

Risk for Constipation: Risk factor: effects of opioids on peristalsis

See Substance Abuse; Substance Withdrawal; Pain Management, Acute; Pain Management, Chronic

OPPORTUNISTIC INFECTION

Delayed Surgical recovery r/t abnormal blood profiles, impaired healing

Risk for Infection: Risk factor: abnormal blood profiles

See AIDS (Acquired Immunodeficiency Syndrome); HIV (Human Immunodeficiency Virus)

OPPOSITIONAL DEFIANT DISORDER (ODD)

See ODD (Oppositional Defiant Disorder)

ORAL MUCOUS MEMBRANE INTEGRITY, IMPAIRED

Impaired Oral Mucous Membrane Integrity (See **Oral Mucous Membrane Integrity,** impaired, Section II)

ORAL THRUSH

See Candidiasis, Oral

ORCHITIS

Readiness for enhanced Health management: follows recommendations for mumps vaccination

See Epididymitis

ORGANIC MENTAL DISORDERS

Chronic Confusion r/t progressive impairment in cognitive functioning

Frail Elderly syndrome r/t alteration in cognitive function

Impaired Social interaction r/t disturbed thought processes

Risk for disturbed personal Identity: Risk factor: delusions/fluctuating perceptions of stimuli

See Dementia

ORTHOPEDIC TRACTION

Ineffective Role performance r/t limited physical mobility

Impaired Social interaction r/t limited physical mobility

Impaired Transfer ability r/t limited physical mobility

Risk for impaired Religiosity: Risk factor: immobility

See Traction and Casts

ORTHOPNEA

Ineffective Breathing pattern r/t inability to breathe with head of bed flat

Decreased Cardiac output r/t inability of heart to meet demands of body

ORTHOSTATIC HYPOTENSION

See Dizziness

OSTEOARTHRITIS

Acute Pain r/t movement

Impaired Walking r/t inflammation and damage to joints

See Arthritis

OSTEOMYELITIS

Decreased Diversional activity engagement r/t prolonged immobilization, hospitalization

Fear: parental r/t concern regarding possible growth plate damage caused by infection, concern that infection may become chronic

Ineffective Health maintenance behaviors r/t continued immobility at home, possible extensive casts, continued antibiotics

Impaired physical Mobility r/t imposed immobility as a result of infected area

Acute Pain r/t inflammation in affected extremity

Ineffective Thermoregulation r/t infectious process

Risk for Constipation: Risk factor: immobility

Risk for Infection: Risk factor: inadequate primary and secondary defenses

Risk for impaired Skin integrity: Risk factor: irritation from splint or cast

See Hospitalized Child

OSTEOPOROSIS

Deficient Knowledge r/t diet, exercise, need to abstain from alcohol and nicotine

Impaired physical Mobility r/t pain, skeletal changes

Imbalanced Nutrition: less than body requirements r/t inadequate intake of calcium and vitamin D

Acute Pain r/t fracture, muscle spasms

Risk for Injury: fracture: Risk factors: lack of activity, risk of falling resulting from environmental hazards, neuromuscular disorders, diminished senses, cardiovascular responses to drugs

Risk for Powerlessness: Risk factor: debilitating disease

Readiness for enhanced Health self-management: expresses desire to manage the treatment of illness and prevent complications

OSTOMY

See Child with Chronic Condition; Colostomy; Ileal Conduit; Ileostomy

OTITIS MEDIA

Acute Pain r/t inflammation, infectious process

Risk for delayed Child Development: speech and language: Risk factor: frequent otitis media

Risk for Infection: Risk factors: eustachian tube obstruction, traumatic eardrum perforation, infectious process

Readiness for enhanced Knowledge: information on treatment and prevention of disease

P

OVARIAN CARCINOMA

Death Anxiety r/t unknown outcome, possible poor prognosis

Fear r/t unknown outcome, possible poor prognosis

Ineffective Health Maintenance Behaviors r/t deficient knowledge regarding self-care, treatment of condition

Readiness for enhanced Family Processes: family functioning meets needs of client

Readiness for enhanced Resilience: participates in support groups

See Chemotherapy; Hysterectomy; Radiation Therapy

P

PACEMAKER

Anxiety r/t change in health status, presence of pacemaker

Death Anxiety r/t worry over possible malfunction of pacemaker

Deficient Knowledge r/t self-care program, when to seek medical attention

Acute Pain r/t surgical procedure

Risk for Bleeding: Risk factor: surgery

Risk for decreased Cardiac tissue perfusion: Risk factor: pacemaker malfunction

Risk for Infection: Risk factors: invasive procedure, presence of foreign body (catheter and generator)

Risk for Powerlessness: Risk factor: presence of electronic device to stimulate heart

Readiness for enhanced Health self-management: appropriate healthcare management of pacemaker

PAGET'S DISEASE

Disturbed Body Image r/t possible enlarged head, bowed tibias, kyphosis

Deficient Knowledge r/t appropriate diet high in protein and calcium, mild exercise

Chronic Sorrow r/t chronic condition with altered body image

Risk for Physical Trauma: fracture: Risk factor: excessive bone destruction

PAIN MANAGEMENT, ACUTE

Acute Pain r/t injury or surgical procedure

Imbalanced Energy Field r/t unpleasant sensory and emotional feelings

PAIN MANAGEMENT, CHRONIC

Chronic Pain (See **Pain,** chronic, Section II)

Chronic Pain Syndrome r/t persistent pain affecting daily living

Risk for Constipation: Risk factor: effects of meds on peristalsis

Readiness for Enhanced Knowledge: expresses a desire to learn alternative methods of non-pharmaceutical pain control

See Substance Abuse

PAINFUL BREASTS, ENGORGEMENT

Acute Pain r/t distention of breast tissue

Ineffective Role performance r/t change in physical capacity to assume role of breastfeeding mother

Impaired Tissue integrity r/t excessive fluid in breast tissues

Risk for ineffective Breastfeeding: Risk factors: pain, infant's inability to latch on to engorged breast

Risk for Infection: Risk factor: milk stasis

PAINFUL BREASTS, SORE NIPPLES

Insufficient Breast Milk Production r/t long breastfeeding time/pain response

Ineffective Breastfeeding r/t pain

Acute Pain r/t cracked nipples

Ineffective Role performance r/t change in physical capacity to assume role of breastfeeding mother

Impaired Skin integrity r/t mechanical factors involved in suckling, breastfeeding management

Risk for Infection: Risk factor: break in skin

PALLOR OF EXTREMITIES

Ineffective peripheral Tissue Perfusion r/t interruption of vascular flow

See Shock; Peripheral Vascular disease (PVD)

PALPITATIONS (HEART PALPITATIONS)

See Dysrhythmia

PANCREATIC CANCER

Death Anxiety r/t possible poor prognosis of disease process

Ineffective family Coping r/t poor prognosis

Fear r/t poor prognosis of the disease

Deficient Knowledge r/t disease-induced diabetes, home management

Spiritual distress r/t poor prognosis

Risk for impaired Liver function: Risk factor: complications from underlying disease

See Cancer; Chemotherapy; Radiation Therapy; Surgery, Perioperative Care; Surgery, Postoperative Care; Surgery, Preoperative Care

PANCREATITIS

Ineffective Breathing pattern r/t splinting from severe pain, disease process and inflammation

Ineffective Denial r/t ineffective coping, alcohol use

Diarrhea r/t decrease in pancreatic secretions resulting in steatorrhea

Deficient Fluid volume r/t vomiting, decreased fluid intake, fever, diaphoresis, fluid shifts

Ineffective Health maintenance behaviors r/t deficient knowledge concerning diet, alcohol use, medication

Nausea r/t irritation of gastrointestinal system

Imbalanced Nutrition: less than body requirements r/t inadequate dietary intake, increased nutritional needs as a result of acute illness, increased metabolic needs caused by increased body temperature, disease process

Acute Pain r/t irritation and edema of the inflamed pancreas

Chronic Sorrow r/t chronic illness

Readiness for enhanced Comfort: expresses desire to enhance comfort

PANIC DISORDER (PANIC ATTACKS)

Ineffective Activity planning r/t unrealistic perception of events

Anxiety r/t situational crisis

Ineffective Coping r/t personal vulnerability

Risk-prone Health behavior r/t low self-efficacy

Disturbed personal Identity r/t situational crisis

Post-Trauma syndrome r/t previous catastrophic event

Social isolation r/t fear of lack of control

Risk for Loneliness: Risk factor: inability to socially interact because of fear of losing control

Risk for Post-Trauma syndrome: Risk factors: perception of the event, diminished ego strength

Risk for Powerlessness: Risk factor: ineffective coping skills

Readiness for enhanced Coping: seeks problem-oriented and emotion-oriented strategies to manage condition

See Anxiety; Anxiety Disorder

PARALYSIS

Disturbed Body Image r/t biophysical changes, loss of movement, immobility

Impaired Comfort r/t prolonged immobility

Constipation r/t effects of spinal cord disruption, inadequate fiber in diet

P

Ineffective Health maintenance behaviors r/t deficient knowledge regarding self-care with paralysis

Ineffective Home Maintenance Behaviors r/t physical disability

Impaired physical Mobility r/t neuromuscular impairment

Impaired wheelchair Mobility r/t neuromuscular impairment

Self-Neglect r/t functional impairment

Powerlessness r/t illness-related regimen

Self-Care deficit: specify r/t neuromuscular impairment

Sexual dysfunction r/t loss of sensation, biopsychosocial alteration

Chronic Sorrow r/t loss of physical mobility

Impaired Transfer ability r/t paralysis

Risk for Autonomic Dysreflexia: Risk factor: cause of paralysis

Risk for Disuse syndrome: Risk factor: paralysis

Risk for Adult Falls: Risk factor: paralysis

Risk for Injury: Risk factors: altered mobility, sensory dysfunction

Risk for Latex Allergic reaction: Risk factor: possible repeated urinary catheterizations

Risk for Post-Trauma syndrome: Risk factor: event causing paralysis

Risk for impaired Religiosity: Risk factors: immobility, possible lack of transportation

Risk for impaired Resilience: Risk factor: chronic disability

Risk for situational low Self-Esteem: Risk factor: change in body image and function

Risk for impaired Skin integrity: Risk factors: altered circulation, altered sensation, immobility

Readiness for enhanced Self-Care: expresses desire to enhance knowledge and responsibility for strategies for self-care

See Child with Chronic Condition; Hemiplegia; Hospitalized Child; Neural Tube Defects (Meningocele, Myelomeningocele, Spina Bifida, Anencephaly); Spinal Cord Injury

PARALYTIC ILEUS

Constipation r/t decreased gastrointestinal motility

Deficient Fluid volume r/t loss of fluids from vomiting, retention of fluid in bowel

Dysfunctional Gastrointestinal motility r/t recent abdominal surgery, electrolyte imbalance

Nausea r/t gastrointestinal irritation

Acute Pain r/t pressure, abdominal distention, presence of nasogastric tube

See Bowel Obstruction

PARANOID PERSONALITY DISORDER

Ineffective Activity planning r/t unrealistic perception of events

Anxiety r/t uncontrollable intrusive, suspicious thoughts

Risk-prone Health behavior r/t intense emotional state

Disturbed personal Identity r/t difficulty with reality testing

Impaired individual Resilience r/t psychological disorder

Chronic low Self-Esteem r/t inability to trust others

Social isolation r/t inappropriate social skills

Risk for Loneliness: Risk factor: social isolation

Risk for other-directed Violence: Risk factor: being suspicious of others and their actions

PARAPLEGIA

See Spinal Cord Injury

PARATHYROIDECTOMY

Anxiety r/t surgery

Risk for ineffective Airway clearance: Risk factors: edema or hematoma formation, airway obstruction

Risk for Bleeding: Risk factor: surgery

Risk for impaired verbal Communication: Risk factors: possible laryngeal damage, edema

Risk for Infection: Risk factor: surgical procedure

See Hypocalcemia

PARENT ATTACHMENT

Risk for impaired Attachment (See **Attachment,** impaired, risk for, Section II)

Readiness for enhanced Childbearing process: demonstrates appropriate care of newborn

See Parental Role Conflict

PARENTAL ROLE CONFLICT

Parental Role conflict (See **Role** conflict, parental, Section II)

Ineffective Relationship r/t unrealistic expectations

Chronic Sorrow r/t difficult parent–child relationship

Risk for Spiritual distress: Risk factor: altered relationships

Readiness for enhanced Parenting: willingness to enhance parenting

PARENTING

Readiness for enhanced Parenting (See **Parenting,** readiness for enhanced, Section II)

PARENTING, IMPAIRED

Impaired Parenting (See **Parenting,** impaired, Section II)

Chronic Sorrow r/t difficult parent–child relationship

Risk for Spiritual distress: Risk factor: altered relationships

PARENTING, RISK FOR IMPAIRED

Risk for impaired Parenting (See **Parenting,** impaired, risk for, Section II)

See Parenting, Impaired

PARESTHESIA

Risk for Injury: Risk factors: inability to feel temperature changes, pain

Risk for impaired Skin integrity: Risk factor: impaired sensation

Risk for Thermal injury: Risk factor: neuromuscular impairment

PARKINSON'S DISEASE

Impaired verbal Communication r/t decreased speech volume, slowness of speech, impaired facial muscles

Constipation r/t weakness of muscles, lack of exercise, inadequate fluid intake, decreased autonomic nervous system activity

Frail Elderly syndrome r/t chronic illness

Imbalanced Nutrition: less than body requirements r/t tremor, slowness in eating, difficulty in chewing and swallowing

Chronic Sorrow r/t loss of physical capacity

Risk for Injury: Risk factors: tremors, slow reactions, altered gait

See Neurologic Disorders

PAROXYSMAL NOCTURNAL DYSPNEA (PND)

See PND (Paroxysmal Nocturnal Dyspnea)

PATENT DUCTUS ARTERIOSUS (PDA)

See Congenital Heart Disease/Cardiac Anomalies

PATIENT-CONTROLLED ANALGESIA (PCA)

See PCA (Patient-Controlled Analgesia)

PATIENT EDUCATION

Deficient Knowledge r/t lack of exposure to information misinterpretation, unfamiliarity with information resources to manage illness

Readiness for enhanced emancipated Decision-Making: expresses desire to enhance understanding of choices for decision-making

Readiness for enhanced Knowledge (specify): interest in learning

Readiness for enhanced Health self-management: expresses desire for information to manage the illness

PCA (PATIENT-CONTROLLED ANALGESIA)

Deficient Knowledge r/t self-care of pain control

Nausea r/t side effects of medication

Risk for Injury: Risk factors: possible complications associated with PCA

Risk for Vascular Trauma: Risk factors: insertion site and length of insertion time

Readiness for enhanced Knowledge: appropriate management of PCA

PECTUS EXCAVATUM

See Marfan Syndrome

PEDICULOSIS

See Lice

PEG (PERCUTANEOUS ENDOSCOPIC GASTROSTOMY)

See Tube Feeding

PELVIC INFLAMMATORY DISEASE (PID)

See PID (Pelvic Inflammatory Disease)

PENILE PROSTHESIS

Ineffective Sexuality pattern r/t use of penile prosthesis

Risk for Surgical Site Infection: Risk factor: invasive surgical procedure

Risk for situational low Self-Esteem: Risk factor: ineffective sexuality pattern

Readiness for enhanced Health self-management: seeks information regarding care and use of prosthesis

See Erectile Dysfunction (ED); Impotence

PEPTIC ULCER

See Ulcer, Peptic (Duodenal or Gastric)

PERCUTANEOUS TRANSLUMINAL CORONARY ANGIOPLASTY (PTCA)

See Angioplasty, Coronary

PERICARDIAL FRICTION RUB

Decreased **Cardiac** output

Acute Pain r/t inflammation, effusion

Risk for decreased Cardiac tissue perfusion: Risk factors: inflammation in pericardial sac, fluid accumulation compressing heart

PERICARDITIS

Decreased activity tolerance r/t reduced cardiac reserve, prescribed bed rest

Decreased Cardiac output r/t impaired cardiac function from inflammation of pericardial sac

Risk for decreased Cardiac tissue perfusion: Risk factor: inflammation in pericardial sac

Deficient Knowledge r/t unfamiliarity with information sources

Risk for imbalanced Nutrition: less than body requirements: Risk factors: fever, hypermetabolic state associated with fever

Acute Pain r/t biological injury, inflammation

PERIODONTAL DISEASE

Risk for impaired Oral Mucous Membrane Integrity (See **Oral Mucous Membrane Integrity,** impaired, risk for, Section II)

PERIOPERATIVE HYPOTHERMIA

Risk for Perioperative Hypothermia (See **Perioperative Hypothermia**, risk for, Section II)

PERIOPERATIVE POSITIONING

Risk for Perioperative Positioning injury (See **Perioperative Positioning** injury, risk for, Section II)

PERIPHERAL NEUROPATHY

See Neuropathy, Peripheral

PERIPHERAL NEUROVASCULAR DYSFUNCTION

Risk for Peripheral Neurovascular dysfunction (See **Peripheral Neurovascular** dysfunction, risk for, Section II)

See Neuropathy, Peripheral; Peripheral Vascular Disease (PVD)

PERIPHERAL VASCULAR DISEASE (PVD)

Ineffective Health maintenance behaviors r/t deficient knowledge regarding self-care and treatment of disease

Chronic Pain: intermittent claudication r/t ischemia

Ineffective peripheral Tissue Perfusion r/t disease process

Risk for Adult Falls: Risk factor: altered mobility

Risk for Injury: Risk factors: tissue hypoxia, altered mobility, altered sensation

Risk for Peripheral Neurovascular dysfunction: Risk factor: possible vascular obstruction

Risk for impaired Tissue integrity: Risk factor: altered circulation or sensation

Readiness for enhanced Health self-management: self-care and treatment of disease

See Neuropathy, Peripheral; Peripheral Neurovascular Dysfunction

PERITONEAL DIALYSIS

Ineffective Breathing pattern r/t pressure from dialysate

Impaired Comfort r/t instillation of dialysate, temperature of dialysate

Ineffective Home Maintenance Behaviors r/t complex home treatment of client

Deficient Knowledge r/t treatment procedure, self-care with peritoneal dialysis

Chronic Sorrow r/t chronic disability

Risk for ineffective Coping: Risk factor: disability requiring change in lifestyle

Risk for unstable blood Glucose level: Risk factors: increased concentrations of glucose in dialysate, ineffective medication management

Risk for imbalanced Fluid volume: Risk factor: medical procedure

Risk for Infection, peritoneal: Risk factors: invasive procedure, presence of catheter, dialysate

Risk for Powerlessness: Risk factors: chronic condition and care involved

See Child with Chronic Condition; Hemodialysis; Hospitalized Child; Renal Failure; Renal Failure, Acute/Chronic, Child

PERITONITIS

Ineffective Breathing pattern r/t pain, increased abdominal pressure

Constipation r/t decreased oral intake, decrease of peristalsis

Deficient Fluid volume r/t retention of fluid in bowel with loss of circulating blood volume

Nausea r/t gastrointestinal irritation

Imbalanced Nutrition: **less than body requirements** r/t nausea, vomiting

Acute Pain r/t inflammation and infection of gastrointestinal system

Risk for dysfunctional Gastrointestinal motility: Risk factor: gastrointestinal disease

PERNICIOUS ANEMIA

Diarrhea r/t malabsorption of nutrients

Fatigue r/t imbalanced nutrition: less than body requirements

Impaired Memory r/t lack of adequate red blood cells

Nausea r/t altered oral mucous membrane; sore tongue, bleeding gums

Imbalanced Nutrition: less than body requirements r/t lack of appetite associated with nausea and altered oral mucous membrane

Impaired Oral Mucous Membrane Integrity r/t vitamin deficiency; inability to absorb vitamin B_{12} associated with lack of intrinsic factor

Risk for Adult Falls: Risk factors: dizziness, lightheadedness

Risk for Peripheral Neurovascular dysfunction: Risk factor: anemia

PERSISTENT FETAL CIRCULATION

See Congenital Heart Disease/Cardiac Anomalies

PERSONAL IDENTITY PROBLEMS

Disturbed personal Identity (See **Identity,** personal, disturbed, Section II)

Risk for disturbed personal Identity (See disturbed personal **Identity,** risk for, Section II)

PERSONALITY DISORDER

Ineffective Activity planning r/t unrealistic perception of events

Impaired individual Resilience r/t psychological disorder

See specific disorder: Antisocial Personality Disorder; Borderline Personality Disorder; OCD (Obsessive-Compulsive Disorder); Paranoid Personality Disorder

PERTUSSIS (WHOOPING COUGH)

Risk for impaired emancipated Decision-Making r/t whether to administer usual childhood vaccinations

See Respiratory Infections, Acute Childhood

PESTICIDE CONTAMINATION

Contamination r/t use of environmental contaminants; pesticides

Risk for Allergic reaction r/t repeated exposure to pesticides

PETECHIAE

See Anticoagulant Therapy; Clotting Disorder; DIC (Disseminated Intravascular Coagulation); Hemophilia

PETIT MAL SEIZURE

Readiness for enhanced Health self-management: wears medical alert bracelet; limits hazardous activities such as driving, swimming, working at heights, operating equipment

See Epilepsy

PHARYNGITIS

See Sore Throat

PHENYLKETONURIA (PKU)

See PKU (Phenylketonuria)

PHEOCHROMOCYTOMA

Anxiety r/t symptoms from increased catecholamines—headache, palpitations, sweating, nervousness, nausea, vomiting, syncope

Ineffective Health maintenance behaviors r/t deficient knowledge regarding treatment and self-care

Insomnia r/t high levels of catecholamines

Nausea r/t increased catecholamines

Risk for decreased Cardiac tissue perfusion: Risk factor: hypertension

See Surgery, Perioperative Care; Surgery, Postoperative Care; Surgery, Preoperative Care

PHLEBITIS

See Thrombophlebitis

PHOBIA (SPECIFIC)

Fear r/t presence or anticipation of specific object or situation

Powerlessness r/t anxiety about encountering unknown or known entity

Impaired individual Resilience r/t psychological disorder

Readiness for enhanced Power: expresses readiness to enhance identification of choices that can be made for change

See Anxiety; Anxiety Disorder; Panic Disorder (Panic Attacks)

PHOTOSENSITIVITY

Ineffective Health maintenance behaviors r/t deficient knowledge regarding medications inducing photosensitivity

Risk for dry Eye: Risk factors: pharmaceutical agents, sunlight exposure

Risk for impaired Skin integrity: Risk factor: exposure to sun

PHYSICAL ABUSE

See Abuse, Child; Abuse, Spouse, Parent, or Significant Other

PICA

Anxiety r/t stress

Imbalanced Nutrition: less than body requirements r/t eating nonnutritive substances

Impaired Parenting r/t lack of supervision, food deprivation

Risk for Constipation: Risk factor: presence of undigestible materials in gastrointestinal tract

Risk for dysfunctional Gastrointestinal motility: Risk factor: abnormal eating behavior

Risk for Infection: Risk factor: ingestion of infectious agents via contaminated substances

Risk for Poisoning: Risk factor: ingestion of substances containing lead

See Anemia

PID (PELVIC INFLAMMATORY DISEASE)

Ineffective Health maintenance behaviors r/t deficient knowledge regarding self-care, treatment of disease

Acute Pain r/t biological injury; inflammation, edema, congestion of pelvic tissues

Ineffective Sexuality pattern r/t medically imposed abstinence from sexual activities until acute infection subsides, change in reproductive potential

Risk for Infection: Risk factors: insufficient knowledge to avoid exposure to pathogens; proper hygiene, nutrition, other health habits

See Maturational Issues, Adolescent; STD (Sexually Transmitted Disease)

PIH (PREGNANCY-INDUCED HYPERTENSION/PREECLAMPSIA)

Anxiety r/t fear of the unknown, threat to self and infant, change in role functioning

Death Anxiety r/t threat of preeclampsia

Decreased Diversional activity engagement r/t bed rest

Interrupted Family processes r/t situational crisis

Ineffective Home Maintenance Behaviors r/t bed rest

Deficient Knowledge r/t lack of experience with situation

Impaired physical Mobility r/t medically prescribed limitations

Impaired Parenting r/t prescribed bed rest

Powerlessness r/t complication threatening pregnancy, medically prescribed limitations

P

Ineffective Role performance r/t change in physical capacity to assume role of pregnant woman or resume other roles

Situational low Self-Esteem r/t loss of idealized pregnancy

Impaired Social interaction r/t imposed bed rest

Risk for imbalanced Fluid volume: Risk factors: hypertension, altered kidney function

Risk for Injury: fetal: Risk factors: decreased uteroplacental perfusion, seizures

Risk for Injury: maternal: Risk factors: vasospasm, high blood pressure

Risk for Unstable Blood Pressure: Risk factors: hypertension, imbalanced fluid volume

Readiness for enhanced Knowledge: exhibits desire for information on managing condition

P

PILOERECTION

Hypothermia r/t exposure to cold environment

PINK EYE

See Conjunctivitis

PINWORMS

Impaired Comfort r/t itching

Ineffective Home Maintenance Behaviors r/t inadequate cleaning of bed linen and toilet seats

Insomnia r/t discomfort

Readiness for enhanced Health management: proper handwashing; short, clean fingernails; avoiding hand, mouth, nose contact with unwashed hands; appropriate cleaning of bed linen and toilet seats

PITUITARY TUMOR, BENIGN

See Cushing's Disease

PKU (PHENYLKETONURIA)

Risk for delayed Child Development: Risk factors: not following strict dietary program; eating foods extremely low in phenylalanine; avoiding eggs, milk, any foods containing aspartame (e.g., NutraSweet)

Readiness for enhanced Health self-management: testing for PKU and following prescribed dietary regimen

PLACENTA ABRUPTIO

Death Anxiety r/t threat of mortality associated with bleeding

Fear r/t threat to self and fetus

Ineffective Health maintenance behaviors r/t deficient knowledge regarding treatment and control of hypertension associated with placenta abruptio

Acute Pain: abdominal/back r/t premature separation of placenta before delivery

Risk for Bleeding: Risk factor: placenta abruptio

Risk for deficient Fluid volume: Risk factor: maternal blood loss

Risk for Powerlessness: Risk factors: complications of pregnancy and unknown outcome

Risk for Shock: Risk factor: hypovolemia

Risk for Spiritual distress: Risk factor: fear from unknown outcome of pregnancy

PLACENTA PREVIA

Death Anxiety r/t threat of mortality associated with bleeding

Disturbed Body Image r/t negative feelings about body and reproductive ability, feelings of helplessness

Ineffective Coping r/t threat to self and fetus

Decreased Diversional activity engagement r/t long-term hospitalization

Interrupted Family processes r/t maternal bed rest, hospitalization

Fear r/t threat to self and fetus, unknown future

Ineffective Home Maintenance Behaviors r/t maternal bed rest, hospitalization

Impaired physical Mobility r/t medical protocol, maternal bed rest

Ineffective Role performance r/t maternal bed rest, hospitalization

Situational low Self-Esteem r/t situational crisis

Spiritual distress r/t inability to participate in usual religious rituals, situational crisis

Risk for Bleeding: Risk factor: placenta previa

Risk for Constipation: Risk factors: bed rest, pregnancy

Risk for deficient Fluid volume: Risk factor: maternal blood loss

Risk for imbalanced Fluid volume: Risk factor: maternal blood loss

Risk for Injury: fetal and maternal: Risk factors: threat to uteroplacental perfusion, hemorrhage

Risk for disturbed Maternal–Fetal dyad: Risk factor: complication of pregnancy

Risk for impaired Parenting: Risk factors: maternal bed rest, hospitalization

Risk for ineffective peripheral Tissue Perfusion: placental: Risk factors: dilation of cervix, loss of placental implantation site

Risk for Powerlessness: Risk factors: complications of pregnancy, unknown outcome

Risk for Shock: Risk factor: hypovolemia

PLANTAR FASCIITIS

Impaired Comfort r/t inflamed structures of feet

Impaired physical Mobility r/t discomfort

Acute Pain r/t inflammation

Chronic Pain r/t inflammation

PLEURAL EFFUSION

Ineffective Breathing pattern r/t pain

Excess Fluid volume r/t compromised regulatory mechanisms; heart, liver, or kidney failure

Acute Pain r/t inflammation, fluid accumulation

PLEURAL FRICTION RUB

Ineffective Breathing pattern r/t pain

Acute Pain r/t inflammation, fluid accumulation

PLEURAL TAP

See Pleural Effusion

PLEURISY

Ineffective Breathing pattern r/t pain

Impaired Gas exchange r/t ventilation perfusion imbalance

Acute Pain r/t pressure on pleural nerve endings associated with fluid accumulation or inflammation

Impaired Walking r/t decreased activity tolerance, inability to "catch breath"

Risk for ineffective Airway clearance: Risk factors: increased secretions, ineffective cough because of pain

Risk for Infection: Risk factor: exposure to pathogens

PMS (PREMENSTRUAL SYNDROME)

Fatigue r/t hormonal changes

Excess Fluid volume r/t alterations of hormonal levels inducing fluid retention

Deficient Knowledge r/t methods to deal with and prevent syndrome

Acute Pain r/t hormonal stimulation of gastrointestinal structures

Risk for Powerlessness: Risk factors: lack of knowledge and ability to deal with symptoms

Risk for impaired Resilience: Risk factor: PMS symptoms

Readiness for enhanced Communication: willingness to express thoughts and feelings about PMS

Readiness for enhanced Health self-management: desire for information to manage and prevent symptoms

PND (PAROXYSMAL NOCTURNAL DYSPNEA)

Anxiety r/t inability to breathe during sleep

Ineffective Breathing pattern r/t increase in carbon dioxide levels, decrease in oxygen levels

Insomnia r/t suffocating feeling from fluid in lungs on awakening from sleep

Sleep deprivation r/t inability to breathe during sleep

Risk for decreased Cardiac tissue perfusion: Risk factor: hypoxia

Risk for Powerlessness: Risk factor: inability to control nocturnal dyspnea

Readiness for enhanced Sleep: expresses willingness to learn measures to enhance sleep

PNEUMONECTOMY

See Thoracotomy

P

PNEUMONIA

Decreased activity tolerance r/t imbalance between oxygen supply and demand

Ineffective Airway clearance r/t inflammation and presence of secretions

Impaired Gas exchange r/t decreased functional lung tissue

Ineffective Health self-management r/t deficient knowledge regarding self-care and treatment of disease

Imbalanced Nutrition: less than body requirements r/t loss of appetite

Impaired Oral Mucous Membrane Integrity r/t dry mouth from mouth breathing, decreased fluid intake

Ineffective Thermoregulation r/t infectious process

Risk for acute Confusion: Risk factors: underlying illness, hypoxia

Risk for deficient Fluid volume: Risk factor: inadequate intake of fluids

Risk for Vascular Trauma: Risk factor: irritation from intravenous antibiotics

See Respiratory Infections, Acute Childhood

PNEUMOTHORAX

Fear r/t threat to own well-being, difficulty breathing

Impaired Gas exchange r/t ventilation-perfusion imbalance, decreased functional lung tissue

Acute Pain r/t recent injury, coughing, deep breathing

Risk for Injury: Risk factor: possible complications associated with closed chest drainage system

See Chest Tubes

POISONING, RISK FOR

Risk for Poisoning (See **Poisoning,** risk for, Section II)

POLIOMYELITIS

See Paralysis

POLYDIPSIA

See Diabetes Mellitus

POLYPHAGIA

Readiness for enhanced Nutrition: knowledge of appropriate diet for diabetes

See Diabetes Mellitus

POLYURIA

See Diabetes Mellitus

POSTOPERATIVE CARE

See Surgery, Postoperative Care

POSTPARTUM DEPRESSION

Anxiety r/t new responsibilities of parenting

Disturbed Body Image r/t normal postpartum recovery

Ineffective Childbearing process r/t depression/lack of support system

Ineffective Coping r/t hormonal changes

Fatigue r/t childbirth, postpartum state, crying child

Risk-prone Health behavior r/t lack of support systems

Ineffective Home Maintenance Behaviors r/t fatigue, care of newborn

Hopelessness r/t stress, exhaustion

Deficient Knowledge r/t lifestyle changes

Impaired Parenting r/t hormone-induced depression

Ineffective Role performance r/t new responsibilities of parenting

Sexual dysfunction r/t fear of another pregnancy, postpartum pain, lochia flow

Sleep deprivation r/t environmental stimulation of newborn

Impaired Social interaction r/t change in role functioning

Risk for disturbed personal Identity r/t role change/depression/inability to cope

Risk for situational low Self-Esteem: Risk factor: decreased power over feelings of sadness

Risk for Spiritual distress: Risk factors: altered relationships, social isolation

Readiness for enhanced Hope: expresses desire to enhance hope and interconnectedness with others

See Depression (Major Depressive Disorder)

POSTPARTUM HEMORRHAGE

Decreased activity tolerance r/t anemia from loss of blood

Death Anxiety r/t threat of mortality associated with bleeding

Disturbed Body Image r/t loss of ideal childbirth

Insufficient Breast Milk Production r/t fluid volume depletion

Interrupted Breastfeeding r/t separation from infant for medical treatment

Decreased Cardiac output r/t hypovolemia

Fear r/t threat to self, unknown future

Deficient Fluid volume r/t uterine atony, loss of blood

Ineffective Home Maintenance Behaviors r/t lack of stamina

Deficient Knowledge r/t lack of exposure to situation

Acute Pain r/t nursing and medical interventions to control bleeding

Ineffective peripheral Tissue Perfusion r/t hypovolemia

Risk for Bleeding: Risk factor: postpartum complications

Risk for impaired Childbearing: Risk factor: postpartum complication

Risk for imbalanced Fluid volume: Risk factor: maternal blood loss

Risk for Infection: Risk factors: loss of blood, depressed immunity

Risk for impaired Parenting: Risk factor: weakened maternal condition

Risk for Powerlessness: Risk factor: acute illness

Risk for Shock: Risk factor: hypovolemia

POSTPARTUM, NORMAL CARE

Anxiety r/t change in role functioning, parenting

Effective Breastfeeding r/t basic breastfeeding knowledge, support of partner and healthcare provider

Fatigue r/t childbirth, new responsibilities of parenting, body changes

Acute Pain r/t episiotomy, lacerations, bruising, breast engorgement, headache, sore nipples, epidural or intravenous site, hemorrhoids

Sexual dysfunction r/t recent childbirth

Impaired Tissue integrity r/t episiotomy, lacerations

Sleep deprivation r/t care of infant

Impaired Urinary elimination r/t effects of anesthesia, tissue trauma

Risk for Constipation: Risk factors: hormonal effects on smooth muscles, fear of straining with defecation, effects of anesthesia

Risk for Infection: Risk factors: tissue trauma, blood loss

Readiness for enhanced family Coping: adaptation to new family member

Readiness for enhanced Hope: desire to increase hope

Readiness for enhanced Parenting: expresses willingness to enhance parenting skills

POST-TRAUMA SYNDROME

Post-Trauma syndrome (See **Post-Trauma** syndrome, Section II)

POST-TRAUMA SYNDROME, RISK FOR

Risk for Post-Trauma syndrome (See **Post-Trauma** syndrome, risk for, Section II)

POST-TRAUMATIC STRESS DISORDER (PTSD)

See PTSD (Post-Traumatic Stress Disorder)

P

POTASSIUM, INCREASE/ DECREASE

See Hyperkalemia; Hypokalemia

POWER/POWERLESSNESS

Powerlessness (See **Powerlessness,** Section II)

Risk for Powerlessness (See **Powerlessness,** risk for, Section II)

Readiness for enhanced Power (See **Power,** readiness for enhanced, Section II)

PREECLAMPSIA

See PIH (Pregnancy-Induced Hypertension/Preeclampsia)

PREGNANCY, CARDIAC DISORDERS

See Cardiac Disorders in Pregnancy

PREGNANCY-INDUCED HYPERTENSION/PREECLAMPSIA (PIH)

See PIH (Pregnancy-Induced Hypertension/Preeclampsia)

PREGNANCY LOSS

Anxiety r/t threat to role functioning, health status, situational crisis

Compromised family Coping r/t lack of support by significant other because of personal suffering

Ineffective Coping r/t situational crisis

Acute Pain r/t surgical intervention

Ineffective Role performance r/t inability to assume parenting role

Ineffective Sexuality pattern r/t self-esteem disturbance resulting from pregnancy loss and anxiety about future pregnancies

Chronic Sorrow r/t loss of a fetus or child

Spiritual distress r/t intense suffering from loss of child

Risk for deficient Fluid volume: Risk factor: blood loss

Risk for maladaptive Grieving: Risk factor: loss of pregnancy

Risk for Infection: Risk factor: retained products of conception

Risk for Powerlessness: Risk factor: situational crisis

Risk for ineffective Relationship: Risk factor: poor communication skills in dealing with the loss

Risk for Spiritual distress: Risk factor: intense suffering

Readiness for enhanced Communication: willingness to express feelings and thoughts about loss

Readiness for enhanced Hope: expresses desire to enhance hope

Readiness for enhanced Spiritual well-being: desire for acceptance of loss

PREGNANCY, NORMAL

Anxiety r/t unknown future, threat to self secondary to pain of labor

Disturbed Body Image r/t altered body function and appearance

Interrupted Family processes r/t developmental transition of pregnancy

Fatigue r/t increased energy demands

Fear r/t labor and delivery

Deficient Knowledge r/t primiparity

Nausea r/t hormonal changes of pregnancy

Imbalanced Nutrition: less than body requirements r/t growing fetus, nausea

Imbalanced Nutrition: more than body requirements r/t deficient knowledge regarding nutritional needs of pregnancy

Sleep deprivation r/t uncomfortable pregnancy state

Impaired Urinary elimination r/t frequency caused by increased pelvic pressure and hormonal stimulation

Risk for Constipation: Risk factor: pregnancy

Risk for Sexual dysfunction: Risk factors: altered body function, self-concept, body image with pregnancy

Readiness for enhanced Childbearing process: appropriate prenatal care

Readiness for enhanced family Coping: satisfying partner relationship, attention to gratification of needs, effective adaptation to developmental tasks of pregnancy

Readiness for enhanced Family processes: family adapts to change

Readiness for enhanced Health self-management: seeks information for prenatal self-care

Readiness for enhanced Nutrition: desire for knowledge of appropriate nutrition during pregnancy

Readiness for enhanced Parenting: expresses willingness to enhance parenting skills

Readiness for enhanced Relationship: meeting developmental goals associated with pregnancy

Readiness for enhanced Spiritual well-being: new role as parent

See Discomforts of Pregnancy

PREMATURE DILATION OF THE CERVIX (INCOMPETENT CERVIX)

Ineffective Activity planning r/t unrealistic perception of events

Ineffective Coping r/t bed rest, threat to fetus

Decreased Diversional activity engagement r/t bed rest

Fear r/t potential loss of infant

Deficient Knowledge r/t treatment regimen, prognosis for pregnancy

Impaired physical Mobility r/t imposed bed rest to prevent preterm birth

Powerlessness r/t inability to control outcome of pregnancy

Ineffective Role performance r/t inability to continue usual patterns of responsibility

Situational low Self-Esteem r/t inability to complete normal pregnancy

Sexual dysfunction r/t fear of harm to fetus

Impaired Social interaction r/t bed rest

Risk for Infection: Risk factor: invasive procedures to prevent preterm birth

Risk for Injury: fetal: Risk factors: preterm birth, use of anesthetics

Risk for Injury: maternal: Risk factor: surgical procedures to prevent preterm birth (e.g., cerclage)

Risk for impaired Resilience: Risk factor: complication of pregnancy

Risk for Spiritual distress: Risk factors: physical/psychological stress

PREMATURE INFANT (CHILD)

Insufficient Breast Milk Production r/t ineffective sucking, latching on of the infant

Impaired Gas exchange r/t effects of cardiopulmonary insufficiency

Disorganized Infant behavior r/t prematurity

Insomnia r/t noisy and noxious intensive care environment

Neonatal Hyperbilirubinemia r/t infant experiences difficulty making transition to extrauterine life

Imbalanced Nutrition: less than body requirements r/t delayed or understimulated rooting reflex, easy fatigue during feeding, diminished endurance

Impaired Swallowing r/t decreased or absent gag reflex, fatigue

Ineffective Thermoregulation r/t large body surface/weight ratio, immaturity of thermal regulation, state of prematurity

Risk for delayed Child Development: Risk factor: prematurity

Risk for Infection: Risk factors: inadequate, immature, or undeveloped acquired immune response

Risk for Injury: Risk factor: prolonged mechanical ventilation, retinopathy of prematurity (ROP) secondary to 100% oxygen environment

Risk for Neonatal Hyperbilirubinemia: Risk factor: late preterm birth

Readiness for enhanced organized Infant behavior: use of some self-regulatory measures

PREMATURE INFANT (PARENT)

Ineffective Breastfeeding r/t disrupted establishment of effective pattern secondary to prematurity or insufficient opportunities

Decisional Conflict r/t support system deficit, multiple sources of information

Compromised family Coping r/t disrupted family roles and disorganization, prolonged condition exhausting supportive capacity of significant persons

Ineffective infant Feeding dynamics r/t insufficient knowledge of nutritional needs

Maladaptive Grieving (prolonged) r/t unresolved conflicts

Parental Role conflict r/t expressed concerns, expressed inability to care for child's physical, emotional, or developmental needs

Chronic Sorrow r/t threat of loss of a child, prolonged hospitalization

Spiritual distress r/t challenged belief or value systems regarding moral or ethical implications of treatment plans

Risk for impaired Attachment: Risk factors: separation, physical barriers, lack of privacy

Risk for disturbed Maternal–Fetal dyad: Risk factor: complication of pregnancy

Risk for Powerlessness: Risk factor: inability to control situation

Risk for impaired Resilience: Risk factor: premature infant

Risk for Spiritual distress: Risk factor: challenged belief or value systems regarding moral or ethical implications of treatment plans

Readiness for enhanced Family process: adaptation to change associated with premature infant

See Child with Chronic Condition; Hospitalized Child

PREMATURE RUPTURE OF MEMBRANES

Anxiety r/t threat to infant's health status

Disturbed Body Image r/t inability to carry pregnancy to term

Ineffective Coping r/t situational crisis

Situational low Self-Esteem r/t inability to carry pregnancy to term

Risk for ineffective Childbearing process: Risk factor: complication of pregnancy

Risk for Infection: Risk factor: rupture of membranes

Risk for Injury: **fetal**: Risk factor: risk of premature birth

PREMENSTRUAL TENSION SYNDROME (PMS)

See PMS (Premenstrual Tension Syndrome)

PRENATAL CARE, NORMAL

Readiness for enhanced Childbearing process: appropriate prenatal lifestyle

Readiness for enhanced Knowledge: appropriate prenatal care

Readiness for enhanced Spiritual well-being: new role as parent

See Pregnancy, Normal

PRENATAL TESTING

Anxiety r/t unknown outcome, delayed test results

Acute Pain r/t invasive procedures

Risk for Infection: Risk factor: invasive procedures during amniocentesis or chorionic villus sampling

Risk for Injury: **fetal** r/t invasive procedures

PREOPERATIVE TEACHING

See Surgery, Preoperative Care

PRESSURE ULCER

Impaired bed Mobility r/t intolerance to activity, pain, cognitive impairment, depression, severe anxiety, severity of illness

Imbalanced Nutrition: **less than body requirements** r/t limited access to food, inability to absorb nutrients because of biological factors, anorexia

Acute Pain r/t tissue destruction, exposure of nerves

Impaired Skin integrity: **stage I or II pressure ulcer** r/t physical immobility, mechanical factors, altered circulation, skin irritants, excessive moisture

Impaired Tissue integrity: **stage III or IV pressure ulcer** r/t altered circulation, impaired physical mobility, excessive moisture

Risk for Infection: Risk factors: physical immobility, mechanical factors (shearing forces, pressure, restraint, altered circulation, skin irritants, excessive moisture, open wound)

Risk for Adult Pressure Injury (See **Pressure injury, risk for adult**, Section II)

PRETERM LABOR

Anxiety r/t threat to fetus, change in role functioning, change in environment and interaction patterns, use of tocolytic drugs

Ineffective Coping r/t situational crisis, preterm labor

Decreased Diversional activity engagement r/t long-term hospitalization

Ineffective Home Maintenance Behaviors r/t medical restrictions

Impaired physical Mobility r/t medically imposed restrictions

Ineffective Role performance r/t inability to carry out normal roles secondary to bed rest or hospitalization, change in expected course of pregnancy

Situational low Self-Esteem r/t threatened ability to carry pregnancy to term

Sexual dysfunction r/t actual or perceived limitation imposed by preterm labor and/or prescribed treatment, separation from partner because of hospitalization

Sleep deprivation r/t change in usual pattern secondary to contractions, hospitalization, treatment regimen

Impaired Social interaction r/t prolonged bed rest or hospitalization

Risk for Injury: **fetal:** Risk factors: premature birth, immature body systems

Risk for Injury: **maternal:** Risk factor: use of tocolytic drugs

Risk for Powerlessness: Risk factor: lack of control over preterm labor

Risk for Vascular Trauma: Risk factor: intravenous medication

Readiness for enhanced Childbearing process: appropriate prenatal lifestyle

Readiness for enhanced Comfort: expresses desire to enhance relaxation

Readiness for enhanced Communication: willingness to discuss thoughts and feelings about situation

PROBLEM-SOLVING DYSFUNCTION

Defensive Coping r/t situational crisis

Impaired Emancipated Decision-Making r/t problem-solving dysfunction

Risk for chronic low Self-Esteem: Risk factor: repeated failures

Readiness for enhanced Communication: willing to share ideas with others

Readiness for enhanced Relationship: shares information and ideas between partners

Readiness for enhanced Resilience: identifies available resources

Readiness for enhanced Spiritual well-being: desires to draw on inner strength and find meaning and purpose to life

PROJECTION

Anxiety r/t threat to self-concept

Defensive Coping r/t inability to acknowledge that own behavior may be a problem, blaming others

Chronic low Self-Esteem r/t failure

Impaired Social interaction r/t self-concept disturbance, confrontational communication style

Risk for Loneliness: Risk factor: blaming others for problems

See Paranoid Personality Disorder

PROLAPSED UMBILICAL CORD

Fear r/t threat to fetus, impending surgery

Ineffective peripheral Tissue Perfusion: fetal r/t interruption in umbilical blood flow

Risk for ineffective Cerebral tissue perfusion: fetal: Risk factor: cord compression

Risk for Injury: maternal: Risk factor: emergency surgery

See TURP (Transurethral Resection of the Prostate)

PROSTATIC HYPERTROPHY

Ineffective Health maintenance behaviors r/t deficient knowledge regarding self-care and prevention of complications

Sleep deprivation r/t nocturia

Urinary Retention r/t obstruction

Risk for Infection: Risk factors: urinary residual after voiding, bacterial invasion of bladder

See BPH (Benign Prostatic Hypertrophy)

PROSTATITIS

Impaired Comfort r/t inflammation

Ineffective Health maintenance behaviors r/t deficient knowledge regarding treatment

Urge urinary Incontinence r/t irritation of bladder

Ineffective Protection r/t depressed immune system

PRURITUS

Impaired Comfort r/t inflammation of skin causing itching

Deficient Knowledge r/t methods to treat and prevent itching

Risk for impaired Skin integrity: Risk factors: scratching, dry skin

PSORIASIS

Disturbed Body Image r/t lesions on body

Impaired Comfort r/t irritated skin

Ineffective Health maintenance behaviors r/t deficient knowledge regarding treatment modalities

Powerlessness r/t lack of control over condition with frequent exacerbations and remissions

Impaired Skin integrity r/t lesions on body

PSYCHOSIS

Ineffective Activity planning r/t compromised ability to process information

Ineffective Health maintenance behaviors r/t cognitive impairment, ineffective individual and family coping

Self-Neglect r/t mental disorder

Impaired individual Resilience r/t psychological disorder

Situational low Self-Esteem r/t excessive use of defense mechanisms (e.g., projection, denial, rationalization)

Risk for disturbed personal Identity: Risk factor: psychosis

Impaired Mood regulation r/t psychosis

Risk for Post-Trauma syndrome: Risk factor: diminished ego strength

See Schizophrenia

PTCA (PERCUTANEOUS TRANSLUMINAL CORONARY ANGIOPLASTY)

See Angioplasty, Coronary

PTSD (POST-TRAUMATIC STRESS DISORDER)

Anxiety r/t exposure to internal or external cues that symbolize or resemble an aspect of the traumatic event

Chronic Sorrow r/t chronic disability (e.g., physical, mental)

Death Anxiety r/t psychological stress associated with traumatic event

Ineffective Breathing pattern r/t hyperventilation associated with anxiety

Ineffective Coping r/t extreme anxiety

Ineffective Impulse control r/t thinking of initial trauma experience

Insomnia r/t recurring nightmares

Post-Trauma syndrome r/t exposure to a traumatic event

Sleep deprivation r/t nightmares interrupting sleep associated with traumatic event

Spiritual distress r/t feelings of detachment or estrangement from others

Risk for Impaired Resilience: Risk factor: chronicity of existing crisis

Risk for Powerlessness: Risk factors: flashbacks, reliving event

Risk for ineffective Relationship: Risk factor: stressful life events

Risk for self- or other-directed Violence: Risk factors: fear of self or others

Readiness for enhanced Comfort: expresses desire to enhance relaxation

Readiness for enhanced Communication: willingness to express feelings and thoughts

Readiness for enhanced Spiritual well-being: desire for harmony after stressful event

PULMONARY EDEMA

Anxiety r/t fear of suffocation

Ineffective Airway clearance r/t presence of tracheobronchial secretions

Decreased Cardiac output r/t increased preload, infective forward perfusion

Impaired Gas exchange r/t extravasation of extravascular fluid in lung tissues and alveoli

Ineffective Health maintenance behaviors r/t deficient knowledge regarding treatment regimen

Sleep deprivation r/t inability to breathe

Risk for acute Confusion: Risk factor: hypoxia

See Heart Failure

PULMONARY EMBOLISM (PE)

Anxiety r/t fear of suffocation

Decreased Cardiac output r/t right ventricular failure secondary to obstructed pulmonary artery

Fear r/t severe pain, possible death

Impaired Gas exchange r/t altered blood flow to alveoli secondary to embolus

Deficient Knowledge r/t activities to prevent embolism, self-care after diagnosis of embolism

Acute Pain r/t biological injury, lack of oxygen to cells

Ineffective peripheral Tissue Perfusion r/t deep vein thrombus formation

See Anticoagulant Therapy

PULMONARY STENOSIS

See Congenital Heart Disease/Cardiac Anomalies

P

PULSE DEFICIT

Risk for Decreased Cardiac output r/t dysrhythmia

See Dysrhythmia

PULSE OXIMETRY

Readiness for enhanced Knowledge: information about treatment regimen

See Hypoxia

PULSE PRESSURE, INCREASED

See Intracranial Pressure, Increased

PULSE PRESSURE, NARROWED

See Shock, Hypovolemic

PULSES, ABSENT OR DIMINISHED PERIPHERAL

Ineffective peripheral Tissue Perfusion r/t interruption of arterial flow

Risk for Peripheral Neurovascular dysfunction: Risk factors: fractures, mechanical compression, orthopedic surgery trauma, immobilization, burns, vascular obstruction

PURPURA

See Clotting Disorder

PYELONEPHRITIS

Ineffective Health maintenance behaviors r/t deficient knowledge regarding self-care, treatment of disease, prevention of further urinary tract infections

Acute Pain r/t inflammation and irritation of urinary tract

Disturbed Sleep pattern r/t urinary frequency

Impaired Urinary elimination r/t irritation of urinary tract

PYLORIC STENOSIS

Imbalanced Nutrition: less than body requirements r/t vomiting secondary to pyloric sphincter obstruction

Acute Pain r/t abdominal fullness

Risk for decreased Fluid volume: Risk factors: vomiting, dehydration

See Hospitalized Child

PYLOROMYOTOMY (PYLORIC STENOSIS REPAIR)

See Surgery, Perioperative Care; Surgery, Postoperative Care; Surgery, Preoperative Care

R

RA (RHEUMATOID ARTHRITIS)

See Rheumatoid Arthritis (RA)

RABIES

Ineffective Health maintenance behaviors r/t deficient knowledge regarding care of wound, isolation, and observation of infected animal

Acute Pain r/t multiple immunization injections

Risk for ineffective Cerebral tissue perfusion: Risk factor: rabies virus

RADIAL NERVE DYSFUNCTION

Acute Pain r/t trauma to hand or arm

See Neuropathy, Peripheral

RADIATION THERAPY

Decreased activity tolerance r/t fatigue from possible anemia

Disturbed Body Image r/t change in appearance, hair loss

Diarrhea r/t irradiation effects

Fatigue r/t malnutrition from lack of appetite, nausea, and vomiting; side effect of radiation

Deficient Knowledge r/t what to expect with radiation therapy, how to do self-care

Nausea r/t side effects of radiation

Imbalanced Nutrition: less than body requirements r/t anorexia, nausea, vomiting, irradiation of areas of pharynx and esophagus

Impaired Oral Mucous Membrane Integrity r/t irradiation effects

Ineffective Protection r/t suppression of bone marrow

Risk for Dry Mouth: Risk factor: Possible side effect of radiation treatments

Risk for impaired Oral Mucous Membrane Integrity: Risk factor: Radiation treatments

Risk for Powerlessness: Risk factors: medical treatment and possible side effects

Risk for impaired Resilience: Risk factor: radiation treatment

Risk for impaired Skin integrity: Risk factor: irradiation effects

Risk for Spiritual distress: Risk factors: radiation treatment, prognosis

RADICAL NECK DISSECTION

See Laryngectomy

RAGE

Risk-prone Health behavior r/t multiple stressors

Labile Emotional Control r/t psychiatric disorders and mood disorders

Impaired individual Resilience r/t poor impulse control

Stress overload r/t multiple coexisting stressors

Risk for Self-Mutilation: Risk factor: command hallucinations

Risk for Suicidal Behavior: Risk factor: desire to kill self

Risk for other-directed Violence: Risk factors: panic state, manic excitement, organic brain syndrome

RAPE-TRAUMA SYNDROME

Rape-Trauma syndrome (See **Rape-Trauma** syndrome, Section II)

Chronic Sorrow r/t forced loss of virginity

Risk for ineffective Childbearing process r/t to trauma and violence

Risk for Post-Trauma syndrome: Risk factor: trauma or violence associated with rape

Risk for Powerlessness: Risk factor: inability to control thoughts about incident

Risk for ineffective Relationship r/t to trauma and violence

Risk for chronic low Self-Esteem r/t perceived lack of respect from others/feeling violated

Risk for Spiritual distress: Risk factor: forced loss of virginity

RASH

Impaired Comfort r/t pruritus

Impaired Skin integrity r/t mechanical trauma

Risk for Infection: Risk factors: traumatized tissue, broken skin

Risk for Latex Allergic reaction: Risk factor: allergy to products associated with latex

RATIONALIZATION

Defensive Coping r/t situational crisis, inability to accept blame for consequences of own behavior

Ineffective Denial r/t fear of consequences, actual or perceived loss

Impaired individual Resilience r/t psychological disturbance

Risk for Post-Trauma syndrome: Risk factor: survivor's role in event

Readiness for enhanced Communication: expresses desire to share thoughts and feelings

Readiness for enhanced Spiritual well-being: possibility of seeking harmony with self, others, higher power, God

RATS, RODENTS IN HOME

Ineffective Home Maintenance Behaviors r/t lack of knowledge, insufficient finances

Risk for Allergic reaction r/t repeated exposure to environmental contamination

See Filthy Home Environment

RAYNAUD'S DISEASE

Deficient Knowledge r/t lack of information about disease process, possible

R

complications, self-care needs regarding disease process and medication

Ineffective peripheral Tissue Perfusion r/t transient reduction of blood flow

Acute Pain r/t transient reduction in blood flow

RDS (RESPIRATORY DISTRESS SYNDROME)

See Respiratory Conditions of the Neonate

RECTAL FULLNESS

Chronic functional Constipation r/t decreased activity level, decreased fluid intake, inadequate fiber in diet, decreased peristalsis, side effects of antidepressant or antipsychotic therapy

Risk for chronic functional Constipation: Risk factor: habitual denial of or ignoring urge to defecate

RECTAL LUMP

See Hemorrhoids

RECTAL PAIN/BLEEDING

Chronic functional Constipation r/t pain on defecation

Deficient Knowledge r/t possible causes of rectal bleeding, pain, treatment modalities

Acute Pain r/t pressure of defecation

Risk for Bleeding: Risk factor: rectal disease

RECTAL SURGERY

See Hemorrhoidectomy

RECTOCELE REPAIR

Chronic functional Constipation r/t painful defecation

Ineffective Health maintenance behaviors r/t deficient knowledge of postoperative care of surgical site, dietary measures, exercise to prevent constipation

Acute Pain r/t surgical procedure

Urinary retention r/t edema from surgery

Risk for Bleeding: Risk factor: surgery

Risk for Surgical Site Infection: Risk factors: surgical procedure, possible contamination of area with feces

REGRESSION

Anxiety r/t threat to or change in health status

Defensive Coping r/t denial of obvious problems, weaknesses

Self-Neglect r/t functional impairment

Powerlessness r/t healthcare environment

Impaired individual Resilience r/t psychological disturbance

Ineffective Role performance r/t powerlessness over health status

See Hospitalized Child; Separation Anxiety

REGRETFUL

Anxiety r/t situational or maturational crises

Death Anxiety r/t feelings of not having accomplished goals in life

Risk for Spiritual distress: Risk factor: inability to forgive

REHABILITATION

Ineffective Coping r/t loss of normal function

Impaired physical Mobility r/t injury, surgery, psychosocial condition warranting rehabilitation

Self-Care deficit: specify r/t impaired physical mobility

Risk for Adult Falls: Risk factor: physical deconditioning

Readiness for enhanced Comfort: expresses desire to enhance feeling of comfort

Readiness for enhanced Self-Concept: accepts strengths and limitations

Readiness for enhanced Health self-Management: expresses desire to manage rehabilitation

RELATIONSHIP

Ineffective Relationship (See ineffective **Relationship,** Section II)

Readiness for enhanced Relationship (See Risk for enhanced **Relationship** see Section II)

RELAXATION TECHNIQUES

Anxiety r/t situational crisis

Readiness for enhanced Comfort: expresses desire to enhance relaxation

Readiness for enhanced Health self-management: desire to manage illness

Readiness for enhanced Religiosity: requests religious materials or experiences

Readiness for enhanced Resilience: desire to enhance resilience

Readiness for enhanced Self-Concept: willingness to enhance self-concept

Readiness for enhanced Spiritual well-being: seeking comfort from higher power

RELIGIOSITY

Impaired Religiosity (See **Religiosity,** impaired, Section II)

Risk for impaired Religiosity (See **Religiosity,** impaired, risk for, Section II)

Readiness for enhanced Religiosity (See **Religiosity,** readiness for enhanced, Section II)

RELIGIOUS CONCERNS

Spiritual distress r/t separation from religious or cultural ties

Risk for impaired Religiosity: Risk factors: ineffective support, coping, caregiving

Risk for Spiritual distress: Risk factors: physical or psychological stress

Readiness for enhanced Spiritual well-being: desire for increased spirituality

RELOCATION STRESS SYNDROME

Relocation stress syndrome (See **Relocation** stress syndrome, Section II)

Risk for Relocation stress syndrome (See **Relocation** stress syndrome, risk for, Section II)

RENAL FAILURE

Decreased activity tolerance r/t effects of anemia, heart failure

Death Anxiety r/t unknown outcome of disease

Decreased Cardiac output r/t effects of heart failure, elevated potassium levels interfering with conduction system

Impaired Comfort r/t pruritus

Ineffective Coping r/t depression resulting from chronic disease

Fatigue r/t effects of chronic uremia and anemia

Excessive Fluid volume r/t decreased urine output, sodium retention, inappropriate fluid Intake

Ineffective Health self-management r/t complexity of healthcare regimen, inadequate number of Cues to action, perceived barriers, powerlessness

Imbalanced Nutrition: less than body requirements r/t anorexia, nausea, vomiting, altered taste sensation, dietary restrictions

Impaired Oral Mucous Membrane Integrity r/t irritation from nitrogenous waste products

Chronic Sorrow r/t chronic illness

Spiritual distress r/t dealing with chronic illness

Impaired urinary Elimination r/t effects of disease, need for dialysis

Risk for Electrolyte imbalance: Risk factor: renal dysfunction

Risk for Infection: Risk factor: altered immune functioning

Risk for Injury: Risk factors: bone changes, neuropathy, muscle weakness

Risk for impaired Oral Mucous Membrane Integrity: Risk factors: dehydration, effects of Uremia

Risk for Powerlessness: Risk factor: chronic illness

Risk for Sepsis: Risk factor: infection

RENAL FAILURE ACUTE/CHRONIC, CHILD

Disturbed Body Image r/t growth retardation, bone changes, visibility of dialysis access devices (shunt, fistula), edema

Deficient Diversional Activity r/t immobility during dialysis

See Child with Chronic Condition; Hospitalized Child

RENAL FAILURE, NONOLIGURIC

Anxiety r/t change in health status

Risk for deficient Fluid volume: Risk factor: loss of large volumes of urine

See Renal Failure

RESPIRATORY ACIDOSIS

See Acidosis, Respiratory

R

RESPIRATORY CONDITIONS OF THE NEONATE (RESPIRATORY DISTRESS SYNDROME [RDS], MECONIUM ASPIRATION, DIAPHRAGMATIC HERNIA)

Ineffective Airway clearance r/t sequelae of attempts to breathe in utero resulting in meconium aspiration

Fatigue r/t increased energy requirements and metabolic demands

Impaired Gas exchange r/t decreased surfactant, immature lung tissue

Dysfunctional Ventilator weaning response r/t immature respiratory system

Risk for Infection: Risk factors: tissue destruction or irritation as a result of aspiration of meconium fluid

See Bronchopulmonary Dysplasia; Hospitalized Child; Premature Infant, Child

RESPIRATORY DISTRESS

See Dyspnea

RESPIRATORY DISTRESS SYNDROME (RDS)

See Respiratory Conditions of the Neonate

RESPIRATORY INFECTIONS, ACUTE CHILDHOOD (CROUP, EPIGLOTTITIS, PERTUSSIS, PNEUMONIA, RESPIRATORY SYNCYTIAL VIRUS)

Decreased activity tolerance r/t generalized weakness, dyspnea, fatigue, poor oxygenation

Ineffective Airway clearance r/t excess tracheobronchial secretions

Ineffective Breathing pattern r/t inflamed bronchial passages, coughing

Fear r/t oxygen deprivation, difficulty breathing

Deficient Fluid volume r/t insensible losses (fever, diaphoresis), inadequate oral fluid intake

Impaired Gas exchange r/t insufficient oxygenation as a result of inflammation or edema of epiglottis, larynx, bronchial passages

Imbalanced Nutrition: less than body requirements r/t anorexia, fatigue, generalized weakness, poor sucking and breathing coordination, dyspnea

Ineffective Thermoregulation r/t infectious process

Risk for Aspiration: Risk factors: inability to coordinate breathing, coughing, sucking

Risk for Infection: **transmission to others:** Risk factor: virulent infectious organisms

Risk for Injury (to pregnant others): Risk factors: exposure to aerosolized medications (e.g., ribavirin, pentamidine), resultant potential fetal toxicity

Risk for Suffocation: Risk factors: inflammation of larynx, epiglottis

See Hospitalized Child

RESPIRATORY SYNCYTIAL VIRUS

See Respiratory Infections, Acute Childhood

RESTLESS LEG SYNDROME

Disturbed Sleep pattern r/t leg discomfort during sleep relieved by frequent leg movement

Chronic Pain r/t leg discomfort

See Stress

RETINAL DETACHMENT

Anxiety r/t change in vision, threat of loss of vision

Deficient Knowledge r/t symptoms, need for early intervention to prevent permanent damage

Vision Loss r/t impaired visual acuity

Risk for impaired Resilience: Risk factor: possible loss of vision

See Vision Impairment

RETINOPATHY, DIABETIC

See Diabetic Retinopathy

RETINOPATHY OF PREMATURITY (ROP)

Risk for Injury: Risk factors: prolonged mechanical ventilation, ROP secondary to 100% oxygen environment

See Retinal Detachment

RH FACTOR INCOMPATIBILITY

Anxiety r/t unknown outcome of pregnancy

Neonatal Hyperbilirubinemia r/t Rh factor incompatibility

Deficient Knowledge r/t treatment regimen from lack of experience with situation

Powerlessness r/t perceived lack of control over outcome of pregnancy

Risk for Injury: fetal: Risk factors: intrauterine destruction of red blood cells, transfusions

Risk for neonatal Hyperbilirubinemia r/t Rh factor incompatibility

Readiness for enhanced Health self-management: prenatal care, compliance with diagnostic and treatment regimen

RHABDOMYOLYSIS

Ineffective Coping r/t seriousness of condition

Impaired physical Mobility r/t myalgia and muscle weakness

Risk for deficient Fluid volume: Risk factor: reduced blood flow to kidneys

Risk for Shock: Risk factor: hypovolemia

Readiness for enhanced Health self-management: seeks information to avoid condition

See Kidney Failure

RHEUMATIC FEVER

See Endocarditis

RHEUMATOID ARTHRITIS (RA)

Imbalanced Nutrition: less than body requirements r/t loss of appetite

Chronic Pain r/t joint inflammation

Disturbed Body Image r/t joint deformity and muscle atrophy

Impaired Physical Mobility r/t pain, impaired joints

Risk for impaired Resilience: Risk factor: chronic, painful, progressive disease

See Arthritis; JRA (Juvenile Rheumatoid Arthritis)

RIB FRACTURE

Ineffective Breathing pattern r/t fractured ribs

Acute Pain r/t movement, deep breathing

Impaired Gas exchange r/t ventilation-perfusion imbalance, decreased depth of ventilation

RIDICULE OF OTHERS

Defensive Coping r/t situational crisis, psychological impairment, substance abuse

Risk for Post-Trauma syndrome: Risk factor: perception of event

RINGWORM OF BODY

Impaired Comfort r/t pruritus

Impaired Skin integrity r/t presence of macules associated with fungus

See Itching; Pruritus

RINGWORM OF NAILS

Disturbed Body Image r/t appearance of nails, removed nails

RINGWORM OF SCALP

Disturbed Body Image r/t possible hair loss (alopecia)

See Itching; Pruritus

ROACHES, INVASION OF HOME WITH

Ineffective Home Maintenance Behaviors r/t lack of knowledge, insufficient finances

See Filthy Home Environment

ROLE PERFORMANCE, ALTERED

Ineffective Role performance (See **Role** performance, ineffective, Section II)

ROP (RETINOPATHY OF PREMATURITY)

See Retinopathy of Prematurity (ROP)

RSV (RESPIRATORY SYNCYTIAL VIRUS)

See Respiratory Infection, Acute Childhood

RUBELLA

See Communicable Diseases, Childhood (e.g., Measles, Mumps, Rubella, Chickenpox, Scabies, Lice, Impetigo)

RUBOR OF EXTREMITIES

Ineffective peripheral Tissue Perfusion r/t interruption of arterial flow

See Peripheral Vascular Disease (PVD)

RUPTURED DISK

See Low Back Pain

S

SAD (SEASONAL AFFECTIVE DISORDER)

Readiness for enhanced Resilience: uses SAD lights during winter months

See Depression (Major Depressive Disorder)

SADNESS

Maladaptive Grieving r/t actual or perceived loss

Impaired Mood regulation r/t chronic illness (See **Mood** regulation, impaired, Section II)

Spiritual distress r/t intense suffering

Risk for Powerlessness: Risk factor: actual or perceived loss

Risk for Spiritual distress: Risk factor: loss of loved one

Readiness for enhanced Communication: willingness to share feelings and thoughts

Readiness for enhanced Spiritual well-being: desire for harmony after actual or perceived loss

See Depression (Major Depressive Disorder); Major Depressive Disorder

SAFE SEX

Readiness for enhanced Health self-management: takes appropriate precautions during sexual activity to keep from contracting sexually transmitted disease

See Sexuality, Adolescent; STD (Sexually Transmitted Disease)

SAFETY, CHILDHOOD

Deficient Knowledge: potential for enhanced health maintenance r/t parental knowledge and skill acquisition regarding appropriate safety measures

Risk for Aspiration (See **Aspiration,** risk for, Section II)

Risk for Injury: Risk factors: developmental age, altered home maintenance

Risk for impaired Parenting: Risk factors: lack of available and effective role model, lack of knowledge, misinformation from other family members (old wives' tales)

Risk for Poisoning: Risk factors: use of lead-based paint; presence of asbestos or radon gas; drugs not locked in cabinet; household products left in accessible area (bleach, detergent, drain cleaners, household cleaners); alcohol and perfume within reach of child; presence of poisonous plants; atmospheric pollutants

Risk for Thermal injury: Risk factor: inadequate supervision

Readiness for enhanced Childbearing process: expresses appropriate knowledge for care of child

SALMONELLA

Ineffective Home Maintenance Behaviors r/t improper preparation or storage of food, lack of safety measures when caring for pet reptile

Risk for Shock: Risk factors: hypovolemia, diarrhea, sepsis

Readiness for enhanced Health self-management: avoiding improperly prepared or stored food, wearing gloves when handling pet reptiles or their feces

See Gastroenteritis; Gastroenteritis, Child

SALPINGECTOMY

Decisional Conflict r/t sterilization procedure

Risk for impaired Urinary elimination: Risk factor: trauma to ureter during surgery

See Hysterectomy; Surgery, Perioperative Care; Surgery, Postoperative Care; Surgery, Preoperative Care

SARCOIDOSIS

Anxiety r/t change in health status

Impaired Gas exchange r/t ventilation-perfusion imbalance

Ineffective Health maintenance behaviors r/t deficient knowledge regarding home care and medication regimen

Acute Pain r/t possible disease affecting joints

Ineffective Protection r/t immune disorder

Risk for decreased Cardiac tissue perfusion: Risk factor: dysrhythmias

Risk for impaired Skin integrity: Risk factor: immunological disorder

SBE (SELF-BREAST EXAMINATION)

Readiness for enhanced Health self-management: desires to have information about SBE

Readiness for enhanced Knowledge: SBE

SCABIES

See Communicable Diseases, Childhood (e.g., Measles, Mumps, Rubella, Chickenpox, Scabies, Lice, Impetigo)

SCARED

Anxiety r/t threat of death, threat to or change in health status

Death Anxiety r/t unresolved issues surrounding end-of-life decisions

Fear r/t hospitalization, real or imagined threat to own well-being

Impaired individual Resilience r/t violence

Readiness for enhanced Communication: willingness to share thoughts and feelings

SCHIZOPHRENIA

Ineffective Activity planning r/t compromised ability to process information

Anxiety r/t unconscious conflict with reality

Impaired verbal Communication r/t psychosis, disorientation, inaccurate perception, hallucinations, delusions

S

Ineffective Coping r/t inadequate support systems, unrealistic perceptions, inadequate coping skills, disturbed thought processes, impaired communication

Decreased Diversional activity engagement r/t social isolation, possible regression

Interrupted Family processes r/t inability to express feelings, impaired communication

Fear r/t altered contact with reality

Ineffective Health maintenance behaviors r/t cognitive impairment, ineffective individual and family coping, lack of material resources

Ineffective family Health self-management r/t chronicity and unpredictability of condition

Ineffective Home Maintenance Behaviors r/t impaired cognitive or emotional functioning, insufficient finances, inadequate support systems

Hopelessness r/t long-term stress from chronic mental illness

Disturbed personal Identity r/t psychiatric disorder

Impaired Memory r/t psychosocial condition

Imbalanced Nutrition: less than body requirements r/t fear of eating, lack of awareness of hunger, disinterest toward food

Impaired individual Resilience r/t psychological disorder

Self-Care deficit: **specify** r/t loss of contact with reality, impairment of perception

Self-Neglect r/t psychosis

Sleep deprivation r/t intrusive thoughts, nightmares

Impaired Social interaction r/t impaired communication patterns, self-concept disturbance, disturbed thought processes

Social isolation r/t lack of trust, regression, delusional thinking, repressed fears

Chronic Sorrow r/t chronic mental illness

Spiritual distress r/t loneliness, social alienation

Risk for Caregiver Role Strain: Risk factors: bizarre behavior of client, chronicity of condition

Risk for compromised Human Dignity: Risk factor: stigmatizing label

Risk for Loneliness: Risk factor: inability to interact socially

Risk for Post-Trauma syndrome: Risk factor: diminished ego strength

Risk for Powerlessness: Risk factor: intrusive, distorted thinking

Risk for impaired Religiosity: Risk factors: ineffective coping, lack of security

Risk for Suicidal Behavior: Risk factor: psychiatric illness

Risk for self-directed Violence: Risk factors: lack of trust, panic, hallucinations, delusional thinking

Risk for other-directed Violence: Risk factor: psychotic disorder

Readiness for enhanced Hope: expresses desire to enhance interconnectedness with others and problem-solve to meet goals

Readiness for enhanced Power: expresses willingness to enhance participation in choices for daily living and health and enhance knowledge for participation in change

SCIATICA

See Neuropathy, Peripheral

SCOLIOSIS

Risk-prone Health behavior r/t lack of developmental maturity to comprehend long-term consequences of noncompliance with treatment procedures

Disturbed Body Image r/t use of therapeutic braces, postsurgery scars, restricted physical activity

Impaired Comfort r/t altered health status and body image

Impaired Gas exchange r/t restricted lung expansion as a result of severe presurgery curvature of spine, immobilization

Ineffective Health maintenance behaviors r/t deficient knowledge regarding treatment modalities, restrictions, home care, postoperative activities

S

Impaired physical Mobility r/t restricted movement, dyspnea caused by severe curvature of spine

Acute Pain r/t musculoskeletal restrictions, surgery, reambulation with cast or spinal rod

Impaired Skin integrity r/t braces, casts, surgical correction

Chronic Sorrow r/t chronic disability

Risk for Perioperative Positioning injury: Risk factor: prone position

Risk for impaired Resilience: Risk factor: chronic condition

Readiness for enhanced Health management: desires knowledge regarding treatment for condition

See Hospitalized Child; Maturational Issues, Adolescent

SEDENTARY LIFESTYLE

Decreased activity tolerance r/t sedentary lifestyle

Sedentary lifestyle (See **Sedentary** lifestyle, Section II)

Obesity (See **Obesity,** Section II)

Overweight (See **Overweight,** Section II)

Risk for Overweight (See **Overweight,** Section II)

Risk for ineffective peripheral Tissue Perfusion: Risk factor: insufficient knowledge of aggravating factors (e.g., immobility, obesity)

Readiness for enhanced Coping: seeking knowledge of new strategies to adjust to sedentary lifestyle

SEIZURE DISORDERS, ADULT

Acute Confusion r/t postseizure state

Social isolation r/t unpredictability of seizures, community-imposed stigma

Risk for ineffective Airway clearance: Risk factor: accumulation of secretions during seizure

Risk for Adult Falls: Risk factor: uncontrolled seizure activity

Risk for Powerlessness: Risk factor: possible seizure

Risk for impaired Resilience: Risk factor: chronic illness

Readiness for enhanced Knowledge: anticonvulsive therapy

Readiness for enhanced Self-Care: expresses desire to enhance knowledge and responsibility for self-care

See Epilepsy

SEIZURE DISORDERS, CHILDHOOD (EPILEPSY, FEBRILE SEIZURES, INFANTILE SPASMS)

Ineffective Health maintenance behaviors r/t lack of knowledge regarding anticonvulsive therapy, fever reduction (febrile seizures)

Social isolation r/t unpredictability of seizures, community-imposed stigma

Risk for ineffective Airway clearance: Risk factor: accumulation of secretions during seizure

Risk for delayed Child Development: Risk factors: effects of seizure disorder, parental overprotection

Risk for Adult Falls: Risk factor: possible seizure

Risk for Injury: Risk factors: uncontrolled movements during seizure, falls, drowsiness caused by anticonvulsants

See Epilepsy

SELF-BREAST EXAMINATION (SBE)

See SBE (Self-Breast Examination)

SELF-CARE

Readiness for enhanced Self-Care (See **Self-Care,** readiness for enhanced, Section II)

SELF-CARE DEFICIT, BATHING

Bathing Self-Care deficit (See **Self-Care** deficit, bathing, Section II)

SELF-CARE DEFICIT, DRESSING

Dressing Self-Care deficit (See **Self-Care** deficit, dressing, Section II)

SELF-CARE DEFICIT, FEEDING

Feeding Self-Care deficit (See **Self-Care** deficit, feeding, Section II)

SELF-CARE DEFICIT, TOILETING

Toileting Self-Care deficit (See **Self-Care** deficit, toileting, Section II)

SELF-CONCEPT

Readiness for enhanced Self-Concept (See **Self-Concept,** readiness for enhanced, Section II)

SELF-DESTRUCTIVE BEHAVIOR

Post-Trauma syndrome r/t unresolved feelings from traumatic event

Risk for Self-Mutilation: Risk factors: feelings of depression, rejection, self-hatred, depersonalization; command hallucinations

Risk for Suicidal Behavior: Risk factor: history of self-destructive behavior

Risk for self-directed Violence: Risk factors: panic state, history of child abuse, toxic reaction to medication

S

SELF-ESTEEM, CHRONIC LOW

Chronic low Self-Esteem (See **Self-Esteem,** low, chronic, Section II)

Risk for disturbed personal Identity: Risk factor: chronic low self-esteem

SELF-ESTEEM, SITUATIONAL LOW

Situational low Self-Esteem (See **Self-Esteem,** low, situational, Section II)

Risk for situational low Self-Esteem (See **Self-Esteem,** low, situational, risk for, Section II)

SELF-MUTILATION

Ineffective Impulse control r/t ineffective management of anxiety

Self-Mutilation (See **Self-Mutilation,** Section II)

Risk for Self-Mutilation (See **Self-Mutilation,** risk for, Section II)

SENILE DEMENTIA

Ineffective Relationship r/t cognitive changes in one partner

Sedentary lifestyle r/t lack of interest in movement

See Dementia

SEPARATION ANXIETY

Ineffective Coping r/t maturational and situational crises, vulnerability related to developmental age, hospitalization, separation from family and familiar surroundings, multiple caregivers

Insomnia r/t separation for significant others

Risk for impaired Attachment: Risk factor: separation

See Hospitalized Child

SEPSIS, CHILD

Impaired Gas exchange r/t pulmonary inflammation associated with disease process

Imbalanced Nutrition: less than body requirements r/t anorexia, generalized weakness, poor sucking reflex

Delayed Surgical recovery r/t presence of infection

Ineffective Thermoregulation r/t infectious process, septic shock

Ineffective peripheral Tissue Perfusion r/t arterial or venous blood flow exchange problems, septic shock

Risk for deficient Fluid volume: Risk factor: inflammation leading to decreased systemic vascular resistance

Risk for impaired Skin integrity: Risk factor: desquamation caused by disseminated intravascular coagulation

See Hospitalized Child; Premature Infant, Child

SEPTICEMIA

Imbalanced Nutrition: less than body requirements r/t anorexia, generalized weakness

Ineffective peripheral Tissue Perfusion r/t decreased systemic vascular resistance

Risk for deficient Fluid volume: Risk factors: vasodilation of peripheral vessels, leaking of capillaries

Risk for Shock: Risk factors: hypotension, hypovolemia

Risk for Unstable Blood Pressure: Risk factor: hypovolemia

See Sepsis, Child; Shock, Septic

SERVICE ANIMAL

Readiness for enhanced Power: expresses desire to enhance independence with actions for change

Readiness for enhanced Resilience: expresses desire to enhance involvement in activities, desire to enhance environmental safety

SEVERE ACUTE RESPIRATORY SYNDROME (SARS)

See Pneumonia

SEXUAL DYSFUNCTION

Sexual Dysfunction (See **Sexual Dysfunction**, Section II)

Ineffective Relationship r/t reported sexual dissatisfaction between partners

Chronic Sorrow r/t loss of ideal sexual experience, altered relationships

Risk for chronic low Self-Esteem

See Erectile Dysfunction (ED)

SEXUAL HARASSMENT VICTIM

Anxiety r/t situational crisis

Risk for Compromised Human Dignity: Risk factors: humiliation, dehumanizing treatment

Risk for Post-Trauma syndrome: Risk factors: perceived traumatic event, insufficient social support

Risk for Spiritual Distress: Risk factors: physical, psychological stress

See Assault Victim

SEXUALITY, ADOLESCENT

Disturbed Body Image r/t anxiety caused by unachieved developmental milestone (puberty) or deficient knowledge regarding reproductive maturation with expressed concerns regarding lack of growth of secondary sex characteristics

Impaired emancipated Decision-Making: sexual activity r/t undefined personal values or beliefs, multiple or divergent sources of information, lack of relevant information

Ineffective Impulse control r/t denial of consequences of actions

Deficient Knowledge: potential for enhanced health maintenance r/t multiple or divergent sources of information or lack of relevant information regarding sexual transmission of disease, contraception, prevention of toxic shock syndrome

See Maturational Issues, Adolescent

SEXUALITY PATTERN, INEFFECTIVE

Ineffective Sexuality pattern (See **Sexuality** pattern, ineffective, Section II)

SEXUALLY TRANSMITTED DISEASE (STD)

See STD (Sexually Transmitted Disease)

SHAKEN BABY SYNDROME

Impaired Parenting r/t stress, history of being abusive

Impaired individual Resilience r/t poor impulse control

Stress overload r/t intense repeated family stressors, family violence

Risk for other-directed Violence: Risk factors: history of violence against others, perinatal complications

See Child Abuse; Suspected Child Abuse and Neglect (SCAN), Child; Suspected Child Abuse and Neglect (SCAN), Parent

SHAKINESS

Anxiety r/t situational or maturational crisis, threat of death

SHAME

Situational low Self-Esteem r/t inability to deal with past traumatic events, blaming of self for events not in one's control

SHINGLES

Acute Pain r/t vesicular eruption along the nerves

Ineffective Protection r/t abnormal blood profiles

Social isolation r/t altered state of wellness, contagiousness of disease

Risk for Infection: Risk factor: tissue destruction

See Itching

SHIVERING

Impaired Comfort r/t altered health status

Fear r/t serious threat to health status

Hypothermia r/t exposure to cool environment

Ineffective Thermoregulation r/t serious infectious process resulting in immune response of fever

See Shock, Septic

SHOCK, CARDIOGENIC

Decreased Cardiac output r/t decreased myocardial contractility, dysrhythmia

SHOCK, HYPOVOLEMIC

Deficient Fluid volume r/t abnormal loss of fluid, trauma, third spacing

SHOCK, SEPTIC

Deficient Fluid volume r/t abnormal loss of intravascular fluid, pooling of blood in peripheral circulation, overwhelming inflammatory response

Ineffective Protection r/t inadequately functioning immune system

See Sepsis, Child; Septicemia

SHOULDER REPAIR

Self-Care deficit: bathing, dressing, feeding r/t immobilization of affected shoulder

Risk for Perioperative Positioning injury: Risk factor: immobility

See Surgery, Preoperative Care; Surgery, Perioperative Care; Surgery, Postoperative Care; Total Joint Replacement (Total Hip/Total Knee/Shoulder)

SICKLE CELL ANEMIA/CRISIS

Decreased activity tolerance r/t fatigue, effects of chronic anemia

Deficient Fluid volume r/t decreased intake, increased fluid requirements during sickle cell crisis, decreased ability of kidneys to concentrate urine

Impaired physical Mobility r/t pain, fatigue

Acute Pain r/t viscous blood, tissue hypoxia

Ineffective peripheral Tissue Perfusion r/t effects of red cell sickling, infarction of tissues

Risk for decreased Cardiac tissue perfusion: Risk factors: effects of red cell sickling, infarction of tissues

Risk for Infection: Risk factor: alterations in splenic function

Risk for impaired Resilience: Risk factor: chronic illness

Risk for ineffective cerebral Tissue perfusion: Risk factors: effects of red cell sickling, infarction of tissues

See Child with Chronic Condition; Hospitalized Child

SIDS (SUDDEN INFANT DEATH SYNDROME)

Anxiety: parental worry r/t life-threatening event

Interrupted Family processes r/t stress as a result of special care needs of infant with apnea

Insomnia: parental/infant r/t home apnea monitoring

Deficient Knowledge: potential for enhanced health maintenance r/t knowledge or skill acquisition of cardiopulmonary resuscitation and home apnea monitoring

Impaired Resilience r/t sudden loss

Risk for Sudden Infant Death (See **Sudden Infant Death**, risk for, Section II)

Risk for Powerlessness: Risk factor: unanticipated life-threatening event

See Terminally Ill Child/Death of Child, Parent

SITTING PROBLEMS

Impaired Sitting (See **Sitting**, impaired, Section II)

SITUATIONAL CRISIS

Imbalanced Energy Field r/t hyperactivity of the energy flow

Ineffective Coping r/t situational crisis

Interrupted Family processes r/t situational crisis

Risk for ineffective Activity planning: Risk factor: inability to process information

Risk for disturbed personal Identity: Risk factor: situational crisis

Readiness for enhanced Communication: willingness to share feelings and thoughts

Readiness for enhanced Religiosity: requests religious material and/or experiences

Readiness for enhanced Resilience: desire to enhance resilience

Readiness for enhanced Spiritual well-being: desire for harmony following crisis

SJS (STEVENS-JOHNSON SYNDROME)

See Stevens-Johnson Syndrome (SJS)

SKIN CANCER

Ineffective Health maintenance behaviors r/t deficient knowledge regarding self-care with skin cancer

Ineffective Protection r/t weakened immune system

Impaired Tissue integrity r/t abnormal cell growth in skin, treatment of skin cancer

Readiness for enhanced Health self-management: follows preventive measures

Readiness for enhanced Knowledge: self-care to prevent and treat skin cancer

SKIN DISORDERS

Impaired Skin integrity (See **Skin** integrity, impaired, Section II)

SKIN TURGOR, CHANGE IN ELASTICITY

Deficient Fluid volume r/t active fluid loss

SLEEP

Readiness for enhanced Sleep (See **Sleep**, readiness for enhanced, Section II)

SLEEP APNEA

Ineffective Breathing pattern r/t obesity, substance abuse, enlarged tonsils, smoking, or neurological pathology such as a brain tumor

Impaired Comfort r/t use of bilevel positive airway pressure (BiPAP)/continuous positive airway pressure (CPAP) machine

SLEEP DEPRIVATION

Fatigue r/t lack of sleep

Sleep deprivation (See **Sleep** deprivation, Section II)

SLEEP PROBLEMS

Insomnia (See **Insomnia**, Section II)

SLEEP PATTERN, DISTURBED, PARENT/CHILD

Insomnia: child r/t anxiety or fear

Insomnia: parent r/t parental responsibilities, stress

See Suspected Child Abuse and Neglect (SCAN), Child; Suspected Child Abuse and Neglect (SCAN), Parent

SLURRING OF SPEECH

Impaired verbal Communication r/t decrease in circulation to brain, brain tumor, anatomical defect, cleft palate

Situational low Self-Esteem r/t speech impairment

See Communication Problems

SMALL BOWEL RESECTION

See Abdominal Surgery

SMELL, LOSS OF ABILITY TO

Risk for Injury: Risk factors: inability to detect gas fumes, smoke smells

See Anosmia (Smell, Loss of Ability to)

SMOKE INHALATION

Ineffective Airway clearance r/t smoke inhalation

Impaired Gas exchange r/t ventilation-perfusion imbalance

Risk for acute Confusion: Risk factor: decreased oxygen supply

Risk for Infection: Risk factors: inflammation, ineffective airway clearance, pneumonia

Risk for Poisoning: Risk factor: exposure to carbon monoxide

Readiness for enhanced Health self-management: functioning smoke detectors and carbon monoxide detectors in home and work, escape route planned and reviewed

See Atelectasis; Burns; Pneumonia

SMOKING BEHAVIOR

Insufficient Breast Milk Production r/t smoking

Risk-prone Health behavior r/t smoking

Ineffective Health maintenance behaviors r/t denial of effects of smoking, lack of effective support for smoking withdrawal

Readiness for enhanced Knowledge: expresses interest in smoking cessation

Risk for dry Eye: Risk factor: smoking

Risk for ineffective peripheral Tissue Perfusion: Risk factor: effect of nicotine

Risk for Thermal injury: Risk factor: unsafe smoking behavior

Readiness for enhanced Health literacy: verbalizes desire to enhance understanding of health information to make healthcare choices

SOCIAL INTERACTION, IMPAIRED

Impaired Social interaction (See **Social** interaction, impaired, Section II)

SOCIAL ISOLATION

Social isolation (See **Social isolation**, Section II)

SOCIOPATHIC PERSONALITY

See Antisocial Personality Disorder

SODIUM, DECREASE/INCREASE

See Hyponatremia; Hypernatremia

SOMATIZATION DISORDER

Anxiety r/t unresolved conflicts channeled into physical complaints or conditions

Ineffective Coping r/t lack of insight into underlying conflicts

Ineffective Denial r/t displaced psychological stress to physical symptoms

Nausea r/t anxiety

Chronic Pain r/t unexpressed anger, multiple physical disorders, depression

Impaired individual Resilience r/t possible psychological disorders

SORE NIPPLES, BREASTFEEDING

Ineffective Breastfeeding r/t deficient knowledge regarding correct feeding procedure

See Painful Breasts, Sore Nipples

SORE THROAT

Impaired Comfort r/t sore throat

Deficient Knowledge r/t treatment, relief of discomfort

Impaired Oral Mucous Membrane Integrity r/t inflammation or infection of oral cavity

Impaired Swallowing r/t irritation of oropharyngeal cavity

Risk for Dry Mouth: Risk factor: painful swallowing

SORROW

Chronic Sorrow (See **Sorrow,** chronic, Section II)

Readiness for enhanced Communication: expresses thoughts and feelings

Readiness for enhanced Spiritual well-being: desire to find purpose and meaning of loss

SPASTIC COLON

See IBS (Irritable Bowel Syndrome)

SPEECH DISORDERS

Anxiety r/t difficulty with communication

Impaired verbal Communication r/t anatomical defect, cleft palate, psychological barriers, decrease in circulation to brain

SPINA BIFIDA

See Neural Tube Defects (Meningocele, Myelomeningocele, Spina Bifida, Anencephaly)

SPINAL CORD INJURY

Decreased Diversional activity engagement r/t long-term hospitalization, frequent lengthy treatments

Fear r/t powerlessness over loss of body function

Disturbed Body Image r/t alteration in body function

Chronic functional Constipation r/t inhibition of reflex arc

Maladaptive Grieving r/t loss of usual body function

Ineffective Coping r/t inability to meet basic needs and insufficient sense of control

Sedentary Lifestyle r/t lack of resources or interest

Impaired physical Mobility r/t neuromuscular impairment

Impaired wheelchair Mobility r/t neuromuscular impairment

Impaired Standing r/t spinal cord injury

Urinary Retention r/t inhibition of reflex arc

Risk for Latex Allergy reaction: Risk factor: continuous or intermittent catheterization

Risk for Autonomic Dysreflexia: Risk factors: bladder or bowel distention, skin irritation, deficient knowledge of patient and caregiver

Risk for ineffective Breathing pattern: Risk factor: neuromuscular impairment

Risk for Infection: Risk factors: chronic disease, stasis of body fluids

Risk for Loneliness: Risk factor: physical immobility

Risk for Powerlessness: Risk factor: loss of function

Risk for Adult Pressure Injury: Risk factors: immobility, decreased sensation

Risk for Thermal Injury: Risk factor: physical immobility

See Child with Chronic Condition; Hospitalized Child, Neural Tube Defects (Meningocele, Myelomeningocele, Spina Bifida, Anencephaly); Paralysis

SPINAL FUSION

Impaired bed Mobility r/t impaired ability to turn side to side while keeping spine in proper alignment

Impaired physical Mobility r/t musculoskeletal impairment associated with surgery, possible back brace

Readiness for enhanced Knowledge: expresses interest in information associated with surgery

See Acute Back Pain; Scoliosis; Surgery, Preoperative Care; Surgery, Perioperative Care; Surgery, Postoperative Care

SPIRITUAL DISTRESS

Spiritual distress (See **Spiritual** distress, Section II)

Risk for chronic low Self-Esteem: Risk factor: unresolved spiritual issues

Risk for Spiritual distress (See **Spiritual** distress, risk for, Section II)

SPIRITUAL WELL-BEING

Readiness for enhanced Spiritual well-being (See **Spiritual** well-being, readiness for enhanced, Section II)

SPLENECTOMY

See Abdominal Surgery

SPRAINS

Acute Pain r/t physical injury

Impaired physical Mobility r/t injury

Impaired Walking r/t injury

STABLE BLOOD PRESSURE, RISK FOR UNSTABLE

Deficient Knowledge r/t inconsistency with medication regiment

(See **Unstable Blood Pressure,** Risk for, Section II)

STANDING PROBLEMS

Impaired Standing (see Impaired **Standing,** Section II)

STAPEDECTOMY

Hearing Loss r/t edema from surgery

Acute Pain r/t headache

Risk for Adult Falls: Risk factor: dizziness

Risk for Infection: Risk factor: invasive procedure

STASIS ULCER

Impaired Tissue integrity r/t chronic venous congestion

Risk for Infection: Risk factor: open wound

See CHF (Congestive Heart Failure); Varicose Veins

STD (SEXUALLY TRANSMITTED DISEASE)

Impaired Comfort r/t infection

Fear r/t altered body function, risk for social isolation, fear of incurable illness

Ineffective Health maintenance behaviors r/t deficient knowledge regarding transmission, symptoms, treatment of STD

Ineffective Sexuality pattern r/t illness, altered body function, need for abstinence to heal

Social isolation r/t fear of contracting or spreading disease

Risk for Infection: spread of infection: Risk factor: lack of knowledge concerning transmission of disease

Readiness for enhanced Knowledge: seeks information regarding prevention and treatment of STDs

See Maturational Issues, Adolescent; PID (Pelvic Inflammatory Disease)

STEMI (ST-ELEVATION MYOCARDIAL INFARCTION)

See MI (Myocardial Infarction)

STENT (CORONARY ARTERY STENT)

Risk for Injury: Risk factor: complications associated with stent placement

Risk for decreased Cardiac tissue perfusion: Risk factor: possible restenosis

Risk for Vascular Trauma: Risk factors: insertion site, catheter width

Readiness for enhanced Decision-Making: expresses desire to enhance risk-benefit analysis, understanding and meaning of choices, and decisions regarding treatment

See Angioplasty, Coronary; Cardiac Catheterization

STERILIZATION SURGERY

Decisional Conflict r/t multiple or divergent sources of information, unclear personal values or beliefs

See Surgery, Preoperative Care; Surgery, Perioperative Care; Surgery, Postoperative Care; Tubal Ligation; Vasectomy

STERTOROUS RESPIRATIONS

Ineffective Airway clearance r/t pharyngeal obstruction

STEVENS-JOHNSON SYNDROME (SJS)

Impaired Oral Mucous Membrane Integrity r/t immunocompromised condition associated with allergic medication reaction

Acute Pain r/t painful skin lesions and painful mucosa lesions

Impaired Skin Integrity r/t allergic medication reaction

Risk for deficient Fluid volume: Risk factors: factors affecting fluid needs (hypermetabolic state, fever), excessive losses through normal routes (vomiting and diarrhea)

Risk for Infection: Risk factor: sloughing skin

Risk for impaired Liver function: Risk factor: impaired immune response

STILLBIRTH

See Pregnancy Loss

STOMA

See Colostomy; Ileostomy

STOMATITIS

Impaired Oral Mucous Membrane Integrity r/t pathological conditions of oral cavity; side effects of chemotherapy

Risk for impaired Oral Mucous Membrane Integrity (See impaired **Oral Mucous Membrane Integrity,** risk for, Section II)

STOOL, HARD/DRY

Chronic functional Constipation r/t inadequate fluid intake, inadequate fiber intake, decreased activity level, decreased gastric motility

STRAINING WITH DEFECATION

Chronic functional Constipation r/t less than adequate fluid intake, less than adequate dietary intake

Risk for decreased Cardiac output: Risk factor: vagal stimulation with dysrhythmia resulting from Valsalva maneuver

STREP THROAT

Risk for Infection: Risk factor: exposure to pathogen

See Sore Throat

STRESS

Anxiety r/t feelings of helplessness, feelings of being threatened

Ineffective Coping r/t ineffective use of problem-solving process, feelings of apprehension or helplessness

Fear r/t powerlessness over feelings

Stress overload r/t intense or multiple stressors

Readiness for enhanced Communication: shows willingness to share thoughts and feelings

Readiness for enhanced Spiritual well-being: expresses desire for harmony and peace in stressful situation

See Anxiety

STRESS URINARY INCONTINENCE

Stress urinary Incontinence r/t degenerative change in pelvic muscles

STRIDOR

Ineffective Airway clearance r/t obstruction, tracheobronchial infection, trauma

STROKE

See CVA (Cerebrovascular Accident)

STUTTERING

Anxiety r/t impaired verbal communication

Impaired verbal Communication r/t anxiety, psychological problems

SUBARACHNOID HEMORRHAGE

Acute Pain: headache r/t irritation of meninges from blood, increased intracranial pressure

Risk for ineffective Cerebral tissue perfusion: Risk factor: bleeding from cerebral vessel

See Intracranial Pressure, Increased

SUBSTANCE ABUSE

Anxiety r/t threat to self-concept, lack of control of drug use

Compromised family Coping r/t codependency issues

Defensive Coping r/t substance abuse

Disabled family Coping r/t differing coping styles between support persons

Ineffective Coping r/t use of substances to cope with life events

Ineffective Denial r/t refusal to acknowledge substance abuse problem

Dysfunctional Family processes r/t substance abuse

Risk-prone Health behavior r/t addiction

S

Deficient community Health r/t prevention and control of illegal substances in community

Ineffective Impulse control r/t addictive process

Insomnia r/t irritability, nightmares, tremors

Imbalanced Nutrition: less than body requirements r/t poor eating habits

Powerlessness r/t feeling unable to change patterns of drug abuse

Ineffective Relationship r/t inability for well-balanced collaboration between partners

Sexual Dysfunction r/t actions and side effects of drugs

Sleep deprivation r/t prolonged psychological discomfort

Impaired Social Interaction r/t disturbed thought processes from drug abuse

Risk for impaired Attachment: Risk factor: substance abuse

Risk for Injury: Risk factors: hallucinations, drug effects

Risk for disturbed personal Identity: Risk factor: ingestion/inhalation of toxic chemicals

Risk for chronic low Self-Esteem: Risk factors: perceived lack of respect from others, repeated failures, repeated negative reinforcement

Risk for Thermal injury: Risk factor: intoxication with drugs or alcohol

Risk for Unstable Blood Pressure: Risk factor: vasoconstriction of cardiac arteries

Risk for Vascular Trauma: Risk factor: chemical irritant self injected into veins

Risk for self-directed Violence: Risk factors: reactions to substances used, impulsive behavior, disorientation, impaired judgment

Risk for other-directed Violence: Risk factor: poor impulse control

Readiness for enhanced Coping: seeking social support and knowledge of new strategies

Readiness for enhanced Self-Concept: accepting strengths and limitations

See Alcoholism

SUBSTANCE ABUSE, ADOLESCENT

See Alcoholism; Maturational Issues, Adolescent; Substance Abuse

SUBSTANCE ABUSE IN PREGNANCY

Ineffective Childbearing process r/t substance abuse

Defensive Coping r/t denial of situation, differing value system

Ineffective Health self-management r/t addiction

Deficient Knowledge r/t lack of exposure to information regarding effects of substance abuse in pregnancy

Risk for impaired Attachment: Risk factors: substance abuse, inability of parent to meet infant's or own personal needs

Risk for Infection: Risk factors: intravenous drug use, lifestyle

Risk for Injury: fetal: Risk factor: effects of drugs on fetal growth and development

Risk for Injury: maternal: Risk factor: drug or alcohol use

Risk for impaired Parenting: Risk factor: lack of ability to meet infant's needs due to addiction with use of alcohol or drugs

See Alcoholism; Substance Abuse

SUBSTANCE WITHDRAWAL

See Acute Substance Withdrawal Syndrome

SUCKING REFLEX

Effective Breastfeeding r/t regular and sustained sucking and swallowing at breast

SUDDEN INFANT DEATH SYNDROME (SIDS)

See SIDS (Sudden Infant Death Syndrome)

SUFFOCATION, RISK FOR

Risk for Suffocation (See **Suffocation**, risk for, Section II)

SUICIDE ATTEMPT

Risk-prone Health behavior r/t low self-efficacy

Ineffective Coping r/t anger, maladaptive grieving

Hopelessness r/t perceived or actual loss, substance abuse, low self-concept, inadequate support systems

Ineffective Impulse control r/t inability to modulate stress, anxiety

Post-Trauma syndrome r/t history of traumatic events, abuse, rape, incest, war, torture

Impaired individual Resilience r/t poor impulse control

Situational low Self-Esteem r/t guilt, inability to trust, feelings of worthlessness or rejection

Social isolation r/t inability to engage in satisfying personal relationships

Spiritual distress r/t hopelessness, despair

Risk for Post-Trauma syndrome: Risk factor: survivor's role in suicide attempt

Risk for Suicidal Behavior (See **Suicidal Behavior,** risk for, Section II)

Readiness for enhanced Communication: willingness to share thoughts and feelings

Readiness for enhanced Spiritual well-being: desire for harmony and inner strength to help redefine purpose for life

See Violent Behavior

SUPPORT SYSTEM, INADEQUATE

Readiness for enhanced family Coping: ability to adapt to tasks associated with care, support of significant other during health crisis

Readiness for enhanced Family processes: activities support the growth of family members

Readiness for enhanced Parenting: children or other dependent person(s) expressing satisfaction with home environment

SUPPRESSION OF LABOR

See Preterm Labor

SURGERY, PERIOPERATIVE CARE

Risk for imbalanced Fluid volume: Risk factor: surgery

Risk for Perioperative Hypothermia: Risk factors: inadequate covering of client, cold surgical room

Risk for Perioperative Positioning injury: Risk factors: predisposing condition, prolonged surgery

SURGERY, POSTOPERATIVE CARE

Decreased activity tolerance r/t pain, surgical procedure

Anxiety r/t change in health status, hospital environment

Deficient Knowledge r/t postoperative expectations, lifestyle changes

Nausea r/t manipulation of gastrointestinal tract, postsurgical anesthesia

Imbalanced Nutrition: less than body requirements r/t anorexia, nausea, vomiting, decreased peristalsis

Ineffective peripheral Tissue Perfusion r/t hypovolemia, circulatory stasis, obesity, prolonged immobility, decreased coughing, decreased deep breathing

Acute Pain r/t inflammation or injury in surgical area

Delayed Surgical recovery r/t extensive surgical procedure, postoperative surgical infection

Urinary retention r/t anesthesia, pain, fear, unfamiliar surroundings, client's position

Risk for Bleeding: Risk factor: surgical procedure

Risk for ineffective Breathing pattern: Risk factors: pain, location of incision, effects of anesthesia or opioids

Risk for Constipation: Risk factors: decreased activity, decreased food or fluid intake, anesthesia, pain medication

Risk for imbalanced Fluid volume: Risk factors: hypermetabolic state, fluid loss during surgery, presence of indwelling tubes, fluids used to distend organ structures being absorbed into body

Risk for Surgical Site Infection: Risk factors: invasive procedure, pain, anesthesia, location of incision, weakened cough as a result of aging

SURGERY, PREOPERATIVE CARE

Anxiety r/t threat to or change in health status, situational crisis, fear of the unknown

Insomnia r/t anxiety about upcoming surgery

Deficient Knowledge r/t preoperative procedures, postoperative expectations

Readiness for enhanced Knowledge: shows understanding of preoperative and postoperative expectations for self-care

SURGICAL RECOVERY, DELAYED

Delayed Surgical recovery (See **Surgical** recovery, delayed, Section II)

Risk for delayed Surgical recovery (See **Surgical** recovery, delayed, risk for, Section II)

SURGICAL SITE INFECTION

Anxiety r/t unforeseen result of surgery

Impaired Comfort r/t surgical site pain

Risk for ineffective Thermoregulation: Risk factor: infectious process

Risk for delayed Surgical Recovery: Risk factor: interrupted healing of surgical site

Readiness for enhanced Knowledge: expresses desire for knowledge of prevention and symptoms of infection

SUSPECTED CHILD ABUSE AND NEGLECT (SCAN), CHILD

Ineffective Activity planning r/t lack of family support

Anxiety: **child** r/t threat of punishment for perceived wrongdoing

Deficient community Health r/t inadequate reporting and follow-up of SCAN

Disturbed personal Identity r/t dysfunctional family processes

Rape-Trauma syndrome r/t altered lifestyle because of abuse, changes in residence

Risk for impaired Resilience: Risk factor: adverse situation

Readiness for enhanced community Coping: obtaining resources to prevent child abuse, neglect

See Child Abuse; Hospitalized Child; Maturational Issues, Adolescent

SUSPECTED CHILD ABUSE AND NEGLECT (SCAN), PARENT

Disabled family Coping r/t dysfunctional family, underdeveloped nurturing parental role, lack of parental support systems or role models

Dysfunctional Family processes r/t inadequate coping skills

S

Ineffective Health maintenance behaviors r/t deficient knowledge of parenting skills as result of unachieved developmental tasks

Ineffective Home Maintenance Behaviors r/t disorganization, parental dysfunction, neglect of safe and nurturing environment

Ineffective Impulse control r/t projection of anger, frustration onto child

Impaired Parenting r/t unrealistic expectations of child; lack of effective role model; unmet social, emotional, or maturational needs of parents; interruption in bonding process

Impaired individual Resilience r/t poor impulse control

Chronic low Self-Esteem r/t lack of successful parenting experiences

Risk for other-directed Violence: parent to child: Risk factors: inadequate coping mechanisms, unresolved stressors, unachieved maturational level by parent

SUSPICION

Disturbed personal Identity r/t psychiatric disorder

Powerlessness r/t repetitive paranoid thinking

Impaired Social interaction r/t disturbed thought processes, paranoid delusions, hallucinations

Risk for self-directed Violence: Risk factor: inability to trust

Risk for other-directed Violence: Risk factor: impulsiveness

SWALLOWING DIFFICULTIES

Impaired Swallowing (See **Swallowing,** impaired, Section II)

SYNCOPE

Anxiety r/t fear of falling

Impaired physical Mobility r/t fear of falling

Ineffective Health self-management r/t lack of knowledge in how to prevent syncope

Social isolation r/t fear of falling

Risk for decreased Cardiac output: Risk factor: dysrhythmia

Risk for Adult Falls: Risk factor: syncope

Risk for Injury: Risk factors: altered sensory perception, transient loss of consciousness, risk for adult falls

Risk for ineffective Cerebral tissue perfusion: Risk factor: interruption of blood flow

SYPHILIS

See STD (Sexually Transmitted Disease)

SYSTEMIC LUPUS ERYTHEMATOSUS

See Lupus Erythematosus

T

T & A (TONSILLECTOMY AND ADENOIDECTOMY)

Ineffective Airway clearance r/t hesitation or reluctance to cough because of pain

Deficient Knowledge: potential for enhanced health maintenance r/t insufficient knowledge regarding postoperative nutritional and rest requirements, signs and symptoms of complications, positioning

Nausea r/t gastric irritation, pharmaceuticals, anesthesia

Acute Pain r/t surgical incision

Risk for Aspiration: Risk factors: postoperative drainage, impaired swallowing

Risk for deficient Fluid volume: Risk factors: decreased intake because of painful swallowing, effects of anesthesia (nausea, vomiting), hemorrhage

Risk for imbalanced Nutrition: less than body requirements: Risk factor: hesitation or reluctance to swallow

TACHYCARDIA

See Dysrhythmia

TACHYPNEA

Ineffective Breathing pattern r/t pain, anxiety, hypoxia

See cause of Tachypnea

TARDIVE DYSKINESIA

Ineffective Health self-management r/t complexity of therapeutic regimen or medication

Deficient Knowledge r/t cognitive limitation in assimilating information relating to side effects associated with neuroleptic medications

Risk for Injury: Risk factor: drug-induced abnormal body movements

TASTE ABNORMALITY

Frail Elderly syndrome r/t chronic illness

TB (PULMONARY TUBERCULOSIS)

Ineffective Airway clearance r/t increased secretions, excessive mucus

Ineffective Breathing pattern r/t decreased energy, fatigue

Fatigue r/t disease state

Impaired Gas exchange r/t disease process

Ineffective Health self-management r/t deficient knowledge of prevention and treatment regimen

Ineffective Home Maintenance Behaviors r/t client or family member with disease

Ineffective Thermoregulation r/t presence of infection

Risk for Infection: Risk factor: insufficient knowledge regarding avoidance of exposure to pathogens

Readiness for enhanced Health management: takes medications according to prescribed protocol for prevention and treatment

TBI (TRAUMATIC BRAIN INJURY)

Interrupted Family processes r/t traumatic injury to family member

Chronic Sorrow r/t change in health status and functional ability

Risk for Post-Trauma syndrome: Risk factor: perception of event causing TBI

Risk for impaired Religiosity: Risk factor: impaired physical mobility

Risk for impaired Resilience: Risk factor: crisis of injury

See Head Injury; Neurologic Disorders

TECHNOLOGY ADDICTION

Decreased Diversional activity engagement r/t insufficient motivation to separate from electronic devices

Impaired Social Interaction r/t lack of desire to engage in personal face-to-face contact with others

Risk for impaired Attachment: Risk factor: preoccupation with electronic devices

Risk for impaired Parenting: Risk factor: insufficient uninterrupted meaningful interaction between parent and child as the result of preoccupation with electronic devices

Risk for ineffective Relationship: Risk factor: ineffective face-to-face communication skills

TEMPERATURE, DECREASED

Hypothermia r/t exposure to cold environment

TEMPERATURE, HIGH

Hyperthermia r/t neurological damage, disease condition with high temperature, excessive heat, inflammatory response

TEMPERATURE REGULATION, IMPAIRED

Ineffective Thermoregulation r/t trauma, illness, cerebral injury

TEN (TOXIC EPIDERMAL NECROLYSIS)

See Toxic Epidermal Necrolysis (TEN)

TENS UNIT (TRANSCUTANEOUS ELECTRICAL NERVE STIMULATION)

Risk for unstable Blood Pressure r/t improper use of TENS unit (front of neck)

Readiness for Enhanced Comfort: expresses desire to enhance resolution of complaints

TENSION

Anxiety r/t threat to or change in health status, situational crisis

Readiness for enhanced Communication: expresses willingness to share feelings and thoughts

See Stress

TERMINALLY ILL ADULT

Death Anxiety r/t unresolved issues relating to death and dying

Imbalanced Energy Field r/t weak energy field patterns

Risk for Spiritual distress: Risk factor: impending death

Readiness for enhanced Religiosity: requests religious material and/or experiences

Readiness for enhanced Spiritual well-being: desire to achieve harmony of mind, body, spirit

See Terminally Ill Child/Death of Child, Parent

TERMINALLY ILL CHILD, ADOLESCENT

Disturbed Body Image r/t effects of terminal disease, already critical feelings of group identity and self-image

Ineffective Coping r/t inability to establish personal and peer identity because of the threat of being different or not being healthy, inability to achieve maturational tasks

Impaired Social interaction r/t forced separation from peers

See Child with Chronic Condition; Hospitalized Child; Terminally Ill Child/ Death of Child, Parent

TERMINALLY ILL CHILD, INFANT/ TODDLER

Ineffective Coping r/t separation from parents and familiar environment from inability to understand dying process

See Child with Chronic Condition; Terminally Ill Child/Death of Child, Parent

TERMINALLY ILL CHILD, PRESCHOOL CHILD

Fear r/t perceived punishment, bodily harm, feelings of guilt caused by magical thinking (i.e., believing that thoughts cause events)

See Child with Chronic Condition; Terminally Ill Child/Death of Child, Parent

TERMINALLY ILL CHILD, SCHOOL-AGE CHILD/PREADOLESCENT

Fear r/t perceived punishment, body mutilation, feelings of guilt

See Child with Chronic Condition; Terminally Ill Child/Death of Child, Parent

TERMINALLY ILL CHILD/DEATH OF CHILD, PARENT

Compromised family Coping r/t inability or unwillingness to discuss impending death and feelings with child or support child through terminal stages of illness

Decisional Conflict r/t continuation or discontinuation of treatment, do-not-resuscitate decision, ethical issues regarding organ donation

Ineffective Denial r/t maladaptive grieving

Interrupted Family processes r/t situational crisis

Hopelessness r/t overwhelming stresses caused by terminal illness

Insomnia r/t grieving process

Impaired Parenting r/t risk for overprotection of surviving siblings

Powerlessness r/t inability to alter course of events

Impaired Social interaction r/t maladaptive grieving

Social isolation: imposed by others r/t feelings of inadequacy in providing support to grieving parents

Social isolation: self-imposed r/t unresolved grief, perceived inadequate parenting skills

Spiritual distress r/t sudden and unexpected death, prolonged suffering before death, questioning the death of youth, questioning the meaning of one's own existence

Risk for maladaptive Grieving: Risk factors: prolonged, unresolved, obstructed progression through stages of grief and mourning

Risk for impaired Resilience: Risk factor: impending death

Readiness for enhanced family Coping: impact of crisis on family values, priorities, goals, or relationships; expressed interest or desire to attach meaning to child's life and death

TETRALOGY OF FALLOT

See Congenital Heart Disease/Cardiac Anomalies

T

TETRAPLEGIA

Autonomic dysreflexia r/t bladder or bowel distention, skin irritation, infection, deficient knowledge of patient and caregiver

Powerlessness r/t inability to perform previous activities

Impaired Sitting r/t paralysis of extremities

Impaired spontaneous Ventilation r/t loss of innervation of respiratory muscles, respiratory muscle fatigue

Risk for Aspiration: Risk factor: inadequate ability to protect airway from neurological damage

Risk for Infection: Risk factor: urinary stasis

Risk for impaired Skin integrity: Risk factor: physical immobilization and decreased sensation

Risk for ineffective Thermoregulation: Risk factors: inability to move to increase temperature, possible presence of infection to increase temperature

THERMOREGULATION, INEFFECTIVE

Ineffective Thermoregulation (See **Thermoregulation,** ineffective, Section II)

Risk for Ineffective Thermoregulation, (See **Ineffective Thermoregulation,** risk for, Section II)

THORACENTESIS

See Pleural Effusion

THORACOTOMY

Decreased activity tolerance r/t pain, imbalance between oxygen supply and demand, presence of chest tubes

Ineffective Airway clearance r/t drowsiness, pain with breathing and coughing

Ineffective Breathing pattern r/t decreased energy, fatigue, pain

Deficient Knowledge r/t self-care, effective breathing exercises, pain relief

Acute Pain r/t surgical procedure, coughing, deep breathing

Risk for Bleeding: Risk factor: surgery

Risk for Surgical Site Infection: Risk factor: invasive procedure

Risk for Injury: Risk factor: disruption of closed-chest drainage system

Risk for Perioperative Positioning injury: Risk factors: lateral positioning, immobility

Risk for Vascular Trauma: Risk factors: chemical irritant; antibiotics

THOUGHT DISORDERS

See Schizophrenia

THROMBOCYTOPENIC PURPURA

See ITP (Idiopathic Thrombocytopenic Purpura)

THROMBOPHLEBITIS

See Deep Vein Thrombosis (DVT)

THYROIDECTOMY

Risk for ineffective Airway clearance r/t edema or hematoma formation, airway obstruction

Risk for impaired verbal Communication: Risk factors: edema, pain, vocal cord or laryngeal nerve damage

Risk for Injury: Risk factor: possible parathyroid damage or removal

See Surgery, Preoperative Care; Surgery, Perioperative Care; Surgery, Postoperative Care

TIA (TRANSIENT ISCHEMIC ATTACK)

Acute Confusion r/t hypoxia

Readiness for enhanced Health management: obtains knowledge regarding treatment prevention of inadequate oxygenation

See Syncope

TIC DISORDER

See Tourette's Syndrome (TS)

TINEA CAPITIS

Impaired Comfort r/t inflammation from skin irritation

See Ringworm of Scalp

TINEA CORPORIS

See Ringworm of Body

TINEA CRURIS

See Jock Itch; Itching; Pruritus

TINEA PEDIS

See Athlete's Foot; Itching; Pruritus

TINEA UNGUIUM (ONYCHOMYCOSIS)

See Ringworm of Nails

TINNITUS

Ineffective Health maintenance behaviors r/t deficient knowledge regarding self-care with tinnitus

Hearing Loss r/t ringing in ears obscuring hearing

TISSUE DAMAGE, INTEGUMENTARY

Impaired Tissue integrity (See **Tissue** integrity, impaired, Section II)

Risk for impaired Tissue integrity (See **Tissue** integrity, impaired, risk for, Section II)

TISSUE PERFUSION, PERIPHERAL

Ineffective peripheral Tissue Perfusion (See **Tissue Perfusion**, peripheral, ineffective, Section II)

Risk for ineffective peripheral Tissue Perfusion (See **Tissue Perfusion,** peripheral, ineffective, risk for, Section II)

TOILETING PROBLEMS

Toileting Self-Care deficit r/t impaired transfer ability, impaired mobility status, intolerance of activity, neuromuscular impairment, cognitive impairment

Impaired Transfer ability r/t neuromuscular deficits

TOILET TRAINING

Deficient Knowledge: **parent** r/t signs of child's readiness for training

Risk for Constipation: Risk factor: withholding stool

Risk for Infection: Risk factor: withholding urination

TONSILLECTOMY AND ADENOIDECTOMY (T & A)

See T & A (Tonsillectomy and Adenoidectomy)

TOOTHACHE

Impaired Dentition r/t ineffective oral hygiene, barriers to self-care, economic barriers to professional care, nutritional deficits, lack of knowledge regarding dental health

Acute Pain r/t inflammation, infection

TOTAL ANOMALOUS PULMONARY VENOUS RETURN

See Congenital Heart Disease/Cardiac Anomalies

TOTAL JOINT REPLACEMENT (TOTAL HIP/TOTAL KNEE/ SHOULDER)

Disturbed Body Image r/t large scar, presence of prosthesis

Impaired physical Mobility r/t musculoskeletal impairment, surgery, prosthesis

Risk for Injury: neurovascular: Risk factors: altered peripheral tissue perfusion, impaired mobility, prosthesis

Risk for Peripheral Neurovascular dysfunction r/t immobilization, surgical procedure

Ineffective peripheral Tissue perfusion r/t surgery

See Surgery, Preoperative Care; Surgery, Perioperative Care; Surgery, Postoperative Care

TOTAL PARENTERAL NUTRITION (TPN)

See TPN (Total Parenteral Nutrition)

TOURETTE'S SYNDROME (TS)

Hopelessness r/t inability to control behavior

Impaired individual Resilience r/t uncontrollable behavior

Risk for situational low Self-Esteem: Risk factors: uncontrollable behavior, motor and phonic tics

See Attention Deficit Disorder

TOXEMIA

See PIH (Pregnancy-Induced Hypertension/Preeclampsia)

TOXIC EPIDERMAL NECROLYSIS (TEN) (ERYTHEMA MULTIFORME)

Death Anxiety r/t uncertainty of prognosis

TPN (TOTAL PARENTERAL NUTRITION)

Imbalanced Nutrition: less than body requirements r/t inability to digest food or absorb nutrients as a result of biological or psychological factors

Risk for Electrolyte imbalance: Risk factor: need for regulation of electrolytes in TPN fluids

Risk for excess Fluid volume: Risk factor: rapid administration of TPN

Risk for unstable blood Glucose level: Risk factor: high glucose levels in TPN to be regulated according to blood glucose levels

Risk for Infection: Risk factors: concentrated glucose solution, invasive administration of fluids

Risk for Vascular Trauma: Risk factors: insertion site, length of treatment time

TRACHEOESOPHAGEAL FISTULA

Ineffective Airway clearance r/t aspiration of feeding because of inability to swallow

Imbalanced Nutrition: less than body requirements r/t difficulties swallowing

Risk for Aspiration: Risk factor: common passage of air and food

Risk for Vascular Trauma: Risk factors: venous medications and site

See Respiratory Conditions of the Neonate; Hospitalized Child

TRACHEOSTOMY

Ineffective Airway clearance r/t increased secretions, mucous plugs

Anxiety r/t impaired verbal communication, ineffective airway clearance

Disturbed Body Image r/t abnormal opening in neck

Impaired verbal Communication r/t presence of mechanical airway

Deficient Knowledge r/t self-care, home maintenance management

Acute Pain r/t edema, surgical procedure

Risk for Aspiration: Risk factor: presence of tracheostomy

Risk for Bleeding: Risk factor: surgical incision

Risk for Surgical Site Infection: Risk factors: invasive procedure, pooling of secretions

TRACTION AND CASTS

Constipation r/t immobility

Decreased Diversional activity engagement r/t immobility

Impaired physical Mobility r/t imposed restrictions on activity because of bone or joint disease injury

Acute Pain r/t immobility, injury, or disease

Self-Care deficit: feeding, dressing, bathing, toileting r/t degree of impaired physical mobility, body area affected by traction or cast

Impaired Transfer ability r/t presence of traction, casts

Risk for Disuse syndrome: Risk factor: mechanical immobilization

See Casts

TRANSFER ABILITY

Impaired Transfer ability (See **Transfer** ability, impaired, Section II)

TRANSIENT ISCHEMIC ATTACK (TIA)

See TIA (Transient Ischemic Attack)

TRANSPOSITION OF GREAT VESSELS

See Congenital Heart Disease/Cardiac Anomalies

TRANSURETHRAL RESECTION OF THE PROSTATE (TURP)

See TURP (Transurethral Resection of the Prostate)

TRAUMA IN PREGNANCY

Anxiety r/t threat to self or fetus, unknown outcome

Deficient Knowledge r/t lack of exposure to situation

Acute Pain r/t trauma

Impaired Skin integrity r/t trauma

Risk for Bleeding: Risk factor: trauma

Risk for deficient Fluid volume: Risk factor: fluid loss

Risk for Infection: Risk factor: traumatized tissue

Risk for Injury: fetal: Risk factor: premature separation of placenta

Risk for disturbed Maternal–Fetal dyad: Risk factor: complication of pregnancy

TRAUMA, PHYSICAL, RISK FOR

Risk for Physical Trauma (See **Physical Trauma**, risk for, Section II)

TRAUMATIC BRAIN INJURY (TBI)

See TBI (Traumatic Brain Injury); Intracranial Pressure, Increased

TRAUMATIC EVENT

Post-Trauma syndrome r/t previously experienced trauma

TRAVELER'S DIARRHEA

Diarrhea r/t travel with exposure to different bacteria, viruses

Risk for deficient Fluid Volume: Risk factor: excessive loss of fluids

Risk for Infection: Risk factors: insufficient knowledge regarding avoidance of exposure to pathogens (water supply, iced drinks, local cheese, ice cream, undercooked meat, fish and shellfish, uncooked vegetables, unclean eating utensils, improper handwashing

TREMBLING OF HANDS

Fear r/t threat to or change in health status, threat of death, situational crisis

TRICUSPID ATRESIA

See Congenital Heart Disease/Cardiac Anomalies

TRIGEMINAL NEURALGIA

Ineffective Health self-management r/t deficient knowledge regarding prevention of stimuli that trigger pain

Imbalanced Nutrition: less than body requirements r/t pain when chewing

Acute Pain r/t irritation of trigeminal nerve

Risk for corneal Injury: Risk factor: possible decreased corneal sensation

TRUNCUS ARTERIOSUS

See Congenital Heart Disease/Cardiac Anomalies

TS (TOURETTE'S SYNDROME)

See Tourette's Syndrome (TS)

TESTICULAR SELF-EXAMINATION

Readiness for enhanced Health management: seeks information regarding self-examination

TUBAL LIGATION

Decisional Conflict r/t tubal sterilization

See Laparoscopy

TUBE FEEDING

Risk for Aspiration: Risk factors: nasogastric tube (NG) improperly administered feeding, improper placement of tube, improper positioning of client during and after feeding, excessive residual feeding or lack of digestion, altered gag reflex

Risk for deficient Fluid volume: Risk factor: inadequate water administration with concentrated feeding

Risk for imbalanced Nutrition: less than body requirements: Risk factors: intolerance to tube feeding, inadequate calorie replacement to meet metabolic needs

TUBERCULOSIS (TB)

See TB (Pulmonary Tuberculosis)

TURP (TRANSURETHRAL RESECTION OF THE PROSTATE)

Deficient Knowledge r/t postoperative self-care, home maintenance management

Acute Pain r/t incision, irritation from catheter, bladder spasms, kidney infection

Urinary retention r/t obstruction of urethra or catheter with clots

Risk for Bleeding: Risk factor: surgery

Risk for deficient Fluid volume: Risk factors: fluid loss, possible bleeding

Risk for urge urinary Incontinence: Risk factor: edema from surgical procedure

Risk for Infection: Risk factors: invasive procedure, route for bacteria entry

U

ULCER, PEPTIC (DUODENAL OR GASTRIC)

Fatigue r/t loss of blood, chronic illness

Ineffective Health maintenance behaviors r/t lack of knowledge regarding health practices to prevent ulcer formation

Nausea r/t gastrointestinal irritation

Acute Pain r/t irritated mucosa from acid secretion

See GI Bleed (Gastrointestinal Bleeding)

ULCERATIVE COLITIS

See Inflammatory Bowel Disease (Child and Adult)

ULCERS, STASIS

See Stasis Ulcer

UNILATERAL NEGLECT OF ONE SIDE OF BODY

Unilateral Neglect (See **Unilateral Neglect,** Section II)

UNSANITARY LIVING CONDITIONS

Ineffective Home Maintenance Behaviors r/t impaired cognitive or emotional functioning, lack of knowledge, insufficient finances, addiction

Risk for Allergic reaction: Risk factor: exposure to environmental contaminants

UPPER RESPIRATORY INFECTION

See Cold, Viral

URGENCY TO URINATE

Urge urinary Incontinence (See **Incontinence,** urinary, urge, Section II)

Risk for urge urinary Incontinence (See **Incontinence,** urinary, urge, risk for, Section II)

URINARY CATHETER

Risk for urinary tract Injury: Risk factors: confused client, long-term use of catheter, large retention balloon or catheter, perirectal burn injured client

URINARY DIVERSION

See Ileal Conduit

URINARY ELIMINATION, IMPAIRED

Impaired Urinary elimination (See **Urinary** elimination, impaired, Section II)

URINARY INCONTINENCE

See Incontinence of Urine

URINARY RETENTION

Urinary Retention (See **Urinary Retention,** Section II)

URINARY TRACT INFECTION (UTI)

See UTI (Urinary Tract Infection)

UROLITHIASIS

See Kidney Stone

UTERINE ATONY IN LABOR

See Dystocia

UTERINE ATONY IN POSTPARTUM

See Postpartum Hemorrhage

UTERINE BLEEDING

See Hemorrhage; Postpartum Hemorrhage; Shock, Hypovolemic

UTI (URINARY TRACT INFECTION)

Ineffective Health maintenance behaviors r/t deficient knowledge regarding methods to treat and prevent UTIs, prolonged use of indwelling urinary catheter

Acute Pain: dysuria r/t inflammatory process in bladder

Impaired Urinary elimination: frequency r/t urinary tract infection

Risk for acute Confusion (in elderly only): Risk factor: infectious process

Risk for urge urinary Incontinence: Risk factor: hyperreflexia from cystitis

V

VAD (VENTRICULAR ASSIST DEVICE)

See Ventricular Assist Device (VAD)

VAGINAL HYSTERECTOMY

Urinary retention r/t edema at surgical site

Risk for urge urinary Incontinence: Risk factors: edema, congestion of pelvic tissues

Risk for Infection: Risk factor: surgical site

Risk for Perioperative Positioning injury: Risk factor: lithotomy position

VAGINITIS

Impaired Comfort r/t pruritus, itching

Ineffective Health maintenance behaviors r/t deficient knowledge regarding self-care with vaginitis

Ineffective Sexuality pattern r/t abstinence during acute stage, pain

VAGOTOMY

See Abdominal Surgery

VALUE SYSTEM CONFLICT

Decisional Conflict r/t unclear personal values or beliefs

Spiritual distress r/t challenged value system

Readiness for enhanced Spiritual well-being: desire for harmony with self, others, higher power, God

VARICOSE VEINS

Ineffective Health maintenance behaviors r/t deficient knowledge regarding healthcare practices, prevention, treatment regimen

Chronic Pain r/t impaired circulation

Ineffective peripheral Tissue Perfusion r/t venous stasis

Risk for impaired Tissue integrity: Risk factor: altered peripheral tissue perfusion

VASCULAR DEMENTIA (FORMERLY CALLED MULTI-INFARCT DEMENTIA)

See Dementia

VASECTOMY

Decisional Conflict r/t surgery as method of permanent sterilization

VENEREAL DISEASE

See STD (Sexually Transmitted Disease)

VENOUS THROMBOEMBOLISM (VTE)

Anxiety r/t lack of circulation to body part

Acute Pain r/t vascular obstruction

Ineffective peripheral Tissue Perfusion r/t interruption of circulatory flow

Risk for Peripheral Neurovascular dysfunction: Risk factor: vascular obstruction

(See **Venous Thromboembolism**, Risk for, Section II)

VENTILATED CLIENT, MECHANICALLY

Ineffective Airway clearance r/t increased secretions, decreased cough and gag reflex

Ineffective Breathing pattern r/t decreased energy and fatigue as a result of possible altered nutrition: less than body requirements, neurological disease or damage

Impaired verbal Communication r/t presence of endotracheal tube, inability to phonate

Fear r/t inability to breathe on own, difficulty communicating

Impaired Gas exchange r/t ventilation-perfusion imbalance

Powerlessness r/t health treatment regimen

Social isolation r/t impaired mobility, ventilator dependence

Impaired spontaneous Ventilation r/t metabolic factors, respiratory muscle fatigue

Dysfunctional Ventilatory weaning response r/t psychological, situational, physiological factors

Risk for Adult Falls: Risk factors: impaired mobility, decreased muscle strength

Risk for Infection: Risk factors: presence of endotracheal tube, pooled secretions

Risk for Adult pressure Injury: Risk factor: decreased mobility

Risk for impaired Resilience: Risk factor: illness

See Child with Chronic Condition; Hospitalized Child; Respiratory Conditions of the Neonate

VENTRICULAR ASSIST DEVICE (VAD)

Anxiety r/t possible failure of device

Risk for Infection: Risk factor: device insertion site

Risk for Vascular Trauma: Risk factor: insertion site

Readiness for enhanced Decision-Making: expresses desire to enhance the understanding of the meaning of choices regarding implanting a VAD

See Open Heart Surgery

VENTRICULAR FIBRILLATION

See Dysrhythmia

VETERANS

Anxiety r/t possible unmet needs, both physical and psychological

Risk for Post-Trauma Syndrome: Risk factors: witnessing death, survivor role, guilt, environment not conducive to needs

Risk for Suicidal Behavior: Risk factors: substance abuse, insufficient social support, physical injury, psychiatric disorder

VERTIGO

See Syncope

VIOLENT BEHAVIOR

Risk for other-directed Violence (See **Violence,** other-directed, risk for, Section II)

Risk for self-directed Violence (See **Violence,** self-directed, risk for, Section II)

VIRAL GASTROENTERITIS

Diarrhea r/t infectious process, Norovirus

Deficient Fluid volume r/t vomiting, diarrhea

Ineffective Health self-management r/t inadequate handwashing

See Gastroenteritis, Child

VISION IMPAIRMENT

Fear r/t loss of sight

Social isolation r/t altered state of wellness, inability to see

Risk for impaired Resilience: Risk factor: presence of new crisis

See Blindness; Cataracts; Glaucoma

VOMITING

Nausea r/t infectious processes, chemotherapy, postsurgical anesthesia, irritation to the gastrointestinal system, stimulation of neuropharmacological mechanisms

Imbalanced Nutrition: less than body requirements r/t inability to ingest food

Risk for Electrolyte imbalance: Risk factor: vomiting

VTE (VENOUS THROMBOEMBOLISM)

See Venous Thromboembolism, Risk for, Section II

W

WALKING IMPAIRMENT

Impaired Walking (See **Walking,** impaired, Section II)

WANDERING

Wandering (See **Wandering,** Section II)

WEAKNESS

Fatigue r/t decreased or increased metabolic energy production

Risk for Adult Falls: Risk factor: weakness

WEIGHT GAIN

Overweight (See **Overweight,** Section II)

WEIGHT LOSS

Imbalanced Nutrition: less than body requirements r/t inability to ingest food because of biological, psychological, economic factors

WELLNESS-SEEKING BEHAVIOR

Readiness for enhanced Health self-management: expresses desire for increased control of health practice

WERNICKE-KORSAKOFF SYNDROME

See Korsakoff's Syndrome

WEST NILE VIRUS

See Meningitis/Encephalitis

WHEELCHAIR USE PROBLEMS

Impaired wheelchair Mobility (See **Mobility,** wheelchair, impaired, Section II)

WHEEZING

Ineffective Airway clearance r/t tracheobronchial obstructions, secretions

WILMS' TUMOR

Chronic functional Constipation r/t obstruction associated with presence of tumor

Acute Pain r/t pressure from tumor

See Chemotherapy; Hospitalized Child; Radiation Therapy; Surgery, Preoperative Care; Surgery, Perioperative Care; Surgery, Postoperative Care

WITHDRAWAL FROM ALCOHOL

See Alcohol Withdrawal

WITHDRAWAL FROM DRUGS

See Acute Substance Withdrawal Syndrome

WOUND DEBRIDEMENT

Acute Pain r/t debridement of wound

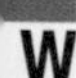

Impaired Tissue integrity r/t debridement, open wound

Risk for Infection: Risk factors: open wound, presence of bacteria

WOUND DEHISCENCE, EVISCERATION

Fear r/t client fear of body parts "falling out," surgical procedure not going as planned

Disturbed Body Image r/t change in body structure and wound appearance

Imbalanced Nutrition: **less than body requirements** r/t inability to digest nutrients, need for increased protein for healing

Risk for deficient Fluid volume: Risk factors: inability to ingest nutrients, obstruction, fluid loss

Risk for Injury: Risk factor: exposed abdominal contents

Risk for delayed Surgical recovery: Risk factors: separation of wound, exposure of abdominal contents

Risk for Surgical Site Infection: Risk factor: open wound after surgical procedure

WOUND INFECTION

Disturbed Body Image r/t open wound

Imbalanced Nutrition: **less than body requirements** r/t biological factors, infection, fever

Ineffective Thermoregulation r/t infection in wound resulting in fever

Impaired Tissue integrity r/t wound, presence of infection

Risk for imbalanced Fluid volume: Risk factor: increased metabolic rate

Risk for Infection: spread of: Risk factor: imbalanced nutrition: less than body requirements

Risk for delayed Surgical recovery: Risk factor: presence of infection

WOUNDS, OPEN

See Lacerations

SECTION

II

Guide to Planning Care

Section II is a listing of nursing diagnosis care plans according to NANDA-I. The care plans are arranged alphabetically by diagnostic concept.

MAKING AN ACCURATE NURSING DIAGNOSIS

Verify the accuracy of the previously suggested nursing diagnoses (from Section I) for the client. To do this:

- Read the definition for the suggested nursing diagnosis and determine if it sounds appropriate.
- Compare the Defining Characteristics with the symptoms that were identified from the client data collected.
- Compare the Risk Factors with the symptoms that were identified from the client data collected (if it is a "Risk for" Nursing Diagnosis, they do not have defining characteristics).

WRITING OUTCOMES, STATEMENTS, AND NURSING INTERVENTIONS

After selecting the appropriate nursing diagnosis, use this section to write outcomes and interventions by using the Client Outcomes/Nursing Interventions as written.

Following these steps, you will be able to write a nursing care plan:

- Follow this care plan to administer nursing care to the client.
- Document all steps and evaluate and update the care plan as needed.

Decreased Activity Tolerance

NANDA-I Definition

Insufficient endurance to complete required or desired daily activities

Defining Characteristics

Abnormal blood pressure response to activity; abnormal heart rate response to activity; anxious when activity is required; electrocardiogram change; exertional discomfort; exertional dyspnea; expresses fatigue; generalized weakness

Related Factors

Decreased muscle strength; depressive symptoms; fear of pain; imbalance between oxygen supply/demand; impaired physical mobility; inexperience with an activity; insufficient muscle mass; malnutrition; pain; physical deconditioning; sedentary lifestyle

At-Risk Population

Individuals with history of decreased activity tolerance; older adults

Associated Conditions

Neoplasms; neurodegenerative diseases; respiration disorders; traumatic brain injuries; vitamin D deficiency

Client Outcomes

Client Will (Specify Time Frame)

- Participate in prescribed physical activity with appropriate changes in heart rate, blood pressure, and breathing rate; maintain monitor patterns (rhythm and ST segment) within normal limits
- State symptoms of adverse effects of exercise and report onset of symptoms immediately
- Maintain normal skin color; skin is warm and dry with activity
- Verbalize an understanding of the need to gradually increase activity based on testing, tolerance, and symptoms
- Demonstrate increased tolerance to activity

Nursing Interventions

- Determine cause of decreased activity tolerance (see Related Factors) and determine whether cause is physical, psychological, or motivational.
- If mainly on bed rest, minimize cardiovascular, neuromuscular, and skeletal deconditioning by positioning the client in an upright position several times daily if possible and performing simple range-of-motion (ROM) techniques (passive or active).
- Assess the client daily for appropriateness of activity and bed rest orders. Mobilize the client as soon as possible.
- If the client is mostly immobile, consider use of a transfer chair or a chair that becomes a stretcher.

- When appropriate, gradually increase activity, allowing the client to assist with positioning, transferring, and self-care as able. Progress the client from sitting in bed to dangling, to standing, to ambulation. Always have the client dangle at the bedside before standing to evaluate for postural hypotension.
- ▲ When getting a client up, observe for symptoms of intolerance such as nausea, pallor, dizziness, visual dimming, and impaired consciousness, as well as changes in vital signs; manual blood pressure monitoring is best.
- If the client has symptoms of postural hypotension, such as dizziness, lightheadedness, or pallor, take precautions, such as dangling the client and applying leg compression stockings before the client stands.
- Perform ROM exercises if the client is unable to tolerate activity or is mostly immobile. See care plan for Risk for **Disuse** syndrome.
- Monitor and record the client's ability to tolerate activity: note pulse rate, blood pressure, respiratory pattern, dyspnea, use of accessory muscles, and skin color before, during, and after the activity. If the following signs and symptoms of cardiac decompensation develop, activity should be stopped immediately:
  - Onset of chest discomfort or pain
  - Dyspnea
  - Palpitations
  - Excessive fatigue
  - Lightheadedness, confusion, ataxia, pallor, cyanosis, nausea, or any peripheral circulatory insufficiency
  - Dysrhythmia
  - Exercise hypotension
  - Excessive rise in blood pressure
  - Inappropriate bradycardia
  - Increased heart rate
  - Decreased oxygen saturation
- ▲ Instruct the client to stop the activity immediately and report to the healthcare provider if the client is experiencing the following symptoms: new or worsened intensity or increased frequency of discomfort; tightness or pressure in chest, back, neck, jaw, shoulders, and/or arms; palpitations; dizziness; weakness; unusual and extreme fatigue; or excessive air hunger.

A

- • Observe and document skin integrity several times a day. Refer to the care plan Risk for impaired **Skin** integrity.
- • Assess for constipation. If present, refer to care plan for **Constipation.**
- ▲ Refer the client to physical therapy to help increase activity levels and strength.
- ▲ Consider a dietitian referral to assess nutritional needs related to **Decreased Activity** tolerance; provide nutrition as indicated. If the client is unable to eat food, use enteral or parenteral feedings as needed.
- • Recognize that malnutrition causes significant morbidity because of the loss of lean body mass.
- • Provide emotional support and encouragement to the client to gradually increase activity. Work with the client to set mutual goals that increase activity levels. Fear of breathlessness, pain, or falling may decrease willingness to increase activity.
- ▲ Observe for pain before activity. If possible, treat pain before activity and ensure that the client is not heavily sedated.
- ▲ Obtain any necessary assistive devices or equipment needed before ambulating the client (e.g., walkers, canes, crutches, portable oxygen).
- ▲ Use a gait-walking belt when ambulating the client.

Decreased Activity Tolerance Due to Respiratory Disease

- • If the client is able to walk and has chronic obstructive pulmonary disease (COPD), use the traditional 6-minute walk distance to evaluate ability to walk.
- ▲ Ensure that the chronic pulmonary client has oxygen saturation testing with exercise. Use supplemental oxygen to keep oxygen saturation 90% or above or as prescribed with activity.
- • Monitor a respiratory client's response to activity by observing for symptoms of respiratory intolerance, such as increased dyspnea, loss of ability to control breathing rhythmically, use of accessory muscles, nasal flaring, appearance of facial distress, and skin tone changes such as pallor and cyanosis.
- • Instruct and assist the client with COPD in using conscious, controlled breathing techniques during exercise, including pursed-lip breathing, and inspiratory muscle use.
- ▲ Evaluate the client's nutritional status. Refer to a dietitian if indicated. Use nutritional supplements to increase nutritional level if needed.

A

▲ For the client in the intensive care unit, consider mobilizing the client with passive exercise.

Decreased Activity Tolerance Due to Cardiovascular Disease

• If the client is able to walk and has heart failure, consider use of the 6-minute walk test to determine physical ability.

• Allow for periods of rest before and after planned exertion periods such as meals, baths, treatments, and physical activity.

▲ Refer to a heart failure program or cardiac rehabilitation program for education, evaluation, and guided support to increase activity and rebuild life.).

▲ Refer to a community support program that includes support of significant others.

• See care plan for Decreased **Cardiac** output for further interventions.

Pediatric

• Focus interview questions toward exercise tolerance specifically including any history of asthma exacerbations.

Geriatric

• Slow the pace of care. Allow the client extra time to perform physical activities.

• Encourage families to help/allow an older client to be independent in whatever activities possible.

▲ Assess for swaying, poor balance, weakness, and fear of falling while older clients stand/walk. Refer to physical therapy if appropriate.

• Refer to the care plan for Risk for **Adult Falls** and Impaired **Walking.**

▲ Initiate ambulation by simply ambulating a patient a few steps from bed to chair, once a healthcare provider's out-of-bed order is obtained.

▲ Evaluate medications the client is taking to see if they could be causing **Decreased Activity** tolerance.

▲ If heart disease is causing **Decreased Activity** tolerance, refer the client for cardiac rehabilitation.

▲ Refer the disabled older client to physical therapy for functional training including gait training, stepping, and sit-to-stand exercises, or for strength training.

Home Care

▲ Begin discharge planning as soon as possible with the case manager or social worker to assess the need for home support systems and the need for community or home health services.

- ▲ Assess the home environment for factors that contribute to decreased activity tolerance such as stairs or distance to the bathroom. Refer the client for occupational therapy, if needed, and to assist the client in restructuring the home and ADL patterns.
- ▲ Refer the client for physical therapy for strength training and possible weight training to regain strength, increase endurance, and improve balance. If the client is homebound, the physical therapist can also initiate cardiac rehabilitation.
- • Encourage progress with positive feedback. The client's experience should be validated within expected norms. Recognition of progress enhances motivation.
- • Teach the client/family the importance of and methods for setting priorities for activities, especially those having a high energy demand (e.g., home/family events). Instruct in realistic expectations.
- • Encourage routine low-level exercise periods such as a daily short walk or chair exercises.
- • Provide the client/family with resources such as senior centers, exercise classes, educational and recreational programs, and volunteer opportunities that can aid in promoting socialization and appropriate activity. Social isolation can be an outcome of and contribute to **Decreased Activity** tolerance.
- • Instruct the client and family in the importance of maintaining proper nutrition.
- • Instruct the client in use of dietary supplements as indicated. Illness may suppress appetite, leading to inadequate nutrition.
- ▲ Refer to medical social services as necessary to assist the family in adjusting to major changes in patterns of living because of **Decreased Activity** tolerance.
- ▲ Assess the need for long-term supports for optimal activity tolerance of priority activities (e.g., assistive devices, oxygen, medication, catheters, massage), especially for a hospice client. Evaluate intermittently.
- ▲ Refer to home health aide services to support the client and family through changing levels of activity tolerance. Introduce aide support early. Instruct the aide to promote independence in activity as tolerated.
- • Allow terminally ill clients and their families to guide care. Control by the client or family respects their autonomy and promotes effective coping.
- • Provide increased attention to comfort and dignity of the terminally ill client in care planning.

- ▲ Institute case management of frail elderly to support continued independent living.

Client/Family Teaching and Discharge Planning

- • Instruct the client on techniques for avoiding **Decreased Activity** tolerance, such as controlled breathing techniques.
- • Teach the client techniques to decrease dizziness from postural hypotension when standing up.
- • Help client with energy conservation and work simplification techniques in ADLs.
- • Describe to the client the symptoms of **Decreased Activity** tolerance, including which symptoms to report to the physician.
- • Explain to the client how to use assistive devices, oxygen, or medications before or during activity.
- • Help the client set up an activity log to record exercise and exercise tolerance.

Risk for Decreased Activity Tolerance

NANDA-I Definition

Susceptible to experiencing insufficient endurance to complete required or desired daily activities.

Risk Factors

Decreased muscle strength; depressive symptoms; fear of pain; imbalance between oxygen supply/demand; impaired physical mobility; inexperience with an activity; insufficient muscle mass; malnutrition; pain; physical deconditioning; sedentary lifestyle

At-Risk Population

Individuals with history of decreased activity tolerance; older adults

Associated Conditions

Neoplasms; neurodegenerative diseases; respiration disorders; traumatic brain injuries; vitamin D deficiency

Client Outcomes, Nursing Interventions, Client/Family Teaching and Discharge Planning

Refer to care plan for **Decreased Activity** tolerance.

Ineffective Activity Planning

NANDA-I Definition

Inability to prepare for a set of actions fixed in time and under certain conditions

Defining Characteristics

Absence of plan; excessive anxiety about a task to be undertaken; fear about task to be undertaken; insufficient organizational skills; insufficient resources; pattern of failure; pattern of procrastination; unmet goals for chosen activity; worried about a task to be undertaken

Related Factors

Flight behavior when faced with proposed solution; hedonism; insufficient information processing ability; insufficient social support; pattern of procrastination; unrealistic perception of event; unrealistic perception of personal abilities

Client Outcomes

Client Will (Specify Time Frame)

- Verbalize need for self-directed activity
- Choose the healthcare option that fits his or her lifestyle within an appropriate amount of time that allows enactment of the choice
- Describe how the chosen option fits into current lifestyle before or after the decision has been made
- Verbalize the need for a behavioral change to improve physical activity
- Offer alternative options to those with barriers to participating in physical activity

Nursing Interventions

- Ask clients how they perceive the situation to gather their personal vision of the problem and how they envisage their self-involvement. Specify the goals.
  - Identify the informational needs of the client: understanding of the client's state of health, supervision of client's treatment if he or she is receiving treatment, diet, and important telephone numbers.
  - Tackle the client's fears and worries and encourage him or her to make a cognitive reconstruction. Use "desire thinking." Drill and repeat: "I can change false ideas that make me believe that I am unable to carry out (achieve) my plan."
- Client verbalizes need for behavioral change for improved physical activity.
- Encourage clients to verbalize the need for physical activity to help reduce role overload.

▲ Determine as fairly as possible the success factors needed for the planning and success of the project: financial resources; the family situation; prior medical, psychiatric, and psychosocial conditions; material resources; and the ability to manage stress.

▲ Older adult patients may be able to delay or prevent problems of chronic diseases by engaging in physical activity (Watson et al., 2016).

Pediatric

- Begin activity planning in preschool-aged children of working parents.
- Establish a contract.
- Provide support to the schools for physical activities in all school venues.
- Support safe neighborhood activity programs.

Geriatric

- Plan activities for older clients.
- Plan activities for older clients with impaired mental function.
- Community-based activities for older adults.

Multicultural

- Provide literature and information in the appropriate language for the client who speaks little to no English.
- Preplanning educational programs for the culturally diverse population needs to be developed.
- Education with support from the physician and family to provide teaching on how exercise can help reduce and/or prevent falls of older adults.

Home Care

- Have a preplanned activity exercise for the home client with a debilitating musculoskeletal disease to help improve functional status.
- Assess the home environment for barriers that can impact the client's motivation to be a participant in the activity planned.
- Home care for the cardiac rehabilitation patient:
- For additional interventions, refer to care plans **Anxiety,** Readiness for enhanced family **Coping,** Readiness for enhanced **Decision-Making, Fear,** Readiness for enhanced **Hope,** Readiness for enhanced **Power,** Readiness for enhanced **Spiritual** well-being, and Readiness for enhanced **Health** management.

Risk for Ineffective Activity Planning

NANDA-I Definition

Susceptible to an inability to prepare for a set of actions fixed in time and under certain conditions, which may compromise health

A

Risk Factors

Flight behavior when faced with proposed solution; hedonism; insufficient information processing ability; insufficient social support; pattern of procrastination; unrealistic perception of event; unrealistic perception of personal abilities

Client Outcomes, Nursing Interventions, Client/Family Teaching and Discharge Planning

Refer to ineffective **Activity** planning.

Ineffective Airway Clearance

NANDA-I Definition

Reduced ability to clear secretions or obstructions from the respiratory tract to maintain a clear airway.

Defining Characteristics

Absence of cough; adventitious breath sounds; altered respiratory rhythm; altered thoracic percussion; altered thoraco-vocal fremitus; bradypena; cyanosis; difficulty verbalizing; diminished breath sounds; excessive sputum; hypoxemia; ineffective cough; ineffective sputum elimination; nasal flaring; orthopnea; psychomotor agitation; subcostal retraction; tachypena; use of accessory muscles of respiration

Related Factors

Dehydration; excessive mucus; exposure to harmful substance; fear of pain; foreign body in airway; inattentive to second-hand smoke; mucus plug; retained secretions; smoking

At Risk Population

Children; infants

Associated Condition

Airway spasm; allergic airway; asthma; chronic obstructive pulmonary disease; congential heart disease; critical illness; exudate in the alveoli; general anesthesia; hyperplasia of the bronchial walls; neuromuscular impairment; respiratory tract infection

Client Outcomes

Client Will (Specify Time Frame)

- Demonstrate effective coughing and clear breath sounds
- Maintain a patent airway at all times
- Explain methods useful to enhance secretion removal
- Explain the significance of changes in sputum to include color, character, amount, and odor
- Identify and avoid specific factors that inhibit effective airway clearance

Nursing Interventions

- • Auscultate breath sounds every 1 to 4 hours. The presence of crackles and wheezes may alert the nurse to airway obstruction, which may lead to or exacerbate existing hypoxia.
- • Monitor respiratory patterns, including rate, depth, and effort.
- • Monitor blood gas values and pulse oxygen saturation levels as available. An oxygen saturation of less than 90% (normal: 95%–100%) or a partial pressure of oxygen of less than 80 mm Hg (normal: 80–100 mm Hg) indicates significant oxygenation problems (Bickley & Szilagyi, 2017; Siela & Kidd, 2017; Lee, 2017).
- ▲ Administer oxygen as ordered.
- • Position the client in a semirecumbent position with the head of the bed at a 30- to 45-degree angle to decrease the aspiration of gastric, oral, and nasal secretions (American Association of Critical Care Nurses, 2016, 2017; Grap, 2009; Siela, 2010; Vollman et al., 2017).
- • Help the client deep breathe and perform controlled coughing. Have the client inhale deeply, hold breath for several seconds, and cough two or three times with mouth open while tightening the upper abdominal muscles.
- • If the client has obstructive lung disease, such as COPD, cystic fibrosis, or bronchiectasis, consider helping the client use the forced expiratory technique called the "huff cough." The client does a series of coughs while saying the word "huff."
- ▲ Encourage the client to use an incentive spirometer. Recognize that controlled coughing and deep breathing may be just as effective as incentive spirometry (Gosselink et al., 2008; GOLD, 2017).
- • Encourage activity and ambulation as tolerated. If the client cannot be ambulated, turn the client from side to side at least every 2 hours. (See interventions for impaired **Gas** exchange for further information on positioning a respiratory client.)
- • Encourage fluid intake of up to 2500 mL/day within cardiac or renal reserve.
- ▲ Administer medications such as bronchodilators or inhaled steroids as ordered. Watch for side effects such as tachycardia or anxiety with bronchodilators, or inflamed pharynx with inhaled steroids.
- ▲ Provide percussion, vibration, and oscillation as appropriate for individual client needs.
- • Observe sputum, noting color, odor, and volume. Normal sputum is clear or gray and minimal, whereas abnormal sputum is green, yellow,

or bloody; malodorous; and often copious. The presence of purulent sputum during a COPD exacerbation can be a sufficient indication for starting empirical antibiotic treatment. Notify healthcare provider of purulent sputum (GOLD, 2017).

Critical Care

- ▲ In intubated clients, body positioning and mobilization may optimize airway secretion clearance. Reposition the client as needed. Use rotational or kinetic bed therapy in clients for whom side-to-side turning is contraindicated or difficult.
- • If the client is intubated, consider use of kinetic therapy. Using a kinetic therapy bed slowly moves the client with 40-degree turns.
- • If the client is intubated and is stable, consider getting the client up to sit at the edge of the bed, transfer to a chair, or walk as appropriate, if an effective interdisciplinary team is developed to keep the client safe (Balas et al., 2012; Costa et al., 2017).
- • When suctioning an endotracheal tube or tracheostomy tube for a client on a ventilator, do the following:
  - Explain the process of suctioning beforehand and ensure the client is not in pain or overly anxious. Suctioning can be a frightening experience; an explanation along with adequate pain relief or needed sedation can reduce stress, anxiety, and pain (Seckel, 2017).
  - Hyperoxygenate before and between endotracheal suction sessions. Studies have demonstrated that hyperoxygenation may help prevent oxygen desaturation in a suctioned client (Seckel, 2017; Vollman et al., 2017; Siela, 2010).
  - Suction for less than 15 seconds. Studies demonstrated that because of a drop in the partial pressure of oxygen with suctioning, preferably there should be no more than 10 seconds of actual suctioning, with the entire procedure taking 15 seconds (Seckel, 2017).
  - Use a closed, in-line suction system. Closed in-line suctioning has minimal effects on heart rate, respiratory rate, tidal volume, and oxygen saturation and may reduce contamination (Seckel, 2017).
  - Avoid saline instillation during suctioning.
  - Use of a subglottic suctioning endotracheal tube reduces the incidence of VAP or ventilator-associated complications (Vollman et al., 2017; Haas et al., 2014).
  - Use of nonstick endotracheal tubes can reduce the formation of biofilm and hence VAP (Haas et al., 2014).

A

- ○ Document results of coughing and suctioning, particularly client tolerance and secretion characteristics such as color, odor, and volume (Seckel, 2017).

Pediatric

- • Educate parents about the risk factors for ineffective airway clearance such as foreign body ingestion and passive smoke exposure.
- • See the care plan Risk for **Suffocation** for more interventions on choking.
- • Educate children and parents on the importance of adherence to peak expiratory flow monitoring for asthma self-management.
- • Educate parents and other caregivers that cough and cold medication bought over the counter are not safe for a child younger than 2 years unless specifically ordered by a healthcare provider.

Geriatric

- • Encourage ambulation as tolerated without causing exhaustion. Immobility is often harmful to older adults because it decreases ventilation and increases stasis of secretions, leading to atelectasis or pneumonia.
- • Actively encourage older adults to deep breathe and cough. Cough reflexes are blunted, and coughing is decreased in older adults.
- • Ensure adequate hydration within cardiac and renal reserves. Older adults are prone to dehydration and therefore more viscous secretions because they frequently use diuretics or laxatives and forget to drink adequate amounts of water.

Home Care

- • Some of the previously mentioned interventions may be adapted for home care use.
- ▲ Begin discharge planning as soon as possible with the case manager or social worker to assess need for home support systems, assistive devices, and community or home health services.
- • Assess home environment for factors that exacerbate airway clearance problems (e.g., presence of allergens, lack of adequate humidity in air, poor air flow, stressful family relationships).
- • Assess affective climate within family and family support system. Refer to care plan for **Caregiver Role Strain.**
- • Refer to GOLD guidelines for management of home care and indications of hospital admission criteria (see http://www.goldcopd .org/).
- • When respiratory procedures are being implemented, explain equipment and procedures to family members and caregivers and provide needed emotional support.

- When electrically based equipment for respiratory support is being implemented, evaluate home environment for electrical safety, proper grounding, and so on. Ensure that notification is sent to the local utility company, the emergency medical team, and police and fire departments.
- Provide family with support for care of a client with chronic or terminal illness.
- Refer to care plan for **Anxiety.** Refer to care plan for **Powerlessness.**
- Instruct the client to avoid exposure to persons with upper respiratory infections, to avoid crowds of people, and wash hands after each exposure to groups of people or public places.

▲ Determine client adherence to medical regimen. Instruct the client and family in importance of reporting effectiveness of current medications to healthcare provider.

- Teach the client when and how to use inhalant or nebulizer treatments at home.
- Teach the client/family the importance of maintaining regimen and having "as-needed" drugs easily accessible at all times.
- Instruct the client and family in the importance of maintaining proper nutrition, adequate fluids, rest, and behavioral pacing for energy conservation and rehabilitation.
- Instruct in use of dietary supplements as indicated.
- Identify an emergency plan, including criteria for use.

▲ Refer for home health aide services for assistance with activities of daily living (ADLs).

▲ Assess family for role changes and coping skills. Refer to medical social services as necessary.

▲ For the client dying at home with a terminal illness, if the "death rattle" is present with gurgling, rattling, or crackling sounds in the airway with each breath, recognize that anticholinergic medications can often help control symptoms, if given early in the process.

▲ For the client with a death rattle, nursing care includes turning to mobilize secretions, keeping the head of the bed elevated for postural drainage of secretions, and avoiding suctioning.

Client/Family Teaching and Discharge Planning

▲ Teach the importance of not smoking. Refer to a smoking cessation program, and encourage clients who relapse to keep trying to quit. Ensure that the client receives appropriate medications to support smoking cessation from the primary healthcare provider.

A

- ▲ Teach the client how to use a flutter clearance device if ordered, which vibrates to loosen mucus and gives positive pressure to keep airways open (Gosselink et al., 2008).
- ▲ Teach the client how to use the peak expiratory flow rate (PEFR) meter if ordered and when to seek medical attention if the PEFR reading drops. Also teach the client how to use metered-dose inhalers and self-administer inhaled corticosteroids as ordered following precautions to decrease side effects.
- • Teach the client how to deep breathe and cough effectively.
- • Teach the client/family to identify and avoid specific factors that exacerbate ineffective airway clearance, including known allergens and especially smoking (if relevant) or exposure to secondhand smoke.
- • Educate the client and family about the significance of changes in sputum characteristics, including color, character, amount, and odor.
- • Teach the client/family the importance of taking antibiotics as prescribed and consuming all tablets until the prescription has run out.
- • Teach the family of the dying client in hospice with a death rattle that rarely are clients aware of the fluid that has accumulated, and help them find evidence of comfort in the client's nonverbal behavior (Twomey & Dowling, 2013; Fielding & Long, 2014).

Risk for Allergy Reaction

NANDA-I Definition

Susceptible to an exaggerated immune response or reaction to substances, which may compromise health

Risk Factors

Exposure to allergen; exposure to environmental allergen; exposure to toxic chemical

At-Risk Population

History of food allergy; history of insect sting allergy; repeated exposure to allergen-producing environmental substance

Client Outcomes

Client Will (Specify Time Frame)

- State risk factors for allergies
- Demonstrate knowledge of plan to treat allergic reaction

A

Nursing Interventions

- • A careful history is important in detecting allergens and avoidance of these allergens.
- • Obtain a precise history of allergies, as well as medications taken and foods ingested before surgery.
- ▲ Teach the client about the correct use of the injectable epinephrine and have the client do a return demonstration.
- ▲ Carefully assess the client for allergies. Below is information that is important for clients with allergies. Refer for immediate treatment if anaphylaxis is suspected.

Causes

Common allergens include animal dander; bee stings or stings from other insects; foods, especially nuts, fish, and shellfish; insect bites; medications; plants; pollens.

Symptoms

Common symptoms of a mild allergic reaction include hives (especially over the neck and face), itching, nasal congestion, rashes, watery, red eyes.

Symptoms of a moderate or severe reaction include cramps or pain in the abdomen, chest discomfort or tightness, diarrhea, difficulty breathing, difficulty swallowing, dizziness or lightheadedness, fear or feeling of apprehension or anxiety, flushing or redness of the face, nausea and vomiting, palpitations, swelling of the face, eyes, or tongue, weakness, wheezing, unconsciousness.

First Aid

For a mild to moderate reaction: calm and reassure the person having the reaction because anxiety can worsen symptoms.

1. Try to identify the allergen and have the person avoid further contact with it. If the allergic reaction is from a bee sting, scrape the stinger off the skin with something firm (e.g., fingernail or plastic credit card). Do not use tweezers; squeezing the stinger will release more venom.
2. Apply cool compresses and over-the-counter hydrocortisone cream for itchy rash.
3. Watch for signs of increasing distress.
4. Get medical help. For a mild reaction, a healthcare provider may recommend over-the-counter medications (e.g., antihistamines).

For a Severe Allergic Reaction (Anaphylaxis)

1. Check the person's airway, breathing, and circulation (the ABCs of Basic Life Support). A warning sign of dangerous throat swelling is a very hoarse or whispered voice or coarse sounds when the person is

breathing in air. If necessary, begin rescue breathing and cardiopulmonary resuscitation.

2. Call 911.
3. Calm and reassure the person.
4. If the allergic reaction is from a bee sting, scrape the stinger off the skin with something firm (e.g., fingernail or plastic credit card). Do not use tweezers; squeezing the stinger will release more venom.
5. If the person has emergency allergy medication on hand, help the person take or inject the medication. Avoid oral medication if the person is having difficulty breathing.
6. Take steps to prevent shock. Have the person lie flat, raise the person's feet about 12 inches, and cover him or her with a coat or blanket. Do NOT place the person in this position if a head, neck, back, or leg injury is suspected or if it causes discomfort.

Do NOT

- Do NOT assume that any allergy shots the person has already received will provide complete protection.
- Do NOT place a pillow under the person's head if he or she is having trouble breathing. This can block the airways.
- Do NOT give the person anything by mouth if the person is having trouble breathing.

When to Contact a Medical Professional

Call for immediate medical emergency assistance if:

- The person is having a severe allergic reaction—always call 911. Do not wait to see if the reaction is getting worse.
- The person has a history of severe allergic reactions (check for a medical ID tag).

Prevention

- Avoid triggers such as foods and medications that have caused an allergic reaction (even a mild one) in the past. Ask detailed questions about ingredients when you are eating away from home. Carefully examine ingredient labels.
- If you have a child who is allergic to certain foods, introduce one new food at a time in limited amounts so you can recognize an allergic reaction.
- People who know that they have had serious allergic reactions should wear a medical ID tag.
- Preoperative patients should be closely assessed for allergies.

A

- ▲ If you have a history of serious allergic reactions, carry emergency medications (e.g., a chewable form of diphenhydramine and injectable epinephrine or a bee sting kit) according to your healthcare provider's instructions.
- • Do not give your injectable epinephrine (or any other personal medication) to anyone else. They may have a condition (e.g., a heart problem) that could be negatively affected by this drug.
- ▲ Refer the client for skin testing to confirm IgE-mediated allergic response.
- • See care plans for **Latex Allergy** response and Risk for **Latex Allergy** response.

Pediatric

- ▲ Teach parents and children with allergies to peanuts and tree nuts to avoid them and to identify them.
- ▲ Teach parents and children with asthma about modifiable risk factors, which include allergy triggers.
- ▲ Counsel parents to limit infant exposure to traffic and cigarette carbon monoxide pollution.
- ▲ Suspect food protein–induced enterocolitis syndrome (FPIES) in formula-fed infants with repetitive emesis, diarrhea, dehydration, and lethargy 1 to 5 hours after ingesting the offending food (the most common are cow's milk, soy, and rice). Remove the offending food.
- ▲ Children should be screened for seafood allergies and, if an allergy is detected, avoid seafood and any foods containing seafood.

Anxiety

NANDA-I Definition

An emotional response to a diffuse threat in which the individual anticipates nonspecific impending danger, catastrophe, or misfortune

Defining Characteristics

Behavioral

Crying; decrease in productivity; expresses anguish; expresses anxiety about life event changes; expresses distress; expresses insecurity; expresses intense dread; helplessness; hypervigilance; increased wariness; insomnia; irritable mood; nervousness; psychomotor agitation; reduced eye contact; scanning behavior; self-focused

Physiological

Altered respiratory pattern; anorexia; brisk reflexes; chest tightness; cold extremities; diarrhea; dry mouth; expresses abdominal pain; expresses feeling faint; expresses muscle weakness; expresses tension; facial flushing; increased blood pressure; increased heart rate; increased sweating; nausea; pupil dilation; quivering voice; reports altered sleep-wake cycle; reports heart palpitations; reports tingling in extremities; superficial vasoconstriction; tremors; urinary frequency; urinary hesitancy; urinary urgency

Cognitive

Altered attention; confusion; decreased perceptual field; expresses forgetfulness; expresses preoccupation; reports of blocking of thoughts; rumination

Related Factors

Conflict about life goals; interpersonal transmission; pain; stressors; substance misuse; unfamiliar situation; unmet needs; value conflict

At-Risk Population

Individuals experiencing developmental crisis; individuals experiencing situational crisis; individuals exposed to toxins; individuals in the perioperative period; individuals with family history of anxiety; individuals with hereditary predisposition

Associated Conditions

Mental disorders

Client Outcomes

Client Will (Specify Time Frame)

- Identify and verbalize symptoms of anxiety
- Identify, verbalize, and demonstrate techniques to control anxiety
- Verbalize absence of or decrease in subjective distress
- Have vital signs that reflect baseline or decreased sympathetic stimulation
- Have posture, facial expressions, gestures, and activity levels that reflect decreased distress
- Demonstrate improved concentration and accuracy of thoughts
- Demonstrate return of basic problem-solving skills
- Demonstrate increased external focus
- Demonstrate some ability to reassure self

Nursing Interventions

- Assess the client's level of anxiety and physical reactions to anxiety (e.g., tachycardia, tachypnea, irritability, restlessness, etc.).
- Rule out withdrawal from alcohol, sedatives, or smoking as the cause of anxiety.
- Use empathy to encourage the client to interpret the anxiety symptoms as normal.

A

- If irrational thoughts or fears are present, offer the client accurate information and encourage him or her to talk about the meaning of the events contributing to the anxiety.
- Encourage the client to use positive self-talk.
- Intervene when possible to remove sources of anxiety.
- Explain all activities, procedures, and issues that involve the client; use nonmedical terms and calm, slow speech, then validate the client's understanding.
- ▲ Use massage therapy to reduce anxiety.
- ▲ Consider massage therapy for preoperative clients.
- Use therapeutic touch and healing touch techniques.
- Use guided imagery to decrease anxiety.
- Suggest yoga to the client.
- Provide clients with a means to listen to music of their choice or audiotapes.

Pediatric

- The previously mentioned interventions may be adapted for the pediatric client.

Geriatric

- ▲ Monitor the client for depression. Use appropriate interventions and referrals.
- Observe for adverse changes if antianxiety drugs are taken.
- Mindfulness meditation is successful in mediating anxiety.

Multicultural

- Assess for the presence of culture-bound anxiety states.
- Identify how anxiety is manifested in the culturally diverse client.
- For diverse clients experiencing preoperative anxiety, provide music of their choice.

Home Care

- The previously mentioned interventions may be adapted for home care use.
- ▲ Assess for suicidal ideation.
- Assess for influence of anxiety on medical regimen.
- Assess for presence of depression.
- Assist family to be supportive of the client in the face of anxiety symptoms.
- ▲ Consider referral for the prescription of antianxiety or antidepressant medications for clients who have panic disorder (PD) or other anxiety-related psychiatric disorders.

A

- ▲ Assist the client/family to institute the medication regimen appropriately. Instruct in side effects and the importance of taking medications as ordered.
- ▲ Refer for psychiatric home healthcare services.

Client/Family Teaching and Discharge Planning

- ▲ Teach use of appropriate community resources in emergency situations (e.g., suicidal thoughts), such as hotlines, emergency departments, law enforcement, and judicial systems.
- • Teach the client/family the symptoms of anxiety.
- • Teach the client techniques to self-manage anxiety.
- • Teach the client to visualize or fantasize about the absence of anxiety or pain, successful experience of the situation, resolution of conflict, or outcome of procedure.
- • Teach the relationship between a healthy physical and emotional lifestyle and a realistic mental attitude.

Death Anxiety

NANDA-I Definition

Emotional distress and insecurity, generated by anticipation of death and the process of dying of oneself or significant others, which negatively effects one's quality of life.

Defining Characteristics

Dysphoria; expresses concern about caregiver strain; expresses concern about the impact of one's death on significant other; expresses deep sadness; expresses fear of developing terminal illness; expresses fear of loneliness; expresses fear of loss of mental abilities when dying; expresses fear of pain related to dying; expresses fear of premature death; expresses fear of prolonged dying process; expresses fear of separation from loved ones; expresses fear of suffering related to dying; expresses fear of the dying process; expresses fear of the unknown; expresses powerlessness; reports negative thoughts related to death and dying

Related Factors

Anticipation of adverse consequences of anesthesia; anticipation of impact of death on others; anticipation of pain; anticipation of suffering; awareness of imminent death; depressive symptoms; discussions on the topic of death; impaired religiosity; loneliness; low self-esteem; nonacceptance of own mortality; spiritual distress; uncertainty about encountering a higher power; uncertainty about life after death; uncertainty about the existence of a higher power; uncertainty of prognosis; unpleasant physical symptoms

A

At-Risk Population

Individuals experiencing terminal care of significant others; individuals receiving terminal care; Individuals with history of adverse experiences with death of significant others; individuals with history of near-death experience; older adults; women; young adults

Associated Condition

Depression; stigmatized illness with high fear of death; terminal illness

Client Outcomes

Client Will (Specify Time Frame)

- State concerns about impact of death on others
- Express feelings associated with dying
- Seek help in dealing with feelings
- Discuss realistic goals
- Use prayer or other religious practice for comfort

Nursing Interventions

▲ Assess the psychosocial maturity of the individual.
▲ Assess clients for pain and provide pain relief measures.
- Assess client for fears related to death.
- Assist clients with life planning: consider and redefine main life goals, focus on areas of strength and/or goals that will provide satisfaction, adopt realistic goals, and recognize those that are impossible to achieve.
- Assist clients with life review and reminiscence.
- Provide music of the client's choosing.
- Provide social support for families: understanding what is most important to families who are caring for clients at the end of life.
- Encourage clients to pray.

Geriatric

- Carefully assess older adults for issues regarding death anxiety.
- Provide back massage for clients who have anxiety regarding issues such as death.

Multicultural

- Assist clients to identify with their culture and its values.
- Refer to care plan for **Anxiety.**

Home Care

- The previously mentioned interventions may be adapted for home care.
- Identify times and places when anxiety is greatest. Provide for psychological support at those times, using such strategies as personal contact, telephone contact, diversionary activities, or therapeutic self.

• = Independent ▲ = Collaborative

A

- Support religious beliefs; encourage the client to participate in services and activities of choice.
- ▲ Refer to appropriate medical services, social services, and/or mental health services, as needed.
- ▲ Identify the client's preferences for end-of-life care; aid in honoring preferences as much as practicable.
- ▲ Assist the client in making contact with death-related planning organizations, if appropriate, such as the Cremation Society and funeral homes.
- Refer to care plan for **Powerlessness.**

Client/Family Teaching and Discharge Planning

- Promote more effective communication to family members engaged in the caregiving role.
- Allow family members to be physically close to their dying loved one, giving them permission, instruction, and opportunities to touch. Keep family members informed.

Risk for Aspiration

NANDA-I Definition

Susceptible to entry of gastrointestinal secretions, oropharyngeal secretions, solids, or fluids to the tracheobronchial passages, which may compromise health

Risk Factors

Barrier to elevating upper body; decrease in gastrointestinal motility; difficulty swallowing; enteral nutrition tube displacement; inadequate knowledge of modifiable factors; increased gastric residue; ineffective airway clearance

At Risk Population

Older adults; premature infants

Associated Condition

Chronic obstructive pulmonary disease; critical illness; decreased level of consciousness; delayed gastric emptying; depressed gag reflex; enteral nutrition; facial surgery; facial trauma; head and neck neoplasms; incompetent lower esophageal sphincter; increased intragastric pressure; jaw fixation techniques; medical devices; neck surgery; neck trauma; neurological diseases; oral surgical procedures; oral trauma; pharmaceutical preparations; pneumonia; stroke; treatment regimen

Client Outcomes

Client Will (Specify Time Frame)

- Maintain patent airway and clear lung sounds

A

- Swallow and digest oral, nasogastric, or gastric feeding without aspiration

Nursing Interventions

- Monitor respiratory rate, depth, and effort. Note any signs of aspiration such as dyspnea, cough, cyanosis, wheezing, hoarseness, foul-smelling sputum, or fever. If new onset of symptoms, then perform oral suction and notify provider immediately.
- Auscultate lung sounds frequently and before and after feedings; note any new onset of crackles or wheezing.
- Take vital signs frequently, noting onset of a fever, increased respiratory rate, and increased heart rate.
- Before initiating oral feeding, check client's gag reflex and ability to swallow by feeling the laryngeal prominence as the client attempts to swallow (Rees, 2013; American Association of Critical Care Nurses, 2016a). If client is having problems swallowing, see nursing interventions for Impaired **Swallowing.**
- If client needs to be fed, feed slowly and allow adequate time for chewing and swallowing.
- When feeding client, watch for signs of impaired swallowing or aspiration, including coughing, choking, and spitting food.
- Have suction machine available when feeding high-risk clients. If aspiration does occur, suction immediately.
- Keep the head of the bed (HOB) elevated at 30 to 45 degrees, preferably with the client sitting up in a chair at 90 degrees when feeding. Keep head elevated for an hour after eating.
- Note presence of nausea, vomiting, or diarrhea. Treat nausea promptly with antiemetics.
- If the client shows symptoms of nausea and vomiting, position on side.
- Assess the abdomen and listen to bowel sounds frequently, noting if they are decreased, absent, or hyperactive.
- Note new onset of abdominal distention or increased rigidity of abdomen.
- If client has a tracheostomy, ask for referral to speech pathologist for swallowing studies before attempting to feed.
- Provide meticulous oral care including brushing of teeth at least two times per day.
- Sedation agents can reduce cough and gag reflexes as well as interfere with the client's ability to manage oropharyngeal secretions.

Enteral Feedings

- Insert nasogastric feeding tube using the internal nares to distal lower esophageal sphincter distance. The ear-to-nose-to-xiphoid-process is often inaccurate.
- Tape the feeding tube securely to the nose using a skin protectant under the tape.
- Check to make sure the initial nasogastric feeding tube placement was confirmed by x-ray, with the openings of the tube in the stomach, not the esophagus or lungs. This is especially important if a small-bore feeding tube is used, although larger tubes used for feedings or medication administration also should be verified by radiography.
- After radiographic confirmation of proper placement of the tube in the intestines, mark the tube's exit site clearly with tape or a permanent marker (Simons & Abdallah, 2012).
- Measure and record the length of the tube that is outside of the body at defined intervals to help ensure correct placement.
- Note the placement of the tube on any chest or abdominal radiographs that are obtained for the client.
- Check the pH of the aspirate.
- Use a number of determinants for verification of correct placement before each feeding or every 4 hours if the client is on continuous feeding. Measure length of tube outside the body, and review recent x-ray results and check pH of the aspirate if relevant and its characteristic appearance. If findings do not ensure correct placement of the tube, obtain a radiograph to verify placement. Do not rely on the air insufflation method to assess correct tube placement.
- Follow unit policy regarding checking for gastric residual volume during continuous feedings or before feedings, and holding feedings if increased residual is present.
- Follow unit protocol regarding returning or discarding gastric residual volume. At this time there is no definitive research base to guide practice.
- Do not use glucose testing to determine correct placement of enteral tube or to identify aspirated enteral feeding.
- Do not use blue dye to tint enteral feedings (Guenter, 2010).
- During enteral feedings, position client with HOB elevated 30 to 45 degrees (American Association of Critical Care Nurses, 2016a; Schallom et al., 2015).

A

- Take actions to prevent inadvertent misconnections with enteral feeding tubes into intravenous (IV) lines or other harmful connections. Safety actions that should be taken to prevent misconnections include:
  - Trace tubing back to origin. Recheck connections at time of client transfer and at change of shift.
  - Label all tubing.
  - Use oral syringes for medications through the enteral feeding; *do not use IV syringes.*
  - Teach nonprofessional personnel to "do not reconnect" if a line becomes dislodged; rather, find the nurse instead of taking the chance of plugging the tube into the wrong place.

Critical Care

- Recognize that critically ill clients are at an increased risk for aspiration because of severe illness and interventions that compromise the gag reflex.
- Recognize that intolerance to feeding as defined by increased gastric residual is more common early in the feeding process.

Geriatric

- Carefully check older client's gag reflex and ability to swallow before feeding.
- Watch for signs of aspiration pneumonia in older adults with cerebrovascular accidents, even if there are no apparent signs of difficulty swallowing or of aspiration.
- Recognize that older adults with aspiration pneumonia have fewer symptoms than younger people; repeat cases of pneumonia in older adults are generally associated with aspiration (Eisenstadt, 2010).
- Use central nervous system depressants cautiously; older clients may have an increased incidence of aspiration with altered levels of consciousness.
- Keep older, mostly bedridden clients sitting upright for 45 minutes to 1 hour after meals.
- Recommend to families that enteral feedings may or may not be indicated for clients with advanced dementia. Instead, if possible, use hand-feeding assistance, modified food consistency as needed, and feeding favorite foods for comfort (Sorrell, 2010).

Home Care

- The previously mentioned interventions may be adapted for home care use.

A

- For clients at high risk for aspiration, obtain complete information from the discharging institution regarding institutional management.
- Assess the client and family for willingness and cognitive ability to learn and cope with swallowing, feeding, and related disorders.
- Assess caregiver understanding and reinforce teaching regarding positioning and assessment of the client for possible aspiration.
- Provide the client with emotional support in dealing with fears of aspiration. Refer to care plan for **Anxiety.**
- Establish emergency and contingency plans for care of the client.
- Have a speech and occupational therapist assess the client's swallowing ability and other physiological factors and recommend strategies for working with the client in the home (e.g., pureeing foods served to the client; providing adequate adaptive equipment for independence in eating).
- Obtain suction equipment for the home as necessary.
- Teach caregivers safe, effective use of suctioning devices. Inform the client and family that only individuals instructed in suctioning should perform the procedure.
- Institute case management of frail elderly to support continued independent living.

Client/Family Teaching and Discharge Planning

- Teach the client and family signs of aspiration and precautions to prevent aspiration.
- Teach the client and family how to safely administer tube feeding.
- Teach the family about proper client positioning to facilitate feeding and reduce risk of aspiration.
- Verify client family/caregiver knowledge about feeding, aspiration precautions, and signs of aspiration.

Risk for Impaired Attachment

NANDA-I Definition

Susceptible to disruption of the interactive process between parent or significant other and child that fosters the development of a protective and nurturing reciprocal relationship

Risk Factors

Anxiety; child's illness prevents effective initiation of parental contact; disorganized infant behavior; inability of parent to meet personal needs;

A

insufficient privacy; parental conflict resulting from disorganized infant behavior; parent-child separation; physical barrier; substance misuse

At-Risk Population

Premature infant

Client Outcomes

Parent(s)/Caregiver(s) Will (Specify Time Frame)

- Be willing to consider pumping breast milk (and storing appropriately) or breastfeeding, if feasible
- Demonstrate behaviors that indicate secure attachment to infant/child
- Provide a safe environment, free of physical hazards
- Provide nurturing environment sensitive to infant/child's need for nutrition/feeding, sleeping, comfort, and social play
- Read and respond contingently to infant/child's distress
- Support infant's self-regulation capabilities, intervening when needed
- Engage in mutually satisfying interactions that provide opportunities for attachment
- Give infant nurturing sensory experiences (e.g., holding, cuddling, stroking, rocking)
- Demonstrate an awareness of developmentally appropriate activities that are pleasurable, emotionally supportive, and growth fostering
- Avoid physical and emotional abuse and/or neglect as retribution for parent's perception of infant/child's misbehavior
- State appropriate community resources and support services

Nursing Interventions

- Establish a trusting relationship with parent/caregiver.
- Support mothers of preterm infants in providing pumped breast milk for their babies until they are ready for oral feedings and transitioning from gavage to breast.
- Identify factors related to postpartum depression (PPD)/major depression and offer appropriate interventions/referrals.
- Identify eating disorders/comorbid factors related to depression and offer appropriate interventions/referrals. **Additional relevant research:** (Emerson et al., 2017).
- Nurture parents so that they in turn can nurture their infant/child.
- Offer parents opportunities to verbalize their childhood fears associated with attachment.
- Suggest journaling or scrapbooking as a way for parents of hospitalized infants to cope with stress and emotions.
- Offer parent-to-parent support to parents of infants in the NICU.

- Encourage parents of hospitalized infants to "personalize the baby" by bringing in clothing, pictures of themselves, toys, and tapes of their voices.
- Encourage physical closeness using skin-to-skin experiences as appropriate.
- Plan ways for parents and their support system to interact/assist with infant/child caregiving.
- Educate parents about the importance of the infant–caregiver relationship as a foundation for the development of the infant's self regulation capacities.
- Assist parents in developing new caregiving competencies and/or revising/extending old ones.
- Educate parents in reading/responding sensitively to their infant's unique "body language" (behavior cues), which communicates approach ("I'm ready to play"), avoidance/stress ("I'm unhappy. I need a change."), and self-calming ("I'm helping myself").
- Educate and support parents' ability to relieve the infant/child's stress/distress/pain.
- Guide parents in adapting their behaviors/activities with infant/child cues and changing needs.
- Attend to both parents and infant/child to strengthen high-quality interactions. **Additional relevant research:** (Strathearn & Kim, 2013).
- Assist parents with providing pleasurable sensory learning experiences (i.e., sight, sound, movement, touch, body awareness).
- Encourage physical closeness using skin-to-skin experiences as appropriate.
- Encourage parents and caregivers to massage their infants and children.
- Identify mothers who may need assistance in enhancing maternal role attainment (MRA).
- Recognize that fathers, compared with mothers, may have different starting points in the attachment process in the NICU because nurses encourage parents to have early skin to skin contact (SSC). **Additional relevant research:** (Arockisamy et al., 2008).

Pediatric

- Recognize and support infant/child's capacity for self regulation and intervene when appropriate.
- Provide lyrical, soothing music in the nursery and at home that is age appropriate (i.e., corrected, in the case of premature infants) and contingent with state/behavioral cues.

- Recognize and support infant/child's attention capabilities.
- Encourage opportunities for mutually satisfying interactions between infant and parent.
- Encourage opportunities for physical closeness.

Multicultural

- Provide culturally sensitive parent support to new immigrant families and other non–native-English-speaking mothers and families.
- Discuss cultural norms with families to provide care that is appropriate for enhancing attachment with the infant/child.
- Promote the attachment process in women who have abused substances by providing a culturally based, women-centered treatment environment.
- Promote attachment process/development of maternal sensitivity in incarcerated women.
- Empower family members to draw on personal strengths in which multiple worldviews/values are recognized, incorporated, and negotiated.
- Encourage positive involvement and relationship development between children and fathers.

Home Care

- The previously mentioned interventions may be adapted for home care use.
- Assess quality of interaction between parent and infant/child.
- Use "interaction coaching" (i.e., teaching mother to let the infant lead) so that the mother will match her interaction style to the baby's cues.
- ▲ Provide supportive care for infants and children whose parents have been deployed during wartime.
- Encourage custodial grandparents to use support groups available for caregivers of children.

Autonomic Dysreflexia

NANDA-I Definition

Life-threatening, uninhibited sympathetic response of the nervous system to a noxious stimulus after a spinal cord injury at the 7th thoracic vertebra (T7) or above

Defining Characteristics

Blurred vision; bradycardia; chest pain; chilling; conjunctival congestion; diaphoresis above the injury; diffuse pain in different areas of the head;

Horner's syndrome; metallic taste in mouth; nasal congestion; pallor below injury; paresthesia; paroxysmal hypertension; pilomotor reflex; red blotches on skin above the injury; tachycardia

Related Factors

Gastrointestinal Stimuli

Constipation; difficult passage of feces; digital stimulation; enemas; fecal impaction; suppositories

Integumentary Stimuli

Cutaneous stimulation; skin irritation

Musculoskeletal-Neurological Stimuli

Irritating stimuli below level of injury; painful stimuli below level of injury; pressure over bony prominence; pressure over genitalia; range of motion exercises; spasm

Regulatory-Situational Stimuli

Constrictive clothing; environmental temperature fluctuations; positioning

Reproductive-Urological Stimuli

Bladder distention; bladder spasm; instrumentation; sexual intercourse

Other

Insufficient caregiver knowledge of disease process; insufficient knowledge of disease process

At-Risk Population

Ejaculation; extremes of environmental temperature; menstruation

Associated Condition

Bowel distention; cystitis; deep vein thrombosis; detrusor sphincter dyssynergia; epididymitis; esophageal reflux disease; fracture; gallstones; gastric ulcer; gastrointestinal system pathology; hemorrhoids; heterotopic bone; labor and delivery period; ovarian cyst; pharmaceutical agent; pregnancy; pulmonary emboli; renal calculi; substance withdrawal; sunburn; surgical procedure; urethritis; urinary catheterization; urinary tract infection; wound

Client Outcomes

Client Will (Specify Time Frame)

- Maintain baseline blood pressure
- Remain free of dysreflexia symptoms
- Explain symptoms, treatment, and prevention of dysreflexia

Nursing Interventions

- Teach spinal cord injury (SCI) patients about potential causes, symptoms, treatment, and prevention of autonomic dysreflexia (AD).

A

- Monitor the client for symptoms of dysreflexia, particularly those with high-level and more complete spinal cord injuries. See Defining Characteristics.
- ▲ Collaborate with providers and caregivers to identify the cause of dysreflexia. AD is triggered by a stimulus from below the level of injury, leading to systemic vasoconstriction. The most common triggers are bladder distension, kidney stones, kink in urinary catheter, urinary tract infection, fecal impaction, pressure ulcer, ingrown toenail, menstruation, hemorrhoids, tight clothing, invasive testing, and sexual intercourse (Caruso et al., 2015; Wan & Krassioukov, 2014).
- If dysreflexia symptoms are present, immediately place client in high Fowler's position, remove all support hoses or binders, loosen clothing, check the urinary catheter for kinks, and attempt to determine the noxious stimulus causing the response. Check the patient's blood pressure every 3 to 5 minutes. If blood pressure cannot be decreased following these initial interventions, notify the provider emergently (i.e., STAT).
    - First, assess bladder function. Check for distention and, if present, catheterize the client using an anesthetic jelly as a lubricant. Do not use the Valsalva maneuver or Crede's method to empty the bladder because this form of reflex voiding could worsen AD. Ensure existing catheter patency and irrigate if necessary. Also assess for signs of urinary tract infection.
    - Second, assess bowel function. Numb the bowel area with a topical anesthetic as ordered and gently check for impaction.
    - Third, assess the skin. Look for any pressure points, wounds, and ingrown toenails.
- ▲ Initiate antihypertensive therapy as soon as ordered and monitor for cardiac dysrhythmias.
- Monitor vital signs every 3 to 5 minutes during an acute event; continue to monitor vital signs after event is resolved (e.g., symptoms resolve and vital signs return to baseline, usually up to 2 hours postevent).
- Watch for complications of dysreflexia, including signs of cerebral hemorrhage, seizures, cardiac dysfunction, or intraocular hemorrhage.
- Accurately and completely record any incidences of dysreflexia; especially note the precipitating stimuli.

- Use the following interventions to prevent dysreflexia:
  - Ensure catheter patency and empty urinary catheter bags frequently. Assess the client for signs and symptoms of urinary tract infection during every shift.
  - Ensure a regular pattern of defecation to prevent fecal impaction.
  - Frequently change position of client to relieve pressure and prevent formation of pressure injuries.
- ▲ Notify all healthcare team members of recurrent AD episodes.
- ▲ For female clients with SCI, assess the client for AD during menstrual cycle. If the client becomes pregnant, collaborate with obstetrical healthcare practitioners to monitor for signs and symptoms of dysreflexia.

Home Care

- The previously mentioned interventions may be adapted for home care use.
- Provide the client and caregiver with written information on common causes of AD and initial treatment.
- Provide resources to clients with any known proclivity toward dysreflexia. Advise them to wear a medical alert bracelet and carry a medical alert wallet card when not accompanied by knowledgeable caregivers.
- ▲ Establish an emergency plan: maintain a current prescription of antihypertensive medication, and administer antihypertensives when dysreflexia is refractory to nonmedicinal interventions. If SBP remains over 150 mm Hg following the previously mentioned interventions, go to the nearest ER and present the AD wallet card on arrival.
- When an episode of dysreflexia has resolved, continue to monitor blood pressure every 30 to 60 minutes for the next 2 hours or admit to an institution for observation.

Client/Family Teaching and Discharge Planning

- Teach recognition of early dysreflexia symptoms, appropriate interventions, and the need to obtain help immediately. Give client a written card describing signs and symptoms of AD and initial actions.
- Teach steps to prevent dysreflexia episodes: routine bladder and bowel care, pressure injury prevention, and preventing other forms of noxious stimuli (e.g., not wearing clothing that is too tight, nail care). Discuss the potential impact of sexual intercourse and pregnancy on AD.

A

Risk for Autonomic Dysreflexia

NANDA-I Definition

Susceptible to life-threatening, uninhibited response of the sympathetic nervous system post-spinal shock, in an individual with spinal cord injury or lesion at the 6th thoracic vertebra (T6) or above (has been demonstrated in patients with injuries at the 7th thoracic vertebra [T7] and the 8th thoracic vertebra [T8]), which may compromise health

Risk Factors

Gastrointestinal Stimuli

Bowel distention; constipation; difficult passage of feces; digital stimulation; enemas; fecal impaction; suppositories

Integumentary Stimuli

Cutaneous stimulations; skin irritation; sunburn; wound

Musculoskeletal-Neurological Stimuli

Irritating stimuli below level of injury; painful stimuli below level of injury; pressure over bony prominence; pressure over genitalia; range of motion exercises; spasm

Regulatory-Situational Stimuli

Constrictive clothing; environmental temperature fluctuations; positioning

Reproductive-Urological Stimuli

Bladder distention; bladder spasm; instrumentation; sexual intercourse

Other

Insufficient caregiver knowledge of disease process; insufficient knowledge of disease process

At-Risk Population

Ejaculation; extremes of environmental temperature; menstruation

Associated Condition

Bowel distention; cystitis; deep vein thrombosis; detrusor sphincter dyssynergia; epididymitis; esophageal reflux disease; fracture; gallstones; gastric ulcer; gastrointestinal system pathology; hemorrhoids; heterotopic bone; labor and delivery period; ovarian cyst; pharmaceutical agent; pregnancy; pulmonary emboli; renal calculi; substance withdrawal; sunburn; surgical procedure; urethritis; urinary catheterization; urinary tract infection; wound

Client Outcomes, Nursing Interventions, Client/Family Teaching and Discharge Planning

Refer to care plan for **Autonomic Dysreflexia.**

Risk for Bleeding

B

NANDA-I Definition

Susceptive to a decrease in blood volume, which may compromise health

Risk Factors

Insufficient knowledge of bleeding precautions

At-Risk Population

History of falls

Associated Condition

Aneurysm; circumcision; disseminated intravascular coagulopathy; gastrointestinal condition; impaired liver function; inherent coagulopathy; postpartum complication; pregnancy complication; trauma; treatment regimen

Client Outcomes

Client Will (Specify Time Frame)

- Discuss precautions to prevent bleeding complications
- Explain actions that should be taken if bleeding happens
- Maintain adherence to agreed on anticoagulant medication and laboratory work regimens
- Monitor for signs and symptoms of bleeding
- Maintain a mean arterial pressure above 70 mm Hg, a heart rate between 60 and 100 beats per minute with a normal rhythm, and urine output greater than 0.5 mL/kg/hr
- Maintain warm, dry skin

Nursing Interventions

- Perform admission fall risk assessment. Safety precautions should be implemented for all at-risk clients.
- Monitor the client closely for hemorrhage, especially in those at increased risk for bleeding. Watch for any signs of bleeding, including bleeding of the gums, nosebleed, blood in sputum, emesis, urine or stool, bleeding from a wound, bleeding into the skin with petechiae, and purpura.
- If bleeding develops, apply pressure over the site or appropriate artery as needed. Apply pressure dressing; if unable to stop the bleeding, then consider a tourniquet if indicated.

▲ Collaborate on an appropriate bleeding management plan, including nonpharmacological and pharmacological measures to stop bleeding based on the antithrombotic used.

▲ Monitor coagulation studies, including prothrombin time, INR, activated partial thromboplastin time (aPTT), fibrinogen, fibrin degradation/split products, and platelet counts as appropriate.

B

▲ Monitor all medications for potential to increase bleeding, including antiplatelets, NSAIDs, selective serotonin reuptake inhibitors (SSRIs), and complementary and alternative therapies such as coenzyme Q10 and ginger.

Safety Guidelines for Anticoagulant Administration: Joint Commission National Patient Safety Goals

Follow approved protocol for anticoagulant administration:

- Use prepackaged medications and prefilled or premixed parenteral therapy as ordered.
- Check laboratory tests (i.e., INR) before administration.
- Use programmable pumps when using parenteral administration
- Ensure appropriate education for client/family and all staff concerning anticoagulants used.
- Notify dietary services when warfarin is prescribed (to provide consistent vitamin K in diet).
- Monitor for any symptoms of bleeding before administration.
- Anticoagulation therapy is complex.

▲ Before administering anticoagulants, assess the clotting profile of the client. If the client is on warfarin, assess the INR. If the INR is outside of the recommended parameters, then notify the provider.

▲ Recognize that vitamin K for vitamin K antagonists (e.g., warfarin, phenprocoumon, Sinthrome, and phenindione) may be given orally or IV as ordered for INR levels greater than 4.5 without signs of bleeding. In the case of major bleeding, prohemostatic therapies may be warranted for the rapid reversal of vitamin K antagonists (tranexamic acid, fresh frozen plasma, cryoprecipitate, platelet transfusion, fibrinogen concentrate, factor IV prothrombin complex concentrate [KCentra], and activated prothrombin complex concentrate) (Makris et al., 2013; Witt et al., 2016).

▲ Manage fluid resuscitation and volume expansion as ordered.

▲ Consider use of permissive hypotension and restrictive transfusion strategies when treating bleeding episodes.

▲ Consider discussing the coadministration of a proton-pump inhibitor alongside traditional NSAIDs, or with the use of a cyclooxygenase 2 inhibitor with the prescriber.

- Ensure adequate nurse staffing to provide a high level of surveillance capability.

Pediatric

- ▲ Recognize that prophylactic vitamin K administration should be used in neonates for vitamin K deficiency bleeding (VKDB).
- ▲ Recognize warning signs of VKDB, including minimal bleeds, evidence of cholestasis (icteric sclera, dark urine, and irritability), and failure to thrive.
- ▲ Monitor children and adolescents for potential bleeding after trauma.
- ▲ Closely monitor children after cardiac surgery for excessive blood loss.

Client/Family Teaching and Discharge Planning

- • Teach client and family or significant others about any anticoagulant medications prescribed, including when to take, how often to have laboratory tests done, signs of bleeding to report, dietary consistency, and need to wear medical alert bracelet and precautions to be followed. Instruct the client to report any adverse side effects to his or her healthcare provider.
- • Instruct the client and family on the disease process and rationale for care. When clients and their family members have sufficient understanding of their disease process, they can participate more fully in care and healthy behaviors. Knowledge empowers clients and family members, allowing them to be active participants in their care.
- • Provide client and family or significant others with both oral and written educational materials that meet the standards of client education and health literacy.

Risk for unstable Blood Pressure

NANDA-I Definition

Susceptible to fluctuating forces of blood flowing through arterial vessels, which may compromise health

Risk Factors

Inconsistency with medication regimen; orthostasis

Associated Condition

Adverse effects of cocaine; adverse effects of nonsteroidal antiinflammatory drugs (NSAIDS); adverse effects of steroids; cardiac dysrhythmia; Cushing syndrome; electrolyte imbalance; fluid retention; fluid shifts; hormonal change; hyperosmolar solutions; hyperparathyroidism; hyperthyroidism; hypothyroidism; increased intracranial pressure; rapid absorption and distribution of antiarrhythmia agent; rapid absorption and distribution of diuretic agent; rapid absorption and distribution of vasodilator agents; sympathetic responses; use of antidepressant agents

B

Client Outcomes

Client Will (Specify Time Frame)

- Maintain vital signs within normal range
- Remain asymptomatic with cardiac rhythm (have absence of arrhythmias, tachycardia, or bradycardia)
- Be free from dizziness with changes in positions (lying to standing)
- Deny fatigue, nausea, vomiting
- Deny chest pain

Nursing Interventions

▲ Hypertension (HTN) is a major risk factor for cardiovascular disease placing the client at increased risk of myocardial infarction and stroke (Whelton et al., 2017).

- Provide client-specific education about the importance of a healthy lifestyle to reduce complications associated with HTN.
- Provide drug- and client-specific education if medications are prescribed to manage the client's HTN.

▲ Screen clients for secondary causes of HTN with abrupt onset or age < 30 years.

▲ Review the client's past medical history.

- Explore the client's subjective statements concerning poor sleep, report of snoring, and daytime fatigue.
- Review the client's history of arrhythmias, especially a history of atrial fibrillation.
- Review the client's current medications, both prescribed and over the counter.
- Steroid agents, administered at higher doses (e.g., 80–200 mg per day), can trigger HTN (Grossman & Messerli, 2012).
- Ask the client if they are prescribed antidepressant agents.
- NSAIDs can induce HTN and/or interfere with antihypertensive therapy.
- Overconsumption of caffeine stimulates sympathetic activity, which causes a rise in blood pressure that can be followed by a decrease in blood pressure once the effects of the caffeine have worn off.
- Licorice consumption may trigger HTN in some patients.
- Some herbal products may induce HTN and/or interfere with antihypertensive treatment.

- Alcohol is known to elevate blood pressure and increases the client's risk of HTN.
- Blood pressure may be unstable with substance abuse disorders (SUDs). Certain drugs have specific effects on the cardiovascular system.
- Cocaine use causes increased alertness and feelings of euphoria, along with dilated pupils, increased body temperature, tachycardia, and increased blood pressure. Tachyarrhythmias and marked elevated blood pressure can be life-threatening.
- Cocaine overdose is a medical emergency because of the risk of cardiac toxicity.
- Opioid intoxication results in changes in heart rate, slowed breathing, and decrease in blood pressure leading to loss of alertness.
- Synthetic cannabinoids are man-made, mind-altering chemicals that may be added to foods or inhaled. There is a growing availability of these designer drugs in which adverse effects are not well known.

Critical Care

- Monitor the client for symptoms associated with chest pain, myocardial infarction, acute HTN, and hypotension.
- Clients with hypertensive crisis will require close monitoring for signs and symptoms consistent with acute renal failure, stroke, myocardial infarction, and acute heart failure.
- Myxedema coma is an acute emergency associated with hypothyroidism that manifests with severe hypotension, bradycardia, hypothermia, seizures, and coma.
- Thyroid storm (thyrotoxicosis) is an acute, life-threatening, hypermetabolic state induced by excessive release of thyroid-stimulating hormone (TSH). Symptoms are severe and include fever, tachycardia, HTN, congestive heart failure leading to hypotension and shock, profuse sweating, respiratory distress, nausea and vomiting, diarrhea, abdominal pain, jaundice, anxiety, seizures, and coma.

Pediatric

- HTN is an underrecognized disease in children. Current recommendations include annual blood pressure monitoring with more focused monitoring in high-risk children.

▲ Secondary causes of HTN should be explored in the absence of childhood obesity, known cardiovascular disease, family history.

B

- Normal ranges for child and adolescent blood pressure measurements were recently updated to reflect age, gender, and weight considerations.

Geriatric

- Risk of cardiac arrhythmias increases with advanced age placing the client at increased risk of HTN and hypotension.
- Comorbid cardiovascular disease risks increase with advanced age.
- Polypharmacy is a risk for both hypotension and HTN in older clients.

Client/Family Teaching and Discharge Planning

- Nutritional education has been found to be an important variable in an individual maintaining cardiovascular health.
- Teach the client to monitor blood pressure and to report changes in blood pressure to the provider and with each healthcare visit.

Disturbed Body Image

NANDA-I Definition

Negative mental picture of one's physical self

Defining Characteristics

Altered proprioception; altered social involvement; avoids looking at one's body; avoids touching one's body; consistently compares oneself with others; depressive symptoms; expresses concerns about sexuality; expresses fear of reaction by others; expresses preoccupation with change; expresses preoccupation with missing body part; focused on past appearance; focused on past function; focused on past strength; frequently weighs self; hides body part; monitors changes in one's body; names body part; names missing body part; neglects nonfunctioning body part; nonverbal response to body changes; nonverbal response to perceived body changes; overexposes body part; perceptions that reflect an altered view of appearance; refuses to acknowledge change; reports feeling one has failed in life; social anxiety; uses impersonal pronouns to describe body part; uses impersonal pronouns to describe missing body part

Related Factors

Body consciousness; conflict between spiritual beliefs and treatment regimen; conflict between values and cultural norms; distrust of body function; fear of disease recurrence; low self efficacy; low self-esteem; obesity; residual limb pain; unrealistic perception of treatment outcome; unrealistic self-expectations

At-Risk Population

Cancer survivors; individuals experiencing altered body weight; individuals experiencing developmental transition; individuals experiencing puberty; individuals with altered body function; individuals with scars; individuals with stomas; women

Associated Condition

Binge-eating disorder; chronic pain; fibromyalgia; human immunodeficiency virus infections; impaired psychosocial functioning; mental disorders; surgical procedures; treatment regimen; wounds and injuries

Client Outcomes

Client Will (Specify Time Frame)

- Demonstrate adaptation to changes in physical appearance or body function as evidenced by adjustment to lifestyle change
- Identify and change irrational beliefs and expectations regarding body size or function
- Recognize health-destructive behaviors and demonstrate willingness to adhere to treatments or methods that will promote health
- Verbalize congruence between body reality and body perception
- Describe, touch, or observe affected body part
- Demonstrate social involvement rather than avoidance and use adaptive coping and/or social skills
- Use cognitive strategies or other coping skills to improve perception of body image and enhance functioning
- Use strategies to enhance appearance (e.g., wig, clothing)

Nursing Interventions

- Incorporate psychosocial questions related to body image as part of nursing assessment to identify clients at risk for body image disturbance.
- Maintain awareness of conditions or changes that are likely to cause a disturbed body image: removal of a body part or change/loss of body function such as blindness or hearing loss, cancer survivors, clients with eating disorders, burns, skin disorders, or those with stomas or other disfiguring conditions, or a loss of perceived attractiveness such as hair loss.
- Be aware of the impact of treatments and surgeries that involve the face and neck and be prepared to address the client's psychosocial needs.
- Maintain understanding that age, gender, and other demographic identifiers may be associated with higher degrees of body image disturbance.
- Consideration should be given to providing counseling for women with breast cancer to assist with acceptance of the reality of the disease and to increase their resilience against breast surgery.

B

- Discuss treatment options and outcomes for women diagnosed with breast cancer. Be prepared to explore options of lumpectomy versus mastectomy and the potential for reconstructive surgery. Include cosmetic and appliance options available to mitigate effects of mastectomy and/or chemotherapy, such as wigs and customized mastectomy bras.
- Nurses and other health professionals should support clients with stomas in problem-focused coping strategies.

Pediatric

- Many of the previously mentioned interventions are appropriate for the pediatric client.
- Educate parents on the role their own attitudes play in a child's body perception and acceptance.
- When caring for teenagers, be aware of the impact of acne vulgaris on quality of life. The impact was proportional to the severity of acne. Assess for symptoms of social withdrawal, limited eye contact, and expressions of low self-esteem. Educate teens on skin care and hygiene, and assist with referrals to a dermatologist when needed.

Geriatric

- Encourage regular exercise for older adults.

Multicultural

- Acknowledge that body image disturbances can affect all individuals regardless of culture, race, or ethnicity. Assess for the influence of cultural beliefs, regional norms, and values on the client's body image.

Home Care

- The previously mentioned interventions may be adapted for home care use.
- Assess client's level of social support. Social support is one of the determinants of the client's recovery and emotional health.
- Assess family/caregiver level of acceptance of the client's body changes.
- Encourage clients to discuss concerns related to sexuality and provide support or information as indicated. Many conditions that affect body image also affect sexuality.
- Teach all aspects of care. Involve clients and caregivers in self-care as soon as possible. Do this in stages if clients still have difficulty looking at or touching a changed body part.

Client/Family Teaching and Discharge Planning

- Advise clients with a stoma about the support available to them.

Insufficient Breast Milk Production

B

NANDA-I Definition

Inadequate supply of maternal breast milk to support nutritional state of an infant or child

Defining Characteristics

Absence of milk production with nipple stimulation; breast milk expressed is less than prescribed volume for infant; delay in milk production; infant constipation; infant frequently crying; infant frequently seeks to suckle at breast; infant refuses to suckle at breast; infant voids small amounts of concentrated urine; infant weight gain < 500 g in a month; prolonged breastfeeding time; unsustained suckling at breast

Related Factors

Ineffective latching on to breast; ineffective sucking reflex; insufficient opportunity for suckling at the breast; insufficient suckling time at breast; maternal alcohol consumption; maternal insufficient fluid volume; maternal malnutrition; maternal smoking; maternal treatment regimen; rejection of breast

Associated Condition

Pregnancy

Client Outcomes

Client Will (Specify Time Frame)

- State knowledge of indicators of adequate milk supply
- State and demonstrate measures to ensure adequate milk supply

Nursing Interventions

- Provide lactation support at all phases of lactation (Neifert & Bunick, 2013; Nielsen et al., 2011).
- Initiate skin-to-skin contact at birth and undisturbed contact for the first hour following birth; the mother should be encouraged to watch the baby, not the clock.
- Encourage postpartum women to start breastfeeding based on infant need as early as possible and reduce formula use to increase breastfeeding frequency. Use nonnarcotic analgesics as early as possible.
- Provide suggestions for mothers on how to increase milk production and how to determine whether there is insufficient milk supply.
- Instruct mothers that breastfeeding frequency, sucking times, and amounts are variable and normal. Assist mothers in optimal milk removal frequency.

B

▲ Consider the use of medication for mothers of preterm infants with insufficient expressed breast milk.

Pediatric

- Provide individualized follow-up with extra home visits or outpatient visits for teen mothers within the first few days after hospital discharge and encourage schools to be more compatible with breastfeeding.

Multicultural

- Provide information and support to mothers on benefits of breastfeeding at antenatal visits.
- Refer to care plans Interrupted **Breastfeeding** and Readiness for enhanced **Breastfeeding** for additional interventions.

Ineffective Breastfeeding

NANDA-I Definition

Difficulty feeding milk from the breasts, which may compromise nutritional status of the infant/child

Defining Characteristics

Inadequate infant stooling; infant arching at breast; infant crying at breast; infant crying within the first hour after breastfeeding; infant fussing within one hour of breastfeeding; infant inability to latch on to maternal breast correctly; infant resisting latching on to breast; infant unresponsive to other comfort measures; insufficient emptying of each breast per feeding; insufficient infant weight gain; insufficient signs of oxytocin release; perceived inadequate milk supply; sore nipples persisting beyond first week; sustained infant weight loss; unsustained suckling at the breast

Related Factors

Delayed stage II lactogenesis; inadequate milk supply; insufficient family support; insufficient opportunity for suckling at breast; insufficient parental knowledge regarding breastfeeding techniques; insufficient parental knowledge regarding importance of breastfeeding; interrupted breastfeeding; maternal ambivalence; maternal anxiety; maternal breast anomaly; maternal fatigue; maternal obesity; maternal pain; pacifier use; poor infant sucking reflex; supplemental feedings with artificial nipple

At-Risk Population

Prematurity; previous breast surgery; previous history of breastfeeding failure; short maternity leave

Associated Condition

Oropharyngeal defect

Client Outcomes

Client Will (Specify Time Frame)

- Achieve effective milk transfer (dyad)
- Verbalize/demonstrate techniques to manage breastfeeding problems (mother)
- Manifest signs of adequate intake at the breast (infant)
- Manifest positive self-esteem in relation to the infant feeding process (mother)
- Explain alternative method of infant feeding if unable to continue exclusive breastfeeding (mother)

Nursing Interventions

- Identify women with risk factors for lower breastfeeding initiation and continuation rates, as well as factors contributing to ineffective breastfeeding (see conditions listed in the section Related Factors) as early as possible in the perinatal experience.
- Provide time for clients to express expectations and concerns, and provide emotional support as needed.
- Encourage skin-to-skin holding, beginning immediately after delivery.
- Use valid and reliable tools to measure breastfeeding performance and to predict early discontinuance of breastfeeding whenever possible/feasible.
- Promote comfort and relaxation to reduce pain and anxiety.
- Avoid supplemental feedings.
- Teach mother to observe for infant behavioral cues and responses to breastfeeding.

▲ Provide necessary equipment/instruction/assistance for milk expression as needed.

▲ Provide referrals and resources: lactation consultants, nurse and peer support programs, community organizations, and written and electronic sources of information.

- See care plan for Readiness for enhanced **Breastfeeding.**

Multicultural

- Assess whether the client's cultural beliefs about breastfeeding are contributing to ineffective breastfeeding.
- Assess the influence of family support on the decision to continue or discontinue breastfeeding.
- See care plan for Readiness for enhanced **Breastfeeding.**

Home Care

The previously mentioned interventions may be adapted for home care use.

- Provide anticipatory guidance in relation to home management of breastfeeding.

▲ Investigate availability of and refer to public health department, hospital home follow-up breastfeeding program, or other postdischarge support.

- See care plan for Risk for impaired **Attachment.**

Client/Family Teaching and Discharge Planning

- Instruct the client on maternal breastfeeding behaviors/techniques (preparation for, positioning, initiation of/promoting latch-on, burping, completion of session, and frequency of feeding) using a variety of strategies such as written materials, videos, and online resources.
- Teach the mother self-care measures (e.g., breast care, management of breast/nipple discomfort, nutrition/fluid, rest/activity).
- Provide information regarding infant feeding cues and behaviors and appropriate maternal responses, as well as measures of infant feeding adequacy.
- Provide education to partner/family/significant others as needed.

Interrupted Breastfeeding

NANDA-I Definition

Break in the continuity of feeding milk from the breasts, which may compromise breastfeeding success and/or nutritional status of the infant/child

Defining Characteristics

Nonexclusive breastfeeding

Related Factors

Maternal employment; maternal-infant separation; need to abruptly wean infant

At-Risk Population

Hospitalization of child; prematurity

Associated Condition

Contraindications to breastfeeding; infant illness; maternal illness

Client Outcomes

Client Will (Specify Time Frame)

Infant

- Receive mother's breast milk if not contraindicated by maternal conditions (e.g., certain drugs, infections) or infant conditions (e.g., galactosemia)

Maternal

- Maintain lactation
- Achieve effective breastfeeding or satisfaction with the breastfeeding experience
- Demonstrate effective methods of breast milk collection and storage

Nursing Interventions

- • Provide information and support to mother and partner/family regarding mother's desire/intention to begin or resume breastfeeding.
- • Clarify that interruption in breastfeeding is truly necessary.
- • Provide anticipatory guidance to the mother/family regarding potential duration of the interruption when possible/feasible, ensuring that measures to sustain or restart lactation and promote parent–infant attachment can make it possible to resume breastfeeding when the condition/situation requiring interruption is resolved.
- • Reassure the mother/family that the infant will benefit from any amount of breast milk provided.
- • Assess mother's concerns, and observe mother performing psychomotor skills (expression, storage, alternative feeding, skin-to-skin care, and/or breastfeeding) and assist as needed.
- • Collaborate with mother/family/healthcare providers (as needed) to develop a plan for skin-to-skin contact.
- • Collaborate with the mother/family/healthcare provider/employer (as needed) to develop a plan for expression/pumping of breast milk and/or infant feeding.
- • Monitor for signs indicating infant's ability to breastfeed and interest in breastfeeding.
- ▲ Use supplementation only as medically indicated.
- • Provide anticipatory guidance for common problems associated with interrupted breastfeeding (e.g., incomplete emptying of milk glands, diminishing milk supply, infant difficulty with resuming breastfeeding, or infant refusal of alternative feeding method).
- ▲ Initiate follow-up and make appropriate referrals.
- • Assist the client to accept and learn an alternative method of infant feeding if effective breastfeeding is not achieved.

• = Independent ▲ = Collaborative

B

- See care plans for Readiness for enhanced **Breastfeeding** and Ineffective **Breastfeeding.**

Multicultural

- Teach culturally appropriate techniques for maintaining lactation.
- See care plans for Readiness for enhanced **Breastfeeding** and Ineffective **Breastfeeding.**

Home Care

- The previously mentioned interventions may be adapted for home care use.

Client/Family Teaching and Discharge Planning

- Teach mother effective methods to express breast milk.
- Teach mother/parents about skin-to-skin care.
- Instruct mother on safe breast milk handling techniques.
- See care plans for Readiness for enhanced **Breastfeeding** and Ineffective **Breastfeeding.**

Readiness for Enhanced Breastfeeding

NANDA-I Definition

A pattern of feeding milk from the breasts to an infant or child, which may be strengthened

Defining Characteristics

Mother expresses desire to enhance ability to exclusively breastfeed; Mother expresses desire to enhance ability to provide breast milk for child's nutritional needs

Client Outcomes

Client Will (Specify Time Frame)

- Maintain effective breastfeeding
- Maintain normal growth patterns (infant)
- Verbalize satisfaction with breastfeeding process (mother)

Nursing Interventions

- Encourage expectant mothers to learn about breastfeeding before and during pregnancy.
- Encourage and facilitate early skin-to-skin contact.
- Encourage rooming-in and breastfeeding on demand.
- Monitor the breastfeeding process, identify opportunities to enhance knowledge and experience, and provide direction as needed.
- Give encouragement and positive feedback to mothers as they learn to breastfeed.

B

- Discuss prevention and treatment of common breastfeeding problems, such as nipple pain and/or trauma.
- Teach mother to observe for infant behavioral cues and responses to breastfeeding.
- Identify current support-person network and opportunities for continued breastfeeding support.
- Use supplementation only as medically indicated, and do not provide samples of formula on discharge from hospital.
- ▲ Provide follow-up contact; as available, provide home visits and/or peer counseling.

Multicultural

- Assess for the influence of cultural beliefs, norms, and values on current breastfeeding practices.

Home Care

- The previously mentioned interventions may be adapted for home care use.

Client/Family Teaching and Discharge Planning

- Include the partner and other family members in education about breastfeeding.
- Teach the client the importance of maternal nutrition.
- Teach mother about the infant's subtle hunger cues (e.g., rooting, sucking, mouthing, hand-to-mouth and hand-to-hand activity) and encourage her to breastfeed whenever signs are apparent.
- Review guidelines for frequency (at least every 2–3 hours, or 8–12 feedings per 24 hours) and duration (until suckling and swallowing slow down and satiety is reached) of feeding times.
- Provide information about common infant behaviors related to breastfeeding, and appropriate maternal responses.
- ▲ Provide referrals and resources: lactation consultants, nurse and peer support programs, community organizations, and written and electronic sources of information.

Ineffective Breathing Pattern

NANDA-I Definition

Inspiration and/or expiration that does not provide adequate ventilation

Defining Characteristics

Abdominal paradoxical respiratory pattern; altered chest excursion; altered tidal volume; bradypnea; cyanosis; decreased expiratory pressure; decreased inspiratory pressure; decreased minute ventilation; decreased vital capacity;

...ercapnia; hyperventilation; hypoventilation; hypoxemia; hypoxia; increased anterior-posterior chest diameter; nasal flaring; orthopnea; prolonged expiration phase; pursed-lip breathing; subcostal retraction; tachypnea; uses accessory muscles to breathe; uses three-point position

Related Factors

Anxiety; body position that inhibits lung expansion; fatigue; increased physical exertion; obesity; pain

At Risk Population

Young women

Associated Condition

Bony deformity; chest wall deformity; chronic obstructive pulmonary disease; critical illness; heart diseases; hyperventilation syndrome; hypoventilation syndrome; increased airway resistance; increased serum hydrogen concentration; musculoskeletal impairment; neurological immaturity; neurological impairment; neuromuscular diseases; reduced pulmonary complacency; sleep-apnea syndromes; spinal cord injuries

Client Outcomes

Client Will (Specify Time Frame)

- Demonstrate a breathing pattern that supports blood gas results within the client's normal parameters
- Report ability to breathe comfortably
- Demonstrate ability to perform pursed-lip breathing and controlled breathing
- Identify and avoid specific factors that exacerbate episodes of ineffective breathing patterns

Nursing Interventions

- Monitor respiratory rate, depth, and ease of respiration.
- Note pattern of respiration. If client is dyspneic, note what seems to cause the dyspnea, the way in which the client deals with the condition, and how the dyspnea resolves or gets worse.
- Note amount of anxiety associated with the dyspnea.
- Attempt to determine if client's dyspnea is physiological or psychological in cause.
- The rapidity of which the onset of dyspnea is noted is also an indicator of the severity of the pathological condition (Croucher, 2014).

Psychological Dyspnea—Hyperventilation

- Monitor for symptoms of hyperventilation including rapid respiratory rate, sighing breaths, lightheadedness, numbness and tingling of hands and feet, palpitations, and sometimes chest pain (Bickley & Szilagyi, 2016).

- Assess cause of hyperventilation by asking client about current emotions and psychological state.
  - Pulmonary rehabilitation programs that contain elements of behavioral, cognitive, or psychosocial components have been shown to improve dyspnea and reduce anxiety and depression, particularly in clients with chronic obstructive pulmonary disease (COPD) (von Leupoldt et al., 2014).
  - Pharmacological treatment to reduce anxiety and panic that likely increase dyspnea are not recommended for clients with asthma and COPD (von Leupoldt et al., 2014).
- Ask the client to breathe with you to slow down respiratory rate.

▲ Consider having the client breathe in and out of a paper bag as tolerated.

▲ If the client has chronic problems with hyperventilation, numbness and tingling in extremities, dizziness, and other signs of panic attacks, refer for counseling or pulmonary rehabilitation (Lareau et al., 2014).

Physiological Dyspnea

▲ Ensure that client in acute dyspneic state has received any ordered medications, oxygen, and any other treatment needed.

- Acute onset of dyspnea is often accompanied by signs of respiratory distress, which include tachypnea, cough, stridor, wheezing, cyanosis, impaired speech, tachycardia, hypotension, peripheral edema, frothy sputum, pursed-lip breathing, accessory respiratory muscle use, crackles, tripod positioning, and other signs (Croucher, 2014).
- Observe color of tongue, oral mucosa, and skin for signs of cyanosis.
- Auscultate breath sounds, noting decreased or absent sounds, crackles, or wheezes.

▲ Monitor oxygen saturation continuously using pulse oximetry. Note blood gas results as available.
  - If a client is both dyspneic and hypoxemic, high-flow oxygen may be more beneficial to relieve the dyspnea.
  - For clients with chronic breathlessness but no hypoxemia, oxygen therapy does not affect the sensation of dyspnea (Siela & Kidd, 2017).

- Using touch on the shoulder, coach the client to slow respiratory rate, demonstrating slower respirations; making eye contact with the client; and communicating in a calm, supportive fashion.
- Support the client in using pursed-lip and controlled breathing techniques.

- • If the client is acutely dyspneic, consider having the client lean forward over a bedside table, resting elbows on the table if tolerated (Mahler, 2014).
- • Position the client in an upright or semi-Fowler's position. See Nursing Interventions and *Rationales* for Impaired **Gas** exchange for further information on positioning.
- • Increased respiratory drive is one of the causes of dyspnea. Pulmonary rehabilitation reduces respiratory drive through endurance exercise training, strength training, restorative therapy with calories and anabolic agents, pacing strategies and pursed-lip breathing techniques, and optimizing bronchodilator therapy (Lareau et al., 2014).
- ▲ Administer oxygen as ordered. Supplemental oxygen may not relieve all dyspnea (Parshall et al., 2012).
- • Altering the central perception of dyspnea may reduce breathlessness through exercise training, reduction in anxiety and fear of dyspnea, and self-management strategies and promotion of self-efficacy (Lareau et al., 2014).
- • Use of music as a distraction may reduce the perception of dyspnea (Mahler, 2014).
- • Inspiratory muscle training likely improves breathlessness during exercise and/or with activities of daily living in clients with COPD and congestive heart failure (CHF) who exhibit inspiratory muscle weakness (Lareau et al., 2014; Mahler, 2014).
- • Increase client's activity to walking three times per day as tolerated. Assist the client to use oxygen during activity as needed. See Nursing Interventions for **Decreased Activity** tolerance. Walking 20 minutes per day is recommended for those unable to be in a structured program (GOLD, 2017).
- • Schedule rest periods before and after activity.
- ▲ Evaluate the client's nutritional status. Refer to a dietitian if needed. Use nutritional supplements to increase nutritional level if needed.
- • Provide small, frequent feedings.
- • Offer a fan to move the air in the environment.
- • Encourage the client to take deep breaths at prescribed intervals and do controlled coughing.
- • Help the client with chronic respiratory disease evaluate dyspnea experience to determine whether previous incidences of dyspnea were similar and to recognize that the client survived those

incidences. Encourage the client to be self-reliant if possible, use problem-solving skills, and maximize use of social support.

- • See Ineffective **Airway** clearance if client has a problem with increased respiratory secretions.
- ▲ Refer the client with COPD for pulmonary rehabilitation.

Geriatric

- • Assess respiratory systems in older adults with the understanding that inspiratory muscles weaken, resulting in a slight barrel chest. Expiratory muscles work harder with use of accessory muscles (Martin-Plank, 2014).
- • Encourage ambulation as tolerated.
- • Encourage older clients to sit upright or stand and to avoid lying down for prolonged periods during the day.

Home Care

- • The previously mentioned interventions may be adapted for home care use.
- • Work with the client to determine what strategies are most helpful during times of dyspnea. Provide education to empower the client to self-manage the disease associated with impaired gas exchange.
- • Assist the client and family in identifying other factors that precipitate or exacerbate episodes of ineffective breathing patterns (i.e., stress, allergens, stairs, activities that have high energy requirements).
- • Assess client knowledge of and compliance with medication regimen.
- ▲ Refer the client for telemonitoring with a pulmonologist as appropriate, with use of an electronic spirometer or an electronic peak flowmeter.
- • Teach the client and family the importance of maintaining the therapeutic regimen and having as-needed drugs easily accessible at all times.
- • Provide the client with emotional support in dealing with symptoms of respiratory difficulty. Provide family with support for care of a client with chronic or terminal illness. Refer to care plan for **Anxiety.** Witnessing breathing difficulties and facing concerns of dealing with chronic or terminal illness can create fear in the caregiver. Fear inhibits effective coping (Campbell, 2017).
- • When respiratory procedures (e.g., apneic monitoring for an infant) are being implemented, explain equipment and procedures to family members, and provide needed emotional support.

C

- When electrically based equipment for respiratory support is being implemented, evaluate home environment for electrical safety, such as proper grounding. Ensure that notification is sent to the local utility company, the emergency medical team, and police and fire departments.
- Refer to GOLD guidelines for management of home care and indications of hospital admission criteria.
- Support clients' efforts at self-care. Ensure they have all the information they need to participate in care.
- Identify an emergency plan including when to call your healthcare provider or 911.
- ▲ Refer to occupational therapy for evaluation and teaching of energy conservation techniques.
- ▲ Refer to home health aide services as needed to support energy conservation.
- ▲ Institute case management of frail elderly to support continued independent living (Martin-Plank, 2014).

Client/Family Teaching and Discharge Planning

- Teach pursed-lip and controlled breathing techniques.
- Teach about dosage, actions, and side effects of medications.
- Teach client progressive muscle relaxation techniques.
- Teach the client to identify and avoid specific factors that exacerbate ineffective breathing patterns, such as exposure to other sources of air pollution, especially smoking. If client smokes, refer to the smoking cessation section in the impaired **Gas** exchange care plan.

Decreased Cardiac Output

NANDA-I Definition

Inadequate blood pumped by the heart to meet the metabolic demands of the body

Defining Characteristics

Altered Heart Rate/Rhythm

Bradycardia; electrocardiogram (ECG) change; heart palpitations; tachycardia

Altered Preload

Decrease in central venous pressure (CVP); decrease in pulmonary artery wedge pressure (PAWP); edema; fatigue; heart murmur; increase in central venous pressure (CVP); increase in pulmonary artery wedge pressure (PAWP); jugular vein distention; weight gain

C

Altered Afterload

Abnormal skin color; alteration in blood pressure; clammy skin; decrease in peripheral pulses; decrease in pulmonary vascular resistance (PVR); decrease in systemic vascular resistance (SVR); dyspnea; increase in pulmonary vascular resistance (PVR); increase in systemic vascular resistance (SVR); oliguria; prolonged capillary refill

Altered Contractility

Adventitious breath sounds; coughing; decreased cardiac index; decrease in ejection fraction; decrease in left ventricular stroke work index (LVSWI); decrease in stroke volume index (SVI); orthopnea; paroxysmal nocturnal dyspnea; presence of S3 heart sound; presence of S4 heart sound

Behavioral/Emotional

Anxiety; restlessness

Related Factors

To be developed

Associated Condition

Alteration in afterload; alteration in contractility; alteration in heart rate; alteration in heart rhythm; alteration in preload; alteration in stroke volume

Client Outcomes

Client Will (Specify Time Frame)

- Demonstrate adequate cardiac output as evidenced by blood pressure, pulse rate, and rhythm within normal parameters for client; strong peripheral pulses; maintained level of mentation, lack of chest discomfort or dyspnea, and adequate urinary output; an ability to tolerate activity without symptoms of dyspnea, syncope, or chest pain
- Remain free of side effects from the medications used to achieve adequate cardiac output
- Explain actions and precautions to prevent primary or secondary cardiac disease

Nursing Interventions

- Recognize characteristics of decreased cardiac output including, but not limited to, fatigue, dyspnea, edema, orthopnea, paroxysmal nocturnal dyspnea, chest pain, decreased exercise capacity, weight gain, hepatomegaly, jugular venous distension, palpitations, lung rhonchi, cough, clammy skin, skin color changes, dysuria, altered mental status, anemia, and hemodynamic changes.
- Monitor and report presence and degree of symptoms including dyspnea at rest, reduced exercise capacity, difficulty with activities of daily living, orthopnea, paroxysmal nocturnal dyspnea, cough,

palpitations, chest pain, distended abdomen, fatigue, presyncope/syncope, or weakness. Monitor and report signs including jugular vein distention, peripheral edema, S3 gallop, rales, positive hepatojugular reflux, ascites, laterally displaced or pronounced point of maximal impact, heart murmur, narrow pulse pressure, cool extremities, tachycardia with pulsus alternans, and irregular heartbeat.

- • Monitor orthostatic blood pressures, oxygenation, hemodynamic values, and daily weights.
- • Recognize that decreased cardiac output can occur in a number of noncardiac disorders such as septic shock and hypovolemia. Expect variation in orders for differential diagnoses related to decreased cardiac output, because orders will be distinct to address the primary cause of the altered cardiac output.
- • Obtain a thorough client-specific and familial history.
- ▲ Monitor pulse oximetry and administer oxygen as needed per healthcare provider's order. Supplemental oxygen increases oxygen availability to the myocardium and can relieve symptoms of hypoxemia. Resting hypoxia or oxygen desaturation may indicate fluid overload or concurrent pulmonary disease.
- • Place client in semi-Fowler's or high Fowler's position with legs down or in a position of comfort. Elevating the head of the bed and legs in the down position may decrease the work of breathing and may also decrease venous return and preload.
- • During acute events, ensure client remains on short-term bed rest or maintains activity level that does not compromise cardiac output.
- • Provide a restful environment by minimizing controllable stressors and unnecessary disturbances. Reducing stressors decreases cardiac workload and oxygen demand.
- ▲ Apply graduated compression stockings or intermittent sequential pneumatic compression (ISPC) leg sleeves as ordered. Ensure proper fit by measuring accurately. Remove stocking at least twice a day, and then reapply. Assess the condition of the extremities frequently. Graduated compression stockings may be contraindicated in clients with peripheral arterial disease (Kahn et al., 2012).
- ▲ Check blood pressure, pulse, and condition before administering cardiac medications (e.g., angiotensin-converting enzyme inhibitors, angiotensin receptor blockers, calcium channel blockers, diuretics, digoxin, and beta-blockers). Notify healthcare provider if heart rate or blood pressure is low before holding medications. It is important

that the nurse evaluate how well the client is tolerating current medications before administering cardiac medications; do not hold medications without healthcare provider input. The healthcare provider may decide to have medications administered even though the blood pressure or pulse rate has lowered.

- • Observe for and report chest pain or discomfort; note location, radiation, severity, quality, duration, and associated manifestations such as nausea, indigestion, or diaphoresis; also note precipitating and relieving factors. Chest pain/discomfort may indicate an inadequate blood supply to the heart, which can further compromise cardiac output.
- ▲ If chest pain is present, refer to the interventions in risk for Decreased **Cardiac** tissue perfusion care plan.
- • Recognize the effect of sleep-disordered breathing in HF and that sleep disorders are common in clients with HF (Yancy et al., 2013, 2017).
- • Administer CPAP or supplemental oxygen at night as ordered for management of suspected or diagnosed sleep disordered breathing.
- ▲ Closely monitor fluid intake, including intravenous lines. Maintain fluid restriction if ordered. In clients with decreased cardiac output, poorly functioning ventricles may not tolerate increased fluid volumes.
- • Monitor intake and output (I&O). If client is acutely ill, measure hourly urine output and note decreases in output. Decreased cardiac output results in decreased perfusion of the kidneys, with a resulting decrease in urine output.
- ▲ Note results of initial diagnostic studies, including electrocardiography, echocardiography, and chest radiography.
- ▲ Note results of further diagnostic imaging studies such as radionuclide imaging, stress echocardiography, cardiac catheterization, or magnetic resonance imaging (MRI).
- ▲ Review laboratory data as needed, including arterial blood gases, complete blood count, serum electrolytes (sodium, potassium, magnesium, and calcium), blood urea nitrogen, creatinine, iron studies, urinalysis, glucose, fasting lipid profile, liver function tests, thyroid-stimulating hormone, B-type natriuretic peptide (BNP assay), or N-terminal pro-B-type natriuretic peptide (NTpro-BNP). Routine blood work can provide insight into the etiology of HF and extent of decompensation.

C

- • Gradually increase activity when the client's condition is stabilized by encouraging slower-paced activities, or shorter periods of activity, with frequent rest periods after exercise prescription; observe for symptoms of intolerance. Take blood pressure and pulse before and after activity and note changes. Activity of the cardiac client should be closely monitored. See **Decreased Activity** tolerance.
- ▲ Encourage a diet that promotes cardiovascular health and reduces risk of hypertension, atherosclerotic disease, renal impairment, insulin resistance, and hypervolemia, within the context of an individual's cultural preferences (Eckel et al., 2013; Van Horn et al., 2016; Whelton et al., 2017).
- ▲ Monitor bowel function. Provide stool softeners as ordered. Caution client not to strain when defecating. Decreased activity, pain medication, and diuretics can cause constipation.
- • Weigh the client at the same time daily (after voiding). Daily weight is a good indicator of fluid balance. Use the same scale if possible when weighing clients for consistency. Increased weight and severity of symptoms can signal decreased cardiac function with retention of fluids.
- ▲ Provide influenza and pneumococcal vaccines as needed before client discharge for those who have yet to receive those inoculations (Centers for Disease Control, 2017).
- • Assess for presence of depression and/or anxiety and refer for treatment if present. See Nursing Interventions for **Anxiety** to facilitate reduction of anxiety in clients and family.
- ▲ Refer to a cardiac rehabilitation program for education and monitored exercise.
- ▲ Refer to an HF program for education, evaluation, and guided support to increase activity and rebuild quality of life. Support for the HF client should be client centered, culturally sensitive, and include family and social support.

Critically Ill

- ▲ Observe for symptoms of cardiogenic shock, including impaired mentation, hypotension, decreased peripheral pulses, cold clammy skin, signs of pulmonary congestion, and decreased organ function. If present, notify the healthcare provider immediately. Cardiogenic shock is a state of circulatory failure from loss of cardiac function associated with inadequate organ perfusion and a high mortality rate.

- ▲ If shock is present, monitor hemodynamic parameters for an increase in pulmonary wedge pressure, an increase in SVR, or a decrease in stroke volume, cardiac output, and cardiac index.
- ▲ Titrate inotropic and vasoactive medications within defined parameters to maintain contractility, preload, and afterload per healthcare provider's order. By following parameters, the nurse ensures maintenance of a delicate balance of medications that stimulate the heart to increase contractility, while maintaining adequate perfusion of the body.
- ▲ Identify significant fluid overload and initiate intravenous diuretics as ordered. Monitor I&Os, daily weight, and vital signs, as well as signs and symptoms of congestion. Watch laboratory data, including serum electrolytes, creatinine, and urea nitrogen.
- ▲ When using pulmonary arterial catheter technology, be sure to appropriately level and zero the equipment, use minimal tubing, maintain system patency, perform square wave testing, position the client appropriately, and consider correlation to respiratory and cardiac cycles when assessing waveforms and integrating data into client assessment.
- ▲ Observe for worsening signs and symptoms of respiratory compromise. Recognize that invasive or noninvasive ventilation may be required for clients with acute cardiogenic pulmonary edema.
- ▲ Monitor client for signs and symptoms of fluid and electrolyte imbalance when clients are receiving ultrafiltration or continuous renal replacement therapy (CRRT). Clients with refractory HF may have ultrafiltration or CRRT ordered as a mechanical method to remove excess fluid volume.
- • Recognize that hypoperfusion from low cardiac output can lead to altered mental status and decreased cognition.
- • Recognize that clients with severe HF may undergo additional therapies, such as internal pacemaker or defibrillator placement, and/or placement of a ventricular assist device (VAD).

Geriatric

- • Recognize that older clients may demonstrate fatigue and depression as signs of HF and decreased cardiac output.
- ▲ If the client has heart disease causing decreased activity tolerance, refer for cardiac rehabilitation.
- ▲ Recognize that edema can present differently in the older population.

C

- ▲ Recognize that blood pressure control is beneficial for older clients to reduce the risk of worsening HF.
- ▲ Recognize that renal function is not always accurately represented by serum creatinine in the older population because of less muscle mass (Yancy et al., 2013).
- ▲ Observe for side effects from cardiac medications. Older adults can have difficulty with metabolism and excretion of medications because of decreased function of the liver and kidneys; therefore toxic side effects are more common.
- ▲ Older adults may require more frequent visits, closer monitoring of medication dose changes, and more gradual increases in medications, because of changes in the metabolism of medications and impaired renal function (Yancy et al., 2013).
- ▲ As older adults approach end of life, clinicians should help to facilitate a comprehensive plan of care that incorporates the client and family's values, goals, and preferences (Allen et al., 2012; National Consensus Project for Quality Palliative Care, 2013).

Home Care

- • Some of the previously mentioned interventions may be adapted for home care use. Home care agencies may use specialized staff and methods to care for chronic HF clients.
- • Assess for fatigue and weakness frequently. Assess home environment for safety, as well as resources/obstacles to energy conservation.
- • Help family adapt daily living patterns to establish life changes that will maintain improved cardiac functioning in the client. Take the client's perspective into consideration and use a holistic approach in assessing and responding to client planning for the future.
- • Assist client to recognize and exercise power in using self-care management to adjust to health change. Refer to care plan for **Powerlessness.**
- ▲ Refer to medical social services, cardiac rehabilitation, telemonitoring, and case management as necessary for assistance with home care, access to resources, and counseling about the impact of severe or chronic cardiac diseases.
- ▲ As the client chooses, refer to palliative care for care, which can begin earlier in the care of the HF client. Palliative care can be used to increase comfort and quality of life in the HF client before end-of-life care.
- ▲ If the client's condition warrants, refer to hospice.

C

Client/Family Teaching and Discharge Planning

- Begin discharge planning as soon as possible on admission to the emergency department (ED) if appropriate with a case manager or social worker to assess home support systems and the need for community or home health services.
- Discharge education should be comprehensive, evidence based, culturally sensitive, and include both the client and family (Yancy et al., 2013).
- Teach the client about any medications prescribed. Medication teaching includes the drug name; its purpose, administration instructions, such as taking it with or without food; and any side effects. Instruct the client to report any adverse side effects to his or her healthcare provider.
- Teach the importance of performing and recording daily weights on arising for the day, and to report weight gain. Ask if client has a scale at home; if not, assist in getting one.
- Teach the types and progression patterns of worsening HF symptoms, when to call a healthcare provider for help, and when to go to the hospital for urgent care (Yancy et al., 2013).
- Stress the importance of ceasing tobacco use (Whelton et al., 2017).

▲ Individuals should be screened for electronic cigarette use (e-cigarette).

- On hospital discharge, educate clients about low-sodium, low–saturated fat diet, with consideration of client education, literacy, and health literacy level.
- Educate clients that comorbidities, including obesity, hypertension, metabolic syndrome, diabetes mellitus, and hyperlipidemia, are common in individuals with HF and can affect clinical outcomes related to HF if not controlled (Bozkurt et al., 2016).
- For clients with diabetes mellitus, educate about the importance of glycemic control.
- Instruct client and family on the importance of regular follow-up care with healthcare providers.

▲ Teach stress reduction (e.g., meditation, imagery, controlled breathing, muscle relaxation techniques).

- Discuss advance directives with the HF client, including resuscitation preferences.
- Clients should be provided with education regarding the influenza vaccine and pneumococcal vaccine prior to discharge.
- Teach the importance of physical activity as tolerated.

Risk for Decreased Cardiac Output

NANDA-I Definition

C

Susceptible to inadequate blood pumped by the heart to meet metabolic demands of the body, which may compromise health

Risk Factors

To be developed

Associated Condition

Alteration in afterload; alteration in contractility; alteration in heart rate; alteration in heart rhythm; alteration in preload; alteration in stroke volume

Client Outcomes, Nursing Interventions, Client/Family Teaching and Discharge Planning

Refer to care plan for Decreased **Cardiac** output

Risk for Decreased Cardiac Tissue Perfusion

NANDA-I Definition

Susceptible to a decrease in cardiac (coronary) circulation, which may compromise health

Risk Factors

Insufficient knowledge of modifiable factors; substance misuse

At-Risk Population

Family history of cardiovascular disease

Associated Condition

Cardiac tamponade; cardiovascular surgery; coronary artery spasm; diabetes mellitus; hyperlipidemia; hypertension; hypovolemia; hypoxemia; hypoxia; increase in C-reactive protein; pharmaceutical agent

Client Outcomes

Client Will (Specify Time Frame)

- Maintain vital signs within normal range
- Retain an asymptomatic cardiac rhythm (have absence of arrhythmias, tachycardia, or bradycardia)
- Be free from chest and radiated discomfort as well as associated symptoms related to acute coronary syndromes (ACSs)
- Deny nausea and be free of vomiting
- Have skin that is dry and of normal temperature

Nursing Interventions

- • Be aware that the primary cause of ACS, which include unstable angina (UA), non–ST-elevation myocardial infarction (NSTEMI), and ST-elevation myocardial infarction (STEMI), is an imbalance between myocardial oxygen consumption and demand that is associated with partially or fully occlusive thrombus development in coronary arteries (Amsterdam et al., 2014).
- • Assess for symptoms of coronary hypoperfusion and possible ACS, including chest discomfort (pressure, tightness, crushing, squeezing, dullness, or achiness), with or without radiation (or originating) in the retrosternum, back, neck, jaw, shoulder, or arm discomfort or numbness; shortness of breath (SOB); associated diaphoresis; abdominal pain; dizziness, lightheadedness, loss of consciousness, or unexplained fatigue; nausea or vomiting with chest discomfort, heartburn, or indigestion; and associated anxiety.
- • Consider atypical presentations of ACS for women, older adults, and individuals with diabetes mellitus, impaired renal function, and dementia.
- • Review the client's medical, surgical, social, and familial history.
- • Perform physical assessments for both coronary artery disease (CAD) and noncoronary findings related to decreased coronary perfusion, including vital signs, pulse oximetry, equal blood pressure in both arms, heart rate, respiratory rate, and pulse oximetry. Check bilateral pulses for quality and regularity. Report tachycardia, bradycardia, hypotension or hypertension, pulsus alternans or pulsus paradoxus, tachypnea, or abnormal pulse oximetry reading. Assess cardiac rhythm for arrhythmias; skin and mucous membrane color, temperature, and dryness; and capillary refill. Assess neck veins for elevated central venous pressure, cyanosis, and pericardial or pleural friction rub. Examine client for cardiac S4 gallop, new heart murmur, lung crackles, altered mentation, pain on abdominal palpation, decreased bowel sounds, or decreased urinary output.
- ▲ Administer supplemental oxygen as ordered and needed for clients presenting with ACS, respiratory distress, or other high-risk features of hypoxemia to maintain a Po_2 of at least 90%.
- ▲ Use continuous pulse oximetry as ordered.
- ▲ Insert one or more large-bore intravenous catheters to keep the vein open. Routinely assess saline locks for patency. Clients who come to the hospital with possible decrease in coronary perfusion or ACS

C

may have intravenous fluids and medications ordered routinely or emergently to maintain or restore adequate cardiac function and rhythm.

- ▲ Observe the cardiac monitor for hemodynamically significant arrhythmias, ST depressions or elevations, T-wave inversions and/or Q-waves as signs of ischemia or injury. Report abnormal findings.
- • Have emergency equipment and defibrillation capability nearby and be prepared to defibrillate immediately if ventricular tachycardia with clinical deterioration or ventricular fibrillation occurs.
- ▲ Perform a 12-lead ECG as ordered to be interpreted within 10 minutes of emergency department arrival and during episodes of chest discomfort or angina equivalent.
- ▲ Administer nonenteric-coated aspirin as ordered, as soon as possible after presentation and for maintenance.
- ▲ Administer nitroglycerin tablets sublingually as ordered, every 5 minutes until the chest pain is resolved while monitoring the blood pressure for hypotension, for a maximum of three doses as ordered. Administer nitroglycerin paste or intravenous preparations as ordered.
- • Do not administer nitroglycerin preparations to individuals with hypotension, or individuals who have received phosphodiesterase type 5 inhibitors, such as sildenafil, tadalafil, or vardenafil, in the last 24 hours (48 hours for long-acting preparations).
- ▲ Administer morphine intravenously as ordered, every 5 to 30 minutes until pain is relieved while monitoring blood pressure when nitroglycerin alone does not relieve chest discomfort.
- ▲ Assess and report abnormal laboratory work results of cardiac enzymes, specifically troponin I or T, B-type natriuretic peptide, chemistries, hematology, coagulation studies, arterial blood gases, finger stick blood sugar, elevated C-reactive protein, or drug screen.
- • Assess for individual risk factors for CAD, such as hypertension, dyslipidemia, cigarette smoking, diabetes mellitus, metabolic syndrome, obesity, or family history of heart disease. Other risk factors including sedentary lifestyle, obesity, or cocaine or amphetamine use. Note age and gender as risk factors.
- ▲ Administer additional heart medications as ordered, including beta-blockers, calcium channel blockers, angiotensin-converting enzyme inhibitors, angiotensin II receptor blockers, aldosterone antagonists, antiplatelet agents, and anticoagulants. Always check blood pressure and pulse rate before administering these medications. If the blood

pressure or pulse rate is low, contact the healthcare provider to establish whether the medication should be withheld. Also check platelet counts, renal function, and coagulation studies as ordered to assess proper effects of these agents.

▲ Administer lipid-lowering therapy as ordered.

▲ Prepare client with education, withholding of meals and/or medications, and intravenous access for early invasive therapy with cardiac catheterization, reperfusion therapy, and possible percutaneous coronary intervention in individuals with refractory angina or hemodynamic or electrical instability, and first medical contact to device time of less than 90 minutes if STEMI is suspected.

▲ Prepare clients with education, withholding of meals and/ or medications, and intravenous access for noninvasive cardiac diagnostic procedures such as echocardiogram, exercise, or pharmacological stress test, and cardiac computed tomography scan as ordered.

▲ Request a referral to a cardiac rehabilitation program.

Geriatric

- Consider atypical presentations of possible ACS in older adults.

▲ Ask the prescriber about possible reduced dosage of medications for older clients, considering weight, creatinine clearance, and glomerular filtration rate.

- Consider issues such as quality of life, palliative care, end-of-life care, and differences in sociocultural aspects for clients and families when supporting them in decisions regarding aggressiveness of care. Ask about living wills, as well as medical and durable power of attorney.

Client/Family Teaching and Discharge Planning

▲ Client and family education regarding a multidisciplinary plan of care should start early. Special attention to client and family education should occur during transitions of care.

- Teach the client and family to call 911 for symptoms of new angina, existing angina unresponsive to rest and sublingual nitroglycerin tablets, or heart attack, or if an individual becomes unresponsive.
- On discharge, instruct clients about symptoms of ischemia, when to cease activity, when to use sublingual nitroglycerin, and when to call 911.
- Teach client about any medications prescribed. Medication teaching includes the drug name, its purpose, administration instructions such as taking it with or without food, and any side effects to be aware of.

Instruct the client to report any adverse side effects to the healthcare provider.

C

- On hospital discharge, educate clients and significant others about discharge medications, including nitroglycerin sublingual tablets or spray, with written, easy-to-understand, culturally sensitive information.
- Provide client education related to risk factors for decreased cardiac tissue perfusion, such as hypertension, hyperlipidemia, metabolic syndrome, diabetes mellitus, tobacco use, obesity, advanced age, and gender (female).
- Instruct the client on antiplatelet and anticoagulation therapy, and about signs of bleeding, need for ongoing medication compliance, and international normalized ratio monitoring.
- After discharge, continue education and support for client blood pressure and diabetes control, weight management, and resumption of physical activity.
- ▲ Clients should be provided with education regarding the influenza vaccine and pneumococcal vaccine before hospital discharge.
- ▲ Stress the importance of ceasing tobacco use (Whelton et al., 2017).
- ▲ Individuals should be screened for electronic cigarette use (e-cigarette).
- ▲ On hospital discharge, educate clients about a low-sodium, low–saturated fat diet, with consideration to client education, literacy, and health literacy level.
- Teach the importance of physical activity as tolerated.

Caregiver Role Strain

NANDA-I Definition

Difficulty in fulfilling care responsibilities, expectations and/or behaviors for family or significant others

Defining Characteristics

Caregiving Activities

Apprehensiveness about future ability to provide care; apprehensiveness about the future health of care receiver; apprehensiveness about possible institutionalization of care receiver; apprehensiveness about well-being of care receiver if unable to provide care; difficulty completing required tasks; difficulty performing required tasks; dysfunctional change in caregiving activities; preoccupation with care routine

Caregiver Health Status

Physiological

Fatigue; gastrointestinal distress; headache; hypertension; rash; weight change

Emotional

Alteration in sleep pattern; anger; depression; emotional vacillation; frustration; impatience; ineffective coping strategies; insufficient time to meet personal needs; nervousness; somatization; stressors

Socioeconomic

Changes in leisure activities; low work productivity; refusal of career advancement; social isolation

Caregiver-Care Receiver Relationship

Difficulty watching care receiver with illness; grieving of changes in relationship with care recipient; uncertainty about changes in relationship with care receiver;

Family Processes

Concerns about family member(s); family conflict

Related Factors

Care Receiver

Condition inhibits conversation; dependency; discharged home with significant needs; increase in care needs; problematic behavior; substance misuse; unpredictability of illness trajectory; unstable health condition

Caregiver

Physical conditions; substance misuse; unrealistic self-expectations; competing role commitments; ineffective coping strategies; inexperience with caregiving; insufficient emotional resilience; insufficient energy; insufficient fulfillment of others' expectations; insufficient fulfillment of self-expectations; insufficient knowledge about community resources; insufficient privacy; insufficient recreation; isolation; not developmentally ready for caregiver role; stressors

Caregiver–Care Receiver Relationship

Abusive relationship; codependency; pattern of ineffective relationships; presence of abuse; unrealistic care receiver expectations; violent relationship

Caregiving Activities

Around-the-clock care responsibilities; change in nature care of activities; complexity of care activities; excessive caregiving activities; extended duration of caregiving required; inadequate physical environment for providing care; insufficient assistance; insufficient equipment for providing care; insufficient respite for caregiver; insufficient time; unpredictability of care situation

Family Processes

C

Family isolation; ineffective family adaptation; pattern of family dysfunction; pattern of family dysfunction prior to the caregiving situation; pattern of ineffective family coping

Socioeconomic

Alienation; difficulty accessing assistance; difficulty accessing community resources; difficulty accessing support; insufficient community resources; insufficient social support; insufficient transportation; social isolation

At-Risk Population

Care receiver's condition inhibits conversation; developmental delay of care receiver; developmental delay of caregiver; exposure to violence; female caregiver; financial crisis; partner as caregiver; prematurity

Associated Condition

Care Receiver

Alteration in cognitive functioning; chronic illness; congenital disorder; illness severity; psychiatric disorder; psychological disorder

Caregiver

Alteration in cognitive functioning; health impairment; psychological disorder

Client Outcomes

Throughout the Care Situation, the Caregiver Will

- Be able to express feelings of strain
- Feel supported by healthcare professionals, family, and friends; feel they have adequate information to provide care
- Report reduced or acceptable feelings of burden or distress
- Take part in self-care activities to maintain own physical and psychological/emotional health; identify resources (family and community) available to help in giving care
- Verbalize mastery of the care activities; feel confident and competent to provide care; have the skills to provide care
- Identify resources to obtain social support
- Ask for help when needed or when feel comprised in ability to provide care
- Not refuse help when needed and offered; ask for help when needed

Throughout the Care Situation, the Care Recipient Will

- Obtain quality and safe physical care and emotional care
- Be treated with respect and dignity

Nursing Interventions

- • Mood management. Regularly monitor signs of depression, anxiety, burden, and deteriorating physical health in the caregiver throughout the care situation if the care demands change frequently, especially if the relationship is poor, the care recipient has cognitive or neuropsychiatric symptoms, there is little social support available, the caregiver becomes enmeshed in the care situation, the caregiver has multiple comorbidities, or has poor preexisting physical or emotional health. Refer to the care plan for **Hopelessness** when appropriate.
- • The impact of providing care on the caregiver's emotional health should be assessed at regular intervals using a reliable and valid instrument such as the Caregiver Strain Risk Index (which was validated with caregivers of clients with diagnosed Parkinson's disease), Caregiver Burden Inventory, Caregiver Reaction Assessment, Screen for Caregiver Burden, Subjective and Objective Scale, and Family Caregiver Self Expectations.
- • Identify potential caregiver personal resources such as mastery, benefit funding, social support, optimism, and positive aspects of care and resilience. Good outcomes can be achieved through resources (Joling et al., 2017).
- • Screen for caregiver role strain at the onset of the care situation, at regular intervals throughout the care situation, at care transitions, and with changes in care recipient status.
- • Assist the client to identify spiritual beliefs and engage in spiritual practices.
- • Regularly monitor social support for the caregiver and help the caregiver identify and use appropriate support systems for varying times in the care situation.
- • Help the caregiver learn mindfulness stress management techniques, which can reduce psychological distress.
- • Encourage the caregiver to share feelings, concerns, uncertainties, and fears. Support groups, even Internet-based ones, can be used to gain support.
- • Observe for any evidence of caregiver or care recipient violence or abuse, particularly verbal abuse and emotional abuse; if evidence is present, identify the conflict and seek help to manage.
- ▲ Encourage regular and open communication with the care recipient and with the healthcare team. Care transitions are a critical point to

ensure that caregivers have adequate information for patient safety and efficient and effective care.

- Assist caregiver to secure and manage finances to meet care recipient's needs.
- Help the caregiver identify competing occupational demands and potential benefits to maintaining work as a way of providing normalcy. Guide caregivers to seek ways to maintain employment through mechanisms such as working remotely, job sharing, or decreasing hours at work.
- Help the caregiver problem solve to meet the care recipient's needs.

Geriatric

- Monitor the caregiver for psychological distress and signs of depression, especially if there was an unsatisfactory family relationship before caregiving.
- Assess the health of caregivers, particularly their control over chronic diseases and comorbid conditions, at regular intervals.
- Implement a telephone-based collaborative care program to provide support.
- Provide medication management to facilitate safe and effective use of medications for self and care recipient by medication reconciliation and education.
- To improve the ability to provide safe care: provide skills training related to direct care, perform complex monitoring tasks, supervise and interpret client symptoms, assist with decision-making, assist with medication adherence.
- Provide emotional support and comfort, and coordinate care. Family members need the resources and support to provide care to the care recipient.
- Insurance authorization: health professionals, such as social workers, assist care recipients to obtain the needed referrals to gain payment for needed health and community services.
- Teach symptom management techniques (assessment, potential causes, aggravating factors, potential alleviating factors, and reassessment), particularly for fatigue, dyspnea, constipation, anorexia, and pain.

Multicultural

- Assess for the influence of cultural beliefs, ethnic and racial norms, and values on the caregiver's ability to provide care as well as the response to care.

- Recognize and understand that culture often plays a role in identifying who will be recognized as a family caregiver.
- Encourage spirituality as a source of support for coping.

Home Care

- Assess the client and caregiver at every visit for the quality of their relationship, and for the quality and safety of the care provided.
- Encourage use of respite care if it seems appropriate to support the caregiver. Allow the caregiver to gain confidence in the respite provider.

▲ Refer the client to home health aide services for assistance with activities of daily living and light housekeeping. Home health aide services can provide physical relief and respite for the caregiver

- Assess preexisting strengths and weaknesses that the caregiver brings to the situation.
- Improving caregiver sense of competency to deal with neuropsychiatric symptoms of dementia patients can prevent or reduce caregiver burden (van der Lee et al., 2014).

Client/Family Teaching and Discharge Planning

- Identify client and caregiver factors that necessitate the use of formal home care services, that may affect provision of care, or that need to be addressed before the client can be safely discharged from home care.
- Collaborate with the caregiver and discuss the care needs of the client, disease processes, medications, and what to expect as part of discharge planning and transition care.
- Use a variety of instructional techniques (e.g., explanations, demonstrations, visual aids) until the caregiver is able to express a degree of comfort with needed care.
- Assess family caregiving skill. The identification of caregiver difficulty with any of a core set of processes highlights areas for intervention.
- Discharge care should be individualized to specific caregiver needs and care situations, and enable them to be prepared.
- Assess the caregiver's need for information such as information on symptom management, disease progression, specific skills, and available support.

▲ Involve the family caregiver in care transitions and discharge from institutions; use a multidisciplinary team to provide medical and social services for detailed instruction and planning specific to the care need. The CARE Act, available in 39 states, requires caregiver instruction at hospital discharge.

▲ Refer to counseling or support groups to assist in adjusting to the caregiver role and periodically evaluate not only the caregiver's emotional response to care but the safety of the care delivered to the care recipient.

Risk for Caregiver Role Strain

NANDA-I Definition

Susceptible to difficulty in fulfilling care responsibilities, expectations, and/or behaviors for family or significant others, which may compromise health

Risk Factors

Care Receiver

Dependency; discharged home with significant needs; increase in care needs; problematic behavior; substance misuse; unpredictability of illness trajectory; unstable health condition

Caregiver

Substance misuse; unrealistic self-expectations; competing role commitments; ineffective coping strategies; inexperience with caregiving; insufficient emotional resilience; insufficient energy; insufficient fulfillment of others' expectations; insufficient fulfillment of self-expectations; insufficient knowledge about community resources; insufficient privacy; insufficient recreation; isolation; not developmentally ready for caregiver role; physical conditions; stressors

Caregiver-Care Receiver Relationship

Abusive relationship; codependency; pattern of ineffective relationships; presence of abuse; unrealistic care receiver expectations; violent relationship

Caregiving Activities

Around-the-clock care responsibilities; change in nature of care activities; complexity of care activities; excessive caregiving activities; extended duration of caregiving required; inadequate physical environment for providing care; insufficient assistance; insufficient equipment for providing care; insufficient respite for caregiver; insufficient time; unpredictability of care situation

Family Processes

Family isolation; ineffective family adaptation; pattern of family dysfunction; pattern of family dysfunction prior to the caregiving situation; pattern of ineffective family coping

Socioeconomic

Alienation; difficulty accessing assistance; difficulty accessing community resources; difficulty accessing support; insufficient community resources; insufficient social support; insufficient transportation; social isolation

At-Risk Population

Care receiver's condition inhibits conversation; developmental delay of care receiver; developmental delay of caregiver; exposure to violence; female caregiver; financial crisis; partner as caregiver; prematurity

Associated Condition

Care Receiver

Alteration in cognitive functioning; chronic illness; congenital disorder; illness severity; psychological disorder; psychiatric disorder

Caregiver

Alteration in cognitive functioning; health impairment; psychological disorder

Client Outcomes, Nursing Interventions, Client/Family Teaching

Refer to care plan for **Caregiver Role Strain.**

Risk for Ineffective Cerebral Tissue Perfusion

NANDA-I Definition

Susceptible to a decrease in cerebral tissue circulation, which may compromise health

Risk Factors

Substance misuse

At-Risk Population

Recent myocardial infarction

Associated Condition

Abnormal partial thromboplastin time (PTT); abnormal prothrombin time (PT); akinetic left ventricular wall segment; aortic atherosclerosis; arterial dissection; atrial fibrillation; atrial myxoma; brain injury; brain neoplasm; carotid stenosis; cerebral aneurysm; coagulopathy; dilated cardiomyopathy; disseminated intravascular coagulopathy; embolism; hypercholesterolemia; hypertension; infective endocarditis; mechanical prosthetic valve; mitral stenosis; pharmaceutical agent; sick sinus syndrome; treatment regimen after sick sinus syndrome

Client Outcomes

Client Will (Specify Time Frame)

- State absence of headache
- Demonstrate appropriate orientation to person, place, time, and situation

- Demonstrate ability to follow simple commands
- Demonstrate equal bilateral motor strength
- Demonstrate adequate swallowing ability
- Maintain (or improve) neurological exam

Nursing Interventions

- To decrease risk of reduced cerebral perfusion related to stroke or transient ischemic attack (TIA):
  - Obtain a family history of hypertension, diabetes, and stroke to identify persons who may be at increased risk of stroke.
  - Monitor BP regularly, because hypertension is a major risk factor for both ischemic and hemorrhagic stroke.
  - Teach hypertensive clients the importance of taking their healthcare provider-ordered antihypertensive agent to prevent stroke.
  - Stress smoking cessation at every encounter with clients, using multimodal techniques to aid in quitting, such as counseling, nicotine replacement, and oral smoking cessation medications. Provide client and family education to reduce lifestyle-associated risk factors for stroke.
  - Teach clients who experience a transient TIA that they are at increased risk for a stroke.
  - Screen clients 65 years of age and older for atrial fibrillation with pulse assessment.
  - Call 911 or activate the rapid response team of a hospital immediately when clients display symptoms of stroke as determined by the Cincinnati Stroke Scale (F: facial drooping; A: arm drift on one side; S: speech slurred) being careful to note the time of symptom appearance. Additional symptoms of stroke include sudden numbness/weakness of face, arm, or leg, especially on one side; sudden confusion; trouble speaking or understanding; sudden difficulty seeing with one or both eyes; sudden trouble walking, dizziness, loss of balance, or coordination; or sudden severe headache (Jauch et al., 2013).
  - Use clinical practice guidelines for glycemic control and BP targets to guide the care of clients with diabetes who have had a stroke or TIA.
  - Maintain head of bed less than 30 degrees in the acute phase (<72 hours of symptom onset) of ischemic stroke.
  - Head of bed may be elevated to sitting position without detrimental effect to cerebral blood flow in clients with ischemic

C

stroke or subarachnoid hemorrhagic at 72 hours after symptom onset.

- ○ Administer oral nimodipine as prescribed by the healthcare provider after subarachnoid hemorrhagic strokes for 21 days.
- ○ Monitor neurological function frequently in the first 2 weeks after subarachnoid hemorrhage, because subtle declines may be related to cerebral vasospasm.
- ○ Maintain cerebral perfusion pressure (CPP) 60 to 70 mm Hg in patients with traumatic brain injury.

▲ To decrease risk of reduced CPP. CPP = Mean arterial pressure – intracranial pressure (CPP = MAP – ICP)

- ○ Maintain euvolemia.

▲ To treat decreased CPP:

- ○ Clients with subarachnoid hemorrhagic stroke experiencing delayed cerebral ischemia, as evidenced by declining neurological exam, should undergo a trial of induced hypertension.
- ○ Administer norepinephrine infusion to raise MAP per collaborative protocol.
- ○ Mobilize patients with subarachnoid hemorrhage as early as 1 day after aneurysm is secured.

Ineffective Childbearing Process

NANDA-I Definition

Inability to prepare for and/or maintain a healthy pregnancy, childbirth process and care of the newborn for ensuring well-being

Defining Characteristics

During Pregnancy

Inadequate prenatal care; inadequate prenatal lifestyle; inadequate preparation of newborn care items; inadequate preparation of the home environment; ineffective management of unpleasant symptoms in pregnancy; insufficient access of support system; insufficient respect for unborn baby; unrealistic birth plan

During Labor and Delivery

Decrease in proactivity during labor and delivery; inadequate lifestyle for stage of labor; inappropriate response to onset of labor; insufficient access of support system; insufficient attachment behavior

C

After Birth

Inadequate baby care techniques; inadequate postpartum lifestyle; inappropriate baby feeding techniques; inappropriate breast care; insufficient access of support system; insufficient attachment behavior; unsafe environment for an infant

Related Factors

Domestic violence; inadequate maternal nutrition; inconsistent prenatal health visits; insufficient cognitive readiness for parenting; insufficient knowledge of child-bearing process; insufficient parental role model; insufficient prenatal care; insufficient support system; low maternal confidence; maternal powerlessness; maternal psychological distress; substance misuse; unrealistic birth plan; unsafe environment

At-Risk Population

Unplanned pregnancy; unwanted pregnancy

Client Outcomes

Client Will (Specify Time Frame)

Antepartum

- Obtain early prenatal care in the first trimester and maintain regular visits
- Demonstrate appropriate care of oneself during pregnancy, including good nutrition and psychological health
- Understand the risks of substance abuse and resources available
- Feel empowered to seek social and spiritual support for emotional well-being during pregnancy
- Prepare home for baby (e.g., crib, diapers, infant car seat, outfits, blankets)
- Use support systems for labor and emotional support
- Develop a realistic birth plan, taking into account any high-risk pregnancy issues
- Understand the labor and delivery process and comfort measures to manage labor pain

Postpartum

- Provide a safe environment for self and infant
- Demonstrate appropriate newborn care and postpartum care of self
- Demonstrate appropriate bonding and parenting skills

Nursing Interventions

- Encourage early prenatal care and regular prenatal visits.

▲ Identify any high-risk factors that may require additional surveillance, such as preterm labor, hypertensive disorders of pregnancy, diabetes, depression, other chronic medical conditions, presence of fetal anomalies, homelessness, or other high-risk factors.

- ▲ Assess and screen for signs and symptoms of depression during pregnancy and in the postpartum period, including history of depression or postpartum depression, poor prenatal care, poor weight gain, hygiene issues, sleep problems, substance abuse, and preterm labor. If depression is present, refer for behavioral-cognitive counseling and/or medication.
- ▲ Observe for signs of alcohol use and counsel women to stop drinking during pregnancy. Give appropriate referral for treatment if needed.
- ▲ Obtain a smoking history and counsel women to stop smoking for the safety of the baby. Give appropriate referral to a smoking cessation program if needed.
- ▲ Monitor for substance abuse with recreational drugs. Refer to a drug treatment program as needed. Refer opiate-dependent women to methadone clinics to improve maternal and fetal pregnancy outcomes.
- ▲ Monitor for psychosocial issues including lack of social support system, loneliness, depression, lack of confidence, maternal powerlessness, and socioeconomic problems.
- ▲ Monitor for signs of domestic violence. Refer to a community program for abused women that provides safe shelter as needed.
- • Provide antenatal education to increase the woman's knowledge needed to make informed choices during pregnancy, labor, and delivery and to promote a healthy lifestyle.
- • Encourage expectant parents to prepare a realistic birth plan or "birth preferences" to prepare for the physical and emotional aspects of the birth process and to plan ahead for how they want various situations handled.
- • Encourage good nutritional intake during pregnancy to facilitate proper growth and development of the fetus. Women should consume an additional 300 calories per day during pregnancy, take a multi-micronutrient supplement containing at least 400 μg folic acid, and achieve a total weight gain of 25 to 30 lb.

Multicultural

- ▲ Provide for a translator if needed. In some cultures a woman prefers to have a female translator.
- ▲ Provide depression screening for clients of all ethnicities.
- • Perform a cultural assessment and provide obstetrical care that is culturally appropriate to ensure a safe and satisfying childbearing experience.

Readiness for Enhanced Childbearing Process

C

NANDA-I Definition

A pattern of preparing for and maintaining a healthy pregnancy, childbirth process and care of the newborn for ensuring well-being which can be strengthened

Defining Characteristics

During Pregnancy

Expresses desire to enhance knowledge of childbearing process; expresses desire to enhance management of unpleasant pregnancy symptoms; expresses desire to enhance prenatal lifestyle; expresses desire to enhance preparation for newborn

During Labor and Delivery

Expresses desire to enhance lifestyle appropriate for stage of labor; expresses desire to enhance proactivity during labor and delivery

After Birth

Expresses desire to strengthen attachment behavior; expresses desire to improve baby care techniques; expresses desire to improve baby feeding techniques; expresses desire to enhance breast care; expresses desire to enhance environmental safety for the baby; expresses desire to enhance postpartum lifestyle; expresses desire to increase use of support system

Client Outcomes

Client Will (Specify Time Frame)

During pregnancy

- Attend all scheduled prenatal visits and attend prenatal education with her significant other or involved family member
- Use appropriate self-care for discomforts of pregnancy
- Make healthy lifestyle choices prenatally: activity and exercise/healthy nutritional practices
- Use strategies to balance activity and rest

During labor and delivery

- Demonstrate appropriate lifestyle choices during labor
- State knowledge of birthing options, signs and symptoms of labor
- Demonstrate effective labor techniques

After birth

- Demonstrate appropriate lifestyle choices postpartum
- Report normal physical sensations after delivery

- State understanding of recommended nutrient intake, strategies to balance activity and rest, appropriate exercise, time frame for resumption of sexual activity, strategies to manage stress
- Demonstrate bonding with infant
- Demonstrate proper handling and positioning of infant/infant safety
- Demonstrate feeding technique and bathing of infant

Nursing Interventions

- Refer to care plans: Risk for impaired **Attachment;** Readiness for enhanced **Breastfeeding;** Readiness for enhanced family **Coping;** Readiness for enhanced **Family** processes; **Growth;** Readiness for enhanced **Nutrition;** Readiness for enhanced **Parenting;** Ineffective **Role** performance.

Prenatal Care

▲ Ensure that pregnant clients have an adequate diet and take multi-micronutrient supplements containing at least 400 μg of folic acid, especially during early pregnancy.

- Assess smoking status of pregnant clients and offer effective smoking cessation interventions.
- See HHS for quitting smoking guidelines (https://betobaccofree.hhs.gov/quit-now/index.html).

▲ Assess all pregnant clients for signs of depression and make appropriate referral for inadequate weight gain, underutilization of prenatal care, increased substance abuse, and premature birth. Assess past personal or family history of depression, being single, poor health functioning, and alcohol use.

- Discuss breastfeeding with a pregnant client, including all the benefits both to the infant and the mother.

Intrapartal Care

- Encourage psychosocial support during labor, especially by the father of the baby or the woman's mother if possible.
- Provide a calm, relaxing, and supportive birth environment.
- Offer the client in labor a clear liquid diet and water if allowed.

Multicultural

Prenatal

▲ Provide for a translator if needed. In some cultures a women prefers to have a female translator.

- Assess the client's beliefs and concerns about prenatal care. Provide culturally appropriate prenatal care for clients.

▲ Refer the client to a centering pregnancy group (8–10 women of similar gestational age receive group prenatal care after initial obstetrical visit) or group prenatal care.

Intrapartal

- Assess client's beliefs and concerns about labor. Consider the client's culture when assisting in labor and delivery.

Postpartal

- Assess client's beliefs and concerns about the postpartum period. Provide culturally appropriate health and nutrition information and guidance on contemporary postpartum practices and take away common misconceptions about traditional dietary and health behaviors (e.g., fruit and vegetables should be restricted because of cold nature). Encourage a balanced diet and discourage unhealthy hygiene taboos.

Home Care

Prenatal

▲ Involve pregnant drug users in drug treatment programs that include coordinated interventions in several areas such as drug use, infectious diseases, mental health, personal and social welfare, and gynecological/obstetric care.

Postpartal

- Suggest parenting websites approved by the medical provider to support new parents with postpartum advice, newborn care, and breastfeeding.

Client/Family Teaching and Discharge Planning

Prenatal

- Provide dietary and lifestyle counseling as part of prenatal care to pregnant women.
- Provide group prenatal care to low-risk pregnant women belonging to high-risk demographic groups.

Postpartal

- Encourage physical activity in postpartum women, after being cleared by the healthcare provider; teach postpartum women that exercise may reduce anxiety and depression, and encourage downloading phone apps that help track exercise, such as Fitbit or Pedometer Master.

▲ Provide breastfeeding mothers contact information for a lactation consultant, phone numbers, and website information for the La

Leche League (http://www.lalecheleague.org), and local breastfeeding support groups.

- Teach mothers of young children principles of a healthy lifestyle: Substitute foods high in saturated fat with foods moderate in PUFAs such as avocados, tuna, walnuts, and olive oil. Include lean protein, fruits and vegetables, and complex carbohydrates. It is also important to increase physical activity.

C

Risk for Ineffective Childbearing Process

NANDA-I Definition

Susceptible to an inability to prepare for and/or maintain a healthy pregnancy, childbirth process and care of the newborn for ensuring well-being

Risk Factors

Domestic violence; inadequate maternal nutrition; inconsistent prenatal health visits; insufficient cognitive readiness for parenting; insufficient knowledge of childbearing process; insufficient parental role model; insufficient prenatal care; insufficient support system; low maternal confidence; maternal powerlessness; maternal psychological distress; substance misuse; unrealistic birth plan; unsafe environment

At-Risk Population

Unplanned pregnancy; unwanted pregnancy

Client Outcomes, Nursing Interventions, Client/Family Teaching

Refer to care plan for Ineffective **Childbearing** process.

Impaired Comfort

NANDA-I Definition

Perceived lack of ease, relief, and transcendence in physical, psychospiritual, environmental, cultural, and/or social dimensions

Defining Characteristics

Alteration in sleep pattern; anxiety; crying; discontent with situation; distressing symptoms; fear; feeling cold; feeling of discomfort; feeling of hunger; feeling warm; inability to relax; irritability; itching; moaning; restlessness; sighing; uneasy in situation

Related Factors

Insufficient environmental control; insufficient privacy; insufficient resources; insufficient situational control; noxious environmental stimuli

C

Associated Condition

Illness-related symptoms; treatment regimen

Client Outcomes

Client Will (Specify Time Frame)

- Provide evidence for improved comfort compared to baseline
- Identify strategies, with or without significant others, to improve and/or maintain acceptable comfort level
- Perform appropriate interventions, with or without significant others, as needed to improve and/or maintain acceptable comfort level
- Evaluate the effectiveness of strategies to maintain/and or reach an acceptable comfort level
- Maintain an acceptable level of comfort when possible

Nursing Interventions

- Assess client's understanding of ranking his or her comfort level.
- Ask about client's current level of comfort. This is the first step in helping clients achieve improved comfort.
- Comfort is a holistic state under which pain management is included.
- Assist clients to understand how to rate their current state of holistic comfort, using the institution's preferred method of documentation.
- Enhance feelings of trust between the client and the healthcare provider. To attain the highest comfort level, clients must be able to trust their nurse.
- Manipulate the environment as necessary to improve comfort.
- Encourage early mobilization and provide routine position changes. Range of motion and weight bearing decrease physical discomforts and disability associated with bed rest.
- Provide simple massage. Massage has many therapeutic effects, including improved relaxation, circulation, and well-being.
- Provide a healing touch, which is well suited for clients who cannot tolerate more stimulating interventions.
- Encourage clients to use relaxation techniques to reduce pain, anxiety, depression, and fatigue.

Geriatric

- Use hand massage for older adults. Most older adults respond well to touch and the healthcare provider's presence. Lines of communication open naturally during hand massage.

C

- Discomfort from cold can be treated with warmed blankets. There are physiological dangers associated with hypothermia.
- Use complementary therapies such as doll therapy in clients with dementia to increase comfort and reduce stress.
- Address any unmet physical, psychological, emotional, spiritual, and environmental needs when attempting to mediate the behavior of an older client with dementia.

Multicultural

- Identify and clarify cultural language used to describe pain and other discomforts. Expressions of pain and discomfort vary across cultures.
- Assess skin for ashy or yellow-brown appearance.
- Use soap sparingly if the skin is dry. Black skin tends to be dry, and soap exacerbates this condition.
- Encourage and allow clients to practice their own cultural beliefs and recognize the impact that diverse cultures have on a client's belief about healthcare, comforting measures, and decision-making.
- Assess for cultural and religious beliefs when providing care.

Client/Family Teaching and Discharge Planning

- Teach techniques to use when the client is uncomfortable, including relaxation techniques, guided imagery, hand massage, and music therapy.
- At end of life, the dying client is comforted by having a companion.
- Instruct the client and family about prescribed medications and complementary therapies that improve comfort.
- Teach the client to follow up with the healthcare provider if discomfort persists. There are many avenues for enhancing comfort.
- Encourage clients to use the Internet as a means of providing education to complement medical care for those who may be homebound or unable to attend face-to-face education.

Mental Health

- Encourage clients to use guided imagery techniques. Guided imagery helps distract clients from stressful situations and facilitates relaxation.
- Provide psychospiritual support and a comforting environment to enhance comfort during emotional crises.
- When nurses attend to the comfort of perioperative clients, the clients' sense of hope for a full recovery increases.
- Providing music and verbal relaxation therapy enhances holistic comfort by reducing anxiety.
- Caregivers should not hesitate to use humor when caring for their clients.

Readiness for Enhanced Comfort

NANDA-I Definition

C

A pattern of ease, relief, and transcendence in physical, psychospiritual, environmental, and/or social dimensions, which can be strengthened

Defining Characteristics

Expresses desire to enhance comfort; expresses desire to enhance feelings of contentment; expresses desire to enhance relaxation; expresses desire to enhance resolution of complaints

During Pregnancy

Expresses desire to enhance knowledge of childbearing process; expresses desire to enhance management of unpleasant pregnancy symptoms; expresses desire to enhance prenatal lifestyle; expresses desire to enhance preparation for newborn

During Labor and Delivery

Expresses desire to enhance lifestyle appropriate for stage of labor; expresses desire to enhance proactivity during labor and delivery

After Birth

Expresses desire to enhance post-partum lifestyle

Client Outcomes

Client Will (Specify Time Frame)

- Assess current level of comfort as acceptable
- Express the need to achieve an enhanced level of comfort
- Identify strategies to enhance comfort
- Perform appropriate interventions as needed for increased comfort
- Evaluate the effectiveness of interventions at regular intervals
- Maintain an enhanced level of comfort when possible

Nursing Interventions

- Assess clients' comfort needs and current level of comfort in various contexts, as outlined in Kolcaba's (2003) comfort theory and practice: physical, psychospiritual, sociocultural, and environmental.
- Educate clients about the various contexts of comfort and help them understand that enhanced comfort is a desirable, positive, and achievable goal.
- Enhance feelings of trust between the client and the healthcare provider to maintain an effective and therapeutic relationship.
- Maintain an open and effective communication with clients and keep them informed about their health, their plan of care, and their environment.

C

- Implement comfort rounds that regularly assess for clients' comfort needs.
- Collaborate with other healthcare professionals, such as healthcare providers, pharmacists, social workers, chaplains, occupational and physical therapists, and dietitians, among others, in planning interventions that address comfort needs in various contexts: physical, psychospiritual, sociocultural, and environmental.
- Educate clients about and encourage the use of various integrative therapies and modalities to provide options that enhance comfort, beyond the traditional plan of care. Institute of Medicine (IOM) and Pain—examples of such modalities include the following and are listed in the following:
    - Therapeutic massage and touch therapy.
    - Guided imagery.
    - Mindfulness and mindfulness-based interventions such as mindfulness-based stress reduction (MBSR), mantra repetition (silent repetition of a sacred word), mindfulness meditation, and mindful breathing and walking, among others).
    - Energy therapy or biofield therapy such as healing touch, therapeutic touch, and Reiki. Biofield therapy seems to be promising in promoting comfort and relaxation, but more sound and systematic research is needed to build a strong body of evidence.
    - Acupuncture and auricular acupuncture.
    - Aromatherapy.
    - Music.
    - Other mind–body therapies such as meditation, yoga, etc.
- Foster and instill hope in clients whenever possible.
- Provide opportunities for and enhance spiritual care activities.
- ▲ Enhance social support and family involvement.
- ▲ Promote participation in creative arts and activity programs.
- ▲ Encourage clients to use health information technology (HIT) as needed.
- Evaluate the effectiveness of all comfort interventions at regular intervals and adjust therapies as necessary.

Geriatric

- Refer to previously mentioned interventions for geriatric interventions.

Pediatric

- Assess and evaluate the child's level of comfort at frequent intervals. With assessment of pain in children, it is best to use input from the parents or a primary care giver.

- Skin-to-skin contact (SSC) in the comfort of newborns, especially those at risk.
- Adjust the environment as needed to enhance comfort.
- Encourage parental presence whenever possible.
- Promote use of alternative comforting strategies such as positioning, presence, massage, spiritual care, music therapy, art therapy, and story telling to enhance comfort when needed.
- Support the child's spirituality.

Multicultural

- Identify cultural beliefs, values, lifestyles, practices, and problem-solving strategies when assessing a client's comfort.
- Enhance cultural knowledge by actively seeking out information regarding different cultural and ethnic groups.

▲ Recognize the impact of culture on communication styles and techniques.

- Provide culturally competent care to clients from different cultural groups.

Home Care

- The nursing interventions described for Readiness for enhanced **Comfort** may be used with clients in the home care setting. When needed, adaptations can be made to meet the needs of specific clients, families, and communities.

▲ Make appropriate referrals to other organizations or healthcare providers as needed to enhance comfort.

▲ Promote an interdisciplinary (home care nurses, physicians, pharmacy, etc.) approach to home care.

- Evaluate regularly if enhanced comfort is attainable in the home care setting.

Client/Family Teaching and Discharge Planning

- Teach client how to regularly assess levels of comfort.
- Instruct client that a variety of interventions may be needed at any given time to enhance comfort.
- Help clients understand that enhanced comfort is an achievable goal.
- Teach techniques to enhance comfort as needed.

▲ When needed, empower clients to seek out other health professionals as members of the interdisciplinary team to assist with comforting measures and techniques.

- Encourage self-care activities and continued self-evaluation of achieved comfort levels to ensure enhanced comfort is maintained.

• = Independent ▲ = Collaborative

Readiness for Enhanced Communication

C

NANDA-I Definition

A pattern of exchanging information and ideas with others, which can be strengthened

Defining Characteristics

Expresses desire to enhance communication

Client Outcomes

Client Will (Specify Time Frame)

- Express willingness to enhance communication
- Demonstrate ability to speak or write a language
- Form words, phrases, and language
- Express thoughts and feelings
- Use and interpret nonverbal cues appropriately
- Express satisfaction with ability to share information and ideas with others

Nursing Interventions

- Establish a therapeutic nurse–client relationship: provide appropriate education for the client, demonstrate caring by being present to the client.
- Assess the client's readiness to communicate, using an individualized creative approach, and avoid making assumptions regarding the client's preferred communication method.
- Assess the client's literacy level so information can be tailored accordingly.
- Use these practical guidelines to assist in communication: Listen attentively and provide a comfortable environment for communicating; slow down and listen to the client's story; use augmentative and alternative communication methods (e.g., lip reading, communication boards, writing, body language, computer/electronic communication devices) as appropriate; repeat instructions if necessary; limit the amount of information given; have the client "teach back" to confirm understanding; avoid asking, "Do you understand?"; and be respectful, caring, and sensitive.

▲ Use interdisciplinary collaboration to ensure continuity of enhanced communication.

▲ Refer couples in maladjusted relationships for psychosocial intervention and social support to strengthen communication; consider nurse specialists.

C

- Consider using music to enhance communication between a client who is dying and his or her family.
- Use social media as a means to facilitate communication.
- Teach clients mindfulness meditation.
- Use photographs as a communication aid.
- Encourage clients with aphasia to sing.
- See care plan for Impaired verbal **Communication.**

Pediatric

- All individuals involved in the care and everyday life of children with learning difficulties need to have a collaborative approach to communication.
- See care plan for Impaired verbal **Communication.**

Geriatric

▲ Assess for hearing and vision impairments, and make appropriate referrals for hearing aids.

- Use touch if culturally acceptable when communicating with older clients and their families.
- Encourage group singing activities and music therapy interventions in clients with dementia.
- Encourage drawing by caregivers of clients with dementia.
- See care plan for Impaired verbal **Communication.**

Multicultural

- See care plan for Impaired verbal **Communication.**

Home Care

- The interventions described previously may be used in home care.
- See care plan for Impaired verbal **Communication.**

Client/Family Teaching and Discharge Planning

- See care plan for Impaired verbal **Communication.**

Impaired Verbal Communication

NANDA-I Definition

Decreased, delayed, or absent ability to receive, process, transmit, and/or use a system of symbols

Defining Characteristics

Absence of eye contact; agraphia; alternative communication; anarthria; aphasia; augmentative communication; decline of speech productivity; decline of speech rate; decreased willingness to participate in social interaction; difficulty comprehending communication; difficulty establishing social interaction; difficulty maintaining communication; difficulty using body expressions;

difficulty using facial expressions; difficulty with selective attention; displays negative emotions; dysarthria; dysgraphia; dyslalia; dysphonia; fatigued by conversation; impaired ability to speak; impaired ability to use body expressions; impaired ability to use facial expressions; inability to speak language of caregiver; inappropriate verbalization; obstinate refusal to speak; slurred speech

Related Factors

Alteration in self-concept; dyspnea; emotional lability; environmental constraints; inadequate stimulation; low self-esteem; perceived vulnerability; psychological barriers; values incongruent with cultural norms

At-Risk Population

Individuals facing physical barriers, individuals in the early postoperative period; individuals unable to verbalize; individuals with communication barriers; individuals without a significant other

Associated Condition

Altered perception; developmental disabilities; flaccid facial paralysis; hemifacial spasm; motor neuron disease; neoplasms; neurocognitive disorders; oropharyngeal defect; peripheral nervous system diseases; psychotic disorders; respiratory muscle weakness; sialorrhea; speech disorders; tongue diseases; tracheostomy; treatment regimen; velopharyngeal insufficiency; vocal cord dysfunction

Client Outcomes

Client Will (Specify Time Frame)

- Use effective communication techniques
- Use alternative methods of communication effectively
- Demonstrate congruency of verbal and nonverbal behavior
- Demonstrate understanding even if not able to speak
- Express desire for social interactions

Nursing Interventions

- Use a comprehensive nursing assessment to determine the language spoken, cultural considerations, literacy level, cognitive level, and use of glasses and/or hearing aids.
- Determine client's own perception of communication difficulties and potential solutions when possible.
- Involve a familiar person when attempting to communicate with a client who has difficulty with communication, if accepted by the client.
- Listen carefully. Validate verbal and nonverbal expressions, particularly when dealing with pain and use appropriate scales for pain when appropriate.
- Use appropriate scales to assess communication and behavior in clients who are nonvocal and mechanically ventilated.

C

- Use therapeutic communication techniques: speak in a well-modulated voice, use simple communication, maintain eye contact at the client's level, get the client's attention before speaking, and show concern for the client.
- Avoid ignoring the client with verbal impairment; be engaged and provide meaningful responses to client concerns. Place call light within reach of client who cannot verbally call for help.
- Validate clients' feelings, focus on their strengths, and assist them in gaining confidence in identifying needs.
- Use touch as appropriate.
- Use presence: spend time with the client and allow time for responses.
- Explain all healthcare procedures, be persistent in deciphering what the client is saying, and do not pretend to understand when the message is unclear.
- Use an individualized and creative multidisciplinary approach to augmentative and alternative communication (AAC) assistance and other communication interventions.
- Use consistent nursing staff for those with communication impairments.

▲ Consult communication specialists from various disciplines as appropriate. Speech language pathologists, audiologists, and interpreters provide comprehensive communication assistance for those with impaired communication.

▲ When the client is having difficulty communicating, assess and refer for audiology consultation for hearing loss. Suspect hearing loss when:
  - Client frequently complains that people mumble, claims that others' speech is not clear, or client hears only parts of conversations.
  - Client often asks people to repeat what they said.
  - Client's friends or relatives state that the client does not seem to hear very well, or plays the television or radio too loudly.
  - Client does not laugh at jokes because of missing too much of the story.
  - Client needs to ask others about the details of a meeting that the client attended.
  - Client cannot hear the doorbell or the telephone.
  - Client finds it easier to understand others when facing them, especially in a noisy environment.
- People with hearing loss do not hear sounds clearly. The loss may range from hearing speech sounds faintly or in a distorted way to profound deafness (American Academy of Audiology, 2017).

- When communicating with a client with a hearing loss:
  - ❍ Obtain client's attention before speaking and face toward his or her unaffected side or better ear while allowing client to see the speaker's face at a reasonably close distance, use gestures as appropriate to aid in communication, do not raise voice or over-enunciate, and minimize extraneous noise.
  - ❍ Provide sufficient light and do not stand in front of a window.
  - ❍ Remove masks if safe to do so, or use see-through masks.
  - ❍ Avoid making assumptions about the communication choice of those with hearing loss or voice impairments.

Pediatric

- Observe behavioral communication cues in infants.
- Identify and define at least two new forms of socially acceptable communication alternatives that may be used by children with significant disabilities.
- Teach children with severe disabilities functional communication skills.

▲ Refer children with primary speech and language delay/disorder for speech and language therapy interventions.

Geriatric

- Carefully assess all clients for hearing difficulty using an audiometer. Healthy People 2020 encouraged early identification of people with hearing loss (Healthy People 2020, 2014).
- Avoid use of "elderspeak," which is a speech style similar to baby talk.
- Initiate communication with the client with dementia, and give client time to respond. Use eye contact, gentle touch as appropriate, and shorter sentences.
- Encourage the client to wear hearing aids, if appropriate.
- Facilitate communication through reminiscing with memory boxes that contain objects, photographs, and writings that have meaning for the client.
- Continue to find means to communicate even with those who are completely nonverbal.

Multicultural

- Attend to the meaning of a culture's nonverbal communication modes such as eye contact, facial expression, touching, and body language.
- Assess for the influence of cultural beliefs, norms, and values on the client's communication process.
- Assess personal space needs, acceptable communication styles, acceptable body language, interpretation of eye contact, perception of

touch, and use of paraverbal modes when communicating with the client.

C

- Assess how language barriers contribute to health disparities among ethnic and racial minorities.
- Although touch is generally beneficial, it is culturally defined, and there may be times when it may not be advisable because of cultural considerations.
- The Office of Minority Health of the US Department of Health and Human Services national standards on culturally and linguistically appropriate services (CLAS) in healthcare should be used as needed.

Home Care

The interventions described previously may be adapted for home care use.

Client/Family Teaching and Discharge Planning

❍ Refer the client to a speech-language pathologist (SLP) or audiologist. Audiological assessment quantifies and qualifies hearing in terms of the degree of hearing loss, the type of hearing loss, and the configuration of the hearing loss. Once a particular hearing loss has been identified, a treatment and management plan can be put into place by an SLP.

❍ Teach the client and family techniques to increase communication, including the use of communication devices and tactile touch. Incorporate multidisciplinary recommendations.

Acute Confusion

NANDA-I Definition

Reversible disturbances of consciousness, attention, cognition, and perception that develop over a short period of time, and which last less than 3 months

Defining Characteristics

Agitation; alteration in cognitive functioning; alteration in level of consciousness; alteration in psychomotor functioning; hallucinations; inability to initiate goal-directed behavior; inability to initiate purposeful behavior; insufficient follow-through with goal-directed behavior; insufficient follow-through with purposeful behavior; misperception; restlessness

Related Factors

Alteration in sleep–wake cycle; dehydration; impaired mobility; inappropriate use of restraints; malnutrition; pain; sensory deprivation; substance misuse; urinary retention

At-Risk Population

Age ≥ 60 years; history of cerebral vascular accident; male gender

Associated Condition

Alteration in cognitive functioning; delirium; dementia; impaired metabolic functioning; infection; pharmaceutical agent

C

Client Outcomes

Client Will (Specify Time Frame)

- Demonstrate restoration of cognitive status to baseline
- Be oriented to time, place, and person
- Demonstrate appropriate motor behavior
- Maintain functional capacity
- Remain free from injury

Nursing Interventions

- Recognize that delirium is characterized by an acute onset, a fluctuating course, inattention, and disordered thinking.
- Identify the three distinct types of delirium: hyperactive (easy to recognize), hypoactive (commonly missed), and mixed (the most commonly occurring) (Downing et al., 2013).
- Hyperactive: delirium characterized by restlessness, agitation, irritability, hypervigilance, hallucinations, and delusions; client may be combative or may attempt to remove tubes, lines.
    - Hypoactive: delirium characterized by decreased motor activity, decreased vocalization, detachment, apathy, lethargy, somnolence, reduced awareness of surroundings, and confusion.
    - Mixed: delirium characterized by the client fluctuating between periods of hyperactivity and agitation and hypoactivity and sedation.
- Obtain an accurate history and perform a mental status examination that includes the following assessment:
    - History from a reliable source that documents an acute and fluctuating change in cognitive function, attention, and behavior from baseline.
    - Cognition as evidenced by level of consciousness; orientation to time, person, and place; thought process (thinking may be disorganized, distorted, fragmented, slow, or accelerated with delirium; conversation may be irrelevant or rambling); and content (perceptual disturbances such as visual, auditory, or tactile delusions or hallucinations).

C

  - ❍ Level of attention (may be decreased or may fluctuate with delirium; may be unable to focus, shift, or sustain attention; may be easily distracted or may be hypervigilant).
  - ❍ Behavior characteristics and level of psychomotor behavior (activity may be increased or decreased and may include restlessness, finger tapping, picking at bedclothes, changing position frequently, spastic movements or tremors, or decreased psychomotor activity such as sluggishness, staring into space, remaining in the same position for prolonged periods).
  - ❍ Level of consciousness (may be easily aroused, lethargic, drowsy, difficult to arouse, unarousable, hyperalert, easily startled, and overly sensitive to stimuli).
  - ❍ Mood and affect (may be paranoid or fearful with delirium; may have rapid mood swings).
  - ❍ Insight and judgment (may be impaired).
  - ❍ Memory (recent and immediate memory is impaired with delirium; unable to register new information).
  - ❍ Language (may have rapid, rambling, slurred, incoherent speech).
  - ❍ Altered sleep–wake cycle (insomnia, excessive daytime sleepiness).
- • Assess the client's behavior and cognition systematically and continually throughout the day and night; use a validated tool to assess presence of delirium, such as the Confusion Assessment Method (CAM) or Delirium Observation Screening Scale (DOS).
- • Recognize that delirium may be superimposed on dementia; the nurse must be aware of the client's baseline cognitive function.
- • Identify predisposing factors that may precede the development of delirium: dementia, cognitive impairment, functional impairment, visual impairment, alcohol misuse, multiple comorbidities, severe illness, history of transient ischemic attack or stroke, depression, history of delirium, and advanced age (older than 70).
- • Identify precipitating factors that may precede the development of delirium, especially for individuals with predisposing factors: use of restraints, indwelling bladder catheter, metabolic disturbances, polypharmacy, pain, infection, dehydration, blood loss, constipation, electrolyte imbalances, immobility, general anesthesia, mechanical ventilation, hospital admission for fractures or hip surgery, anticholinergic medications, anxiety, sleep deprivation, lack of use of vision and/or hearing aids, and environmental factors.
- • Facilitate appropriate extended visitation for clients at risk of delirium.

C

- ▲ Assess for and report possible physiological alterations (e.g., sepsis, hypoglycemia, hypoxia, hypotension, infection, changes in temperature, fluid and electrolyte imbalance, use of medications with known cognitive and psychotropic side effects).
  - ❍ Treat the underlying risk factors or the causes of delirium in collaboration with the healthcare team: establish/maintain normal fluid and electrolyte balance, normal body temperature, normal oxygenation (if the client experiences low oxygen saturation, deliver supplemental oxygen), normal blood glucose levels, and normal blood pressure, and address malnutrition and anemia.
- ▲ Conduct a medication review and eliminate unnecessary medications; potentially inappropriate medications for older adults at risk for delirium include anticholinergics, benzodiazepines, corticosteroids, H_2 receptor antagonists, sedative hypnotics, and tricyclic antidepressants (American Geriatrics Society, 2015).
  - ❍ Communicate client status, cognition, and behavioral manifestations to all necessary healthcare providers.
  - ❍ Monitor for any trends occurring in these manifestations, including laboratory tests.
- • Identify, evaluate, and treat pain quickly and adequately (see care plans for Acute **Pain** or Chronic **Pain**).
- • Facilitate sleep hygiene.
- • Promote regulation of bowel and bladder function; use bladder scanning to identify retention, avoid prolonged insertion of urinary catheters, and remove catheters as soon as possible.
- • Ensure adequate nutritional and fluid intake.
- • Promote early mobilization and rehabilitation in a progressive manner.
- • Promote continuity of care; avoid frequent changes in staff and surroundings.
- • Plan care that allows for an appropriate sleep–wake cycle. Refer to the care plan for **Sleep** deprivation.
- • Facilitate appropriate sensory input by having clients use aids (e.g., glasses, hearing aids, dentures) as needed; check for impacted ear wax.
- • Modulate sensory exposure; eliminate excessive noise, use appropriate lighting based on the time of day, and establish a calm environment.
- • Provide cognitive stimulation through conversation about current events, viewpoints, and relationships and encourage reminiscence or word games.

- Allow appropriate visitation.
- Provide reality orientation, including identifying self by name at each encounter with the client, calling the client by their preferred name, and the gentle use of orientation techniques; when reorientation is not effective, use distraction.
- Provide clocks and calendars, update dry erase white boards each shift, encourage family to visit regularly and to bring familiar objects from home, such as family photos or an afghan, and gently correct misperceptions.
- Use gentle, caring communication; provide reassurance of safety; and give simple explanations of procedures.
- Provide supportive nursing care, including meeting basic needs, such as feeding, regular toileting, and ensuring adequate hydration; closely observe behaviors that provide clues as to what might be distressing the client. Delirious clients are unable to care for themselves because of their confusion (Rubin et al., 2011).

▲ Recognize that delirium is frequently treated with antipsychotic medications or sedatives; if there is no other way to keep the client safe, administer these medications cautiously, as ordered, while monitoring for medication side effects.
  - For clients nearing the end of life, for whom delirium may be irreversible, focus on relief of symptoms by increasing supervision, reducing invasive lines and devices that restrict movement, keeping the bed in low position, and placing mats on the floor; support of family, caregivers, and the healthcare team is also of prime importance.
  - Choose the appropriate medication and consider the type and reversibility of the delirium; titrate the medication to control the symptoms and minimize side effects.

Critical Care

- Recognize admission risk factors for delirium.
- Obtain an accurate history regarding cognitive impairment and mental health, including history of anxiety and depression, alcohol use, medication use, chronic pain, and use of benzodiazepines.
- Assess level of arousal using the Richmond Agitation Sedation Scale; clients receiving a score of –5 to –4 are comatose and unable to be assessed for delirium.
- Assess for pain every 2 to 3 hours or more frequently as needed with a standardized assessment tool, which includes either a numerical

rating scale or one with behavioral indicators, such as the Behavioral Pain Scale (BPS) or Critical Care Pain Observation Tool (CPOT).

C

- ▲ Incorporate the Awakening and Breathing Coordination, Delirium Monitoring and Management, and Early Mobility (ABCDE) ICU delirium and weakness prevention bundle in conjunction with the interdisciplinary team.
  - ❍ Assess safety and implementation of a spontaneous awakening trial (SAT) using an established protocol.
  - ❍ Assess safety and implementation of a spontaneous breathing trial (SBT).
  - ❍ Assess sedation and agitation level using a valid and reliable tool; titrate sedation to target sedation level.
  - ❍ Screen for delirium using a reliable and valid monitoring tool once per shift or more often if delirium is present, and recognize that hypoactive delirium is the form most often present in the ICU; communicate and discuss results with the interdisciplinary team.
  - ❍ Assess safety to begin mobilization; collaborate with physical therapy (PT), occupational therapy (OT), and respiratory therapy (RT) to implement an early mobility plan using a progressive approach.
- • Encourage visits from families and educate families about delirium if it occurs.
- • Promote uninterrupted sleep by grouping cares at night to avoid sleep interruption, offering eye mask, soft music, and earplugs; optimizing room temperature; by reducing noise and light after 10 p.m.; and by avoiding excessive daytime napping.

Geriatric

- • The interventions described previously are relevant to the geriatric client.
- • Reorient high-risk clients frequently, answer questions, and discuss concerns; use a white board, clock, watch, and calendar, and encourage family members to bring familiar objects from home such as family photos or afghan to assist with orientation.
- • Provide cognitive stimulation by discussing current events, reading the newspaper, promoting reminiscence, or using games.
- • Promote use of glasses, assistive hearing devices, hearing aids, and dentures.
- • Provide feeding assistance as needed. See care plan for Imbalanced **Nutrition:** less than body requirements.

- ▲ Determine whether the client is adequately nourished; watch for protein–calorie malnutrition. Consult with healthcare provider or dietitian as needed.
- • Promote adequate hydration; keep a glass of water within easy reach of the client and offer fluids frequently.
- • Avoid use of restraints; remove all nonessential equipment such as telemetry, blood pressure cuffs, catheters, and intravenous lines as soon as possible.
- • Consider use of music to decrease the development of delirium, especially in surgical patients.
- • Evaluate all medications for potential to cause or exacerbate delirium; potentially inappropriate medications for older adults at risk for delirium include tricyclic antidepressants, anticholinergics, antipsychotics, benzodiazepines, corticosteroids, H_2 receptor antagonists, and sedative hypnotics.
- • Assess pain frequently and treat pain with the lowest dose of regularly scheduled medication as well as with nonpharmacological approaches; use client self-report or a validated behavioral pain scale to assess pain accurately.
- ▲ Assess risk for falls and implement fall prevention strategies.
- • Recognize that delirium may be superimposed on dementia; determine client's baseline cognitive status.
- ▲ Determine whether the client is nourished; watch for protein–calorie malnutrition. Consult with healthcare provider or dietitian as needed.
- • Explain hospital routines and procedures slowly and in simple terms; repeat information as necessary.
- • Provide continuity of care when possible, avoid room changes, and encourage frequent visits from family members or significant others.
- • Educate family members about delirium assessment and strategies to use to prevent and lessen delirium; use the Family Confusion Assessment Method (FAM-CAM) assessment tool to solicit accurate information from caregivers regarding the presence of delirium.
- • If clients know that they are not thinking clearly, acknowledge the concern. Fear is frequently experienced by people with delirium.

Home Care

- • The interventions described previously are relevant to home care use. Assess and monitor for acute changes in cognition and behavior.
- • Recognize that delirium is reversible but can become chronic if untreated in a multidisciplinary fashion; the client may be

discharged from the hospital to home care in a state of undiagnosed delirium.

- Avoid preconceptions about the source of acute confusion; assess each occurrence on the basis of available evidence.
- ▲ Institute case management of frail elderly clients to support continued independent living if possible once delirium has resolved.

Client/Family Teaching and Discharge Planning

- ▲ Teach the family to recognize signs of early confusion and seek medical help.
- Counsel the client and family regarding the management of delirium and its sequelae. Increased care requirements at discharge may be needed for clients who have experienced delirium; frailty and delirium can lead to functional decline and institutionalization (Quinlan et al., 2011).

C

Chronic Confusion

NANDA-I Definition

Irreversible, progressive, insidious disturbances of consciousness, attention, cognition, and perception, which last more than 3 months.

Defining Characteristics

Altered personality; difficulty retrieving information when speaking; difficulty with decision-making; impaired executive functioning skills; impaired psychosocial functioning; inability to perform at least one daily activity; incoherent speech; long-term memory loss; marked change in behavior; short-term memory loss

Related Factors

Chronic sorrow; sedentary lifestyle; substance misuse

At Risk Population

Individuals aged ≥ 60 years

Associated Condition

Human immunodeficiency virus infections; mental disorders; neurocognitive disorders; stroke

Client Outcomes

Client Will (Specify Time Frame)

- Remain content and free from harm
- Function at maximal cognitive level
- Participate in activities of daily living at the maximum of functional ability
- Have minimal episodes of agitation (agitation occurs in up to 70% of clients with dementia)

C

Nursing Interventions

Note: Nursing science has a rich history of conceptualizing behavioral and psychological symptoms of dementia (including agitation and vocalizations) as expressions of unmet pathophysiological and psychological needs related to environmental and caregiver factors (Kolanowski et al., 2017).

- Assess the client for delirium (physiological causes of delirium include acute hypoxia, pain, medication effects, malnutrition, and infections such as urinary tract infection, fatigue, electrolyte disturbances, constipation, and urinary retention).
- Assess for pain using a method appropriate to the level of cognition.
- Assess the client for signs of depression and anxiety (including sadness, irritability, agitation, somatic complaints, tension, loss of concentration, insomnia, poor appetite, apathy, flat affect, and withdrawn behavior) with an instrument appropriate for the cognitive level.
- Assess the for psychological stressors, including changes in the environment, caregiver, or routine; demands to perform beyond capacity; or multiple competing stimuli, including discomfort; and encourage communication by addressing the client in a calm, gentle tone of voice, using appropriate body language, facial expressions, and gestures.
- Promote person-centered care through supporting, encouraging, educating, and supervising staff and other caregivers.
- Begin each interaction with the client by gaining and maintaining eye contact, identifying yourself, and calling the client by name. Approach the client with a caring, accepting, and empathetic attitude, and speak calmly and slowly.
- Enhance communication with a calm approach; avoid distractions; show interest; keep communication simple; give clear choices and one-step instructions; give the client time with word finding; use repetition and rephrasing; and use gestures, prompts, and cues or visual aids.
- Facilitate the use of music therapy; identify the client's music preferences and interview family members if necessary.
- Promote regular, supervised physical activity and exercise.
- Facilitate the use of doll therapy for patients with advanced dementia and challenging behaviors.
- Obtain information about the client's life history, interests, routines, needs, and preferences from the family or significant others; collaborate with family members to engage in reminiscence.

- Provide opportunities for contact with nature gardens or nature-based stimuli, such as facilitating time spent outdoors or indoor gardening.
- Provide animal-assisted activities when possible.
- Use individual or group reminiscence therapy.
- Use the Environmental Audit Tool to evaluate and optimize living environment (provide unobtrusive safety features, reduce unnecessary stimulation, enhance useful stimulation, provide for wandering, etc.).
- Use lighting to support regulation of sleep–wake patterns and associated behavioral issues.
- Engage volunteers and family caregivers in one-on-one activities with the client, such as folding, sorting, or stacking activities; arranging flowers; or other hobbies or routines the individual enjoyed before the onset of dementia.
- Provide information to the patient/resident/client and family regarding advance directives, palliative and hospice care options, and discuss/document goals of care.
- For clients with memory impairment concerns, refer to the **Impaired Memory** care plan.
- For clients who wander, refer to the **Wandering** care plan.
- For care of clients with self-care deficits, see the appropriate care plan (Feeding **Self-Care** deficit; Dressing **Self-Care** deficit; Toileting **Self-Care** deficit; Bathing **Self-Care** deficit, etc.).

Geriatric

Note: All interventions are appropriate for geriatric clients.

Multicultural

- Provide culturally and linguistically appropriate care.
- Assess for the influence of cultural beliefs, norms, and values on the patient and the family's understanding of chronic confusion or dementia; assist the family or caregiver in identifying and accessing available social services or other supportive services.

Home Care

Note: Because community-based care is usually less structured than institutional care, in the home setting the goal of maintaining safety for the client takes on primary importance.

- The interventions described previously may be adapted for home care use.
- Assess the home for safety features and client needs for assistive devices. Refer to the care plans for Feeding **Self-Care** deficit;

Dressing **Self-Care** deficit; Toileting **Self-Care** deficit; Bathing **Self-Care** deficit, etc., as needed.

C

- Provide education and support to the family regarding effective communication, home safety, fall prevention, engagement in meaningful activities, ways to manage cognitive and behavioral changes, and comprehensive healthcare including screening for depression. Be prepared to offer support and information to family members who also live at a distance.
- Provide information about respite care to family caregivers.
- Reinforce the use of therapeutic communication guidelines.
- Assess family caregivers for caregiver stress, loneliness, and depression. Refer to the care plan for **Caregiver Role Strain.**

Client/Family Teaching and Discharge Planning

- In the client's early stages of dementia, provide the caregiver with information on illness processes, needed care, available services, role changes, and importance of advance directives discussion; facilitate family cohesion.
- Provide education and support to the family regarding effective communication, home safety, fall prevention, engagement in meaningful activities, ways to manage cognitive and behavioral changes, and comprehensive healthcare including screening for depression. Be prepared to offer support and information to family members who also live at a distance.

Risk for Acute Confusion

NANDA-I Definition

Susceptible to reversible disturbances of consciousness, attention, cognition and perception that develop over a short period of time, which may compromise health

Risk Factors

Alteration in sleep–wake cycle; dehydration; impaired mobility; inappropriate use of restraints; malnutrition; pain; sensory deprivation; substance misuse; urinary retention

At-Risk Population

Age ≥ 60 years; history of cerebral vascular accident; male gender

Associated Condition

Alteration in cognitive functioning; delirium; dementia; impaired metabolic functioning; infection; pharmaceutical agent

Client Outcomes, Nursing Interventions, Client/Family Teaching

Refer to care plan for Acute **Confusion.**

Constipation

NANDA-I Definition

Infrequent or difficult evacuation of feces.

Defining Characteristics

Evidence of symptoms in standardized diagnostic criteria; hard stools; lumpy stools; need for manual maneuvers to facilitate defecation; passing fewer than three stools a week; sensation of anorectal obstruction; sensation of incomplete evacuation; straining with defecation

Related Factors

Altered regular routine; average daily physical activity is less than recommended for age and gender; communication barriers; habitually suppresses urge to defecate; impaired physical mobility; impaired postural balance; inadequate knowledge of modifiable factors; inadequate toileting habits; insufficient fiber intake; insufficient fluid intake; insufficient privacy; stressors; substance misuse

At Risk Population

Individuals admitted to hospital; individuals experiencing prolonged hospitalization; individuals in aged care settings; individuals in the early postoperative period; older adults; pregnant women; women

Associated Conditions

Blockage in the colon; blockage in the rectum; depression; developmental disabilities; digestive system diseases; endocrine system diseases; heart diseases; mental disorders; muscular diseases; nervous system diseases; neurocognitive disorders; pelvic floor disorders; pharmaceutical preparations; radiotherapy; urogynecological disorders

Client Outcomes

Client Will (Specify Time Frame)

Maintain passage of soft, formed stool every 1 to 3 days without straining; State relief from discomfort of constipation; Identify measures that prevent or treat constipation

Nursing Interventions

- Introduce yourself to the client and any companions and inform them of your role. Introducing yourself to a client helps establish and develop a therapeutic relationship that recognizes the person within the client and forms the basis for building trust on which to base the provision of care (Howatson-Jones et al., 2012).

- Gain consent to perform care before proceeding further with the assessment. Clients have the right of autonomy both legally and morally and therefore should be fully involved in the decision-making process (Avery, 2013).
- Wash hands using a recognized technique.
- Assess usual pattern of defecation and establish the extent of the constipation problem.
- Assess the client's bowel habits:
  - Time of day of bowel evacuation
  - Amount and frequency of stool
  - Consistency of stool (using the Bristol Stool Scale)
  - Bleeding/passing mucus on defecation
  - History of bowel habits and/or laxative use
- Assess the client's lifestyle factors that may influence constipation:
  - Fiber content in diet
  - Daily fluid intake
  - Exercise patterns
  - Personal remedies for constipation
  - Recently stopped smoking
  - Alcohol consumption/recreational drug use
- Review the client's past medical history:
  - Obstetrical/gynecological/urological history and surgeries
  - Diseases that affect bowel motility
  - Bleeding/passing mucous on defecation
  - Current medications
- Assess the client for emotional influences that may be contributing to constipation:
  - Anxiety and depression
  - Long-term defecation issues
  - Stress
- Complete a physical examination (palpation for abdominal distention, percussion for dullness, and auscultation for bowel sounds).
- Encourage the client or family to keep a 7-day diary of bowel habits to include time of day, length of time spent on the toilet, consistency, amount and frequency of stool, and any straining (using the Bristol Stool Scale).

C

- Encourage the client or family to keep a 7-day diary of lifestyle issues in relation to bowel habits to include fluid consumption, fiber content in diet, usual bowel stimulus, and exercise regimen.
- Use the Bristol Stool Scale to assess stool consistency.
- ▲ Review the client's current medications.
- Discuss with clients already taking opioids (temporarily or long term) that constipation is a common side effect. Advise them to contact their healthcare provider for a prescription of an appropriate laxative.
- ▲ Recognize that opioids cause constipation. If the client is receiving temporary opioids (e.g., for acute postoperative pain), request an order for routine stool softeners from the primary care provider, monitor bowel movements, and request a laxative for the client if constipation develops. If the client is receiving around-the-clock opiates (e.g., for palliative care), laxatives, then softeners, stimulants, or osmotics should be requested.
- ▲ If the client is terminally ill and is receiving around-the-clock opioids for palliative care, speak with the prescribing healthcare provider about ordering low-dose naloxone, which is a drug that blocks opioid effects on the gastrointestinal tract without interfering with analgesia (Sanders et al., 2015).
- If new onset of constipation, determine whether the client has recently stopped smoking.
- Palpate for abdominal distention, percuss for dullness, and auscultate bowel sounds.
- ▲ Check for impaction; if present, then use a combination of oral laxatives and enemas initially to remove fecal loading and impaction (National Institute for Health and Care Excellence, 2015). Clients with neurogenic bowel dysfunction (e.g., spinal cord injury) commonly require manual evacuation of stool (McClurg & Norton, 2016).
- ▲ Advise a fiber intake of 18 to 25 g daily and suggest foodstuffs high in fiber (e.g., prune juice, leafy green vegetables, whole meal bread and pasta).
- Add fiber gradually to the diet to decrease bloating and flatus.
- Provide prune or prune juice daily. Each 100 g of prunes contains about 6 g of fiber, 15 g of sorbitol, and 184 mg of polyphenol, which all have laxative effects (Attaluri et al., 2011).

- • Advise a fluid intake of 1.5 to 2 L of fluid per day (ideally, 6–8 glasses of water), unless contraindicated by comorbidities, such as kidney or heart disease.
- ▲ If the client is uncomfortable or in pain because of constipation or has acute or chronic constipation that does not respond to increased fiber, fluid, activity, and appropriate toileting, refer the client to the primary care provider for an evaluation of bowel function and health status.
- • Encourage physical activity within the client's current ability to mobilize. Encourage turning and changing position in bed if immobile. For clients with reduced mobility, encourage knee-to-chest raises, waist twists, and stretching the arms away from the body. For fully mobile clients, encourage walking and swimming.
- • Demonstrate the use of gentle external abdominal massage, using aroma therapy oils, following the direction of colon activity.
- • Recommend that clients establish a regular elimination routine. If required, assist clients to the bathroom at the same time every day; always be mindful of the need for privacy (closing of bathroom doors).
- • Provide privacy for defecation. If not contraindicated, help the client to the bathroom and close the door.
- • Help clients onto a bedside commode or toilet so they can either squat or lean forward while sitting. Recognize that it is difficult to impossible to defecate in the lying supine position. Sitting upright allows gravity to aid defecation.
- • Educate the client about how to adopt the best posture for defecation. Keep knees slightly higher than hips, keep feet flat on the floor, and lean forward putting elbows onto knees.
- • Teach clients about the importance of responding promptly to the urge to defecate.
- • Consider the use of laxatives, suppositories, enemas, and bowel irrigation as required if other, more natural interventions are not effective.
- • Discourage the use of long-term laxatives and enemas and advise clients to gradually reduce their use if taken regularly.

Geriatric

- • Assess older adults for the presence of factors that contribute to constipation, including dietary fiber and fluid intake (less than 1.5 L/

day), physical activity, use of constipating medications, and diseases that are associated with constipation.

- Explain the importance of adequate fiber intake, fluid intake, activity, and established toileting routines to ensure soft, formed stool.
- Determine the client's perception of normal bowel elimination and laxative use; promote adherence to a regular schedule.
- Explain why straining (Valsalva maneuver) should be avoided.
- Respond quickly to the client's call for assistance with toileting.
- Offer food, fluids, activity, and toileting opportunities to older clients who are cognitively impaired.
- Avoid regular use of enemas in older adults.
- Advise the client against attempting to remove impacted feces on his or her own.
- ▲ Use opioids cautiously. Opioids cause constipation (Andrews & Morgan, 2013).
- Position the client on the toilet or commode and place a small footstool under the feet. Placing a small footstool helps the client assume a squatting posture to facilitate defecation.

Home Care

- The interventions described previously may be adapted for home care use.
- Take complaints seriously and evaluate claims of constipation in a matter-of-fact manner.
- Assess the self-care management activities the client is already using.
- Offer the following treatment recommendations:
  - ❍ Acknowledge the client's lifelong experience of bowel function; respect beliefs, attitudes, and preferences, and avoid patronizing responses.
  - ❍ Make available comprehensive, useful written information about constipation and possible solutions.
  - ❍ Make available empathetic and accessible professional care to provide treatment and advice; a multidisciplinary approach (including healthcare provider, nurse, and pharmacist) should be used.
  - ❍ Institute a bowel management program.
  - ❍ Consider affordability when suggesting solutions to constipation; discuss cost-effective strategies.
  - ❍ Discuss a range of solutions to constipation and allow the client to choose the preferred options.

C

- ○ Have orders in place for a suppository and enema as needed. As part of a bowel management program, suppositories or enemas may become necessary.
- • Although the use of a bedside commode may be necessitated by the client's condition, allow the client to use the toilet in the bathroom when possible and provide assistance.
- • In older clients, routinely advise consumption of fluids, fruits, and vegetables as part of the diet, and ambulation if the client is able.
- ▲ Refer for consideration of the use of polyethylene glycol 3350 (PEG-3350) for constipation.
- • When using a bowel program, establish a pattern that is very regular and allows the client to be part of the family unit.

Client/Family Teaching and Discharge Planning

- • Instruct the client on normal bowel function and the need for adequate fluid and fiber intake, activity, and a defined toileting pattern in a bowel program.
- • Encourage the client to heed defecation warning signs and develop a regular schedule of defecation by using a stimulus such as a warm drink or prune juice.
- • Encourage the client to avoid long-term use of laxatives and enemas and to gradually withdraw from their use if they are used regularly.
- • If not contraindicated, teach the client how to do bent-leg sit-ups to increase abdominal tone; also encourage the client to contract the abdominal muscles frequently throughout the day. Help the client develop a daily exercise program to increase peristalsis.
- • Provide client with comprehensive written information about constipation and its management.
- ▲ Collaborate with members of the interprofessional team to provide treatment and advice to clients and caregivers. Teamwork is a central process in healthcare organizations. It increases the capacity of teams to absorb and develop new knowledge, which will improve patient health and well-being (Ortega et al., 2013).
- • Formalize all advice by providing a bowel management program reiterating the mechanism of normal bowel function and the need for adequate fluid and fiber intake, physical activity, and a defined toileting pattern in an agreed bowel program.
- • Document all care and advice given in a factual and comprehensive manner.

Risk for Constipation

NANDA-I Definition

Susceptible to a decrease in normal frequency of defecation accompanied by difficult or incomplete passage of stool, which may compromise health

Risk Factors

Altered regular routine; average daily physical activity is less than recommended for age and gender; communication barriers; habitually suppresses urge to defecate; impaired physical mobility; impaired postural balance; inadequate knowledge of modifiable factors; inadequate toileting habits; insufficient fiber intake; insufficient fluid intake; insufficient privacy; stressors; substance misuse

At Risk Population

Individuals admitted to hospital; individuals experiencing prolonged hospitalization; individuals in aged care settings; individuals in the early postoperative period; older adults; pregnant women; women

Associated Conditions

Blockage in the colon; blockage in the rectum; depression; developmental disabilities; digestive system diseases; endocrine system diseases; heart diseases; mental disorders; muscular diseases; nervous system diseases; neurocognitive disorders; pelvic floor disorders; pharmaceutical preparations; radiotherapy; urogynecological disorders

Client Outcomes, Nursing Interventions, Client/Family Teaching

Refer to care plans for **Constipation.**

Perceived Constipation

NANDA-I Definition

Self-diagnosis of infrequent or difficult evacuation of feces combined with abuse of methods to ensure a daily bowel movement.

Defining Characteristics

Enema misuse; expects a daily bowel movement at the same time every day; laxative misuse; suppository misuse

Related Factors

Cultural health beliefs; deficient knowledge about normal evacuation patterns; family health beliefs; disturbed thought process

Client Outcomes

Client Will (Specify Time Frame)

- Regularly defecate soft, formed stool without use of aids
- Explain the need to decrease or eliminate the use of stimulant laxatives, suppositories, and enemas

- Identify alternatives to stimulant laxatives, enemas, and suppositories for ensuring defecation
- Explain that defecation does not have to occur every day

Nursing Interventions

- Introduce yourself to the client and any companions, and inform them of your role.
- Gain consent before proceeding further with the assessment.
- Wash hands using a recognized technique.
- Assess usual pattern of defecation and establish the extent of the perceived constipation problem to include:
  - Assess the client's bowel habits
    - Time of day
    - Amount and frequency of stool
    - Consistency of stool (using the Bristol Stool Scale)
    - Bleeding/passing mucus on defecation
    - Patient history of bowel habits and/or laxative use
    - Family history of bowel habits and/or laxative use
  - Assess the client's lifestyle that may impact bowel function
    - Fiber content in diet
    - Daily fluid intake
    - Exercise patterns
    - Personal remedies for constipation
    - Cultural remedies for constipation
    - Recently stopped smoking
    - Alcohol consumption/recreational drug use
  - Review the client's past medical history
    - Obstetrical/gynecological/urological history and surgeries
    - Diseases that affect bowel motility
    - Bleeding/passing mucus on defecation
    - Current medications
  - Emotional Influences
    - Anxiety and depression/psychological disorders
    - History of eating disorders
    - History of physical/or sexual abuse
    - Long-term defecation issues
    - Stress
- Encourage the client or family to keep a 7-day diary of bowel habits to include time of day, length of time spent on the toilet, consistency, amount and frequency of stool, and any straining (using the Bristol Stool Scale).

- Encourage the client or family to keep a 7-day diary of lifestyle issues in relation to bowel habits to include fluid consumption, fiber content in diet, usual bowel stimulus, and exercise regimen.
- Educate the client that it is not necessary to have a daily bowel movement.
- Encourage the client to record use of laxatives, suppositories, or enemas, and suggest replacing them with an increase in fluid and fiber intake.
- Advise a fiber intake of 18 to 30 g daily in adults and suggest foodstuffs high in fiber (e.g., prune juice, leafy green vegetables, whole meal bread and pasta).
- Advise a fluid intake of 1.5 to 2 L of fluid per day (ideally, 6–8 glasses of water), unless contraindicated by comorbidities, such as kidney or heart disease.
- Obtain a referral to a dietitian for analysis of the client's diet and fluid intake to provide strategies to improve diet and nutrition.
- Encourage physical activity within the client's current ability to mobilize. Encourage turning and changing position in bed if immobile. For clients with reduced mobility, encourage knee-to-chest raises, waist twists, and stretching the arms away from the body. For fully mobile clients, encourage walking and swimming.
- Demonstrate the use of gentle external abdominal massage, using aroma therapy oils, following the direction of colon activity.
- Recommend clients establish a regular elimination routine. If required, assist clients to the bathroom at the same time every day being mindful of the need for privacy (closing of bathroom doors).
- Observe for the presence of an eating disorder by using laxatives to control or decrease weight; refer for counseling if needed.
- Observe family cultural patterns related to eating and bowel habits. Cultural patterns may control bowel habits.

Client/Family Teaching and Discharge Planning

- Provide education to the client on ways to adopt the best posture for defecation. Keep knees slightly higher than hips, keep feet flat on the floor, and lean forward putting elbows onto knees.
- Teach clients the importance of responding promptly to the urge to defecate.
- Discourage the use of long-term laxatives and enemas and explain the potential harmful effects of the continual use of defecation aids such as laxatives and enemas.

- Advise clients to gradually reduce their use of laxatives, if taken regularly, which may take months to achieve.
- Provide client with comprehensive written information about constipation and its management.
- Collaborate with members of the interprofessional team to provide treatment and advice to clients and caregivers.
- Formalize all advice by providing a bowel management program reiterating the mechanism of normal bowel function and the need for adequate fluid and fiber intake, physical activity, and a defined toileting pattern in an agreed bowel program.
- Document all care and advice given in a factual and comprehensive manner.

Chronic Functional Constipation

NANDA-I Definition

Infrequent or difficult evacuation of feces, which has been present for at least 3 of the prior 12 months

Defining Characteristics

Adult: Presence of ≥ 2 of the following symptoms on the Rome III classification system:

Lumpy or hard stools in ≥ 25% defecations; straining during ≥ 25% defecations; sensation of incomplete evacuation for ≥ 25% defecations; sensation of anorectal obstruction/blockage for ≥ 25% defecations; manual maneuvers to facilitate ≥ 25% defecations (digital manipulation, pelvic floor support); ≤ 3 evacuations per week

Child > 4 years; Presence of ≥ 2 criteria on the Rome III pediatric classification system for ≥ 2 months:

≤ 2 defecations per week; ≥ 1 episode of fecal incontinence per week; stool retentive posturing; painful or hard bowel movements; presence of large fecal mass in the rectum; large diameter stools that may obstruct the toilet

Child ≤ 4 years; Presence of ≥ 2 criteria on the Rome III pediatric classification system for ≥ 1 month:

≤ 2 defecations per week; ≥ 1 episode of fecal incontinence per week; stool retentive posturing; painful or hard bowel movements; presence of large fecal mass in the rectum; large diameter stools that may obstruct the toilet

General

Distended abdomen; fecal impaction; leakage of stool with digital stimulation; pain with defecation; palpable abdominal mass; positive fecal occult blood test; prolonged straining; type 1 or type 2 on Bristol Stool Chart

Related Factors

Decrease in food intake; dehydration; depression; diet disproportionally high in fat; diet disproportionally high in protein; frail elderly syndrome; habitually suppresses urge to defecate; impaired mobility; insufficient dietary intake; insufficient fluid intake; insufficient knowledge of modifiable factors; low caloric intake; low-fiber diet; sedentary lifestyle

Associated Condition

Amyloidosis; anal fissure; anal stricture; autonomic neuropathy; cerebral vascular accident; chronic intestinal pseudoobstruction; chronic renal insufficiency; colorectal cancer; dementia; dermatomyositis; diabetes mellitus; extra intestinal mass; hemorrhoids; Hirschsprung's disease; hypercalcemia; hypothyroidism; inflammatory bowel disease; ischemic stenosis; multiple sclerosis; myotonic dystrophy; panhypopituitarism; paraplegia; Parkinson's disease; pelvic floor dysfunction; perineal damage; pharmaceutical agent; polypharmacy; porphyria; postinflammatory stenosis; pregnancy; proctitis; scleroderma; slow colon transit time; spinal cord injury; surgical stenosis

Client Outcomes

Client Will (Specify Time Frame)

- Maintain passage of soft, formed stool every 1 to 3 days without straining
- State relief from discomfort of constipation
- Identify measures that prevent or treat constipation

Nursing Interventions

All Client Ages

- Introduce yourself to the client and anyone accompanying him or her and inform them of your role. Introducing yourself to a client helps establish and develop a therapeutic relationship that recognizes the person within the client and forms the basis for building trust on which to base the provision of care (Howatson-Jones et al., 2012).
- Gain consent to provide care before proceeding further with the assessment. Clients have the right of autonomy both legally and morally and therefore should be fully involved in the decision-making process (Avery, 2013).

- Wash hands using a recognized technique. Strict hand hygiene regimens significantly reduce the incidence of methicillin-resistant Staphylococcus aureus and Clostridium difficile infection (Goldberg, 2017).
- Assess usual pattern of defecation and establish the extent of the constipation problem to include:
  - Assess Bowel habits
    - Time of day
    - Amount and frequency of stool
    - Consistency of stool (using the Bristol Stool Scale)
    - Bleeding/passing mucus on defecation
    - History of bowel habits and/or laxative use
    - Assess children younger than 4 years using the Rome III pediatric classification (for at least 1 month)
    - Assess children older than age 4 years using the Rome III pediatric classification (for at least 2 months)
  - Assess the client's lifestyle that may impact bowel function
    - Fiber content in diet
    - Daily fluid intake
    - Exercise patterns
    - Personal remedies for constipation
    - Recently stopped smoking
    - Alcohol consumption/recreational drug use
    - Personal habits related to defecation
  - Review the client's past medical history
    - Obstetrical/gynecological/urological history and surgeries
    - Existing anatomical anomalies (e.g., anal fissures, anal strictures, and hemorrhoids)
    - Diseases that affect bowel motility (e.g., colorectal cancer, chronic intestinal pseudoobstruction, and Hirschsprung's disease)
    - Bleeding/passing mucus on defecation
    - Current medications
  - Emotional influences
    - Anxiety and depression
    - Long-term defecation issues
    - Stress

- Complete a physical assessment (palpation for abdominal distention; percussion for dullness; auscultation for bowel sounds; and observation for anal fissures, anal strictures, and hemorrhoids).
- Encourage the client or family to keep a 7-day diary of bowel habits to include time of day, length of time spent on the toilet, consistency, amount and frequency of stool, and any straining (using the Bristol Stool Scale).
- Encourage the client or family to keep a 7-day diary of lifestyle issues in relation to bowel habits to include fluid consumption, fiber content in diet, usual bowel stimulus, and exercise regime.
- Actively encourage the use of reward/star charts with children when establishing regular bowel routines.
- Discuss with clients already taking opioids (temporarily or long term) that constipation is a common side effect. Advise the client to contact their primary healthcare provider for a prescription of an appropriate laxative.
- Advise a fiber intake of 18 to 30 g daily in adults and suggest foodstuffs to facilitate this diet (e.g., prune juice, leafy green vegetables, whole meal bread and pasta).
- Advise a fluid intake of 1.5 to 2 L of fluid per day (ideally, 6–8 glasses of water), unless this is contraindicated by comorbidities such as renal or heart disease.
- Encourage physical activity within the client's current ability to mobilize. Encourage turning and changing position in bed if immobile. For reduced mobility clients, encourage knee-to-chest raises, waist twists, and stretching the arms away from the body. For fully mobile clients, encourage walking and swimming.
- Demonstrate the use of gentle external abdominal massage, following the direction of colon activity.
- Recommend clients establish a regular elimination routine. If required, assist clients to the bathroom at the same time every day, being mindful of the need for privacy (closing of bathroom doors).
- Educate the client in how to adopt the best posture for defecation: keep knees slightly higher than hips, keep feet flat on the floor and lean forward, putting elbows onto knees.
- Consider the teaching of biofeedback therapy to encourage a "new normal" bowel routine for clients to adopt.
- Teach clients about the need to respond promptly to the defecation urge.

C

- Consider the use of laxatives, suppositories, enemas, and bowel irrigation as required when other more natural interventions are not effective.
- Discourage the use of long-term laxatives and enemas and advise clients to gradually reduce their use if taken regularly.
- Provide client with comprehensive written information about constipation and its management.
- Provide written instructions for children about taking their medication and about how the bowel works.
- Liaise with members of the interprofessional team as appropriate to provide treatment and advice to clients and caregivers.
- Educate the client on the mechanism of normal bowel function and the need for adequate fluid and fiber intake, physical activity, and a defined toileting pattern in an agreed-on bowel management program.
- Document all care and advice given in a factual and comprehensive manner.

Risk for Chronic Functional Constipation

NANDA-I Definition

Susceptible to infrequent or difficult evacuation of feces, which has been present nearly 3 of the prior 12 months, which may compromise health

Risk Factors

Decrease in food intake; dehydration; depression; diet disproportionally high in fat; diet disproportionally high in protein; frail elderly syndrome; habitually suppresses urge to defecate; impaired mobility; insufficient dietary intake; insufficient fluid intake; insufficient knowledge of modifiable factors; low caloric intake; low-fiber diet; sedentary lifestyle

Associated Condition

Amyloidosis; anal fissure; anal stricture; autonomic neuropathy; cerebral vascular accident; chronic intestinal pseudoobstruction; chronic renal insufficiency; colorectal cancer; dementia; dermatomyositis; diabetes mellitus; extra intestinal mass; hemorrhoids; Hirschsprung's disease; hypercalcemia; hypothyroidism; inflammatory bowel disease; ischemic stenosis; multiple sclerosis; myotonic dystrophy; panhypopituitarism; paraplegia; Parkinson's disease; pelvic floor dysfunction; perineal damage; pharmaceutical agen polypharmacy; porphyria; postinflammatory stenosis; pregnancy; proctitis; scleroderma; slow colon transit time; spinal cord injury; surgical stenosis

Client Outcomes, Nursing Interventions, Client/Family Teaching and Discharge Planning

Refer to care plan for Chronic functional **Constipation.**

Contamination

NANDA-I Definition

Exposure to environmental contaminants in doses sufficient to cause adverse health effects

Defining Characteristics

Pesticides

Dermatological effects of pesticide exposure; gastrointestinal effects of pesticide exposure; neurological effects of pesticide exposure; pulmonary effects of pesticide exposure; renal effects of pesticide exposure

Chemicals

Dermatological effects of chemical exposure; gastrointestinal effects of chemical exposure; immunological effects of chemical exposure; neurological effects of chemical exposure; pulmonary effects of chemical exposure; renal effects of chemical exposure

Biologicals

Dermatological effects of biological exposure; gastrointestinal effects of biological exposure; neurological effects of biological exposure; pulmonary effects of biological exposure; renal effects of biological exposure

Pollution

Neurological effects of pollution exposure; pulmonary effects of pollution exposure

Waste

Dermatological effects of waste exposure; gastrointestinal effects of waste exposure; hepatic effects of waste exposure; pulmonary effects of waste exposure

Radiation

Genetic effects of radiation exposure; immunological effects of radiation exposure; neurological effects of radiation exposure; oncological effects of radiation exposure

Related Factors

External

Carpeted flooring; chemical contamination of food; chemical contamination of water; flaking; peeling surface in presence of young children; inadequate breakdown of contaminant; inadequate household hygiene practices; inadequate municipal services; inadequate personal hygiene practices; inadequate protective clothing; inappropriate use of protective clothing; ingestion of contaminated material; playing where environmental contaminants are used; unprotected exposure to chemical; unprotected exposure to heavy metal; unprotected exposure to radioactive material; use of environmental contaminates in the home; use of noxious material in insufficiently ventilated area; use of noxious material without effective protection

Internal

Concomitant exposure; inadequate nutrition; smoking

Associated Condition

Pre-existing disease; pregnancy

At-Risk Population

Children < 5 years; economically disadvantaged; exposure to areas with high contamination level; exposure to atmospheric pollutants; exposure to bioterrorism; exposure to disaster; exposure to radiation; female gender; gestational age during exposure; older adults; previous exposure to contaminant

Client Outcomes

Client Will (Specify Time Frame)

- Have minimal health effects associated with contamination
- Cooperate with appropriate decontamination protocol
- Participate in appropriate isolation precautions

Community Will (Specify Time Frame)

- Use health surveillance data system to monitor for contamination incidents
- Use disaster plan to evacuate and triage affected members
- Have minimal health effects associated with contamination
- Use measures to reduce household environmental risks

Nursing Interventions

▲ Help individuals cope with contamination incident by doing the following:
  - ❍ Use groups that have survived terrorist attacks as a useful resource for victims.
  - ❍ Provide accurate information on risks involved, preventive measures, use of antibiotics and vaccines.
  - ❍ Assist to deal with feelings of fear, vulnerability, and grief.
  - ❍ Encourage individuals to talk to others about their fears.
  - ❍ Assist victims to think positively and to move toward the future.

• Triage, stabilize, transport, and treat affected community members.

C

- Prioritize mental healthcare for highly vulnerable risk groups or those with special needs (deeply affected groups, women, older persons, children and adolescents, displaced persons—especially those living in shelters, persons with preexisting mental health disorders, including those living in institutions) (Pan American Health Organization, 2012).
- Collaborate with members of the healthcare delivery system and outside agencies (local health department, emergency medical services [EMS], state and federal agencies).
- Use approved procedures for decontamination of persons, clothing, and equipment. Victims may first require decontamination before entering health facility to receive care to prevent the spread of contamination (US Army Medical Research Institute of Infectious Diseases, 2014).
- Use appropriate isolation precautions: universal, airborne, droplet, and contact isolation to prevent cross-contamination by contaminating agents (US Army Medical Research Institute of Infectious Diseases, 2014).
- Monitor individuals for therapeutic effects, side effects, and compliance with postexposure drug therapy that may extend over a long period of time and require monitoring for compliance and for therapeutic and side effects (Veenema, 2013; Adalja et al., 2015).
- Perform effective handwashing before and after handling medical charts, entering case notes, touching clients, and performing procedures, especially in intensive care unit environments.
- Prevent cross-contamination by systematically disinfecting stethoscopes (diaphragm and tubing) after each use.
- Minimize occupational exposure to antineoplastic agents by following National Institute of Occupational Safety and Health (NIOSH) guidelines regarding personal protective equipment and correct handling of hazardous drugs.

Geriatric

- Help the client identify age-related factors that may affect response to contamination incidents.
- Advise older adults to follow public notices related to drinking water.
- Encourage older adults to receive influenza vaccination when it is available, beginning as early as late August and continuing through the end of February.

- Instruct older adults with special needs or chronic conditions to create and share a plan with family and friends for emergencies and keep medications, prescriptions, and special devices on hand.

Pediatric

- Provide environmental health hazard information.
- Reduce risks from exposure to environmental contaminants by identifying the ages and life stages of children.
- Screen newly arrived immigrant and refugee children for elevated blood lead levels secondary to lead hazards in older housing.
- Be aware that the risk for lead exposure is much higher in many countries from which children are adopted than in the United States; screening should then be conducted for those identified from 6 months and up to 16 years of age (CDC, 2014b).
- The current reference level of 5 μg/dL is used to identify children and environments associated with lead exposure hazards.

Multicultural

- Ask about use of imported or culture-specific products that contain lead, such as greta and azarcon (Hispanic folk medicine for upset stomach and diarrhea), ghasard (Indian folk medicine tonic), ba-baw-san (Chinese herbal remedy), and daw-tay (Thai and Myanmar remedy).
- Nurses need to consider the cultural and social factors that impact access to and understanding of the healthcare system, particularly for groups such as migrant workers who do not have consistent healthcare providers.

Home Care

- Assess current environmental stressors and identify community resources.
- Recognize that relocated and unemployed individuals/families are at risk for psychological distress.
- Support policy and program initiatives that provide emergency mental health services following large-scale contamination events.
- Instruct community members concerned about lead in drinking water from plumbing pipes and fixtures to have the water tested by calling the Environmental Protection Agency (EPA) drinking water hotline at 800-426-4791.
- Educate community members to reduce exposure to lead by inquiring about lead-based paint before buying a home or renting an

apartment built before 1978; federal law requires disclosure of known information about lead-based paint (EPA, 2017).
- Instruct individuals and families that food contamination occurs through a variety of mechanisms and that food safety is associated with proper washing of hands, surfaces, and utensils; prompt refrigeration of food; and cooking foods at the correct temperature.

Client/Family Teaching and Discharge Planning

- Provide truthful information to the person or family affected.
- Discuss signs and symptoms of contamination.
- Explain decontamination protocols.
- Explain need for isolation procedures.
- Emphasize the importance of preexposure and postexposure treatment of contamination. *Early treatment decreases associated complications related to contamination* (ATSDR, 2014).
- Provide parents with actionable information to reduce environmental contamination in the home.

Risk for Contamination

NANDA-I Definition

Susceptible to exposure to environmental contaminants, which may compromise health

Risk Factors

External

Carpeted flooring; chemical contamination of food; chemical contamination of water; flaking; peeling surface in presence of young children; inadequate breakdown of contaminant; inadequate household hygiene practices; inadequate municipal services; inadequate personal hygiene practices; inadequate protective clothing; inappropriate use of protective clothing; ingestion of contaminated material; playing where environmental contaminants are used; unprotected exposure to chemical; unprotected exposure to heavy metal; unprotected exposure to radioactive material; use of environmental contaminant in the home; use of noxious material in insufficiently ventilated area; use of noxious material without effective protection

Internal

Concomitant exposure; inadequate nutrition; smoking

At-Risk Population

Children < 5 years; economically disadvantaged; exposure to areas with high contaminant level; exposure to atmospheric pollutants; exposure to bioterrorism; exposure to disaster; exposure to radiation; female gender; gestational age during exposure; older adults; previous exposure to contaminant

Associated Condition

Preexisting disease; pregnancy

Client Outcomes, Nursing Interventions, Client/Family Teaching

Refer to care plans for **Contamination.**

Risk for Adverse Reaction to Iodinated Contrast Media

NANDA-I Definition

Susceptible to noxious or unintended reaction associated with the use of iodinated contrast media that can occur within seven days after contrast agent injection, which may compromise health

Risk Factors

Dehydration; Generalized weakness

At-Risk Population

Extremes of age; history of allergy; history of previous adverse effect from iodinated contrast media

Associated Condition

Chronic illness; concurrent use of pharmaceutical agents; contrast media precipitates adverse event; fragile vein; unconsciousness

Client Outcomes

Client Will (Specify Time Frame)

- Maintain normal blood urea nitrogen and serum creatinine levels
- Maintain urine output of 0.5 mL/kg/hr
- Maintain serum electrolytes (K^+, PO_4, Na^+) within normal limits

Nursing Interventions

Recognize that iodinated contrast media can be harmful to clients in a number of ways, including onset of contrast-induced nephropathy (CIN), allergic reactions to the dye, and damage to veins and vascular access devices.

Contrast-Induced Nephropathy

Protect clients from contrast media-induced nephropathy by taking the following actions:

▲ Assess clients for low body mass index (BMI), history of heart failure, or repeated administration of contrast material.

- ▲ In nondiabetic clients with acute coronary syndrome, assess for presence of hyperglycemia on admission and report to healthcare provider.
- • Identify clients who have had multiple doses of iodinated contrast media in less than 24 hours and report to healthcare provider.
- • Communicate information about at-risk clients to provider and procedure team in the hand-off report and electronic medical record.
- ▲ Ensure that clients having diagnostic testing with contrast are well hydrated with isotonic intravenous (IV) fluids as ordered before and after the examination.
- ▲ Verify that a baseline serum creatinine has been drawn from clients at risk for CIN.
- • Be vigilant for signs of CIN in clients who have cancer.
- ▲ Monitor for and report signs of acute kidney injury for 48 hours after iodinated contrast administration in clients at risk: absolute serum creatinine increase ≥0.3 mg/dL, percentage increase in serum creatinine ≥50%, or urine output reduced to ≤0.5 mL/kg/hr for at least 6 hours. (Refer to your institution policy for specific clinical parameters).
- ▲ Clients taking metformin may increase client risk of developing lactic acidosis should CIN develop after contrast administration.

Allergic Reaction to Contrast Media

- ▲ Previous allergic reactions to contrast material, history of asthma, and other allergies are factors that may increase the client's risk of developing an adverse reaction. Discuss premedication with methylprednisolone or diphenhydramine with the provider for clients who have had previous reactions to contrast media or known asthma or allergies.
- ▲ Monitor carefully for symptoms of a reaction, which can be mild, moderate, or severe. Report all symptoms to the provider because symptoms can advance rapidly from mild to severe.
  - ❍ *Mild reactions*: Nausea, vomiting, headache, itching, flushing, mild skin rash, or hives
  - ❍ *Moderate reactions*: Severe skin rash or hives, wheezing, abnormal heart rhythms, high or low blood pressure, shortness of breath, or difficulty breathing
  - ❍ *Severe reactions:* Difficulty breathing, cardiac arrest, swelling of throat or other parts of the body, convulsion, or profound low blood pressure)

Vein Damage and Damage to Vascular Access Devices

C

- Recognize that *only* vascular access devices labeled "power injectable" can be used to administer power-injected contrast media. These include a power port, a power peripherally inserted central catheter (PICC) line, and a power central venous catheter (Radiology and Biomedical Imaging, 2017a).
- Reduce the risk of vein and vascular access device damage with the following:
  - Maintain constant communication with the client during the injection and monitor client for report of pain or swelling at the injection site.
  - Monitor access site for extravasation during and after the procedure; be vigilant for clients at increased risk of extravasation.
  - Assess for venous backflow before injecting contrast.
  - Directly monitor and palpate the venipuncture site during the first 15 seconds of injection.

Geriatric

- Screen the older client thoroughly before diagnostic testing using contrast media.

Pediatric

"When the proper technique is used, contrast medium can be safely administered intravenously by power injector at high flow rates of up to 2 mls/second (depending on size of patient). A short peripheral IV catheter in the antecubital or forearm is the preferred route for intravenous contrast administration" (Radiology & Biomedical Imaging, 2017b).

Client/Family Teaching and Discharge Teaching

Provide patient/family teaching on the importance of keeping appointments with provider for monitoring kidney status, reporting symptoms of fluid retention or decrease in urine output, and awareness of increased risk for CIN with repeat exposure to contrast media (Jorgensen, 2013).

Readiness for Enhanced Community Coping

NANDA-I Definition

A pattern of community activities for adaptation and problem-solving for meeting the demands or needs of the community, which can be strengthened

C

Defining Characteristics

Expresses desire to enhance availability of community recreation programs; expresses desire to enhance availability of community relaxation programs; expresses desire to enhance communication among community members; expresses desire to enhance communication between groups and larger community; expresses desire to enhance community planning for predictable stressors; expresses desire to enhance community resources for managing stressors; expresses desire to enhance community responsibility for stress management; expresses desire to enhance problem-solving for identified issue

Community Outcomes

Community Will (Specify Time Frame)

- Develop enhanced coping strategies
- Maintain effective coping strategies for management of stress

Nursing Interventions

Note: Interventions depend on the specific aspects of community coping that can be enhanced (e.g., planning for stress management, communication, development of community power, community perceptions of stress, community coping strategies).

▲ Establish a collaborative partnership with the community.
- Assess community needs with the use of concept mapping methodology.
- Encourage participation in faith-based organizations that want to improve community stress management.

▲ Identify the health services and information resources that are currently available in the community through network analysis.
- Work with community members to increase problem-solving abilities.
- Provide support to the community and help community members identify and mobilize additional supports.
- Advocate for the community in multiple arenas (e.g., multimedia, social media, and governmental agencies).
- Work with communities to ensure that vulnerable individuals with access and functional needs are included in preparations for, response to, and recovery from disasters.
- Write grant proposals to help community members obtain funds for programs that reduce stress or improve coping (Anderson & McFarlane, 2011).

C

- Work with members of the community to identify and develop coping strategies that promote a sense of power (e.g., obtaining sources for funding, collaborating with other communities) (Anderson & McFarlane, 2011).

Pediatric

- Protect children and adolescents from exposure to community violence.
- Assess children and adolescents for the effects of direct and indirect crime exposure rather than only focusing solely on violent victimization.

Multicultural

- Acknowledge the stressors unique to racial/ethnic communities.
- Identify community strengths with community members.
- Use an empowerment approach to address health behaviors in diverse communities. An empowerment approach includes education, sharing of information, and health volunteerism.
- Work with members of the community to prioritize and target health goals specific to the community.
- Establish and sustain partnerships with key individuals within communities when developing and implementing programs.
- Use mentoring strategies for community members.
- Use community church settings as a forum for advocacy, teaching, and program implementation.

Client/Family Teaching and Discharge Planning

- Review coping skills, power for coping, and the use of power resources.

Defensive Coping

NANDA-I Definition

Repeated projection of falsely positive self-evaluation based on a self-protective pattern that defends against underlying perceived threats to positive self-regard

Defining Characteristics

Alteration in reality testing; denial of problems; denial of weaknesses; difficulty establishing relationships; difficulty maintaining relationships; grandiosity; hostile laughter; hypersensitivity to a discourtesy; hypersensitivity to criticism; insufficient follow-through with treatment; insufficient participation in treatment; projection of blame; projection of responsibility;

rationalization of failures; reality distortion; ridicule of others; superior attitude toward others

Related Factors

Conflict between self-perception and value system; fear of failure; fear of humiliation; fear of repercussions; insufficient confidence in others; insufficient resilience; insufficient self-confidence; insufficient support system; uncertainty; unrealistic self-expectations

Client Outcomes

Client Will (Specify Time Frame)

- Acknowledge need for change in coping style
- Accept responsibility for own behavior
- Establish realistic goals with validation from caregivers
- Solicit caregiver validation in decision-making

Nursing Interventions

- Assess for possible symptoms associated with defensive coping: depressive symptoms, excessive self-focused attention, negativism and anxiety, hypertension, post-traumatic stress disorder (e.g., exposure to terrorism), substance use symptoms, unjust world beliefs.
- ▲ Use cognitive behavioral interventions.
- Ask appropriate questions to assess whether denial (defensive coping) is being used in association with health problems including alcoholism, myocardial infarction (MI), or rheumatoid arthritis.
- Promote interventions with multisensory stimulation environments.
- Empower the client/caregiver's self-knowledge.

Geriatric

- ▲ Identify problems with alcohol in older adults with the appropriate tools and make suitable referrals.
- Encourage exercise for positive coping.
- Stimulate individual reminiscence therapy.
- Stimulate group reminiscence therapy.

Multicultural

- Acknowledge racial/ethnic differences at the onset of care.
- Assess an individual's sociocultural backgrounds in teaching self-management and self-regulation.
- Encourage the client to use spiritual coping mechanisms such as faith and prayer.
- Encourage spirituality as a source of support for coping.

Home Care

- ▲ Refer the client for programs that teach coping skills.

Client/Family Teaching and Discharge Planning

- Teach coping skills to clients and caregivers.
- Teach reflexive and expressive writing to address emotions.

Ineffective Coping

NANDA-I Definition

A pattern of invalid appraisal of stressors, with cognitive and/or behavioral efforts, that fails to manage demands related to well-being

Defining Characteristics

Alteration in concentration; alteration in sleep pattern; change in communication pattern; destructive behavior toward others; destructive behavior toward self; difficulty organizing information; fatigue; frequent illness; inability to ask for help; inability to attend to information; inability to deal with a situation; inability to meet basic needs; inability to meet role expectation; ineffective coping strategies; insufficient access of social support; insufficient goal-directed behavior; insufficient problem resolution; insufficient problem-solving skills; risk-taking behavior; substance misuse

Related Factors

High degree of threat; inability to conserve adaptive energies; inaccurate threat appraisal; inadequate confidence in ability to deal with a situation; inadequate opportunity to prepare for stressor; inadequate resources; ineffective tension release strategies; insufficient sense of control; insufficient social support

At-Risk Population

Maturational crisis; situational crisis

Client Outcomes

Client Will (Specify Time Frame)

- Use effective coping strategies
- Use behaviors to decrease stress
- Remain free of destructive behavior toward self or others
- Report decrease in physical symptoms of stress
- Report increase in psychological comfort
- Seek help from a healthcare professional as appropriate

Nursing Interventions

- Observe for contributing factors of ineffective coping such as poor self-concept, grief, lack of problem-solving skills, lack of support, recent change in life situation, maturational or situational crises.

- Use verbal and nonverbal therapeutic communication approaches including empathy, active listening, and confrontation to encourage the client and family to express emotions such as sadness, guilt, and anger (within appropriate limits); verbalize fears and concerns; and set goals.
- Collaborate with the client to identify strengths such as the ability to relate the facts and to recognize the source of stressors.
- Encourage the client to describe previous stressors and the coping mechanisms used.
- Provide opportunities for the client to discuss the meaning the situation might have for the client.
- Assist the client to set realistic goals and identify personal skills and knowledge.
- Provide information regarding care before care is given.
- Discuss changes with the client before making them.
- Provide mental and physical activities within the client's ability (e.g., reading, television, radio, crafts, outings, movies, dinners out, social gatherings, exercise, sports, games).
- Discuss the power of the client and family to change a situation or the need to accept a situation.
- Offer instruction regarding alternative coping strategies.
- Encourage use of spiritual resources as desired.
- Encourage use of social support resources.

▲ Refer for additional or more intensive therapies as needed.

Pediatric

- Monitor the client's risk of harming self or others and intervene appropriately. **QSEN:** See care plan for risk for **Suicidal Behavior.**
- Monitor adolescents for exposure to community violence.

Geriatric

▲ Assess and report possible physiological alterations (e.g., sepsis, hypoglycemia, hypotension, infection, changes in temperature, fluid and electrolyte imbalances, use of medications with known cognitive and psychotropic side effects).

- Screen for elder neglect or other forms of elder mistreatment.
- Encourage the client to make choices (as appropriate) and participate in planning care and scheduled activities.
- Target selected coping mechanisms for older persons based on client features, use, and preferences.

C

- Increase and mobilize support available to older persons by encouraging a variety of mechanisms involving family, friends, peers, and healthcare providers.
- Actively listen to complaints and concerns.
- Engage the client in reminiscence.

Multicultural

- Assess for the influence of cultural beliefs, norms, and values on the client's perceptions of effective coping.
- Assess for intergenerational family problems that can overwhelm coping abilities.
- Negotiate with the client regarding aspects of coping behavior that will need to be modified.
- Encourage moderate aerobic exercise or other forms of physical activity (as appropriate).
- Identify which family members the client can count on for support.
- Support the inner resources that clients use for coping.
- Use an empowerment framework to redefine coping strategies.

Home Care

- The interventions described previously may be adapted for home care use.
- ▲ **QSEN:** Assess for suicidal tendencies. Refer for mental healthcare immediately if indicated.
- ▲ **QSEN:** Identify an emergency plan should the client become suicidal. Ineffective coping can occur in a crisis situation and can lead to suicidal ideation if the client sees no hope for a solution. A suicidal client is not safe in the home environment unless supported by professional help. Refer to the care plan for risk for **Suicidal Behavior.**
- Discuss preferred coping strategies of family caregivers.
- Encourage the client to participate knowingly in their care. Refer to the care plan for **Powerlessness.**
- ▲ Refer the client and family to support groups.
- ▲ If monitoring medication use, contract with the client or solicit assistance from a responsible caregiver.
- ▲ Institute case management for frail elderly clients to support continued independent living.

Client/Family Teaching and Discharge Planning

- Teach the client to problem solve. Have the client define the problem and cause, and list the advantages and disadvantages of the options.

- Teach relaxation techniques.
- Work closely with the client to develop appropriate educational tools that address individualized needs.
- ▲ Teach the client about available community resources (e.g., therapists, ministers, counselors, self-help groups).

Readiness for Enhanced Coping

NANDA-I Definition

A pattern of valid appraisal of stressors with cognitive and/or behavioral efforts to manage demands related to well-being, which can be strengthened

Defining Characteristics

Awareness of possible environmental change; expresses desire to enhance knowledge of stress management strategies; expresses desire to enhance management of stressors; expresses desire to enhance social support; expresses desire to enhance use of emotion-oriented strategies; expresses desire to enhanced use of problem-oriented strategies; expresses desire to enhance use of spiritual resource

Client Outcomes

Client Will (Specify Time Frame)

- Acknowledge personal power
- State awareness of possible environmental changes that may contribute to decreased coping
- State that stressors are manageable
- Seek new effective coping strategies
- Seek social support for problems associated with coping
- Demonstrate ability to cope, using a broad range of coping strategies
- Use spiritual support of personal choice

Nursing Interventions

- Assess and support positive psychological strengths: that is, hope, optimism, self-efficacy, resiliency, and social support.
- Be physically and emotionally present for the client while using a variety of therapeutic communication techniques.
- Empower the client to set realistic goals and to engage in problem-solving.
- Encourage expression of positive thoughts and emotions.

- Encourage the client to use spiritual coping mechanisms such as faith and prayer.
- Help the client with serious and chronic conditions such as depression, cancer diagnosis, and chemotherapy treatment to maintain social support networks or assist in building new ones.
- ▲ Refer for cognitive-behavioral therapy (CBT) to enhance coping skills.

Pediatric

- Encourage children and adolescents to engage in diversional activities and exercise to promote self-esteem, enhance coping, and prevent behavioral and other physical and psychosocial problems.
- Provide families of children with chronic illness with education, transitional assistance, and psychosocial support to enhance coping.

Geriatric

- Encourage active, meaning-based coping strategies for older adults with chronic illness.
- Consider the use of Web-based and technological resources for older adults in the community.
- Refer the older client to self-help support groups that address health, psychosocial, and/or social support.

Multicultural

- Assess an individual's sociocultural backgrounds to identify factors that support coping.
- Encourage spirituality as a source of support for coping.
- Facilitate positive ethnocultural identity to enhance coping.
- Foster family support.

Home Care

- The interventions described previously may be adapted for home care use.
- Engage both clients and their caregivers as a dyad.
- ▲ Institute case management for frail elderly clients to support continued independent living.
- Refer the client and family to support groups.
- Refer prostate cancer clients and their spouses to family programs that include family-based interventions of communication, hope, coping, uncertainty, and symptom management.
- ▲ Refer military members, veterans, and family members for appropriate health services.

Client/Family Teaching and Discharge Planning

- Teach the client about available community resources (e.g., therapists, ministers, counselors, self-help groups, family education groups).
- Teach caregivers using a variety of interventions that contribute to coping.
- Teach expressive writing, journaling, and education about emotions.

Ineffective Community Coping

NANDA-I Definition

A pattern of community activities for adaptation and problem-solving that is unsatisfactory for meeting the demands or needs of the community

Defining Characteristics

Community does not meet expectations of its members; deficient community participation; elevated community illness rate; excessive community conflict; excessive stress; high incidence of community problems; perceived community powerlessness; perceived community vulnerability

Related Factors

Inadequate resources for problem-solving; insufficient community resources; nonexistent community systems

At-Risk Population

Exposure to disaster; history of disaster

Community Outcomes

A Broad Range of Community Members Will (Specify Time Frame)

- Participate in community actions to improve power resources
- Develop improved communication among community members
- Participate in problem-solving
- Demonstrate cohesiveness in problem-solving
- Develop new strategies for problem-solving
- Express power to deal with change and manage problems

Nursing Interventions

Note: The diagnosis of Ineffective **Coping** does not apply and should not be used when stress is being imposed by external sources or circumstance. If the community is a victim of circumstances, using the nursing diagnosis Ineffective **Coping** is equivalent to blaming the victim. See the care plan for Readiness for enhanced community **Coping.**

C

- ▲ Establish a collaborative partnership with the community (see the care plan for Readiness for enhanced community **Coping** for additional references).
- • Assess community needs with the use of concept mapping methodology.
- • Encourage participation in faith-based organizations that want to improve community stress management.
- ▲ Identify the health services and information resources that are currently available in the community through network analysis.
- • Work with community members to increase problem-solving abilities.
- • Provide support to the community and help community members identify and mobilize additional supports.
- • Advocate for the community in multiple arenas (e.g., multimedia, social media, governmental agencies).
- • Work with communities to ensure that vulnerable individuals with access and functional needs are included in preparations for, response to, and recovery from disasters.
- • Write grant proposals to help community members obtain funds for programs that reduce stress or improve coping (Anderson & McFarlane, 2011).
- • Work with members of the community to identify and develop coping strategies that promote a sense of power (e.g., obtaining sources for funding, collaborating with other communities) (Anderson & McFarlane, 2011).

Pediatric

- • Protect children and adolescents from exposure to community violence.
- • Assess children and adolescents for the effects of direct and indirect crime exposure rather than only focusing solely on violent victimization.

Multicultural

- • Acknowledge the stressors unique to racial/ethnic communities.
- • Identify community strengths with community members.
- • Use an empowerment approach to address health behaviors in diverse communities.
- • Work with members of the community to prioritize and target health goals specific to the community.

- Establish and sustain partnerships with key individuals within communities when developing and implementing programs.
- Use mentoring strategies for community members.
- Use community church settings as a forum for advocacy, teaching, and program implementation.

Community Teaching

- Teach strategies for stress management.
- Explain the relationship between enhancing power resources and coping.

C

Compromised Family Coping

NANDA-I Definition

An usually supportive primary person (family member, significant other, or close friend) provides insufficient, ineffective, or compromised support, comfort, assistance, or encouragement that may be needed by the client to manage or master adaptive tasks related to his or her health challenge

Defining Characteristics

Assistive behaviors by support person produce unsatisfactory results; client complaint about support person's response to health problems; client concern about support person's response to health problem; limitation in communication between support person and client; protective behavior by support person incongruent with client's abilities; protective behavior by support person incongruent with client's need for autonomy; support person reports inadequate understanding that interferes with effective behaviors; support person reports insufficient knowledge that interferes with effective behaviors; support person reports preoccupation with own reaction to client's need; support person withdraws from client

Related Factors

Coexisting situations affecting the support person; exhaustion of support person's capacity; family disorganization; insufficient information available to support person; insufficient reciprocal support; insufficient support given by client to support person; insufficient understanding of information by support person; misinformation obtained by support person; preoccupation by support person with concern outside of family

At-Risk Population

Developmental crisis experienced by support person; family role change; prolonged disease that exhausts capacity of support person; situational crisis faced by support person

Client Outcomes

Family/Significant Person Will (Specify Time Frame)

C

- Verbalize internal resources to help deal with the situation
- Verbalize knowledge and understanding of illness, disability, or disease
- Provide support and assistance as needed
- Identify need for and seek outside support

Nursing Interventions

- Assess the strengths and deficiencies of the family system. Consider using Family Systems Nursing to focus on the entire family as a unit of care.
- Establish rapport with families by providing accurate communication.
- Assist family members to recognize the need for help and teach them how to ask for it.
- Encourage family members to verbalize feelings. Spend time with them, sit down and make eye contact, and offer refreshments and other nourishment.
- Provide family support interventions in situations in which caregiving is involved in the family.
- Provide privacy during family visits. If possible, maintain flexible visiting hours to accommodate more frequent family visits. If possible, arrange staff assignments so the same staff members have contact with the family. Familiarize other staff members with the situation in the absence of the usual staff member. Providing privacy, maintaining flexible hours, and arranging consistent staff assignments reduces stress, enhances communication, and facilitates the building of trust.
- Provide education to clients regarding active coping strategies to use in situations involving chronic illnesses.
- Provide psychoeducation interventions and support for families providing palliative care to help reduce caregiver stress and burden.
- Refer the family with ill family members to appropriate resources for assistance as indicated (e.g., counseling, psychotherapy, financial assistance, spiritual support).

Pediatric

- Provide screening for postpartum depression (PPD) during the prenatal period and during the 6-week postpartum checkup to identify symptoms of depression in mothers.

C

- ▲ Consider medication management and psychosocial interventions, including individual therapy, group therapy, support groups, and brief psychotherapy.
- ▲ Use preventive strategies, such as screening, psychoeducation, postpartum debriefing, and companionship in the delivery room (e.g., community volunteer).
- • Use technology-based education to help increase knowledge and support for parents performing care procedures for their children.
- • Make communication and environmental adaptations when interacting with children with autism spectrum disorder (ASD) to enhance communication, improve quality of care, and reduce frustration.
- • Effectively engaging and collaborating with parents is essential for supporting parents of children with long-term health conditions, and it may enhance the parent–professional relationship and communication.
- • Provide evidence-based psychological therapies for parents with children with chronic conditions.
- • When performing pediatric diabetes care, be attentive to the mother's experience, including burnout experienced as a result of caregiving for the child.
- • Provide options for home-based interventions when severe childhood illnesses make it difficult for children and families to participate in interventions. In-home visits, assessments, and interventions may help improve self-management among the patient and family and reduce emergency room (ER) visits and inpatient hospitalizations

Geriatric

- ▲ Perform a holistic assessment of all needs of informal family caregivers.
- ▲ Provide caregivers with options for Internet-based support strategies to enhance coping.
- • In situations in which familial caregiving is being provided, assess current coping strategies utilized within the family. Provide interventions for family caregivers that are designed specifically to enhance coping skills, including problem-solving strategies and emotional support.
- • Assist informal caregivers with reducing unmet needs by helping them obtain the information and education necessary for caring for an older adult with a chronic health condition.

C

Multicultural

- Acknowledge sociocultural differences and healthcare disparities at the onset of care.
- Use valid and culturally competent assessment tools and procedures when working with families with different racial/ethnic backgrounds.
- Assess for the influence of cultural beliefs, norms, and values on the individual/family/community's perceptions of coping.
- Provide opportunities for families to discuss spirituality.
- Ensure culturally responsive approaches to end-of-life care.

Home Care

- The interventions described previously may be adapted for home care use.
- Assess the reason behind the breakdown of family coping.
- ▲ During the time of compromised coping, increase visits to ensure the safety of the client, support of the family, and reassurance regarding expectations for prognosis as appropriate.
- ▲ Assess the needs of the caregiver in the home, and intervene to meet needs as appropriate; explore all available resources that may be used to provide adequate home care (e.g., parish nursing as an effective adjunct, home health aide services to relieve the caregiver's fatigue).
- ▲ Encourage caregivers to attend to their own physical, mental, and spiritual health, and give more specific information about the client's needs and ways to meet them.
- ▲ Refer the family to medical social services for evaluation and supportive counseling. Serve as an advocate, mentor, and role model for caregiving; provide written information for the care needed by the client.
- ▲ A positive approach and caring by the nurse and concrete task definition and assignment reinforce positive coping strategies and allow caregivers to feel less guilty when tasks are delegated to multiple caregivers.
- ▲ When a terminal illness is the precipitating factor for ineffective coping, offer hospice services and support groups as possible resources.
- Encourage the client and family to discuss changes in daily functioning and routines created by the client's illness, and validate discomfort resulting from changes.
- Support positive individual and family coping efforts.

C

- Screen for mental health disorders (MHDs) in the elderly home care population.
- During home care visits and assessments, provide individuals and families with information for Internet-based interventions, including information on using social media as a health communications tool.

Client/Family Teaching and Discharge Planning

- Assess grief in parents who have lost a child to help determine parental needs, especially in the first year after the death of a child.
- ▲ Refer women with breast cancer and their family caregivers to support groups (including social network sites and online communities) and to other services that provide assistance with daily coping.
- ▲ For families dealing with childhood illnesses or other psychosocial stressors, refer parents to support and education groups to provide opportunities for parents to access support, learn new parenting skills, and obtain additional coping resources.
- Provide comprehensive discharge planning for individuals with a mental health diagnosis to help improve quality of life at home.
- Children of parents with dual diagnoses (e.g., psychiatric illness and addiction) require more extensive support and resources.
- Nurses can help type II diabetes patients with self-management education and support (DSME/S), which includes the facilitation of knowledge, skills, and abilities necessary to manage diabetes, as well as obtaining the support necessary for executing and maintaining the coping and behavioral skills needed for self-management.
- Involve informal caregivers of older adults in the discharge process.

Disabled Family Coping

NANDA-I Definition

Behavior of primary person (family member, significant other, or close friend) that disables his or her capacities and the client's capacities to effectively address tasks essential to either person's adaptation to the health challenge

Defining Characteristics

Abandonment; adopts illness symptoms of client; aggression; agitation; client dependence; depression; desertion; disregard for client's needs; distortion of reality about client's health problem; family behaviors detrimental to well-being; hostility; impaired ability to structure a meaningful life;

impaired individualism; intolerance; neglect of basic needs of client; neglect of relationship with family member; neglect of treatment regimen; performing routines without regard for client's needs; prolonged hyperfocus on client; psychosomatic symptoms; rejection

C

Related Factors

Ambivalent family relationships; chronically unexpressed feelings by support person; differing coping styles between support person and client; differing coping styles between support persons; inconsistent management of family's resistance to treatment

Client Outcomes

Family/Significant Person Will (Specify Time Frame)

- Identify normal family routines that will need to be adapted
- Participate positively in the client's care within the limits of his or her abilities
- Identify responses that may be harmful
- Acknowledge and accept the need for assistance with circumstances
- Identify appropriate activities for affected family member

Nursing Interventions

- Families dealing with acute trauma are susceptible to mild to very severe levels of anxiety. Support should be offered through necessary channels, which are appropriate to the situation, such as providing frequent information, offering social services, or counseling.
- Assess coping strategies of both the patient and the spouse when managing women with breast cancer and men with prostate cancer.
- Cancer caregiving interventions should include communication skill building, including strategies for self-care.
- Provide ideas for positive child coping and consider collaboration with mental health providers for children with chronic illnesses who are facing emotional problems.
- Assess social support of family members caring for survivors of traumatic brain injuries (TBIs). Facilitate realistic expectations about caregiving.
- Respect and promote the spiritual needs of the client and family.

Pediatric

- Assist parents and children suffering from chronic illness to develop accommodative coping skills (adapting to stressors rather than attempting to change the stressors).
- Assess educational level of parents of ill children and construct parent teaching to address educational attainment.

Geriatric

- Assess the emotional well-being of family members who are caring for clients with long-term illnesses, such as stroke.
- Be aware of age-related deterioration in coping skills.

Multicultural

- Be sensitive to the stigma attached to particular illness in various cultures.

Home Care

The interventions described previously may be adapted for home care use:

- Assess for strain in family caregivers.
- Assess for "caregiver fatigue" and provide information related to available respite care.
- Consult social services for available home resources related to the client's age and illness.

Client/Family Teaching and Discharge Planning

- Involve the client and family in the planning of care as often as possible.
- Recognize that family decision-makers may need additional psychosocial support services.
- Educate family members regarding stress management techniques including massage and alternative therapies.

Readiness for Enhanced Family Coping

NANDA-I Definition

A pattern of management of adaptive tasks by primary person (family member, significant other, or close friend) involved with the client's health challenge, which can be strengthened

Defining Characteristics

Expresses desire to acknowledge growth impact of crisis; expresses desire to choose experiences that optimize wellness; expresses desire to enhance connection with others who have experienced a similar situation; expresses desire to enhance enrichment of lifestyle; expresses desire to enhance health promotion

Client Outcomes

Client Will (Specify Time Frame)

State a plan indicating coping strengths, abilities, and resources, as well as areas for growth and change; perform tasks and engage resources needed for growth and change; evaluate changes and continually reevaluate plan for continued growth

Nursing Interventions

C

- ▲ Assess the structure, resources, and coping abilities of families and use these assessments in selecting interventions and formulating care plans.
- ▲ Acknowledge, assess, and support the spiritual needs and resources of families and clients.
- ▲ Establish rapport with families and empower their decision-making through effective communication and patient/family-centered care.
- ▲ Provide family members with educational and skill-building interventions to alleviate caregiving stress and to facilitate adherence to prescribed plans of care.
- ▲ Develop, provide, and encourage family members to use counseling services and interventions.
- ▲ Identify and refer to support programs that discuss experiences and challenges similar to those faced by the family (e.g., cancer support groups).
- ▲ Incorporate the use of emerging technologies to increase the reach of interventions to support family coping.
- ▲ Refer to Compromised family **Coping** for additional interventions.

Pediatric

- ▲ Identify and assess the management styles of families and facilitate the use of more effective ways of coping with childhood illness.
- ▲ Provide educational and supportive interventions for families caring for children with illness and disability.

Geriatric

- ▲ Encourage family caregivers to participate in counseling and support groups.
- ▲ Provide educational and therapeutic interventions to family caregivers that focus on knowledge and skill building.

Multicultural

- ▲ Acknowledge and understand the importance of cultural influences in families and ensure that assessments and assessment tools account for such cultural differences.
- ▲ Understand and incorporate cultural differences into interventions to enhance the impact of family interventions.

Readiness for Enhanced Decision-Making

NANDA-I Definition

A pattern of choosing a course of action for meeting short- and long-term health-related goals, which can be strengthened

Defining Characteristics

Expresses desire to enhance congruency of decisions with sociocultural goal; expresses desire to enhance congruency of decisions with sociocultural value; expresses desire to enhance congruency of decisions with goal; expresses desire to enhance congruency of decisions with values; expresses desire to enhance decision-making; expresses desire to enhance risk-benefit analysis of decisions; expresses desire to enhance understanding of choices for decision-making; expresses desire to enhance understanding of meaning of choices; expresses desire to enhance use of reliable evidence for decisions

Client Outcomes

Client Will (Specify Time Frame)

- Review treatment options with providers
- Ask questions about the benefits and risks of treatment options
- Communicate decisions about treatment options to providers in relation to personal preferences, values, and goals

Nursing Interventions

- Support and encourage clients and their representatives to engage in healthcare decisions.
- Provide information that is appropriate, relevant, and timely.
- Determine the health literacy of clients and their representatives before helping with decision-making.
- Tailor information to the specific needs of individual clients, according to principles of health literacy.
- Motivate clients to be as independent as possible in decision-making.
- Facilitate communication between the client and family members regarding the final decision; offer support to the person actually making the decision.
- Design educational interventions for decision support.

Geriatric

- The previously mentioned interventions may be adapted for geriatric use.
- Facilitate collaborative decision-making.

Multiculural

- Use existing decision aids for particular types of decisions or develop decision aids as indicated.

D

Home Care

- The previously mentioned interventions may be adapted for home care use.
- Develop clinical practice guidelines that include shared decision-making.

Client/Family Teaching and Discharge Planning

- Instruct the client and family members to provide advance directives in the following areas:
  - Person to contact in an emergency
  - Preference (if any) to die at home or in the hospital
  - Desire to initiate advanced directives, such as a living will or medical power of attorney
  - Desire to donate an organ
  - Funeral arrangements (i.e., burial, cremation)

Decisional Conflict

NANDA-I Definition

Uncertainty about course of action to be taken when choice among competing actions involves risk, loss, or challenge to values and beliefs

Defining Characteristics

Delay in decision-making; distress while attempting a decision; physical sign of distress; physical sign of tension; questioning of moral principle while attempting a decision; questioning of moral rule while attempting a decision; questioning of moral values while attempting a decision; questioning of personal beliefs while attempting a decision; questioning of personal values while attempting a decision; recognizes undesired consequences of actions being considered; self-focused; uncertainty about choices; vacillating among choices

Related Factors

Conflict with moral obligation; conflicting information sources; inexperience with decision-making; insufficient information; insufficient support system; interference in decision-making; moral principle supports mutually inconsistent actions; moral rule supports mutually inconsistent actions; moral value supports mutually inconsistent actions; perceived threat to value system; unclear personal beliefs unclear personal values

Client Outcomes

Client Will (Specify Time Frame)

- State the advantages and disadvantages of choices
- Share fears and concerns regarding choices and responses of others
- Seek resources and information necessary for making an informed choice
- Make an informed choice

Nursing Interventions

- Observe for factors causing or contributing to conflict (e.g., value conflicts, fear of outcome, poor problem-solving skills).
- Provide emotional support.
- Use decision aids or computer-based decision aids to assist clients in making decisions.
- Initiate health teaching and referrals when needed.
- Facilitate communication between the client and family members regarding the final decision; offer support to the person actually making the decision.

Geriatric

- Carefully assess clients with dementia regarding ability to make decisions.
- Discuss the purpose of advance directives such as a living will or medical power of attorney.

Multicultural

- Assess for the influence of cultural beliefs, norms, and values on the client's decision-making conflict.
- Provide support for client's decision-making.

Home Care

- The interventions described previously may be adapted for home care use.

Client/Family Teaching and Discharge Planning

- Instruct the client and family members to provide advance directives in the following areas:
  - Person to contact in an emergency
  - Preference (if any) to die at home or in the hospital
  - Desire to initiate advanced directives, such as a living will or medical power of attorney
  - Desire to donate an organ
  - Funeral arrangements (i.e., burial, cremation)
- Inform the family of treatment options; encourage and defend self-determination.

- Recognize and allow the client to discuss the selection of complementary therapies available, such as spiritual support, relaxation, imagery, exercise, lifestyle changes, diet (e.g., macrobiotic, vegetarian), and nutritional supplementation.
- ▲ Provide the Physician Orders for Life-Sustaining Treatment (POLST) form for clients and families faced with end-of-life choices across the healthcare continuum.

Impaired Emancipated Decision-Making

NANDA-I Definition

A process of choosing a healthcare decision that does not include personal knowledge and/or consideration of social norms, or does not occur in a flexible environment, resulting in decisional dissatisfaction

Defining Characteristics

Delay in enacting chosen healthcare option; distress when listening to other's opinion; excessive concern about what others think is the best decision; excessive fear of what others think about a decision; feeling constrained in describing own opinion; inability to choose a healthcare option that best fits current lifestyle; inability to describe how option will fit into current lifestyle; limited verbalization about healthcare option in others' presence

Related Factors

Decrease in understanding of all available healthcare options; inability to adequately verbalize perceptions about healthcare options; inadequate time to discuss healthcare options; insufficient confidence to openly discuss healthcare options; insufficient information regarding healthcare options; insufficient privacy to openly discuss healthcare options; insufficient self-confidence in decision-making

At-Risk Population

Limited decision-making experience; traditional hierarchical family; traditional hierarchical healthcare system

Client Outcomes

Client Will (Specify Time Frame)

- Verbalize option outcomes freely before making a healthcare decision
- Freely verbalize own opinion with healthcare providers before making a healthcare decision
- Choose the healthcare option that fits his or her lifestyle within an appropriate amount of time that allows enactment of the choice

- Describe how the chosen option fits into his or her current lifestyle before or after the decision has been made
- Verbalizes appropriate concern about others' opinions before making the healthcare choice
- Remains stress-free when listening to others' opinions before making the healthcare choice
- Arrives at a decision in a timely manner

D

Nursing Interventions

- Assess client's readiness to openly discussing the decision-making process.
- Use active listening in a nonjudgmental manner to provide the client with a flexible decision-making environment.
- Use anticipatory guidance by proactively providing the client with information.
- Establish a purposeful provider–client relationship.
- ▲ Refer to counseling as needed.
- Provide decision-making support.
- Provide a flexible environment by encouraging others to accept the client's choice.
- Encourage the client to use personal knowledge as part of the decision-making process to increase decisional satisfaction.

Pediatric

- When able, involve the client in healthcare decision-making when possible.
- Enhance client decision-making in critical care setting.

Geriatric

- Include geriatric clients in the decisional process.

Multicultural

- Consider cultural influences on decision-making.

Home Care

- Use open communication to assist clients to develop healthcare plans to which they can adhere.

Readiness for Enhanced Emancipated Decision-Making

NANDA-I Definition

A process of choosing a healthcare decision that includes personal knowledge and/or consideration of social norms, which can be strengthened

Defining Characteristics

Expresses desire to enhance ability to choose healthcare options that best fit current lifestyle; expresses desire to enhance ability to enact chosen healthcare option; expresses desire to enhance ability to understand all available healthcare options; expresses desire to enhance ability to verbalize own opinion without constraint; expresses desire to enhance comfort to verbalize healthcare options in the presence of others; expresses desire to enhance confidence in decision-making; expresses desire to enhance confidence to discuss healthcare options openly; expresses desire to enhance decision-making; expresses desire to enhance privacy to discuss healthcare options

Client Outcomes

Client Will (Specify Time Frame)

- Verbalize option of outcomes freely before making a healthcare decision
- Freely verbalize own opinion with healthcare providers before making a healthcare decision
- Choose the healthcare option that best fits his or her lifestyle within an appropriate amount of time that allows enactment of the choice
- Describe how the chosen option fits into his or her current lifestyle before or after the decision has been made
- Verbalizes appropriate concern about others' opinions before making the healthcare choice
- Remains stress free when listening to others' opinions before making the healthcare choice
- Arrives at a decision in a timely manner

Nursing Interventions

- • Assess client's readiness to choose through active listening.
- • Use anticipatory guidance by proactively providing the client with information. (Refer to Impaired emancipated **Decision-Making.**)
- • Establish a purposeful provider–client relationship.
- ▲ Include interdisciplinary healthcare professionals as needed to increase knowledge of chosen option.
- • Provide decision-making support. (Refer to Impaired emancipated **Decision-Making.**)
- • Continue to provide a flexible environment for client to enact choice.
- • Encourage the client to use personal knowledge as part of the decision-making process to increase decisional satisfaction.

Pediatric

- Understand interventions that parents prefer when in the decision-making process.

Multicultural

- Use open communication to assist clients to develop healthcare plans to which they can adhere.

Home Care/Nursing Home Care

- Optimize self-care personal knowledge for home care.
- Refer to care plan Impaired emancipated **Decision-Making** for additional interventions for pediatric, critical care, geriatric, and multicultural care.

D

Risk for Impaired Emancipated Decision-Making

NANDA-I Definition

Susceptible to a process of choosing a healthcare decision that does not include personal knowledge and/or consideration of social norms, or does not occur in a flexible environment, resulting in decisional dissatisfaction

Risk Factors

Decrease in understanding of all available healthcare options; inability to adequately verbalize perceptions about healthcare options; inadequate time to discuss healthcare options; insufficient confidence to openly discuss healthcare options; insufficient information regarding healthcare options; insufficient privacy to openly discuss healthcare options; insufficient self-confidence in decision-making

At-Risk Population

Limited decision-making experience; traditional hierarchical family; traditional hierarchical healthcare systems

Client Outcomes

Client Will (Specify Time Frame)

- Verbalize option outcomes freely before making a healthcare decision in a private setting within which he or she feels comfortable
- Freely verbalize own opinion with healthcare providers before making a healthcare decision
- Discuss how options fit or hinder his or her lifestyle within an appropriate amount of time that allows enactment of the choice
- Discuss concerns about others' opinions before making the healthcare choice

- Decrease stress about others' opinions by placing options in perspective through informational resources
- Discuss the time frame in which the decision needs to be made

Nursing Interventions

- Assess client's vulnerability for an impaired decision-making process.
- Assess the client's experience with decision-making.
- Recognize the traditional hierarchical family and healthcare system.
- Provide privacy to discuss healthcare options.
- Allow the client time to choose.

▲ Understand the primary care providers' role in the decision-making process.

- Provide informational resources.
- Provide encouragement so clients increase their confidence in the decision-making process.

Pediatric

- Understand the parent/guardian's vulnerability when making healthcare decisions for their children.
- Understand the adolescent decision-making processes.
- Refer to care plan Impaired emancipated **Decision-Making** for additional interventions for critical care, geriatric, multicultural care, and home care.

Ineffective Denial

NANDA-I Definition

Conscious or unconscious attempt to disavow the knowledge or meaning of an event to reduce anxiety and/or fear, leading to the detriment of health

Defining Characteristics

Delay in seeking healthcare; denies fear of death; denies fear of invalidism; displaces fear of impact of the condition; displaces source of symptoms; does not admit impact of disease on life; does not perceive relevance of danger; does not perceive relevance of symptoms; inappropriate affect; minimizes symptoms; refusal of healthcare; use of dismissive comments when speaking of distressing event; use of dismissive gestures when speaking of distressing event; use of treatment not advised by healthcare professional

Related Factors

Anxiety; excessive stress; fear of death; fear of losing autonomy; fear of separation; ineffective coping strategies; insufficient emotional support;

insufficient sense of control; perceived inadequacy in dealing with strong emotions; threat of unpleasant reality

Client Outcomes

Client Will (Specify Time Frame)

- Seek out appropriate healthcare attention when needed
- Use home remedies only when appropriate
- Display appropriate affect and verbalize fears
- Actively engage in treatment program related to identified "substance" of abuse
- Remain substance free
- Demonstrate alternate adaptive coping mechanism

Nursing Interventions

- Assess the client's and family's understanding of the illness, the treatments, and expected outcomes.
- Allow client time for adjustment to his or her situation.
- Aid the client in making choices regarding treatment and actively involve him or her in the decision-making process.
- Allow the client to express and use denial as a coping mechanism if appropriate to treatment.
- Support the client's spiritual coping measures.
- Develop a trusting, therapeutic relationship with the client/family.
- Assist the client in using existing and additional sources of support.
- Refer to care plans for Defensive **Coping** and Dysfunctional **Family** processes.

Geriatric

- Allow the client to explain his or her concepts of healthcare needs, and then use reality-focused techniques whenever possible to provide feedback.
- Encourage communication among family members.
- Recognize denial and be aware that grieving may prolong denial.

Multicultural

- Assess for the influence of cultural beliefs, norms, and values involved in the client's understanding of and ability to acknowledge health status.
- Discuss with the client those aspects of his or her health behavior/lifestyle that will remain unchanged by health status and those aspects of health behavior that need to be modified to improve health status.

- Assess the role of fatalism in the client's ability to acknowledge health status.

Home Care

D

- Previously mentioned interventions may be adapted for home care utilization.
- Observe family interaction and roles. Refer the client/family for follow-up if prolonged denial is a risk.

Encourage communication between family members, particularly when dealing with the loss of a significant person.

Client/Family Teaching and Discharge Planning

- Instruct client and family to recognize the signs and symptoms of recurring illness and the appropriate responses to alteration in client's health status.
- Consider the client's belief in and use of complementary therapies in self-managing his or her disease.
- Teach family members that denial may continue throughout the adjustment to treatment and they should not be confrontational.

▲ Inform family of available community support resources.

Impaired Dentition

NANDA-I Definition

Disruption in tooth development/eruption pattern or structural integrity of individual teeth

Defining Characteristics

Absence of teeth; abraded teeth; dental caries; enamel discoloration; erosion of enamel; excessive oral calculus; excessive oral plaque; facial asymmetry; halitosis; incomplete tooth eruption for age; loose tooth; malocclusion; premature loss of primary teeth; root caries; tooth fracture; tooth misalignment; toothache

Related Factors

Barrier to self-care; difficulty accessing dental care; excessive intake of fluoride; excessive use of abrasive oral cleaning agents; habitual use of staining substance; inadequate dietary habits; inadequate oral hygiene; insufficient knowledge of dental health; malnutrition

At-Risk Population

Economically disadvantaged; genetic predisposition

Associated Condition

Bruxism; chronic vomiting; oral temperature sensitivity; pharmaceutical agent

Client Outcomes

Client Will (Specify Time Frame)

- Have clean teeth, healthy pink gums
- Be free of halitosis
- Explain and demonstrate how to perform oral care
- Demonstrate ability to masticate foods without difficulty
- State absence of pain in mouth

Nursing Interventions

▲ Inspect oral cavity/teeth/gingiva at least once daily and note any discoloration, presence of debris, amount of plaque buildup, presence of lesions such as white lesions or patches, edema, or bleeding, and intactness of teeth. Refer to a dentist or periodontist as appropriate.

- If the client is free of bleeding disorders and able to swallow, encourage toothbrushing with a soft toothbrush using fluoride-containing toothpaste at least two times per day. Do not use foam swabs or lemon glycerin swabs to clean the teeth.
- Encourage the client to perform interdental hygiene by flossing or cleaning between teeth with interdental brushes, woodsticks, or oral irrigation at least once per day if free of a bleeding disorder. If the client is unable to floss, assist with flossing or encourage the use of an oral irrigator (i.e., "water flossing").
- Use a rotation-oscillation power toothbrush for removal of dental plaque.
- Determine the client's mental status and manual dexterity; if the client is unable to care for self, nursing personnel must provide dental hygiene. The nursing diagnosis Bathing **Self-Care** deficit is then applicable.
  - If the client is unable to brush his or her own teeth, follow this procedure:

1. Position the client sitting upright or on side.
2. Use a soft bristle baby toothbrush.
3. Use fluoride toothpaste and tap water or saline as a solution.
4. Brush teeth in an up-and-down manner.
5. Suction as needed.

- Monitor the client's nutritional and fluid status to determine if adequate. Recommend the client eat a balanced diet and limit between-meal snacks.
- Recommend that the client maintain a healthy diet with limited sugar intake; in particular, the client should limit sugary beverages and snacks.
- Instruct the client with halitosis to clean the tongue when performing oral hygiene. Brush tongue with a tongue scraper or toothbrush and follow with a mouth rinse.
- Determine the client's usual method of oral care. Whenever possible, build on the client's existing knowledge base and current practices to develop an individualized plan of care.
- Instruct the client to use a soft-bristled toothbrush, which should be replaced every 3 to 4 months. Angle the toothbrush at a 45-degree angle to the gums and use short lateral strokes. Brush all surfaces of each tooth. Use short, vertical strokes to clean inner tooth surfaces (ADA, 2017c).
- Therapeutic mouthwashes help prevent or reduce periodontal disease symptoms including plaque, gingivitis, and caries. Cosmetic mouthwashes can provide comfort and reduce halitosis, but are otherwise ineffective (ADA, 2017d). Avoid the use of hydrogen peroxide or alcohol-based mouthwashes.
- ▲ Recommend client see a dentist at prescribed intervals, generally two times per year if teeth are in satisfactory condition.
- ▲ If there are any signs of bleeding when the teeth are brushed, refer the client to a dentist. If bleeding accompanies apparently inflamed gums, refer client to a periodontist. Bleeding in the presence of halitosis is associated with gingivitis. If platelet numbers are decreased, or if the client is edentulous, use moistened Toothettes or a customized extra soft toothbrush for oral care.
- Recognize that meticulous dental care/oral care can be effective in preventing hospital-acquired (or extended care–acquired) pneumonia.
- Provide scrupulous dental care to critically ill clients, including ventilated clients to prevent ventilator-associated pneumonia.
- If teeth are nonfunctional for chewing, modification of oral intake (e.g., edentulous diet, soft diet) may be necessary. The nursing diagnosis Imbalanced **Nutrition:** less than body requirements may apply.

- If the client is unable to swallow, keep suction nearby when providing oral care.
- See care plan for impaired **Oral Mucous Membrane.**

Pregnant Client

- Encourage the expectant mother to eat a healthy, balanced diet that is rich in calcium. The teeth usually start to form in the gums during the second trimester of pregnancy.
- Pregnancy is associated with increased risk of oral health complications including gingivitis, caries, erosion, and granulomas. Meticulous, twice-daily oral care is critical to maternal health and pregnancy outcomes.
- Advise the pregnant mother not to smoke.
- Advise the expectant mother to practice good care of her teeth, and to protect her child's teeth once born.

Infant Oral Hygiene

- Gently wipe the infant's gums with a clean washcloth or sterile gauze at least once a day.
- Never allow the infant to fall asleep with a bottle containing milk, formula, fruit juice, or sweetened liquids. If the infant needs a comforter between regular feedings, at night, or during naps, fill a bottle with cool water or provide a clean pacifier recommended by the dentist or healthcare provider. Never give an infant a pacifier dipped in any sweet liquid. Avoid filling the infant's bottle with liquids such as sugar water and soft drinks.

▲ When multiple teeth appear, brush the child's teeth with a small toothbrush with a small (pea-size) amount of fluoride toothpaste. Application of either a fluoride gel or fluoride varnish is recommended.

- Advise parents to begin dental visits at 1 year of age.

Older Children

▲ Encourage the family to talk with the dentist about dental sealants, which can help prevent cavities in permanent teeth.

- Teach to brush teeth twice a day.
- Recommend the child use dental floss to help prevent gum disease. The dentist will give guidelines on when to start using floss.
- Recommend that parents should not allow the child to smoke or chew tobacco, and stress the importance of setting a good example by not using tobacco products themselves.

D

- Recommend the child drink fluoridated water when possible. Fluoride in drinking water is one of several available fluoride resources.
- Recommend the child use toothpaste containing fluoride.

Geriatric

- Provide dentists with accurate medication history to avoid drug interactions and client harm. If the client is taking anticoagulants, laboratory values should be reviewed before providing dental care.
- Help clients brush their own teeth, or provide dental care after breakfast and before bed every day.
- If the client has dementia or delirium and exhibits care-resistant behavior such as fighting, biting, or refusing care, then use the following method:
  - Ensure client is in a quiet environment such as his or her own bathroom, and sitting or standing at the sink to prime memory for appropriate actions.
  - Approach the client at eye level within his or her range of vision.
  - Approach with a smile, and begin conversation with a touch of the hand and gradually move up.
  - Use mirror–mirror technique, standing behind the client, and brush and floss teeth.
  - Use respectful adult speech. Do not use "elderspeak," which is a sing-song voice, or diminutive terms such as "deary" or "honey."
  - Promote self-care when client brushes own teeth if possible.
  - Use distractors when needed: talking, reminiscing, singing.

▲ Ensure that dentures are removed and cleaned regularly, after each meal and before bedtime. Brush and rise dentures to remove debris and soak overnight in a peroxide-based cleaning solution. Dentures left in the mouth at night impede circulation to the palate and predispose the client to oral lesions.

▲ Support other caregivers providing oral hygiene. Physical and cognitive impairment in older adults can interfere with the client's ability to perform oral hygiene, and oral hygiene should be provided by a caregiver. If no caregiver is available, the client is prone to dental problems such as dental caries, tooth abscess, tooth fracture, and gingival and periodontal disease.

Multicultural

- Assess for the influence of cultural beliefs, norms, and values on the client's understanding of dental care.

- Assess for barriers to access to dental care, such as lack of insurance. Minority groups may have limited access to dental care (Da Fonseca & Avenetti, 2017).

Home Care

- Assess client patterns for daily and professional dental care and related patterns (e.g., smoking, nail biting). Assess for environmental influences on dental status (e.g., fluoride).
- Assess client facilities and financial resources for providing dental care.
- Request dietary log from the client, adding column for type of food (i.e., soft, pureed, regular).
- Observe a typical meal to assess firsthand the effect of impaired dentition on nutrition.
- Assist the client with accessing financial or other resources to support optimum dental and nutritional status.

Client/Family Teaching and Discharge Planning

- Teach how to inspect the oral cavity and monitor for problems with the teeth and gums.
- Teach how to implement a personal plan of dental hygiene, including appropriate brushing of teeth and tongue and use of dental floss. Use motivational interviewing sessions to facilitate increased compliance in dental care.
- Advise the clients to change their toothbrush every 3 to 4 months, because after that toothbrushes are less effective in removing plaque and are a source of bacterial contamination of the mouth and teeth (ADA, 2017c).
- Teach the client the value of having an optimal fluoride concentration in drinking water, and to brush teeth twice daily with toothpaste containing fluoride.
- Teach clients of all ages about the need to decrease intake of sugary foods and to brush teeth regularly.
- Inform individuals who are considering tongue piercing of the potential complications such as chipping and cracking of teeth and possible trauma to the gingiva. If piercing is done, teach the client how to care for the wound and prevent complications.

Risk for Delayed Child Development

NANDA-I Definition

Child who is susceptible to failure to achieve developmental milestones within the expected timeframe.

D

Risk Factors

Infant or Child Factors

Inadequate access to health care provider; inadequate attachment behavior; inadequate stimulation; unaddressed psychological neglect

Caregiver Factors

Anxiety; decreased emotional support availability; depressive symptoms; excessive stress; unaddressed domestic violence

At-Risk Population

Children aged 0-9 years; children born to economically disadvantaged families; children exposed to community violence; children exposed to environmental pollutants; children whose caregivers have developmental disabilities; children whose mothers had inadequate prenatal care; children with below normal growth standards for age and gender; institutionalized children; low birth weight infants; premature infants

Associated Conditions

Antenatal pharmaceutical preparations; congenital disorders; depression; inborn genetic diseases; maternal mental disorders; maternal physical illnesses; prenatal substance misuse; sensation disorders

Client Outcomes

Client/Parents/Primary Caregiver Will (Specify Time Frame)

- Infant/Child/Adolescent will achieve expected milestones in all areas of development (physical, cognitive, and psychosocial)
- Parent/Caregiver will verbalize understanding of potential impediments to normal development and demonstrate actions or environmental/lifestyle changes necessary to provide appropriate care in a safe, nurturing environment

Nursing Interventions

Preconception/Pregnancy

- Assess for alcohol/drug use during pregnancy. Expectant mothers should be instructed that no amount of alcohol consumption is safe during pregnancy.
- Be aware of state legislation requiring mandatory reporting of maternal prenatal drug use. Be aware that mandatory reporting may further hamper prenatal care in that drug-addicted mothers may delay or defer care for fear of legal action.

D

- Advise expectant mothers to stop smoking and assist with methods of smoking cessation. Smoking is a known precursor to low birth weight and other significant prenatal issues.
- Recommend that women of childbearing age take 400 µg of folic acid daily to reduce the risk of neural tube defects.

Neonate/Infant

- Encourage mother–baby interactions when caring for premature infants.
- Encourage caution regarding use of glucocorticoids in premature and term infants.

Toddler/Preschooler/School-Age

- Provide support and education to parents of toddlers with developmental disabilities (i.e., Down's syndrome [DS], cerebral palsy).
- Be aware of the role maternal eating disorders plays in childhood development.
- Encourage parents of toddlers to obtain age-appropriate developmental screenings to detect early problems.
- Toddlers who are underweight should be offered solid foods first rather than juices.
- Teach parents the importance of avoiding lead-based paints in the home and other sources of lead in the environment.
- Understand the role premature birth plays in the development of speech.
- Teach new mothers the importance of breastfeeding.

Diarrhea

NANDA-I Definition

Passage of three or more loose or liquid stools per day

Defining Characteristics

Abdominal cramping; abdominal pain; bowel urgency; dehydration; hyperactive bowel sounds

Related Factors

Anxiety; early formula feeding; inadequate access to safe drinking water; inadequate access to safe food; inadequate knowledge about rotavirus vaccine; inadequate knowledge about sanitary food preparation; inadequate knowledge about sanitary food storage; inadequate personal hygiene practices; increased stress level; laxative misuse; malnutrition; substance misuse

At-Risk Population

Frequent travelers; individuals at extremes of age; individuals exposed to toxins

Associated Condition

Critical illness; endocrine system diseases; enteral nutrition; gastrointestinal diseases; immunosuppression; infections; pharmaceutical preparations; treatment regimen

D

Client Outcomes

Client Will (Specify Time Frame)

- Defecate formed, soft stool every 1 to 3 days
- Maintain the perirectal area free of irritation
- State relief from cramping and less or no diarrhea
- Explain cause of diarrhea and rationale for treatment
- Maintain good skin turgor and weight at usual level
- Have negative stool cultures

Nursing Interventions

- • Assess pattern of defecation or have the client keep a diary that includes the following: time of day defecation occurs; usual stimulus for defecation; consistency, amount, and frequency of stool; type of, amount of, and time food consumed; fluid intake; history of bowel habits and laxative use; diet; exercise patterns; obstetrical/gynecological, medical, and surgical histories; medications; alterations in perianal sensations; and present bowel regimen.
- • Recommend use of standardized tool to consistently assess, quantify, and then treat diarrhea.
- • Inspect, auscultate, palpate, and percuss the abdomen, in that order.
- ▲ Use an evidence-based bowel management protocol that includes identifying and treating the cause of the diarrhea, obtaining a stool specimen if infectious etiology is suspected, evaluate current medications and osmolality of enteral feedings, assess and treat hydration status of client, review and stop ordered and/or over-the-counter (OTC) laxatives, assess food preparation practices, asses home environment, provide good skin care and apply barrier creams to prevent skin irritation from diarrhea, and evaluate need for antidiarrheal agents and possible fecal containment device with provider.
- ▲ Identify the cause of diarrhea if possible based on history (e.g., infection, gastrointestinal inflammation, medication effect, malnutrition or malabsorption, laxative abuse, osmotic enteral feedings, anxiety, stress).
- ▲ Testing for diarrhea may consist of laboratory work such as a complete blood count with differential and blood cultures if the client is febrile. Also obtain stool specimens as ordered, to either rule out

or diagnose an infectious process (e.g., ova and parasites, *Clostridium difficile* infection, bacterial cultures for food poisoning).

▲ Consider the possibility of *C. difficile* infection if the client has any of the following: watery diarrhea, low-grade fever, abdominal cramps, history of antibiotic therapy, history of gastrointestinal tract surgery, and if the client is taking medications that reduce gastric acid, including proton-pump inhibitors (PPIs).

• Use standard precautions when caring for clients with diarrhea to prevent spread of infectious diarrhea; use gloves and handwashing. *C. difficile* and viruses causing diarrhea have been shown to be highly contagious. *C. difficile* is difficult to eradicate because of spore formation (Martin et al., 2014).

▲ Antibiotic stewardship is an important aspect in the prevention of *C. difficile* infections. *Antibiotics should be used judiciously* (Vardakas, Trigkidis, & Boukouvala, 2016; Centers for Disease Control and Prevention, 2017). If the client has diarrhea associated with antibiotic therapy, consult with the healthcare provider regarding the use of probiotics, such as yogurt with active cultures, to treat diarrhea, or probiotic dietary supplements, or preferably use probiotics to prevent diarrhea when first beginning antibiotic therapy.

▲ If a probiotic is ordered, administer it with food. Recommend that it be taken through the antibiotic course and 10 to 14 days afterward.

▲ Recognize that *C. difficile* can commonly recur and that reculturing of stool is often required before initiating retreatment.

• Have the client complete a diet diary for 7 days and monitor the intake of high-fructose corn syrup and fructose sweeteners in relation to onset of diarrhea symptoms. If diarrhea is associated with fructose ingestion, intake should be limited or eliminated.

▲ If the client has infectious diarrhea, consider avoiding use of medications that slow peristalsis.

• Assess for dehydration by observing skin turgor over sternum and inspecting for longitudinal furrows of the tongue. Watch for excessive thirst, fever, dizziness, lightheadedness, palpitations, excessive cramping, bloody stools, hypotension, and symptoms of shock.

• Refer to care plans for Deficient **Fluid** volume and Risk for **Electrolyte** imbalance if appropriate.

▲ If the client has frequent or chronic diarrhea, consider suggesting use of dietary fiber after consultation with a nutritionist and/or provider.

- ▲ If diarrhea is chronic and there is evidence of malnutrition, consult with the provider for a dietary consult and possible nutrition supplementation to maintain nutrition while the gastrointestinal system heals (Schiller & Sellin, 2016).
- • Encourage the client to eat small, frequent meals, eating foods that are easy to digest at first (e.g., bananas, crackers, pretzels, rice, potatoes, clear soups, applesauce), but switch to a regular diet as soon as tolerated. Also recommend avoiding milk products, foods high in fiber, and caffeine (dark sodas, tea, coffee, chocolate). *The bananas, rice, applesauce, toast (BRAT) diet has been traditionally recommended but may be nutritionally incomplete (International Foundation for Functional Gastrointestinal Disorders, 2014; Schiller, Pardi, & Sellin, 2017).*
- • Provide a readily available bathroom, commode, or bedpan.
- • Thoroughly cleanse and dry the perianal and perineal skin daily as needed using a cleanser capable of stool removal. Apply skin moisture barrier cream as needed. Refer to perirectal skin care in the care plan for **Impaired Bowel Continence.**
- ▲ If the client has enteral tube feedings and diarrhea, consider infusion rate; position of feeding tube; tonicity of formula; possible formula contamination; and excessive intake of hyperosmolar medications, such as sorbitol commonly found in the liquid version of medications (Taylor et al., 2016). Consider changing the formula to a lower-osmolarity, lactose-free, or high-fiber feeding.
- • Avoid administering bolus enteral feedings into the small bowel. The stomach has a larger capacity for large fluid volumes, whereas the small bowel can usually only tolerate up to 150 mL/hr (Taylor et al., 2016).
- ▲ Dilute liquid medications before administration through the enteral tube and flush the enteral feeding tube with sufficient water before and after medication administration.
- • Teach clients with cancer the types of diarrhea they may encounter, emphasizing not only chemotherapy- and radiation-induced diarrhea but also *C. difficile,* along with associated signs and symptoms, and treatments.
- ▲ For chemotherapy-induced diarrhea (CID) and radiation-induced diarrhea (RID), review rationale for pharmacological interventions, along with soluble fiber and probiotic supplements. Consult a registered dietitian to assist with recommendations to alleviate diarrhea, decrease dehydration, and maintain nutritional status.

▲ Acute traveler's diarrhea is the most common illness affecting individuals traveling to, usually, low-income regions of the world.

Pediatric

▲ Assess for mild or moderate signs of dehydration with both acute and persistent diarrhea: mild (increased thirst and dry mouth or tongue) and moderate (decreased urination; no wet diapers for 3+ hours; feeling of weakness/lightheadedness, irritability, or listlessness; few or no tears when crying) (Gupta, 2016). Refer to primary care provider for treatment.

▲ Recommend that parents give the child oral rehydration fluids to drink in the amounts specified by the healthcare provider, especially during the first 4 to 6 hours to replace lost fluid. Once the child is rehydrated, an orally administered maintenance solution should be used along with food. Continue even if child vomits.

- Recommend the mother resumes breastfeeding as soon as possible.
- Recommend parents avoid giving the child flat soda, fruit juices, gelatin dessert, or instant fruit drink.
- Recommend parents give children foods with complex carbohydrates, such as potatoes, rice, bread, cereal, yogurt, fruits, and vegetables. Avoid fatty foods, foods high in simple sugars, and milk products.

▲ Recommend rotavirus vaccine within the child's vaccination schedule.

Geriatric

▲ Evaluate medications the client is taking. Recognize that many medications can result in diarrhea, including digitalis, propranolol, angiotensin-converting enzyme inhibitors, histamine-receptor antagonists, nonsteroidal antiinflammatory drugs, anticholinergic agents, oral hypoglycemia agents, antibiotics, and so forth.

▲ Monitor the client closely to detect whether an impaction is causing diarrhea; remove impaction as ordered. Clients with fecal impaction commonly experience leakage of mucus or liquid stool from the rectum, rectal irritation, distention, and impaired anal sensation (Schiller, Pardi, & Sellin, 2017; Schiller & Sellin, 2016).

▲ Seek medical attention if diarrhea is severe or persists for more than 24 hours, or if the client has a history of dehydration or electrolyte disturbances, such as lassitude, weakness, or prostration.

- Provide emotional support for clients who are having trouble controlling unpredictable episodes of diarrhea. Diarrhea can be a great source of embarrassment to older clients and can lead to social isolation and a feeling of powerlessness.

Home Care

D

Previously mentioned interventions may be adapted for home care use to keep the client well hydrated.

- • Assess the home for general sanitation and methods of food preparation. Reinforce principles of sanitation for food handling.
- • Assess for methods of handling soiled laundry if the client is bed bound or has been incontinent. Instruct or reinforce universal precautions with family and bloodborne pathogen precautions with agency caregivers.
- • When assessing medication history, include OTC drugs, both general and those currently being used to treat the diarrhea. Instruct clients not to mix OTC medications when self-treating.
- • Evaluate current medications for indications that specific interventions are warranted.
- ▲ Evaluate the need for a home health aide or homemaker service referral. Caregiver may need support for maintaining client cleanliness to prevent skin breakdown.
- • Evaluate the need for durable medical equipment in the home. The client may need a bedside commode, call bell, or raised toilet seat to facilitate prompt toileting.

Client/Family Teaching and Discharge Planning

- • Encourage avoidance of coffee, spices, milk products, and foods that irritate or stimulate the gastrointestinal tract.
- • Teach the appropriate method of taking ordered antidiarrheal medications; explain side effects.
- • Explain how to prevent the spread of infectious diarrhea (e.g., careful handwashing, appropriate handling and storage of food, and thoroughly cleaning the bathroom and kitchen).
- • Help the client determine stressors and set up an appropriate stress reduction plan, if stress is the cause of diarrhea.
- • Teach signs and symptoms of dehydration and electrolyte imbalance.
- • Teach perirectal skin care.
- ▲ Consider teaching clients about complementary therapies, such as probiotics, after consultation with primary care provider.

Risk for Disuse Syndrome

NANDA-I Definition

Susceptible to deterioration of body systems as the result of prescribed or unavoidable musculoskeletal inactivity, which may compromise health

D

Risk Factors

Pain

Associated Condition

Alteration in level of consciousness; mechanical immobility; paralysis; prescribed immobility

Client Outcomes

Client Will (Specify Time Frame)

- Express pain level that is tolerable to allow for desired mobility
- Maintain full range of motion in joints
- Maintain intact skin, good peripheral blood flow, and normal pulmonary function
- Maintain normal bowel and bladder function
- Express feelings about imposed immobility
- Explain methods to prevent complications of immobility

Nursing Interventions

- Screen for mobility skills in the following order: (1) bed mobility; (2) supported and unsupported sitting; (3) transitional movements such as sit to stand, stand to sit, and transfers to chair from bed, from chair to bed, and so forth; and (4) standing and walking activities. Use a mobility assessment tool such as the Banner Mobility Assessment Tool (Boynton et al., 2014) or the Perme ICU Mobility Score (Perme et al., 2014).
- Assess the level of assistance needed by the client and express in terms of amount of effort expended by the person assisting the client. The range is as follows: total assist, meaning client performs 0% to 25% of task and, if client requires the help of more than one caregiver, it is referred to as a dependent transfer; maximum assist, meaning client gives 25% of effort while the caregiver performs the majority of the work; moderate assist, meaning client gives 50% of effort; minimal assist, meaning client gives 75% of effort; contact guard assist, meaning no physical assist is given but caregiver is physically touching client for steadying, guiding, or in case of loss of balance; stand-by assist, meaning caregiver's hands are up and ready in case needed; supervision, meaning supervision of task is needed

D

even if at a distance; modified independent, meaning client needs assistive device or extra time to accomplish task; and independent, meaning client is able to complete task safely without instruction or assistance.

- ▲ Request a referral to a physical therapist (PT) as needed so that client's range of motion, muscle strength, balance, coordination, endurance, and early mobilization can be part of the initial evaluation. The PT may provide the client with bed exercises, including stretching, flexing/extending muscle groups, or using bands to maintain muscle strength and tone. Collaboration with nursing staff, therapy, and respiratory therapy as needed to mobilize patients as early and as safely possible.
- • Passive range of motion can be done as the client tolerates.
- • Use specialized boots to prevent pressure injury on the heels and foot drop; remove boots twice daily to assess the skin and to provide foot care as needed. Elevate heels off the bed as the client tolerates when boots are not in place.
- • When positioning a client on the side, tilt client 30 degrees or less while lying on the side.
- • Assess skin condition every shift and more frequently if needed. Use a risk assessment tool such the Braden Scale or the Norton Scale to predict the risk of developing pressure ulcers (now referred to as pressure injury).
- • Discuss with staff and management a "safe patient handling" policy that may include a "no lift" policy to prevent staff injury.
- • Turn clients at high risk for pressure/shear/friction frequently. Turn clients at least every 2 to 4 hours on a pressure-reducing mattress and every 2 hours on standard foam mattress.
- • Provide the client with a pressure-relieving horizontal support surface. For further interventions on skin care, refer to the care plan for Impaired **Skin** integrity.
- • Help the client out of bed as soon as able.
- • When getting the client up after bed rest, do so slowly and watch for signs and symptoms of postural (orthostatic) hypotension, including dizziness, tachycardia, nausea, diaphoresis, or syncope.
- • Obtain assistive devices such as braces, crutches, or canes to help the client reach and maintain as much mobility as possible.
- ▲ Apply graduated compression stockings as ordered, if indicated for orthostatic hypotension. Ensure proper fit by measuring accurately.

Remove the stockings at least twice a day, in the morning with the bath and in the evening to assess the condition of the extremity, and then reapply. Knee length is preferred, rather than thigh length.
- Observe for signs of DVT, including pain, tenderness, redness, and swelling in the calf and thigh. Also observe for signs and symptoms of pulmonary embolism, including sudden onset of dyspnea, chest pain, syncope, dizziness, tachycardia, or tachypnea.
- Have the client cough and deep breathe or use incentive spirometry every 2 hours while awake.
- Monitor respiratory functions, noting breath sounds, work of breathing, and respiratory rate. Percuss for new onset of dullness in lungs.
- Note bowel function daily. Provide fluids, fiber, and natural laxatives such as prune juice as needed.
- Increase fluid intake to 2000 mL/day within the client's cardiac and renal reserve.
- Encourage intake of a balanced diet with adequate amounts of fiber and protein.

Critical Care

▲ Recognize that the client who has been in an intensive care environment may develop a neuromuscular dysfunction acquired in the absence of causative factors other than the underlying critical illness and its treatment, resulting in intensive care unit–acquired weakness, with an approximate incidence of 40% requiring more than 1 week of mechanical ventilation (Appleton, Kinsella, & Quasim, 2015). The client may need a workup to determine the cause before satisfactory ambulation can begin.

▲ Consider the use of a continuous lateral rotation therapy bed.

▲ For the stable client in the intensive care unit, consider mobilizing the client in a four-phase method from dangling at the side of the bed to walking if there is sufficient knowledgeable staff available to protect the client from harm.

Geriatric

- Get the client out of bed as early as possible and ambulate frequently after consultation with the healthcare provider.
- Consider physical and occupational therapy referrals to guide with environmental safety assessment and home exercise program.
- Monitor nutrition status in the elderly to prevent malnutrition.

- Monitor for signs of depression: flat affect, poor appetite, insomnia, and many somatic complaints.
- Keep careful track of bowel function in older adults; do not allow the client to become constipated.

Home Care

- Some of the previous interventions may be adapted for home care use.
- ▲ Begin discharge planning at time of admission with case manager or social worker and input from physical and occupational therapy as appropriate to assess need for home support systems and community or home health services.
- ▲ Become oriented to all programs of care for the client before discharge from institutional care.
- ▲ Confirm the immediate availability of all necessary assistive devices for home.
- Perform complete physical assessment and recent history at initial home visit.
- ▲ Refer to physical and occupational therapies for immediate evaluations of the client's potential for independence and functioning in the home setting and for follow-up care.
- Allow the client to have as much input and control of the plan of care as possible. Client perception of control increases self-esteem and motivation to follow medical plan of care.
- Assess knowledge of all care with caregivers. Review as necessary. Having the necessary knowledge and skills to perform care decreases caregiver role strain and supports safety of the client.
- ▲ Support the family of the client in the assumption of caregiver activities. Refer for home health aide services for assistance and respite as appropriate. Refer to medical social services as appropriate.
- ▲ Institute case management of frail elderly to support continued independent living, if possible in the home environment.

Client/Family Teaching and Discharge Planning

- Teach client/family how to perform range-of-motion exercises in bed if not contraindicated; this is referred to as a Home Exercise Program.
- Teach the family how to turn and position the client and provide all care necessary.

Note: Nursing diagnoses that are commonly relevant when the client is on bed rest include **Constipation,** risk for Impaired **Skin** integrity, Disturbed **Sleep** pattern, **Frail Elderly** syndrome, and **Powerlessness.**

Decreased Diversional Activity Engagement

NANDA-I Definition

Decreased stimulation, interest, or participation in recreational or leisure activities

Defining Characteristics

Alteration in mood; boredom; discontent with situation; flat affect; frequent naps; physical deconditioning

Related Factors

Current setting does not allow engagement in activity; impaired mobility; environmental barrier; insufficient energy; insufficient motivation; physical discomfort; insufficient diversional activity

At-Risk Population

Extremes of age; prolonged hospitalization; prolonged institutionalization

Associated Condition

Prescribed immobility; psychological stress; therapeutic isolation

Client Outcomes

Client Will (Specify Time Frame)

- Engage in personally satisfying diversional activities

Nursing Interventions

- Observe ability to engage in activities that require good vision and use of hands.
- Discuss activities with clients that are interesting and feasible in the present environment.
- Encourage the client to share feelings about situation of inactivity.
- Encourage the client to participate in any available social or recreational opportunities in the healthcare environment.
- Encourage a mix of physical and mental activities if possible (e.g., crafts, crossword puzzles).
- Provide videos and/or DVDs of movies for recreation and distraction.
- Provide magazines and books of interest.
- Provide books on CD and CD player, and electronic versions of books for listening or reading as available.

- Set up a puzzle in a community space, or provide individual puzzles as desired.
- Provide access to a portable computer so that the client can access e-mail and the Internet. Give client a list of interesting websites, including games and directions on how to perform Web searches if needed.
- Encourage the client to schedule visitors so that they are not all present at once or at inconvenient times.
- ▲ Request recreational or art therapist to assist with activities.
- ▲ Refer to occupational therapy.
- Provide a change in scenery; get the client out of the room as much as possible.
- Help the client experience nature through looking at a nature scene from a window, or walking through a garden if possible.
- Structure the environment as needed to promote optimal comfort and sensory diversity (e.g., have family bring in posters, banners, or photos; change lighting; change arrangement of furniture).
- Work with family or music therapist to provide music that is enjoyable to the client.
- Use art making and music listening.
- Structure the client's schedule around personal wishes for time of care, relaxation, and participation in fun activities.
- Spend time with the client when possible, giving the client full attention and being present in the moment, or arrange for a friendly visitor.
- Be creative, for example, use of the activity pillowcases with soft fabric pieces, plastic zipper, and a pouch to hold a picture as a diversional intervention that could be used in inpatient and hospice care settings.
- Engage clients in physical activity or exercise programs as an adjunct treatment modality for a variety of mental illnesses, e.g., depression, schizophrenia, anxiety, disorders, post-traumatic stress disorders, and substance abuse.

Pediatric

- ▲ Request an order for a child life specialist or, if not available, a play therapist for children. Child life therapists provide opportunities for self-expression and play for hospitalized children and may help normalize the environment.
- Engage preschool children in play therapy.

- Engage school-age children in play activities during hospitalization.
- Promote a referral to a music therapist.
- Consider art therapy for children living with chronic illness who have activity restrictions.
- Provide opportunities for children to connect with family and friends through technology.
- Provide animal-assisted therapy for hospitalized children.
- Provide computer games and virtual reality experiences for children, which can be used as distraction techniques during venipuncture, wound care, or other procedures.

Geriatric

- Assess the interests of older adults and the types of activities that they enjoy; encourage creative expression such as storytelling, drama, dance, art, writing, or music.
- If the client is able, arrange for him or her to attend group senior citizen activities.
- Promote activity for older adults through the use of exergames (video games combined with exercise).
- Encourage involvement in dance.
- Encourage clients to use their ability to help others by volunteering.
- Provide an environment that promotes activity (e.g., one that has adequate lighting for crafts, large-print books, and adequate acoustics).
- Provide opportunities for storytelling and life review.
- For clients who love gardening but who may have difficulty being outside, bring in seeds, soil, and pots for indoor gardening experiences. Use seeds such as sunflower, pumpkin, and zinnia that grow rapidly.
- For hospitalized clients with cognitive impairment, engage the assistance of volunteers to provide diversional activities.
- For clients in assisted-living facilities, provide leisure educational programs and pleasant dining experiences.
- For clients who are interested in reading and writing, promote book or writing groups or journaling, and creative or expressive writing.
- Prescribe activities to engage passive dementia clients based on their former interests and hobbies.
- Initiate opportunities for creative expression such as a TimeSlips storytelling group or Memories in the Making project to foster meaningful activities for clients with dementia.

Home Care

- Many of the previously listed interventions may be administered in the home setting.
- Explore with the client previous interests; consider related activities that are within the client's capabilities.
- ▲ Assess the client for depression. Refer for mental health services as indicated.
- Assess the family's ability to respond to the client's psychosocial needs for stimulation. Assist as able.
- ▲ Refer to occupational therapy.
- Introduce (or continue) friendly volunteer visitors if the client is willing and able to have the company. If transportation is an issue or if the client does not want visitors in the home, consider alternatives (e.g., telephone contacts, computer messaging).
- If the client is approaching the end of life, and is interested, assist in making a videotape, audiotape, or memory book for family members with treasured stories, memoirs, pictures, and video clips.

Client/Family Teaching and Discharge Planning

- Work with the client and family on learning diversional activities in which the client is interested (e.g., knitting, hooking rugs, writing memoirs).
- If the client is in isolation, give the client complete information on why isolation is needed and how it should be accomplished, especially guidelines for visitors; provide diversional activities and encourage visitation.

Ineffective Adolescent Eating Dynamics

NANDA-I Definition

Altered eating attitudes and behaviors resulting in over and under eating patterns that compromise nutritional health

Defining Characteristics

Avoids participation in regular mealtimes; complains of hunger between meals; food refusal; frequent snacking; frequently eating from fast food restaurants; frequently eating poor-quality food; frequently eating processed food; overeating; poor appetite; undereating

Related Factors

Altered family dynamics; anxiety; changes to self-esteem on entering puberty; depression; eating disorder; eating in isolation; excessive family mealtime control; excessive stress; inadequate choice of food; irregular mealtime; media influence on eating behaviors of high caloric unhealthy foods; media influence on knowledge of high caloric unhealthy foods; negative parental influences on eating behaviors; psychological abuse; psychological neglect; stressful mealtimes

Associated Condition

Physical challenge with eating; physical challenge with feeding; physical health issue of parents; psychological health issues of parents

Client Outcomes

Client Will (Specify Time Frame)

- Maintain weight within normal range for height and age
- Eat breakfast daily
- Participate in meal planning and preparation
- Consume healthy and nutritious foods

Nursing Interventions

- • Assess for goals and motives related to eating behaviors.
- ▲ Assess the adolescent client for comorbid psychological disorders and make appropriate referrals for treatment.
- • Assess the adolescent for experiences of cyberbullying and the strength of friendship dynamics.
- • Offer obese or overweight adolescents healthy methods for weight loss.
- • Offer families of obese or overweight children prejudice-free, individually accepting, and supportive interventions to address weight loss.
- • Recommend that families eat together for at least one meal per day.
- • Recommend involving the adolescents in planning family meals and food preparation.
- • Assist parents at being good role models of healthy eating.
- • Recommend that the family try new foods, such as either a new food or recipe every week.
- • Frame healthy eating as consistent with the adolescent values of autonomy from adult control and the pursuit of social justice.
- • Explore the adolescent's friendship dynamics.

Multicultural

- Assess racial-ethnic minority overweight adolescents for disordered eating behaviors.
- Assess racial-ethnic minority adolescents for experiences of harassment.

E

Home Care

- The interventions previously described may be adapted for home care use.

Client/Family Teaching and Discharge Planning

▲ Refer the adolescent and family to family treatment-behavior (FT-B) for treatment of eating disorders.

▲ Teach the family that hospitalization of the adolescent may be indicated for medical stabilization of serious physical complications and refer as needed.

Ineffective Child Eating Dynamics

NANDA-I Definition

Altered attitudes, behaviors, and influences on child eating patterns resulting in compromised nutritional health

Defining Characteristics

Avoids participation in regular mealtimes; complains of hunger between meals; food refusal; frequent snacking; frequently eating from fast food restaurants; frequently eating poor quality food; frequently eating processed food; overeating; poor appetite; undereating

Related Factors

Eating Habit

Bribing child to eat; consumption of large volumes of food in a short period of time; disordered eating habits; eating in isolation; excessive parental control over child's eating experience; excessive parental control over family mealtime; forcing child to eat; inadequate choice of food; lack of regular mealtimes; limiting child's eating; rewarding child to eat; stressful mealtimes; unpredictable eating patterns; unstructured eating of snacks between meals

Family Process

Abusive relationship; anxious parent–child relationship; disengaged parenting style; hostile parent–child relationship; insecure parent–child relationship; over-involved parenting style; tense parent–child relationship; under-involved parenting style

Parental

Anorexia; depression; inability to divide eating responsibility between parent and child; inability to divide feeding responsibility between parent and child; inability to support healthy eating patterns; ineffective coping strategies; lack of confidence in child to develop healthy eating habits; lack of confidence in child to grow appropriately; substance misuse

Environmental

Media influence on eating behaviors of high caloric unhealthy foods; media influence on knowledge of high caloric unhealthy foods

At-Risk Population

Economically disadvantaged; homeless; involvement with the foster care system; life transition; parental obesity

Associated Condition

Physical challenge with eating; physical challenge with feeding; physical health issue of parents; psychological health issues of parents

Client Will (Specify Time Frame)

Client Outcomes

- Identify hunger and satiety cues
- Consume healthy and nutritious foods
- Consume adequate calories to support growth and development
- Engage in positive interactions with caregiver during meals

Nursing Interventions

▲ Use a nutritional screening tool designed for nurses such as Subjective Global Nutrition Assessment (SGNA), and refer to a dietician for scores of moderate or severe.

- Assess parents for food or eating concerns, aberrant feeding behavior, or inappropriate feeding practices.
- Assess child for type of eating difficulty. Children can present with limited appetite, food selectivity, and fear of feeding.
- Assess the caregivers feeding style by asking three questions: How anxious are you about your child's eating? How would you describe what happens during mealtime? What do you do when your child will not eat?
- Assess the child for persistent picky eating with three questions/answers: Is your child a picky eater? (yes). Does she or he have strong likes with regard to food? (yes). Does your child accept new foods readily? (no).
- Assess child for symptoms of malnutrition including short stature, thin arms and legs, poor condition of skin and hair, visible vertebrae

and rib cage, wasted buttocks, wasted facial appearance, lethargy, and in extreme cases, edema.

- • Assess weight and height of the child and use a growth chart to help determine growth pattern, which reflects nutrition. Age-related growth charts are available from www.cdc.gov/growthcharts/ (Centers for Disease Control and Prevention, 2016).
- • Recommend that families eat together for at least one meal per day.
- • Encourage parent–child interactions that promote attachment.
- • Recommend that the child eats an appropriate size breakfast daily.
- • Recommend involving the family in planning meals and food preparation. Children can learn about nutrition as they help plan and make meals.
- • Assist parents at being good role models of healthy eating.
- • Recommend that the family try new foods, either a new food or recipe every week.
- ▲ Refer children with highly selective food behaviors and sensory food aversion to a nutritional specialist.
- ▲ Refer children with feeding difficulties caused by a medical condition to the appropriate specialist.

Multicultural

- • Assess for the meanings, attitudes, and behaviors related to feeding practices in culturally diverse families.
- • Assess the feeding styles of Hispanic and African American mothers for congruence with current child feeding recommendations.

Home Care

- • The interventions previously described may be adapted for home care use.

Client/Family Teaching and Discharge Planning

- • Provide parents with the following guidelines: avoid distractions during mealtimes (television, cell phones, etc.), maintain a pleasant neutral attitude throughout meal, feed to encourage appetite, limit meal duration (20–30 minutes), 4 to 6 meals/snacks a day with only water in between, serve age-appropriate foods, systematically introduce new foods (up to 8–15 times), encourage self-feeding, and tolerate age-appropriate mess.
- • Teach families to use positive family- and parent-level interpersonal dynamics (i.e., warmth, group enjoyment, parental positive reinforcement) and positive family- and parent-level food-related

dynamics (i.e., food warmth, food communication, parental food positive reinforcement) at family meals.
- Teach parents to recognize the difference between hunger and satiety in their children.
- Teach parents of children with limited appetites to establish a feeding schedule with a maximum of five meals per day and nothing but water in between. Parents must be taught to model healthy eating, adhere to the established feeding schedule, and set limits/consequences for mealtime behavior.
- Teach parents of children with food selectivity to refrain from coercive and indulgent feeding practices.
- Teach parents the concept of being a responsive feeder, in which the parent determines where, when, and what the child is fed and the child determines how much to eat. Responsive feeders guide the child's eating, set limits, model appropriate eating, talk positively about food, and respond appropriately to the child's feeding cues.

E

Ineffective Infant Eating Dynamics

NANDA-I Definition

Altered parental feeding behaviors resulting in over- or undereating patterns

Defining Characteristics

Food refusal; inappropriate transition to solid foods; overeating; poor appetite; undereating

Related Factors

Abusive relationship; attachment issues; disengaged parenting style; lack of confidence in child to develop healthy eating habits; lack of confidence in child to grow appropriately; lack of knowledge of appropriate methods of feeding infant for each stage of development; lack of knowledge of infant's developmental stages; lack of knowledge of parent's responsibility in infant feeding; media influence on feeding infant high caloric; unhealthy foods; media influence on knowledge of high caloric; unhealthy foods; multiple caregivers; over-involved parenting style; under-involved parenting style

At-Risk Population

Abandonment; economically disadvantaged; history of unsafe eating and feeding experiences; homeless; involvement with the foster care system; life transition; neonatal intensive care experiences; prematurity; prolonged hospitalization; small for gestational age

Associated Condition

Chromosomal disorders; cleft lip; cleft palate; congenital heart disease; genetic disorder; neural tube defects; physical challenge with eating; physical health issues of parents; prolonged enteral feedings; psychological health issues of parents; sensory integration problems

E

Client Outcomes

Client Will (Specify Time Frame)

- Infant will consume adequate calories to support growth and development
- Caregiver will follow healthy infant feeding practices
- Caregiver will identify infant behavioral cues related to hunger and satiety
- Caregiver and infant will engage in positive interactions during feeding

Nursing Interventions

- Assess weight and height of the infant and use a growth chart to help determine growth pattern, which reflects nutrition. Age-related growth charts are available from www.cdc.gov/growthcharts/ (Centers for Disease Control and Prevention, 2016).
- Assess mothers for symptoms of postpartum depression.
- Encourage parent–child interactions that promote attachment.
- Encourage overweight and obese mothers to follow current infant feeding guidelines.
- Encourage breastfeeding as appropriate.
- Teach infant caregivers to recognize the following infant communication: infants signal appetite through interest or disinterest in food; infants use rapid and transient facial expressions to signal liking; and they use subtle or potent gestures, body movements, and vocalizations to express wanting.
- Provide teaching and resources during pregnancy about recommended infant feeding practices.
- Provide caregivers of infants with teaching to encourage the early development of healthy eating patterns.
- Provide caregivers of infants with teaching about the strong association between sugar-sweetened beverages, obesity, and related chronic diseases.
- Assist mothers to identify infant engagement and disengagement cues during breastfeeding or formula feeding.
- Provide mothers with unconditional positive regard in their choice of breast, formula, or mixed feeding of their infant.

Multicultural

- Assess for cultural beliefs, values, and practices related to the feeding of infants.
- Identify the support persons of the infant caregiver and extend healthy infant feeding education and information to those support persons.

Home Care

- The interventions previously described may be adapted for home care use.

Client/Family Teaching and Discharge Planning

- Many of the interventions previously described involve teaching.

E

Risk for Electrolyte Imbalance

NANDA-I Definition

Susceptible to changes in serum electrolyte levels, which may compromise health

Risk Factors

Diarrhea; excessive fluid volume; insufficient fluid volume; insufficient knowledge of modifiable factors; vomiting

Associated Condition

Compromised regulatory mechanism; endocrine regulatory dysfunction; renal dysfunction; treatment regimen

Client Outcomes

Client Will (Specify Time Frame)

- Maintain a normal sinus heart rhythm with a regular rate
- Have a decrease in edema
- Maintain an absence of muscle cramping
- Maintain normal serum potassium, sodium, calcium, magnesium and phosphorus
- Maintain normal serum pH

Nursing Interventions

▲ Monitor vital signs at least three times a day, or more frequently as needed. Notify healthcare provider of significant deviation from baseline.

▲ Monitor cardiac rate and rhythm. Report changes to provider.

- Monitor intake and output and daily weights using a consistent scale.
- Monitor the client's respiratory status and muscle strength.

- Assess cardiac status and neurological alterations.
- ▲ Review laboratory data as ordered and report deviations to provider.
- Review the client's medical and surgical history for possible causes of altered electrolytes.
- ▲ Complete pain assessment. Assess and document the onset, intensity, character, location, duration, aggravating factors, and relieving factors. Notify the provider for any increase in pain or discomfort or if comfort measures are not effective.
- ▲ Monitor the effects of ordered medications such as diuretics and heart medications.
- ▲ Administer parenteral fluids as ordered and monitor their effects.

Geriatric

- Monitor electrolyte levels carefully, including sodium levels and potassium levels, with both increased and decreased levels possible.

Client/Family Teaching and Discharge Planning

- Teach client/family the signs of low potassium and the risk factors.
- Teach client/family the signs of high potassium and the risk factors.
- Teach client/family the signs of low sodium and the risk factors.
- Teach client/family the signs of high sodium and the risk factors.
- Teach client/family the importance of hydration during exercise. Dehydration occurs when the amount of water leaving the body is greater than the amount consumed.
- Teach client/family the warning signs of dehydration. Early signs of dehydration include thirst and decreased urine output. As dehydration increases, symptoms may include dry mouth, muscle cramps, nausea and vomiting, lightheadedness, and orthostatic hypotension.
- Teach client about any medications prescribed. Medication teaching includes the drug name, its purpose, administration instructions such as taking it with or without food, and any side effects.
- ▲ Instruct the client to report any adverse medication side effects to his or her healthcare provider. Assessing and instructing clients about medications and focusing on important details can help prevent client medication errors.

Imbalanced Energy Field

NANDA-I Definition

A disruption in the vital flow of human energy that is normally a continuous whole and is unique, dynamic, creative and nonlinear

• = Independent ▲ = Collaborative

Defining Characteristics

Arrhythmic energy field patterns; blockage of energy flow; congested energy field patterns; congestion of the energy flow; dissonant rhythms of the energy field patterns; energy deficit of the energy flow; expression of the need to regain the experience of the whole; hyperactivity of the energy flow; irregular energy field patterns; magnetic pull to an area of the energy field; pulsating to pounding frequency of the energy field patterns; pulsations sensed in the energy flow; random energy field patterns; rapid energy field patterns; slow energy field patterns; strong energy field patterns; temperature differentials of cold in the energy flow; temperature differentials of heat in the energy flow; tingling sensed in the energy flow; tumultuous energy field patterns; unsynchronized rhythms sensed in the energy flow; weak energy field patterns

Related Factors

Anxiety; discomfort; excessive stress; interventions that disrupt the energetic pattern or flow; pain

At-Risk Population

Crisis states; life transition

Associated Condition

Illness; injury

Nursing Interventions

- Consider using complementary health approaches (CHAs)–energy medicine (TT/healing touch, hope inspiration, and reiki) for clients with anxiety, tension, pain, or other conditions that indicate a disruption in the flow of energy.
- Refer to care plans for **Anxiety, Acute Pain,** and **Chronic Pain.**

Guidelines for Complementary Health Approaches

- CHA may be practiced by anyone with the requisite preparation, desire, and commitment.
- Volunteers who are not licensed healthcare professionals may practice in the home, but not in the healthcare setting unless they undertake a rigorous training program.

Pediatric

- Consider using CHAs for pediatric clients with adjunct therapies to decrease stress, anxiety, and pain.

Geriatric

- Consider CHAs for elderly with pain.

Multicultural

- Assess for the influence of cultural beliefs, norms, and values on the client's use of CAM.

Home Care

- Help the client and family accept CAMS as natural healing interventions.
- ▲ In the presence of a psychiatric disorder, refer for psychiatric home healthcare services for client reassurance and implementation of therapeutic regimens.

Client/Family Teaching and Discharge Planning

- Teach the client how to use guided imagery.
- Consider the use of progressive muscle relaxation, autogenic training, relaxation response, biofeedback, emotional freedom technique, guided imagery, diaphragmatic breathing, transcendental meditation, cognitive behavioral therapy, mindfulness-based stress reduction, and emotional freedom technique.

Risk for Dry Eye

NANDA-I Definition

Susceptible to inadequate tear film, which may cause eye discomfort and/or damage ocular surface, which may compromise health

Risk Factors

Air conditioning; air pollution; caffeine intake; decreased blinking frequency; excessive wind; inadequate knowledge of modifiable factors; inappropriate use of contact lenses; inappropriate use of fans; inappropriate use of hairdryer; inattentive to second-hand smoke; insufficient fluid intake; low air humidity; omega-3 fatty acids deficiency; smoking; sunlight exposure; use of products with benzalkonium chloride preservatives; vitamin A deficiency

At-Risk Population

Contact lens wearer; individuals experiencing prolonged intensive care unit stay; individuals with history of allergy; older adults; women

Associated Condition

Artificial respiration; autoimmune diseases; chemotherapy; decreased blinking; decreased level of consciousness; hormonal change; incomplete eyelid closure; leukocytosis; metabolic diseases; neurological injury with sensory or motor reflex loss; neuromuscular blockade; oxygen therapy; pharmaceutical preparations; proptosis; radiotherapy; reduced tear volume; surgical procedures

Client Outcomes

Client Will (Specify Time Frame)

- State eyes are comfortable with no itching, burning, or dryness
- Have corneal surface that is intact and without injury

- Demonstrate self-administration of eye drops if ordered
- State vision is clear

Nursing Interventions

- ▲ Assess for symptoms of dry eyes, such as "irritation, tearing, burning, stinging, dry or foreign body sensation, mild itching, photophobia, blurry vision, contact lens intolerance, redness, mucus discharge, increased frequency of blinking, eye fatigue, diurnal fluctuation, symptoms that worsen later in the day" (American Academy of Ophthalmology [AAO], 2015, 2018).
- ▲ If symptoms are present, then refer client to an ophthalmologist for diagnosis and treatment.
- ▲ Administer ordered eye drops.
- • Consider use of eyeglass side shields or moisture chambers.
- ▲ Watch for symptoms of blepharitis, including crusting and irritation at the base of the lashes and adjacent redness of the eyelid, which may accompany dry eye; refer for treatment as needed.
- ▲ Discuss use of caffeine with client's healthcare provider.
- • Provide education to the client about how limiting screen time, computers, smart devices, and television can assist with eyestrain and dry eyes.

Geriatric

- • Recognize that symptoms of dry eye are more common in menopausal women and geriatric clients.

Critical Care

- ▲ Provide regular cleaning of the eyes, lubricating eye drops and ointments, and consultation with an ophthalmologist if infection is suspected in clients in the intensive care unit (ICU).
- • Avoid using adhesive tape to keep eyes closed in sedated patients.

Client/Family Teaching and Discharge Planning

- • Teach client conditions that can exacerbate dry eye symptoms.
- • Teach client good eye hygiene:
  - ❍ Apply warm compresses for 10-minute intervals using a clean cloth and water that has been boiled and cooled (or sterile water).
  - ❍ Gently massage around eyelids.
  - ❍ Gently clean eyelids to remove excess oil, crusts, and bacteria. Use a few drops of baby shampoo in water that has been boiled and cooled, or in sterile water.
  - ❍ Good hygiene can help improve dry eyes, especially dry eye associated with blepharitis (NHS, 2014).

- Teach clients methods to decrease problems with dry eye including the following:
  - Avoid drafty (e.g., ceiling fans) and low-humidity environments.
  - Avoid smoking and exposure to secondhand smoke.
- ▲ Discuss avoidance of offending medications with healthcare provider.
- Drink plenty of water to keep well hydrated.
- Teach client to lower the computer screen to below eye level and to blink more frequently.
- ▲ Teach client to consult with the healthcare provider regarding use of omega-3 supplements to decrease dry eye.
- Teach client how to self-administer eye drops.
- Warn clients with dry eyes that driving at night can be dangerous.

Labile Emotional Control

NANDA-I Definition

Uncontrollable outbursts of exaggerated and involuntary emotional expression

Defining Characteristics

Absence of eye contact; crying; difficulty in use of facial expressions; embarrassment regarding emotional expression; excessive crying without feeling sadness; excessive laughing without feeling happiness; expression of emotion incongruent with triggering factor; involuntary crying; involuntary laughing; uncontrollable crying; uncontrollable laughing; withdrawal from occupational situation; withdrawal from social situation

Related Factors

Alteration in self-esteem; emotional disturbance; fatigue; insufficient knowledge about symptom control; insufficient knowledge of disease; insufficient muscle strength; social distress; stressors; substance misuse

Associated Condition

Brain injury; functional impairment; mood disorder; musculoskeletal impairment; pharmaceutical agent; physical disability; psychiatric disorder

Client Outcomes

Client Will (Specify Time Frame)

- Improve coping strategies
- Improve knowledge about disease process, signs and symptoms, triggers, symptom control
- Use mechanisms to control impulses and ask for help when feeling impulses

- Improve feelings of dignity
- Enhance and improve response to social and environmental stimuli

Nursing Interventions

- Identify clients at risk of having labile emotional control.
- Assess clients with the Pathological Laughter and Crying Scale (PLACS) to identify pathological laughing and crying or related disorders (e.g., Involuntary Emotional Expression Disorder (IEED), PBA).
- Assess clients for use of experiential avoidance, which is the process of negatively evaluating, escaping, or avoiding unwanted thoughts, emotions, or sensations.
- Offer the client choices, when possible, in emotional situations.
- Provide progressive muscle relaxation (PMR) exercise and guided imagery (GI) techniques.
- Offer instruction regarding alternative coping strategies such as mindfulness and breath awareness.
- Consider using cognitive-behavioral therapy (CBT).
- Provide music therapy.

Pediatric

- Assess adolescents with high emotional dysregulation for substance use disorders.
- Teach parents that their reactions to their children's emotions play a critical role in teaching children effective emotion regulation.
- Provide parents with emotion coaching strategies to manage their children's emotional outbursts. Emotion coaching includes fostering parental awareness and acceptance of their children's emotions with behaviors that acknowledge their children's emotions, and teaches understanding, coping with, and appropriately expressing emotion.

▲ Refer adolescent clients to a dialectical behavior therapy (DBT) group.

Geriatric

- Many of the previous interventions may be adapted for geriatric use.
- Evaluate geriatric clients suspected of PBA with the following three-step model: (1) crying inconsistent with environment/stimuli; (2) diagnosis of any of the following neurological disorders, such as TBI, PD, MS, ALS; or (3) at least two of the following disorders, such as stroke, schizophrenia (including schizoaffective and schizophreniform disorders), or documentation of spinal cord injury (SCI) as most closely associated with the PBA diagnosis.

Multicultural, Home Care

- The previous interventions may be adapted for multicultural and home care.

Client/Family Teaching and Discharge Planning

- Inform client and family about the emotional lability and talk with them about how to cope with the situation.
- Use verbal and nonverbal therapeutic communication approaches including empathy, active listening, and confrontation to encourage the client and family to express emotions such as sadness, guilt, and anger (within appropriate limits); verbalize fears and concerns; and set goals.
- Provide psychoeducation for stress-related variables to client and family.

Risk for Adult Falls

NANDA-I Definition

Adult susceptible to experiencing an event resulting in coming to rest inadvertently on the ground, floor, or other lower level, which may compromise health.

Risk Factors

Physiological Factors

Chronic musculoskeletal pain; decreased lower extremity strength; dehydration; diarrhea; faintness when extending neck; faintness when turning neck; hypoglycemia; impaired physical mobility; impaired postural balance; incontinence; obesity; sleep disturbances; vitamin D deficiency

Psychoneurological Factors

Agitated confusion; anxiety; depressive symptoms; fear of falling; persistent wandering; substance misuse

Unmodified Environmental Factors

Cluttered environment; elevated bed surface; exposure to unsafe weather-related condition; inadequate anti-slip material in bathroom; inadequate anti-slip material on floors; inadequate lighting; inappropriate toilet seat height; inattentive to pets; lack of safety rails; objects out of reach; seats without arms; seats without backs; uneven floor; unfamiliar setting; use of throw rugs

Other Factors

Factors identified by standardized, validated screening tool; getting up at night without help; inadequate knowledge of modifiable factors; inappropriate clothing for walking; inappropriate footwear

At-Risk Population

Economically disadvantaged individuals; individuals aged ≥60 years; individuals dependent for activities of daily living; individuals dependent for instrumental activities of daily living; individuals experiencing prolonged hospitalization; individuals in aged care settings; individuals in palliative care settings; individuals in rehabilitation settings; individuals in the early postoperative period; individuals living alone; individuals receiving home-based care; individuals with history of falls; individuals with low educational level; individuals with restraints

Associated Conditions

Anemia; assistive devices for walking; depression; endocrine system diseases; lower limb prosthetics; major injury; mental disorders; musculoskeletal diseases; neurocognitive disorders; orthostatic hypotension; pharmaceutical preparations; sensation disorders; vascular diseases

Client Outcomes

Client Will (Specify Time Frame)

- Remain free of falls
- Have a decreased risk of injury if sustains a fall
- Adapt environment to minimize the incidence of falls
- Explain methods to prevent injury

Nursing Interventions

- Safety Guidelines. Complete a fall-risk assessment for older adults in any healthcare setting with national guidelines and action plans such as the Falls Free: 2015 National Falls Prevention Action Plan (National Council on Aging, 2015).
- Use a valid and reliable fall risk assessment tool to assess the client risk for falling, for example, in the acute care setting the Hendrich II Model (Hendrich, Bender, & Nyhuis, 2016). Recognize that risk factors for falling include recent history of falls, fear of falling, confusion, depression, altered elimination patterns, cardiovascular/respiratory disease impairing perfusion or oxygenation, postural hypotension, dizziness or vertigo, primary cancer diagnosis, and altered mobility (National Council on Aging, 2015; Gray-Miceli, 2016).
- Screen all clients for balance and mobility skills (i.e., supine to sit, sitting supported and unsupported, sit to stand, standing, walking and turning around, transferring, stooping to floor and recovering, and sitting down). Use tools such as the Balance Scale by Tinetti or the Timed Up & Go Test.
- Carefully assist a mostly immobile client up. Be sure to lock the bed and wheelchair and have sufficient personnel to protect the client from falls. When rising from a lying position, have the client change

positions slowly, dangle legs, and stand next to the bed before walking to prevent orthostatic hypotension.

- Use a "high-risk fall" armband/bracelet and "fall risk" room sign to alert staff for increased vigilance and mobility assistance.
- ▲ Evaluate the client's medications to determine whether medications increase the risk of falling. Consult with healthcare provider regarding the client's need for medication if appropriate.

- Orient the client to the environment. Place the call light within reach and show how to call for assistance; answer call light promptly.
- Use one-fourth to one-half length side rails only, and maintain bed in a low position. Ensure that wheels are locked on the bed and commode. Keep dim light in the room at night.
- Keep the path to the bathroom clear, label the bathroom, and leave the door open.
- ▲ Avoid use of restraints if possible. Obtain healthcare provider's order if restraints are deemed necessary, and use the least restrictive device.
- In place of restraints, use the following:
  - Well-staffed and educated nursing personnel with frequent client contact with careful consideration during shift changes
  - Nursing units designed to care for clients with cognitive and/or functional impairments
  - Nonskid footwear, sneakers preferable
  - Glasses and/or hearing aids, as needed
  - Adequate lighting, night-light in bathroom
  - Frequent toileting
  - Frequently assess need for invasive devices, tubes, intravenous (IV) access
  - Hide tubes with bandages to prevent pulling of tubes
  - Consider alternative IV placement site to prevent pulling out IV line
  - Alarm systems with ankle, above-the-knee, or wrist sensors
  - Bed or wheelchair alarms
  - Wedge cushions on chairs to prevent slipping
  - Increased observation of the client
  - Locked doors to unit
  - Low- or very-low-height beds
  - Border-defining pillow/mattress to cue the client to stay in bed
- If the client has an acute change in mental status (delirium), recognize that the cause is usually physiological and is a medical emergency. Consider possible causes for delirium. Consult with the

healthcare provider immediately. See interventions for Acute **Confusion.**

- If the client has chronic confusion caused by dementia, implement individualized strategies to enhance communication.
- Ask family to stay with the client to assist with activities of daily living and prevent the client from accidentally falling or pulling out tubes.

▲ If the client is unsteady on his or her feet, have two nursing staff members alongside when walking the client. Use facility-approved mobility devices to assist with client ambulation (e.g., gait belts, walkers). Consider referral to physical therapy for gait training and strengthening.

- Place a fall-prone client in a room that is near the nurses' station.
- Help clients sit in a stable chair with armrests. Avoid use of wheelchairs except for transportation as needed.

▲ Refer to physical therapy or other programs for exercise programs that target strength, balance, flexibility, or endurance.

Geriatric

- Assess mobility and gait speed using the Timed Up & Go Test. Ask the client to stand up from a standard arm chair, walk 10 feet (or 3 meters), turn around, walk back to the chair, and sit down (Podsiadlo & Richardson, 1991). This should be done with the client wearing usual footwear.
- Complete a fall risk assessment for older adults in acute care using a valid and reliable tool, such as the Hendrich II Fall Risk Model.

▲ If there is new onset of falling, assess for laboratory abnormalities, signs and symptoms of infection and dehydration, blood glucose level for diabetics, and check blood pressure and pulse rate with client in supine, sitting, and standing positions for hypotension and orthostatic hypotension. If the client has borderline high blood pressure, the risk of falling because of the administration of antihypertensives may outweigh the benefits of the antihypertensive medication. Discuss with the healthcare provider on a client-to-client basis.

- Complete a fear-of-falling assessment for older adults. This includes measuring fear of falling, or the level of concern about falling, and falls self-efficacy, which is the degree of confidence a person has in performing common activities of daily living without falling. Fear of falling may be measured by a single-item question asking about the presence of fear of falling or rating severity of fear of falling on a 1 to 4 Likert scale as is commonly done in studies. Falls self-efficacy may be measured using a valid and reliable tool such as the Falls Efficacy Scale-International (Yardley et al., 2005; Greenberg, 2011, 2012; Greenberg et al., 2016).

- • Encourage the client to wear glasses and use walking aids when ambulating.
- • If the client experiences dizziness because of orthostatic hypotension when getting up, teach methods to decrease dizziness, such as rising slowly, remaining seated several minutes before standing, flexing feet upward several times while sitting, sitting down immediately if feeling dizzy, and trying to have someone present when standing.
- ▲ If the client is experiencing syncope, determine symptoms that occur before syncope, and note medications that the client is taking. Refer for medical care. The circumstances surrounding syncope often suggest the cause.
- ▲ Observe client for signs of anemia, and refer to healthcare provider for testing if appropriate.
- • Evaluate client for chronic alcohol intake and mental health and neurological function.
- ▲ Refer to physical therapy for strength training, using free weights or machines, and suggest participation in exercise programs.
- ▲ Evidence-based guidelines for preventing falls in older adults were published by the American Geriatrics Society (AGS) and British Geriatrics Society (BGS) collaboratively and specify recommendations for all clinical settings. These recommendations include screening and assessment and interventions. Examples of interventions include: (1) exercise for balance and for gait and strength training, such as tai chi or physical therapy; (2) environmental adaptation to reduce fall risk factors in the home and in daily activities; (3) cataract surgery when indicated; (4) medication reduction with particular attention to medications that affect the brain such as sleeping medications and antidepressants; (5) assessment and treatment of postural hypotension; (6) identification and appropriate treatment of foot problems; and (7) vitamin D supplementation for those with vitamin D (The American Geriatrics Society, 2011).

Home Care

- • Some of the previously mentioned interventions may be adapted for home care use.

- Implement evidence-based fall prevention practices in community settings and home healthcare programs for older adults (National Council on Aging, 2015).
- ▲ If delirium is present, assess for cause of delirium and/or falls with the use of an interprofessional team. Consult with the healthcare provider immediately. Assess and monitor for acute changes in cognition and behavior.
- Assess home environment for threats to safety including clutter, slippery floors, scatter rugs, and other potential hazards. Additionally, assess external environment (e.g., uneven pavement, unleveled stairs/steps).
- ▲ Institute a home-based, nurse-delivered exercise program to reduce falls or refer to physical therapy services for client and family education of safe transfers and ambulation and for strengthening exercises for the client (Grabiner, 2013; National Council on Aging, 2015).
- ▲ Instruct the client and family or caregivers on how to correct identified hazards for those with visual impairment. Refer to physical and occupational therapy services for assistance if needed.
- ▲ Use a multifactorial assessment along with interventions targeted to the identified risk factors. Key components of the interventions include evaluating need for all medications, balance, gait and strength training, use of strategies to deal with postural hypotension if present, home safety evaluation with needed modifications, and any needed cardiovascular treatment.
- If the client lives alone or spends a great deal of time alone, teach the client what to do if he or she falls and cannot get up, and make sure he or she has a personal emergency response system or a mobile phone that is available from the floor (Tinetti, 2003; The American Geriatrics Society, 2011; National Council on Aging, 2015).
- Ensure appropriate nonglare lighting in the home. Ask the client to install indoor strip or "runway" type of lighting to baseboards to help clients balance. Install motion-sensitive lighting that turns on automatically when the client gets out of bed to go to the bathroom.
- Have the client wear supportive, low-heeled shoes with good traction when ambulating. Avoid use of slip-on footwear. Wear appropriate footwear in inclement weather.
- Provide a signaling device for clients who wander or are at risk for falls.

- Provide medical identification bracelet for clients at risk for injury from dementia, diabetes, seizures, or other medical disorders.
- Suggest a tai chi class designed for older adults and selected clients who have sufficient balance to participate.

Client/Family Teaching and Discharge Planning

- Safety Guidelines. Teach the client and the family about the fall reduction measures that are being used to prevent falls (The Joint Commission, 2017).
- Teach the client how to safely ambulate at home, including using safety measures such as handrails in bathroom, reaching for items on high shelves, and avoiding carrying things or performing other tasks while walking.
- Teach the client the importance of maintaining a regular exercise program. If the client is afraid of falling while walking outside, suggest that he or she walk the length of a local mall.

Dysfunctional Family Processes

NANDA-I Definition

Family functioning which fails to support the well-being of its members

Defining Characteristics

Behavioral

Agitation; alteration in concentration; blaming; broken promises; chaos; maladaptive grieving; conflict avoidance; contradictory communication pattern; controlling communication pattern; criticizing; decrease in physical contact; denial of problems; dependency; difficulty having fun; difficulty with intimate relationship; difficulty with life-cycle transition; disturbance in academic performance in children; enabling substance use pattern; escalating conflict; failure to accomplish developmental tasks; harsh self-judgment; immaturity; inability to accept a wide range of feelings; inability to accept help; inability to adapt to change; inability to deal constructively with traumatic experiences; inability to express wide range of feelings; inability to meet the emotional needs of its members; inability to meet the security needs of its members; inability to meet the spiritual needs of its members; inability to receive help appropriately; inappropriate anger expression; ineffective communication skills; insufficient knowledge about substance misuse; insufficient problem-solving skills; lying; manipulation; nicotine addiction; orientation favors tension relief rather than goal attainment; paradoxical communication pattern; power struggles; rationalization;

refusal to get help; seeking of affirmation; seeking of approval; self-blame; social isolation; special occasions centered on substance use; stress-related physical illness; substance misuse; unreliable behavior; verbal abuse of children; verbal abuse of parent; verbal abuse of partner

Feelings

Abandonment; anger; anxiety; confuses love and pity; confusion; depression; dissatisfaction; distress; embarrassment; emotional isolation; emotionally controlled by others; failure; fear; feeling different from others; feeling misunderstood; feeling unloved; frustration; guilt; hopelessness; hostility; hurt; insecurity; lack of identity; lingering resentment; loneliness; loss; loss of identity; low self-esteem; mistrust; moodiness; powerlessness; rejection; repressed emotions; shame; taking responsibility for substance misuser's behavior; tension; unhappiness; vulnerability; worthlessness

Roles and Relationships

Change in role function; chronic family problems; closed communication system; conflict between partners; deterioration in family relationships; diminished ability of family members to relate to each other for mutual growth and maturation; disruption in family rituals; disruption in family roles; disturbance in family dynamics; family denial; inconsistent parenting; ineffective communication with partner; insufficient cohesiveness; insufficient family respect for autonomy of its members; insufficient family respect for individuality of its members; insufficient relationship skills; neglect of obligation to family member; pattern of rejection; perceived insufficient parental support; triangulating family relationships

Related Factors

Addictive personality; ineffective coping strategies; insufficient problem-solving skills; substance misuse

At-Risk Population

Economically disadvantaged; family history of resistance to treatment; family history of substance misuse; genetic predisposition to substance misuse

Associated Condition

Biological factors; Intimacy dysfunction; surgical procedure

Client Outcomes

Family/Client Will (Specify Time Frame)

- State one way that alcoholism has affected the health of the family
- Identify three healthy coping behaviors that family members can use to facilitate a shift toward improved family functioning
- Identify one Al-Anon meeting from the Al-Anon meeting schedule that family members express a desire to attend

- Attend different types of meetings (lead, big book, discussion, beginner's meeting) to find a good match and commit to attending that group regularly

Nursing Interventions

- • Refer to care plans for Ineffective **Denial** and Defensive **Coping** for additional interventions.
- ▲ Behavioral screening and intervention (BSI) should be integrated into all healthcare settings. Different terminology has evolved for screening, intervention, and referral for various behavioral issues. The five As—ask, advise, assess, assist, and arrange—apply to tobacco use. Screening, brief intervention, and referral to treatment (SBIRT) pertains to alcohol and drug use.
- • Screen clients for at-risk drinking during routine primary care visits and before surgery using the Alcohol Use Disorders Identification Test (AUDIT).
- • Provide brief education and individual counsel as a routine part of primary care.
- • Refer for family therapy and other family oriented resources.
- ▲ Refer for possible use of medication-assisted treatment to address substance use.

Pediatric

- ▲ Encourage early intervention. When parental depression, childhood exposure to conflict and violence, and childhood experience with abuse and neglect coexist with parental substance abuse, their children are more likely to engage in increased teacher-rated unfavorable student behavioral problems.
- • Encourage parent communication about alcohol use with adolescents.
- ▲ Consider the Community Reinforcement Approach (CRA), which encourages clients to become progressively involved in alternative non–substance-related pleasant social activities and to work on enhancing the enjoyment they receive within the "community" of their family and job.
- ▲ Educate family members about available educational and support programs and encourage no/limited alcohol use in the home.
- • Encourage adolescents to attend a 12-step program.
- • Provide interactive school-based drug prevention program to middle school students.

Geriatric

- • Include the assessment of possible alcohol abuse when assessing older family members.

Multicultural

- Acknowledge racial/ethnic differences at the onset of care.
- Use a family-centered approach when working with Latino, Asian American, African American, and Native American clients.
- Some less acculturated Latino families may be unwilling to discuss family issues with healthcare providers until they perceive a close personal relationship with the provider.
- Work with families in a way that incorporates cultural elements.

Home Care

Note: In the community setting, alcoholism as a cause of dysfunctional family processes must be considered in two categories: (1) when the client suffers personally from the illness, and (2) when a significant other suffers from the illness, that is, the client is not the active alcoholic but may depend on the alcoholic for caregiving. The following considerations apply to both situations with appropriate adaptation for the circumstances.

- The previous interventions may be adapted for home care use.
- Work with family members to support a sense of valued fit on their part; include them in treatment planning and identify the importance of their roles in the client's care. At the same time, encourage the pursuit of positive outside activities that enhance their sense of belonging.
- Educate client and family regarding the interactions of alcohol use with medications and the therapeutic regimen.
- ▲ Refer for psychiatric home healthcare services for client reassurance and implementation of therapeutic regimen.
- ▲ Consider the use of a smartphone-based intervention for alcohol use disorders.

Client/Family Teaching and Discharge Planning

- Suggest that the client complete a confidential Internet self-screening test for identification of problems and suggestions for treatment if a problem with alcohol is suspected. Many tools are available.
- Provide education for the family.
- Facilitate participation in mutual help groups (MHGs).

Interrupted Family Processes

NANDA-I Definition

Break in the continuity of family functioning which fails to support the well-being of its members

Defining Characteristics

Change in availability for affective responsiveness; change in family conflict resolution; change in family satisfaction; change in intimacy; change in participation for problem-solving; assigned tasks change; change in communication pattern; change in somatization; change in stress-reduction behavior; changes in expressions of conflict with community resources; changes in expressions of isolation from community resources; changes in participation for decision-making; changes in relationship pattern; decrease in available emotional support; decrease in mutual support; ineffective task completion; power alliance change; ritual change

Related Factors

Changes in interaction with community; power shift among family members; shift in family roles

At-Risk Population

Change in family finances; change in family social status; developmental crisis; developmental transition; situational crisis; situational transitions

Associated Condition

Shift in health status of a family member

Client Outcomes

Family/Client Will (Specify Time Frame)

- Express feelings (family)
- Identify ways to cope effectively and use appropriate support systems (family)
- Treat impaired family member as normally as possible to avoid overdependence (family)
- Meet physical, psychosocial, and spiritual needs of members or seek appropriate assistance (family)
- Demonstrate knowledge of illness or injury, treatment modalities, and prognosis (family)
- Participate in the development of the plan of care to the best of ability (significant person)

Nursing Interventions

- Recognize informal roles in medical decision-making by family members.
- Acknowledge the range of emotions and feelings that may be experienced when the health status of a family member changes.
- Encourage family members to list their personal strengths and available resources.

- Establish relationships among clients, their families, and healthcare professionals.
- Encourage family to visit the client; adjust visiting hours to accommodate the family's schedule.
- Allow and encourage family members to assist in the client's treatment.
- Support family members during emotional and conflict type situations in the clinical setting.
- Anticipate and implement family reunification efforts after a disaster.
- Refer to the care plan Readiness for enhanced **Family** processes for additional interventions.

Pediatric

- Carefully assess potential for reunifying children placed in foster care with their birth parents.
- Provide prebirth risk assessments to identify prebirth and postbirth supports for high-risk pregnant women.
- Provide parents with both general information and professional support by family-centered early childhood intervention services to their families.
- Encourage and support parents/family to assist in client's care.
- Assess military families for the influence of deployment on family functioning.
- ▲ Refer parents and other primary caregivers to a mindfulness-based stress reduction (MBSR) program.

Geriatric

- Encourage family members to be involved in the care of relatives who are in residential care settings.
- Support group problem-solving among family caregivers and include the older member.
- ▲ Refer family for counseling with a psychotherapist who is knowledgeable about gerontology.
- Refer to care plan for readiness for Enhanced **Family** processes for additional interventions.

Multicultural

- Motivate family members to speak openly about illnesses, keeping in mind the importance of ethnic origin.
- Assess LGBTQ youth for factors that contribute to family rejection.
- Refer to the care plan readiness for Enhanced **Family** processes for additional interventions.

Home Care
- The nursing interventions described in the care plan for Compromised family **Coping** should be used in the home environment with adaptations as necessary.
- Encourage family members to find meaning in life with a serious illness.

Client/Family Teaching and Discharge Planning
- Refer to Client/Family Teaching and Discharge Planning in Compromised family **Coping** and Readiness for enhanced family **Coping** for suggestions that may be used with minor adaptations.

Readiness for Enhanced Family Processes

NANDA-I Definition

A pattern of family functioning to support the well-being of its members, which can be strengthened

Defining Characteristics

Expresses desire to enhance balance between autonomy and cohesiveness; expresses desire to enhance communication pattern; expresses desire to enhance energy level of family to support activities of daily living; expresses desire to enhance family adaptation to change; expresses desire to enhance family dynamics; expresses desire to enhance family resilience; expresses desire to enhance growth of family members; expresses desire to enhance interdependence with community; expresses desire to enhance maintenance of boundaries between family members; expresses desire to enhance respect for family members; expresses desire to enhance safety of family members

Client Outcomes

Family/Client Will (Specify Time Frame)

- Identify ways to cope effectively and use appropriate support systems (family)
- Meet physical, psychosocial, and spiritual needs of members or seek appropriate assistance (family)
- Demonstrate knowledge of potential environmental, lifestyle, and genetic risks to health and use appropriate measures to decrease possibility of risk (family)
- Focus on wellness, disease prevention, and maintenance (family and individual)

- Seek balance among exercise, work, leisure, rest, and nutrition (family and individual)

Nursing Interventions

- Assess the family's stress level and coping abilities during the initial nursing assessment.
- Consider the use of family-centered theory as the conceptual foundation to help guide interventions.
- Use family-centered care and role modeling for holistic care of families.
- Discuss with family members and identify the perceptions of the healthcare experience.
- Support family needs, strengths, and resourcefulness through family interviews.
- Spend time with family members; allow them to verbalize their feelings.
- Encourage family members to find meaning in a serious illness.
- Provide family-centered care to explore and use all available resources appropriate for the situation (e.g., counseling, social services, self-help groups, pastoral care).
- Consider focus groups to provide insight into family perceptions of illness and/or disease prevention.

Pediatric

- Provide a parenting class series based on individual and couple changes in meaning and identity, roles, and relationships and interaction during the transition to parenthood. Address mother and father roles, infant communication abilities, and patterns of the first 3 months of life in a mutually enjoyable, possibility-focused manner.
- Encourage families with adolescents to have family meals.

Geriatric

- Carefully listen to residents and family members in the long-term care facility.
- Support caregivers' awareness of the positive effects of their contribution to the well-being of parents.
- Teach family members about the effect of developmental events (e.g., retirement, death, change in health status, and household composition).
- Encourage social networks; social integration; social engagement and internet social networking with friends, children, and relatives of older adults.

Multicultural

- Assess for the influence of cultural beliefs, norms, and values on the family's perceptions of normal functioning.
- Identify and acknowledge the stresses unique to racial/ethnic families.
- Assess and support spiritual needs of families.
- With the client's consent, facilitate a group meeting for family members to discuss how the family is functioning.
- Facilitate modeling and role playing for the client and family regarding healthy ways to start a discussion about the client's prognosis.
- Encourage family mealtimes.

Home Care

- The previous nursing interventions should be used in the home environment with adaptations as necessary.

▲ Encourage virtual support groups to family caregivers.

Client/Family Teaching and Discharge Planning

- Refer to Client/Family Teaching and Discharge Planning for readiness for enhanced family **Coping** for suggestions that may be used with minor adaptations.

Fatigue

NANDA-I Definition

An overwhelming, sustained sense of exhaustion and decreased capacity for physical and mental work at the usual level

Defining Characteristics

Altered attention; apathy; decreased aerobic capacity; decreased gait velocity; difficulty maintaining usual physical activity; difficulty maintaining usual routines; disinterested in surroundings; drowsiness; expresses altered libido; expresses demoralization; expresses frustration; expresses lack of energy; expresses nonrelief through usual energy-recovery strategies; expresses tiredness; expresses weakness; inadequate role performance; increased physical symptoms; increased rest requirement; insufficient physical endurance; introspection; lethargy; tiredness

Related Factors

Altered sleep-wake cycle; anxiety; depressive symptoms; environmental constraints; increased mental exertion; increased physical exertion; malnutrition; nonstimulating lifestyle; pain; physical deconditioning; stressors

At-Risk Population

Individuals exposed to negativelife event; individuals with demanding occupation; pregnant women; women experiencing labor

Associated Conditions

Anemia; chemotherapy; chronic disease; chronic inflammation

Client Outcomes

Client Will (Specify Time Frame)

- Identify potential etiology of fatigue
- Identify potential factors that aggravate and relieve fatigue
- Describe ways to assess and track patterns of fatigue over set periods of time (e.g., within a day, a few days, a week, a month)
- Describe ways in which fatigue affects the ability to accomplish activities of daily living (ADLs)
- Verbalize increased energy and improved vitality
- Explain energy conservation plan to offset fatigue
- Explain energy restoration plan to offset fatigue
- Verbalize ability and capacity to concentrate
- Verbalize strategies for restorative activities

Nursing Interventions

- Assess severity of fatigue on a scale of 0 to 10 (average fatigue, worst and best levels); assess frequency of fatigue (number of days per week and time of day), activities and symptoms associated with increased fatigue (e.g., pain), activities that relieve, ability to perform ADLs and instrumental ADLs, interference with social and role function, times of the day for increased energy, ability to concentrate, mood, usual pattern of physical activity, and interference with sleep cycles. Consider use of instruments such as the Profile of Mood State Short Form Fatigue Subscale, the Multidimensional Assessment of Fatigue, the Lee Fatigue Scale, the Multidimensional Fatigue Inventory, the HIV-Related Fatigue Scale, or the Brief Fatigue Inventory, Short Form Vitality Subscale, Piper Fatigue Scale, Chalder Fatigue Scale, or Nottingham of Chronic Illness Therapy Fatigue Scale, and Fatigue Severity Scale.
- Evaluate adequacy of nutrition and sleep hygiene (napping throughout the day, inability to fall asleep or stay asleep). Encourage the client to get adequate rest; limit naps (particularly in the late afternoon or evening); use a routine sleep/wake schedule; plan and prioritize for daily activities as tolerated; allow exposure to sunlight during daytime hours by going outside or opening shades and curtains in the home; use relaxation techniques before bedtime such as meditation, music therapy, or guided imagery (Kwekkeboom & Bratzke, 2016); avoid caffeine in the late afternoon or evening; and

eat a well-balanced diet that includes fresh fruits, vegetables, and lean meats. Mindfulness interventions also result in improved sleep quality (Black et al., 2015). Refer to Imbalanced **Nutrition:** less than body requirements or **Insomnia** if appropriate.

- • Evaluate fluid status and assess for dehydration. Encourage at least eight glasses of water a day. Avoid caffeine, which can cause further dehydration.
- ▲ Collaborate with the primary care provider to identify physiological and/or psychological causes of fatigue that could be treated, such as anemia, pain, electrolyte imbalance (e.g., altered potassium levels), dehydration, thyroid disorders, anemia, arthritis, depression, anxiety, sleep disturbances (insomnia/sleep deprivation), acute or chronic infection, medication use or side effects, alcohol use/abuse, metabolic disorders (diabetes), or a preexisting comorbidity or disease (multiple sclerosis, cancer or cancer treatment, respiratory disease, fibromyalgia, cardiac disease, renal disease, Parkinson's disease) (Berger et al., 2015).
- ▲ Work with the primary care provider to determine if the client has chronic fatigue syndrome.
- • Encourage the client to express feelings, attribution of cause and behaviors about fatigue, including potential causes of fatigue, and possible interventions to alleviate fatigue. Such interventions could include setting small, easily achieved short-term goals and developing energy management and energy conservation techniques; use active listening techniques to help identify sources of hope. Retroactive activities should be considered. Assess client's level of motivation and willingness to adopt new behaviors that can improve symptoms of fatigue.
- • Encourage the client to keep a journal of activities (or record using one of the many apps available) that contribute to symptoms of fatigue, patterns of symptoms across days/weeks/months, and feelings, including how fatigue affects the client's normal daily activities and roles.
- • Help the client identify sources of support and prioritize essential and nonessential tasks to determine which tasks need to be completed and which can be delegated and to whom. Give the client permission to limit or change social and role demands if needed (e.g., switch to part-time employment, give up activities for a short period, hire cleaning service).

- ▲ Collaborate with the primary care provider regarding the appropriateness of referrals to physical therapy for carefully monitored aerobic exercise program and possible physical aids, such as a walker or cane if client has a disability.
- • Encourage the client to try complementary and alternative therapy such as guided imagery, massage therapy, relaxation, mediation, mindfulness, and acupressure (Heo et al., 2017).
- ▲ Refer the client to diagnosis-appropriate support groups such as the National Chronic Fatigue Syndrome Association, National Parkinson Foundation, PatientsLikeMe, Multiple Sclerosis Association, American Cancer Society, or the National Comprehensive Cancer Network.
- ▲ For a person with cardiac disease, recognize that fatigue is common with myocardial infarction, congestive heart failure (CHF), or chronic cardiac insufficiency. Refer to cardiac rehabilitation for a carefully prescribed and monitored exercise and rehabilitation program.
- • If fatigue is associated with cancer or cancer-related treatment, assess for other symptoms that may enhance fatigue (e.g., pain, insomnia, anemia, emotional distress, electrolyte imbalance [nausea, vomiting, diarrhea], or depression).
- ▲ Collaborate with the primary care provider to identify attentional fatigue, which may manifest itself as the inability to direct attention necessary to perform usual activities. Attentional fatigue is associated with sleep disturbances, depressive symptoms, anxiety, and psychosocial stressors, which can lead to inability to concentrate, inability to plan goals, and inability to control emotions or social interactions.
- ▲ Collaborate with primary care providers to identify potential pharmacological treatment for fatigue.

Geriatric

- • Evaluate fatigue in geriatric clients routinely, particularly in clients with limited physical function and lower levels of social support. Chronic conditions related to age can contribute to fatigue in the geriatric client, such as cancer, dyspnea, anemia, multiple medication usage and side effects from medication, depression, insomnia (Keles et al., 2016), nutritional deficiencies, electrolyte imbalance, and comorbidities such as chronic obstructive pulmonary disease (COPD) (Kentson et al., 2016) and cardiac disease (Nasiri et al., 2016).
- • Review medications to determine possible side effects or interaction effects that could cause fatigue.

F

- Review comorbid conditions that may contribute to fatigue, such as CHF, pulmonary disease, cardiac disease, multiple sclerosis, arthritis, obesity, anemia, depression, Parkinson's disease, insomnia, and cancer.
- Identify recent losses and even loss of function; monitor for depression or loneliness as a possible contributing factor to fatigue.
- Review other symptoms the client may be experiencing. Fatigue is often associated with other symptom clusters such as depression and sleep disturbances.
- ▲ Review medications for side effects. Certain medications (e.g., diuretics with associated loss of potassium, antihypertensives, antihistamines, pain medications [Rich & Nienaber, 2014], anticonvulsants, chemotherapeutic agents, psychiatric medications, and corticosteroids) may cause fatigue in older adults. Fatigue is a major component of FRAILTY Scales (Gleason et al., 2017).

Home Care

The previously mentioned interventions may be adapted for home care use as well.

- Assess the client's history and current patterns of fatigue as they relate to the home environment and environmental and behavioral triggers of increased fatigue.
- ▲ Encourage planned exercise regimens or physical activities such as walking or light aerobic exercises. This activity can be organized in the home or in a setting such as senior centers or wellness facilities.
- ▲ Refer to occupational and/or physical therapy if substantial intervention is needed to assist the client in adapting to home and daily patterns.
- For clients receiving chemotherapy, intervene to:
  - Relieve symptom distress (anxiety, nausea and vomiting, diarrhea, lack of appetite, emotional distress, difficulty sleeping).
  - Encourage as much physical activity as possible with a specific recommendation (Hoffman et al., 2017).
- Teach the client and family the importance of and methods for setting priorities for activities, especially those with high energy demand (e.g., home or family events). Instruct in realistic expectations and behavioral pacing.
  - Identify with the client ways in which he or she continues to be a valued part of his or her social environment.
  - Identify with the client ways in which he or she continues to participate in preferred daily activity or social activities.

- ❍ Encourage the client to maintain regular family routines (e.g., meals, sleep patterns) as much as possible.

Client/Family Teaching and Discharge Planning

- Help the client reframe cognitively; share information about fatigue and how to live with it, including need for positive self-talk.
- Teach strategies for energy conservation (e.g., sitting instead of standing during showering, storing items at waist level).
- Teach the client to carry a pocket calendar, make lists of required activities, and post reminders around the house.
- Teach the importance of following a healthy lifestyle with adequate nutrition, fluids, and rest; pain relief; insomnia correction; and appropriate exercise to decrease fatigue (i.e., energy restoration).
- See **Hopelessness** care plan if appropriate.

Fear

NANDA-I Definition

Basic, intense emotional response aroused by the detection of imminent threat, involving an immediate alarm reaction (American Psychological Association).

Defining Characteristics

Physiological Factors

Anorexia; diaphoresis; diarrhea; dyspnea; increased blood pressure; increased heart rate; increased respiratory rate; increased sweating; increased urinary frequency; muscle tension; nausea; pallor; pupil dilation; vomiting, xerostomia

Behavioral/Emotional

Apprehensiveness; concentration on the source of fear; decreased self-assurance; expresses alarm; expresses fear; expresses intense dread; expresses tension; impulsive behaviors; nervousness; psychomotor agitation

Related Factors

Communication barriers; learned response to threat; response to phobic stimulus; unfamiliar situation

At Risk Population

Children; individuals exposed to traumatic situation; individuals living in areas with increased violence; individuals receiving terminal care; individuals separated from social support; individuals undergoing surgical procedure; individuals with family history of post-traumatic shock; individuals with history of falls; older adults; pregnant women; women; women experiencing childbirth

Associated Condition

Sensation disorders

Client Outcomes

Client Will (Specify Time Frame)

- Verbalize known fears
- State accurate information about the situation
- Identify, verbalize, and demonstrate those coping behaviors that reduce own fear
- Report and demonstrate reduced fear

Nursing Interventions

- Assess source of fear with the client.
- Assess for a history of anxiety.
- Assess for presence of fear avoidance beliefs.
- Have the client draw the object of his or her fear.
- Stay with clients when they express fear; provide verbal and nonverbal (touch and hug with permission and if culturally acceptable) reassurances of safety if safety is within control.
- Explore coping skills previously used by the client to deal with fear; reinforce these skills and explore other outlets. Provide backrubs and massage for clients to decrease anxiety.

▲ Refer for cognitive behavior therapy.

▲ Animal-assisted therapy can be incorporated into the care of clients in hospice situations.

- Encourage clients to express their fears in narrative form.
- Enhance client's self-efficacy when a client is experiencing initial fear of disease progression.
- Engage client in a mindfulness-based stress reduction program.
- Provide brief psychoeducation to client who has fear about surgery.

Pediatric

- Incorporate play therapy as an intervention to reduce fears.

Geriatric

- Provide a protective and safe environment, use consistent caregivers, and maintain the accustomed environmental structure.
- Assess for fear of falls in hospitalized clients with hip fractures to determine risk of poor health outcomes.
- Pair cognitive-behavioral strategies with exercises to improve physical skills and mobility to decrease fear of falling.
- Assist the client in identifying and reducing risk factors for falls, including environmental hazards in and out of the home, the importance of good nutrition and activity, proper footwear, and how to stand up after a fall.

Multicultural

- Identify what triggers fear response.
- Assess for fears of racism in culturally diverse clients.
- Explore client's meaning of illness, including a fear of illness.
- Provide education, support, and guidance.

Home Care

- The previous interventions may be adapted for home care use.
- Refer to care plan for **Anxiety**.
- ▲ Encourage the client to seek or continue appropriate counseling to reduce fear associated with stress or resolve alterations in irrational thought processes.
- ▲ Offer to sit quietly with a terminally ill client as needed by the client or family, or provide hospice volunteers to do the same.

Client/Family Teaching and Discharge Planning

- Teach the client the difference between warranted and excessive fear.
- Teach clients to use guided imagery when they are fearful; have them use all senses to visualize a place that is "comfortable and safe" for them.
- Teach use of appropriate community resources in emergency situations (e.g., hotlines, emergency departments, law enforcement, judicial systems).
- If fear is associated with bioterrorism, provide accurate information and ensure that healthcare personnel have appropriate training and preparation.

Ineffective Infant Suck-Swallow Response

NANDA-I Definition

Impaired ability of an infant to suck or coordinate the suck-swallow response.

Defining Characteristics

Arrhythmia; bradycardic events; choking; circumoral cyanosis; excessive coughing; finger splaying; flaccidity; gagging; hiccups; hyperextension of extremities; impaired ability to initiate an effective suck; impaired ability to sustain an effective suck; impaired motor tone; inability to coordinate sucking, swallowing, and breathing; irritability; nasal flaring; oxygen desaturation; pallor; subcostal retraction; time-out signals; use of accessory muscles of respiration

Related Factors

Hypoglycemia; hypothermia; hypotonia; inappropriate positioning; unsatisfactory sucking behavior

At-Risk Population

Infants born to mothers with substance misuse; infants delivered using obstetrical forceps; infants delivered using obstetrical vacuum extraction; infants experiencing prolonged hospitalization; premature infants

Associated Condition

Convulsive episodes; gastroesophageal reflux; high flow oxygen by nasal cannula; lacerations during delivery; low appearance, pulse, grimace, activity, & respiration (APGAR) scores; neurological delay; neurological impairment; oral hypersensitivity; oropharyngeal deformity; prolonged enteral nutrition

Client Outcomes

Infant Will (Specify Time Frame)

- Consume adequate calories that will result in appropriate weight gain and optimal growth and development
- Have opportunities for skin-to-skin (kangaroo care) experiences
- Have opportunities for "trophic" (i.e., small volume of breast milk/formula) enteral feedings prior to full oral feedings
- Progress to stable, neurobehavioral organization (i.e., motor, state, self-regulation, attention-interaction)
- Demonstrate presence of mature oral reflexes that are necessary for safe feeding
- Progress to safe, self-regulated oral feedings
- Coordinate the suck-swallow-breathe sequence while nippling
- Display clear behavioral cues related to hunger and satiety
- Display approach/engagement cues, with minimal avoidance/disengagement cues
- Have opportunities to pace own feeding, taking breaks as needed
- Display evidence of being in the "quiet-alert" state while nippling
- Progress to and engage in mutually positive parent/caregiver–infant/child interactions during feedings

Parent/Family Will (Specify Time Frame)

- Recognize necessity of adequate calories for appropriate weight gain and optimal growth and development
- Learn to read and respond contingently to infant's behavioral cues (e.g., hunger, satiety, approach/engagement, stress/avoidance/disengagement)
- Learn strategies that promote organized infant behavior
- Learn appropriate positioning and handling techniques
- Learn effective ways to relieve stress behaviors during nippling
- Learn ways to help infant coordinate suck-swallow-breathe sequence (i.e., external pacing techniques)
- Engage in mutually positive interactions with infant during feeding

- Recognize ways to facilitate effective feedings: feed in quiet-alert state; keep length of feeding appropriate; burp; prepare/structure environment; recognize signs of sensory overload; encourage self-regulation; respect need for breaks and breathing pauses; avoid pulling and twisting nipple during pauses; allow infant to resume sucking when ready; provide oral support (cheek and/or jaw) as needed; use appropriate nipple hole size and flow rate

Nursing Interventions

F

- • Refer to care plans for Disorganized **Infant** behavior, Risk for disorganized **Infant** behavior, Ineffective and Interrupted **Breastfeeding,** and Insufficient **Breast Milk** and assess as needed.
- • Interventions follow a sequential pattern of implementation that can be adapted as appropriate.
- • Assess coordination of infant's suck, swallow, and gag reflex.
- ▲ Provide developmentally supportive neonatal intensive care for preterm infants.
- • Provide opportunities for kangaroo (i.e., skin-to-skin) care.
- ▲ Before the infant is ready for oral feedings, implement gavage feedings (or other alternative) as ordered, using breast milk whenever possible.
- • Provide a naturalistic environment for tube feedings (nasoorogastric, gavage, or other) that approximates a pleasurable oral feeding experience: hold infant in semiupright/flexed position; offer nonnutritive sucking; pace feedings; allow for semidemand feedings contingent with infant cues; offer rest breaks; burp, as appropriate.
- • Foster direct breastfeeding as early as possible and enable the first oral feed to be at the breast in the neonatal intensive care unit (NICU).
- • Allow parents to feed the infant when possible.
- • Position infant in semiupright position, with head, shoulders, and hips in a straight line facing the mother with the infant's nose level with the mother's nipple.
- • Feed infant in the quiet-alert state.
- • Determine the appropriate shape, size, and hole of nipple to provide flow rate for preterm infants.
- • Implement pacing for infants having difficulty coordinating breathing with sucking and swallowing.
- • Provide infants with jaw and/or cheek support, as needed.
- • Allow the stable newborn to breastfeed within the first half hour after birth.
- • Allow appropriate time for nipple feeding to ensure infant's safety, limiting to 15 to 20 minutes for bottle feeding.

- Monitor length of breastfeeding so that it does not exceed 30 minutes. Breast milk transfer may last from as little as 5 to 20 minutes during breastfeeding depending on variations in milk supply during a 24-hour day (Flaherman et al., 2012).
- Encourage transitioning from scheduled to semidemand feedings, contingent with infant behavior cues.

- ▲ Refer to a multidisciplinary team (e.g., neonatal/pediatric nutritionist, physical or occupational therapist, speech pathologist, lactation specialist) as needed.

Home Care

- The previously mentioned appropriate interventions may be adapted for home care use.
- ▲ Infants with risk factors and clinical indicators of feeding problems present before hospital discharge should be referred to appropriate community early-intervention service providers (e.g., community health nurses, early learning programs [individualized per states], occupational therapy, speech pathologists, feeding specialists) to facilitate adequate weight gain for optimal growth and development.

Client/Family Teaching and Discharge Planning

- Provide anticipatory guidance for infant's expected feeding course.
- Teach various effective feeding methods and strategies to parents.
- Teach parents how to read, interpret, and respond contingently to infant cues.
- Help parents identify support systems before hospital discharge.
- Provide anticipatory guidance for the infant's discharge.

Risk for Female Genital Mutilation

NANDA-I Definition

Susceptible to full or partial ablation of the female external genitalia and other lesions of the genitalia, whether for cultural, religious, or any other non-therapeutic reasons, which may compromise health.

Risk Factors

Lack of family knowledge about impact of practice on physical health; lack of family knowledge about impact of practice on reproductive health; lack of family knowledge about impact of practice on psychosocial health

At-Risk Population

Residing in country where practice is accepted; family leaders belong to ethnic group in which practice is accepted; belonging to family in which any female member has been subjected to practice; favorable attitude of family towards practice; female gender; belonging to ethnic group in which practice is accepted; planning to visit family's country of origin

Client/Family Outcomes

Client Will (Specify Time Frame)

- Express effects of family/culture on beliefs about female genital mutilation
- Demonstrate evidence that female genital mutilation has not occurred
- Express/implement a plan for avoiding female genital mutilation
- Maintain safety of female children
- Demonstrate the ability to make decisions independent of cultural group
- Demonstrate self-advocacy skills

F

Nursing Interventions

- Identify the decision-making process related to the practice of female genital mutilation (FGM).
- Identify the type of FGM the female client is at risk for.
- Assess and identify geographic, environmental, familial, religious, and/or other cultural factors that increase risk for FGM.
- Encourage the mothers of at-risk daughters to express their beliefs and attitudes toward FGM.
- Assess the mothers of at-risk daughters for positive affect (expression of feelings) and attitudes toward FGM.
- In a respectful and nonjudgmental manner, convey accurate and clear information about FGM, using language and methods that can be readily understood by clients.
- In a respectful and nonjudgmental manner, provide the client, client's parents, and family with information that FGM is not a universal practice and that it is an illegal practice in many parts of the world.

In a respectful and nonjudgmental manner, provide the client, client's parents, and family with health education to address false beliefs about female and clitoral anatomy and the physiology of women.

- In a respectful and nonjudgmental manner, provide the client, client's parents, and family with health education to inform about the negative health outcomes associated with FMG.
- In a respectful and nonjudgmental manner, provide the client, client's parents, and family with health education to inform about the negative birth outcomes associated with mothers who have had FMG.
- Use therapeutic and culturally competent communication to focus on the current and future safety of the female child at risk for FGM.

- Utilize a cultural mediator to interpret cross-cultural norms about FGM.
- In a respectful and nonjudgmental manner, provide fathers with health education to address beliefs about FGM and provide information about the negative health outcomes associated with FGM.
- ▲ Refer families to counseling services.
- See care plans for Post-Trauma syndrome, Impaired parenting, and Social isolation.

Pediatric

- Identify a system for assessment and referral of female infants at risk of female genital mutilation born to mothers who have undergone FGM.
- For female children that may be a victim of FGM, or are at risk of female genital mutilation, notify Child Protective Services and other law enforcement authorities.

Risk for Imbalanced Fluid Volume

NANDA-I Definition

Susceptible to a decrease, increase, or rapid shift from one to the other of intravascular, interstitial, and/or intracellular fluid, which may compromise health. This refers to body fluid loss, gain, or both

Risk Factors

Altered fluid intake; difficulty accessing water; excessive sodium intake; inadequate knowledge about fluid needs; ineffective medication self-management; insufficient muscle mass; malnutrition

At Risk Population

Individuals at extremes of weight; individuals with external conditions affecting fluid needs; individuals with internal conditions affecting fluid needs; women

Associated Condition

Active fluid volume loss; deviations affecting fluid absorption; deviations affecting fluid elimination; deviations affecting fluid intake; deviations affecting vascular permeability; excessive fluid loss through normal route; fluid loss through abnormal route; pharmaceutical preparations; treatment regimen

Client Outcomes

- Lung sounds clear, respiratory rate 12 to 20 and free of dyspnea
- Urine output greater than 0.5 mL/kg/hr
- Blood pressure, pulse rate, temperature, and oxygen saturation within expected range
- Laboratory values within expected range: that is, normal serum sodium, hematocrit, and osmolarity

- Extremities and dependent areas free of edema
- Mental orientation appropriate based on previous condition

Nursing Interventions

Surgical Clients

- Monitor the fluid balance. If there are symptoms of hypovolemia, refer to the interventions in the care plan for Deficient **Fluid** volume. If there are symptoms of hypervolemia, refer to the interventions in the care plan for Excess **Fluid** volume.

Preoperative

- Collect a thorough history and perform a preoperative assessment to identify clients with increased risk for hemorrhage or hypovolemia: that is, clients who take herbal supplements, those with recent traumatic injury, abnormal bleeding or altered clotting times, complicated kidney or liver disease, diabetes, cardiovascular disease, major organ transplant, history of aspirin and/or nonsteroidal antiinflammatory drug (NSAID) use, anticoagulant therapy, or history of hemophilia, von Willebrand's disease, or disseminated intravascular coagulation. Assess the client's use of over-the-counter agents to include herbal products.
- Recognize that nothing by mouth (NPO) at midnight may or may not be appropriate for each surgical client. Guidelines from the American Society of Anesthesiologists (2011) recommended that healthy clients having elective surgery should be allowed to have clear liquids up to 2 hours before surgery.
- Determine length of time the client has been without normal intake, been NPO, or experienced fluid loss (e.g., vomiting, diarrhea, bleeding).
- Assess and document the client's mental status.
- Recognize that there is conflicting evidence regarding liberal intraoperative fluid management versus restrictive fluid management. Fluid administration during surgery is more restrictive to prevent pulmonary complications associated with excessive fluid administration (Assaad, Popescu & Perrino, 2013).
- Recognize that an individualized fluid management plan would be developed incorporating client-specific assessment parameters (e.g., existing comorbid diseases, age) and type of surgical procedure (Allison & George, 2014).
- Recognize the effects of general anesthetics, inhalational agents, and regional anesthesia on perfusion in the body and the potential for decreasing the blood pressure.

F

- Monitor for signs of intraoperative hypovolemia such as dry skin, dry mucous membranes, tachycardia, decreased urinary output, decreased CVP, hypotension, increased pulse, and/or deep rapid respirations.
- Monitor for signs of intraoperative hypervolemia such as dyspnea, coarse crackles, increased pulse and respirations, decreased oxygenation, and decreased urinary output, all of which could progress to pulmonary edema.
- In the critically ill surgical client a pulmonary artery catheter or other minimally invasive CO monitoring device may be used to determine fluid balance and guide fluid and vasoactive intravenous (IV) drip administration.
- Monitor the client for hyponatremia with symptoms such as headache, anorexia, nausea and vomiting, diarrhea, tachycardia, general malaise, muscle cramps, weakness, lethargy, change in mental status, disorientation, seizures, and death.
- Monitor clients undergoing laparoscopic or hysteroscopic procedures for the development of hyponatremia, hypervolemia, and pulmonary edema when an irrigation fluid is used.
- Monitor clients undergoing transurethral resection of the prostate (TURP) procedures for development of hyponatremia and hypervolemia with symptoms of TURP syndrome including headache, visual changes, agitation, lethargy, vomiting, muscle twitching, bradycardia, diminished pupillary reflexes, hypertension, and respiratory distress.
- Measure the irrigation fluid used during urological and gynecological procedures accurately for volume deficit such as amount of irrigation used minus amount of irrigation recovered via suction.
- Monitor intraoperative intake and output including blood loss, urine output, and third-space losses to provide an estimate of fluid volume.
- Observe the surgical client for hyperkalemia with symptoms including dysrhythmias, heart block, asystole, abdominal distention, and weakness.
- Maintain the client's core temperature at normal levels, using warming devices as needed. **EB:** Hypothermia (body temperature (<36°C) is present in the postoperative period in 26% to 90% of all patients who have undergone elective surgery. The risk of

hypothermia is particularly high in patients over 60 years of age with poor nutritional status and preexisting disease, which impairs thermoregulation (e.g., diabetes mellitus with polyneuropathy), and in those who have had major or lengthy surgery. Lower temperatures in the operating room also increase the risk of hypothermia: the lower the temperature, the higher the risk (Torossian et al., 2015).

- Fluids administration during surgery can increase risk of hypothermia

Postoperative

- Continue to monitor fluids postoperatively.
- Assess the client for development of tissue edema, especially after cataract surgery in patients with comorbidities such as diabetes.
- Recognize that IV fluid replacement decisions incorporate multiple assessment parameters such as hourly urine output, blood pressure, heart rate, respiratory rate, lung sounds, output from drains, and changes in laboratory results (e.g., hemoglobin/hematocrit, serum electrolytes).

Geriatric

- Check skin turgor of older clients on the forehead, subclavian area, or inner thigh; also look for the presence of longitudinal furrows on the tongue and dry mucous membranes.
- Closely monitor urine output, concentration of urine, and serum BUN/creatinine results.
- Monitor older clients for excess fluid volume during the treatment of deficient fluid volume: auscultate lung sounds, assess for edema, and trend vital signs.
- Assess the older client's cognitive status.

Pediatric

- Assess the pediatric client's weight, length of NPO status, underlying illness, and the surgical procedure to be performed.
- Recognize that newborns require very little fluid replacement when undergoing major surgical procedures during the first few days of life.
- Monitor pediatric surgical clients closely for signs of fluid loss.
- Administer fluids preoperatively until NPO status must be initiated so that fluid deficit is decreased.
- Perform an assessment for signs of fluid responsiveness in the pediatric client.

Deficient Fluid Volume

NANDA-I Definition

Decreased intravascular, interstitial, and/or intracellular fluid. This refers to dehydration, water loss alone without change in sodium

Defining Characteristics

F

Altered mental status; altered skin turgor; decreased blood pressure; decreased pulse pressure; decreased pulse volume; decreased tongue turgor; decreased urine output; decreased venous filling; dry mucous membranes; dry skin; increased body temperature; increased heart rate; increased serum hematocrit levels; increased urine concentration; sudden weight loss; sunken eyes; thirst; weakness

Related Factors

Difficulty meeting increased fluid volume requirement; inadequate access to fluid; inadequate knowledge about fluid needs; ineffective medication self-management; insufficient fluid intake; insufficient muscle mass; malnutrition

At-Risk Population

Individuals at extremes of weight; individuals with external conditions affecting fluid needs; individuals with internal conditions affecting fluid needs; women

Associated Conditions

Active fluid volume loss; deviations affecting fluid absorption; deviations affecting fluid elimination; deviations affecting fluid intake; excessive fluid loss through normal route; fluid loss through abnormal route; pharmaceutical preparations; treatment regimen

Client Outcomes

Client Will (Specify Time Frame)

- Maintain urine output of 0.5 mL/kg/hr or at least more than 1300 mL/day
- Maintain normal blood pressure, heart rate, and body temperature
- Maintain elastic skin turgor; moist tongue and mucous membranes; and orientation to person, place, and time
- Explain measures that can be taken to treat or prevent fluid volume loss
- Describe symptoms that indicate the need to consult with healthcare provider

Nursing Interventions

- Watch for early signs of hypovolemia, including thirst, restlessness, headaches, and inability to concentrate.
- Recognize symptoms of cyanosis, cold clammy skin, weak thready pulse, confusion, and oliguria as late signs of hypovolemia.

- Monitor pulse, respiration, and blood pressure of clients with deficient fluid volume every 15 minutes to 1 hour for the unstable client and every 4 hours for the stable client.
- Check orthostatic blood pressures with the client lying, sitting, and standing.
- Note skin turgor over bony prominences such as the hand or shin.
- Monitor for the existence of factors causing deficient fluid volume (e.g., hypovolemia from vomiting, diarrhea, difficulty maintaining oral intake, fever, uncontrolled type 2 diabetes, diuretic therapy).
- Observe for dry tongue and mucous membranes, and longitudinal tongue furrows.
- Recognize that checking capillary refill may not be helpful in identifying fluid volume deficit.
- Weigh client daily and watch for sudden decreases, especially in the presence of decreasing urine output or active fluid loss.
- Monitor total fluid intake and output every 4 hours (or every hour for the unstable client or the client who has urine output equal to or less than 0.5 mL/kg/hr).
- A urine output of less than 0.5 mL/kg/hr may be indicative of acute kidney injury (Prowle et al., 2011). Nevertheless, in any condition of hypovolemia, renal perfusion pressure falls. If it falls below the level of autoregulation (blood pressure [BP] <80 mm Hg), then renal blood flow and glomerular filtration will fall (Andeucchi et al., 2017)
- Note the color of urine, urine osmolality, and specific gravity.
- Provide fresh water and oral fluids preferred by the client (distribute over 24 hours [e.g., 1200 mL during days, 800 mL during evenings, and 200 mL during nights]), provide prescribed diet, offer snacks (e.g., frequent drinks, fresh fruits, fruit juice), and instruct significant other to assist the client with feedings as appropriate).

▲ Provide oral replacement therapy as ordered and tolerated with a hypotonic glucose-electrolyte solution when the client has acute diarrhea or nausea/vomiting. Provide small, frequent quantities of slightly chilled solutions.

▲ Administer antidiarrheals and antiemetics as ordered and appropriate. Consider what the client is eating to prevent further diarrhea (Bolen, 2017).

- If the client is on enteral feedings, research has shown either continuous or intermittent feedings had similar results regarding diarrhea and nausea (deAraujo et al., 2014).

- ▲ Hydrate the client with isotonic IV solutions as prescribed.
- • Assist with ambulation if the client has postural hypotension. Hypovolemia causes orthostatic hypotension, which can result in syncope when the client goes from a sitting to standing position (Wagner & Hardin-Pierce, 2014).

Critically Ill

- ▲ Monitor stroke volume, passive leg lift, and ultrasound as trends for more accurate fluid volume status.
- ▲ Monitor serum and urine osmolality blood urea nitrogen (BUN)/ creatinine ratio and hematocrit for elevations.
- ▲ Insert an indwelling urinary catheter if ordered and measure urine output hourly. Notify healthcare provider if urine output is less than 0.5 mL/kg/hr.
- ▲ When ordered, initiate a fluid challenge of crystalloids (e.g., 0.9% normal saline or lactated Ringer's) for replacement of intravascular volume.
- ▲ Monitor the client's response to prescribed fluid therapy and fluid challenge, especially noting vital signs (mean arterial pressure (MAP) > 65 in the first 6 hours of treatment, systolic blood pressure > 100 mm Hg) (Singer et al., 2016; Rhodes et al., 2017), urine output, blood lactate concentrations, and lung sounds.
- • Position the client flat with legs elevated when hypotensive, if not contraindicated.
- ▲ Monitor trends in serum lactic acid levels and base deficit obtained from blood gases as ordered.
- ▲ Consult provider if signs and symptoms of deficient fluid volume persist or worsen.

Pediatric

- • Monitor the child for signs of deficient fluid volume, including sunken eyes, decreased tears, dry mucous membranes, poor skin turgor, and decreased urine output (Graves, 2013).
- ▲ Reinforce the healthcare provider recommendation for the parents to give the child oral rehydration fluids to drink in the amounts specified, especially during the first 4 to 6 hours to replace fluid losses. Consider using diluted oral rehydration fluids. Once the child is rehydrated, an orally administered maintenance solution should be used along with food.
- • Recommend that the mother resume breastfeeding as soon as possible.

- Recommend that parents not give the child carbonated soda, fruit juices, gelatin dessert, or instant fruit drink mix; instead, give the child oral rehydration fluids ordered and, when tolerated, food.
- Once the child has been rehydrated, begin feeding regular food but avoid milk products (Guandalini et al., 2017).

F

Geriatric

- Monitor older clients for deficient fluid volume carefully, noting new onset of headache, weakness, dizziness, and postural hypotension.
- Implement fall precautions for clients experiencing weakness, dizziness, and/or postural hypotension.
- Evaluate the risk for dehydration using the Dehydration Risk Appraisal Checklist.
- Check skin turgor of older clients on the forehead and axilla; check for dry mucous membranes and dry tongue.
- Encourage fluid intake by offering fluids regularly to cognitively impaired clients.
- Because older clients have low water reserves, they should be encouraged to drink regularly even when not thirsty. Frequent and varied beverage offerings should be made available by hydration assistants to routinely offer increased beverages to clients in extended care.
- Flag the food tray of clients with chronic dehydration to indicate if the client is identified as having chronic dehydration and indicate that they should finish 75% to 100% of their food and fluids. Offering beverages in brightly colored cups may improve fluid intake.
- Recognize that lower blood pressures and monitoring of an intake record over 24 hours is recommended to track oral intake and possible dehydration (Oates et al., 2015).
- A higher BUN/creatinine ratio can be significant signs of dehydration in older adults.
- Monitor older clients for excess fluid volume during the treatment of deficient fluid volume: auscultate lung sounds, assess for edema, and note vital signs.

Home Care

- Teach family members how to monitor output in the home (e.g., use of commode "hat" in the toilet, urinal, or bedpan, or use of catheter and closed drainage system). Instruct them to monitor both intake and output. Use common terms such as "cups" or "glasses of water a day" when providing education.

- When weighing the client, use same scale each day. Be sure scale is on a flat, not cushioned, surface. Do not weigh the client with a scale placed on any type of rug, because scales provide more accurate readings when used on a hard surface.
- Teach family about complications of deficient fluid volume and when to call the healthcare provider.
- Teach the family the signs of hypovolemia, especially in older adults, and how to monitor for dizziness or unsteady gait.
- If the client is receiving IV fluids, there must be a responsible caregiver in the home. Teach caregiver about administration of fluids, complications of IV administration (e.g., fluid volume overload, development of phlebitis, speed of medication reactions), and when to call for assistance. Assist caregiver with administration for as long as necessary to maintain client safety.
- Identify an emergency plan, including when to call 911.
- Deficient fluid volume may be a symptom of impending death in terminally ill clients. In palliative care situations, treatment of deficient fluid volume should be determined based on client/family goals. Information and support should be provided to assist the client/family in this decision. Support the family/client in a palliative care situation to decide if it is appropriate to intervene for deficient fluid volume or to allow the client to die without fluids.

Client/Family Teaching and Discharge Planning

- Instruct the client to avoid rapid position changes, especially from supine to sitting or standing.
- Teach the client and family about appropriate diet and fluid intake.
- Teach the client and family how to measure and record intake and output accurately.
- Teach the client and family about measures instituted to treat hypovolemia and to prevent or treat fluid volume loss.
- Instruct the client and family about signs of deficient fluid volume that indicate they should contact healthcare provider.

Excess Fluid Volume

NANDA-I Definition

Surplus intake and/or retention of fluid

Defining Characteristics

Adventitious breath sounds; altered blood pressure; altered mental status; altered pulmonary artery pressure; altered respiratory pattern; altered urine specific gravity; anxiety; azotemia; decreased serum hematocrit levels; decreased serum hemoglobin level; edema; hepatomegaly; increased central venous pressure; intake exceeds output; jugular vein distension; oliguria; pleural effusion; positive hepatojugular reflex; presence of S3 heart sound; psychomotor agitation; pulmonary congestion; weight gain over short period of time

Related Factors

Excessive fluid intake; excessive sodium intake; ineffective medication self-management

Associated Conditions

Deviations affecting fluid elimination; pharmaceutical preparations

Client Outcomes

Client Will (Specify Time Frame)

- Remain free of edema, effusion, anasarca
- Maintain body weight appropriate for the client
- Maintain clear lung sounds; no evidence of dyspnea or orthopnea
- Remain free of jugular vein distention, positive hepatojugular reflex, and S3 heart sound
- Maintain normal CVP, PAP, cardiac output, and vital signs
- Maintain urine output of 0.5 mL/kg/hr or more with normal urine osmolality and specific gravity
- Explain actions that are needed to treat or prevent excess fluid volume including fluid and dietary restrictions, and medications
- Describe symptoms that indicate the need to consult with healthcare provider

Nursing Interventions

- Monitor location and extent of edema using the 1+ to 4+ scale to quantify edema; also measure the legs using a millimeter tape in the same area at the same time each day. Note differences in measurement between extremities.
- Monitor daily weight for sudden increases; use same scale and type of clothing at same time each day, preferably before breakfast.

- Monitor intake and output; note trends reflecting decreasing urine output in relation to fluid intake.
- Chronic HF is characterized by neurohormonal activation and sodium retention that leads to excessive fluid accumulation in the systemic and pulmonary circulations.
- Auscultate lung sounds for crackles, monitor respiration effort, and determine the presence and severity of orthopnea.
- Monitor serum and urine osmolality, serum sodium, blood urea nitrogen (BUN)/creatinine ratio, and hematocrit for abnormalities.
- BUN and creatinine are monitored currently as biomarkers of kidney injury and failure.
- With head of bed elevated 30 to 45 degrees, monitor jugular veins for distention with the client in the upright position; assess for positive hepatojugular reflex.
- Monitor the client's behavior for restlessness, anxiety, or confusion; use safety precautions if symptoms are present.
- ▲ Monitor for the development of conditions that increase the client's risk for excess fluid volume, including HF, kidney failure, and liver failure, all of which result in decreased glomerular filtration rate and fluid retention.
- ▲ Provide a restricted-sodium diet as appropriate if ordered.
- ▲ Monitor serum albumin level and provide protein intake as appropriate.
- ▲ Administer prescribed diuretics as appropriate; ensure adequate blood pressure before administration. If diuretic is administered intravenously, note and record the blood pressure and urine output after the dose. Monitor serum sodium for hyponatremia.
- Monitor for side effects of diuretic therapy including orthostatic hypotension (especially if the client is also receiving angiotensin-converting enzyme [ACE] inhibitors), hypovolemia, and electrolyte imbalances (hypokalemia and hyponatremia).
- ▲ Implement fluid restriction as ordered, especially when serum sodium is low; include all routes of intake. Schedule limited intake of fluids around the clock, and include the type of fluids preferred by the client.
- Maintain the rate of all IV infusions, using an IV pump.
- Turn clients with dependent edema at least every 2 hours and monitor for areas that may develop pressure ulcers.

- ▲ Provide ordered care for edematous extremities including compression, elevation, and muscle exercises.
- • Promote a positive body image and good self-esteem. *Visible edema may alter the client's body image.* Refer to the care plan for Disturbed **Body Image.**
- ▲ Consult with the healthcare provider if signs and symptoms of excess fluid volume persist or worsen.

Critically Ill

- • Insert an indwelling urinary catheter if ordered and measure urine output hourly. Notify healthcare provider if output is less than 0.5 mL/kg/hr.
- ▲ Monitor blood pressure, heart rate, passive leg lift, mean arterial pressure, CVP, PAP, and cardiac output/index; note and report trends of increasing or decreasing pressures over time.
- ▲ Monitor the effects of infusion of diuretic drips. Perform continuous renal replacement therapy (CRRT) as ordered if the client is critically ill and hemodynamically unstable and excessive fluid must be removed.

Geriatric

- • Recognize that the presence of fluid volume excess is particularly serious in older adults.
- • Monitor electrolyte levels carefully, including sodium levels and potassium levels, with both increased and decreased levels possible.
- • Refer to the care plan for risk for **Electrolyte** imbalance and the care plan for **Sexual Dysfunction.**

Home Care

- • Assess client and family knowledge of disease processes causing excess fluid volume.
- ▲ Teach about disease process and complications of excess fluid volume, including when to contact the healthcare provider.
- • Assess client and family knowledge and compliance with medical regimen, including medications, diet, rest, and exercise. Assist family with integrating restrictions into daily living.
- ▲ Teach and reinforce knowledge of medications. Instruct the client not to use over-the-counter (OTC) medications (e.g., diet medications) without first consulting the provider.
- ▲ Instruct the client to make the primary healthcare provider aware of medications ordered by other healthcare providers.

- • Identify emergency plan for rapidly developing or critical levels of excess fluid volume when diuresing is not safe at home.
- ▲ Teach about signs and symptoms of both excess and deficient fluid volume, such as darker urine, dry mouth, and peripheral edema, and when to call the healthcare provider.

Client/Family Teaching and Discharge Planning

- • Describe signs and symptoms of excess fluid volume and actions to take if they occur.
- ▲ Teach client on diuretics to weigh self daily in the morning and to notify the healthcare provider if there is a 2.2 pound (1 kg) or more weight gain (Wagner & Hardin-Pierce, 2014).
- ▲ Teach the importance of fluid and sodium restrictions. Help the client and family devise a schedule for intake of fluids throughout the entire day. Refer to a dietitian concerning implementation of a low-sodium diet.
- • Teach clients how to measure and document intake and output with common household measurements, such as cups.
- ▲ Teach how to take diuretics correctly: take one dose in the morning and second dose (if taken) no later than 4 p.m. Adjust potassium intake as appropriate for potassium-losing or potassium-sparing diuretics. Note the appearance of side effects such as weakness, muscle cramps, hypertension, or palpitations (Wagner & Hardin-Pierce, 2014).
- • For the client undergoing hemodialysis, teach client the required restrictions in dietary electrolytes, protein, and fluid. Spend time with the client to detect any factors that may interfere with the client's compliance with the fluid restriction or restrictive diet.

Risk for Deficient Fluid Volume

NANDA-I Definition

Susceptible to experiencing decreased intravascular, interstitial, and/or intracellular fluid volumes, which may compromise health

Risk Factors

Difficulty meeting increased fluid volume requirement; inadequate access to fluid; inadequate knowledge about fluid needs; ineffective medication self-management; insufficient fluid intake; insufficient muscle mass; malnutrition

At-Risk Population

Individuals at extremes of weight; individuals with external conditions affecting fluid needs; individuals with internal conditions affecting fluid needs; women

Associated Conditions

Active fluid volume loss; deviations affecting fluid absorption; deviations affecting fluid elimination; deviations affecting fluid intake; excessive fluid loss through normal route; fluid loss through abnormal route; pharmaceutical preparations; treatment regimen

Client Outcomes, Nursing Interventions, Client/Family Teaching

Refer to care plan for Deficient **Fluid** volume

Frail Elderly Syndrome

NANDA-I Definition

Dynamic state of unstable equilibrium that affects the older individual experiencing deterioration in one or more domains of health (physical, functional, psychological, or social) and leads to increased susceptibility to adverse health effects, in particular disability

Defining Characteristics

Decreased Activity tolerance (00298); bathing self-care deficit (00108); decreased cardiac output (00029); dressing self-care deficit (00109); fatigue (00093); feeding self-care deficit (00102); hopelessness (00124); imbalanced nutrition: less than body requirements (00002); impaired memory (00131); impaired physical mobility (00085); impaired walking (00088); impaired social isolation (00053); toileting self-care deficit (00110)

Related Factors

Decreased activity tolerance; anxiety; average daily physical activity is less than recommended for gender and age; decrease in energy; decrease in muscle strength; depression; exhaustion; fear of falling; immobility; impaired balance; impaired mobility; insufficient social support; malnutrition; muscle weakness; obesity; sadness; sedentary lifestyle; social isolation

At-Risk Population

Age >70 years; constricted living space; economically disadvantaged; ethnicity other than Caucasian; female gender; history of falls; living alone; low educational level; prolonged hospitalization; social vulnerability

Client Outcomes

Client Will (Specify Time Frame)

- Remain living as independently as possible in the home or care setting of his or her choice
- Maintain safety when engaging in activities of daily living and ambulation
- Increase exercise and/or daily physical activity to build muscle strength
- Maintain a healthy weight

Nursing Interventions

- Assess frailty with a tool such as the Frailty Index or the Edmonton Frail Scale.
- Recognize that balance and gait impairment are features of frailty and are risk factors for falls.
- Preserve physical functioning through individualized physical activity plans.
- Assess falls using a falls risk assessment tool such as the Hendrich II Fall Risk Model.
- Assess risk of fracture using tools such as the Cardiovascular Health Study (CHS) or Study of Osteoporotic Fracture (SOF) indicators.
- Evaluate the client's medications to determine whether medications increase the risk of frailty and/or are potentially inappropriate mediations (PIM), and if appropriate, consult with the client's healthcare provider regarding the client's medications.
- ▲ Refer to a dietitian for an individualized therapeutic diet.
- Refer to care plan for Readiness for enhanced **Nutrition** for additional interventions.
- Monitor weight loss.
- Encourage clients to engage in active lifestyles.
- Provide an exercise-training program.
- Promote the benefits of home-based exercise to older clients who are frail.
- Use an Interprofessional and person-centered approach for supporting frail older adults.
- Develop a trusting and responsive relationship with frail clients.

Multicultural, Home Care, Client/Family Teaching

- The previously mentioned interventions may be adapted for multicultural, home care, and client family teaching.

Risk for Frail Elderly Syndrome

NANDA-I Definition

Susceptible to a dynamic state of unstable equilibrium that affects the older individual experiencing deterioration in one or more domain of health (physical, functional, psychological, or social) and leads to increased susceptibility to adverse health effects in particular disability

Risk Factors

Decreased activity tolerance; anxiety; average daily physical activity is less than recommended for gender and age; decrease in energy; decrease in muscle strength; depression; exhaustion; fear of falling; immobility; impaired balance; impaired mobility; insufficient knowledge of modifiable factors; insufficient social support; malnutrition; muscle weakness; obesity; sadness; sedentary lifestyle; social isolation

At-Risk Population

Age >70 years; constricted living space; economically disadvantaged; ethnicity other than Caucasian; female gender; history of falls; living alone; low educational level; prolonged hospitalization; social vulnerability

Associated Condition

Alteration in cognitive functioning; altered clotting process; anorexia; chronic illness; decrease in serum 25-hydroxyvitamin D concentration; endocrine regulatory dysfunction; psychiatric disorder; sarcopenia; sarcopenic obesity; sensory deficit; suppressed inflammatory response; unintentional loss of 25% of body weight over 1 year; unintentional weight loss >10 pounds (>4.5 kg) in 1 year; walking 15 feet requires >6 seconds (4 m > 5 seconds)

Client Outcomes, Nursing Interventions

Refer to care plan for **Frail Elderly** syndrome

Impaired Gas Exchange

NANDA-I Definition

Excess or deficit in oxygenation and/or carbon dioxide elimination

Defining Characteristics

Abnormal arterial pH; abnormal skin color; altered respiratory depth; altered respiratory rhythm; bradypnea; confusion; decreased carbon dioxide level; diaphoresis; headache upon awakening; hypercapnia; hypoxemia; hypoxia; irritable mood; nasal flaring; psychomotor agitation; somnolence; tachycardia; tachypnea; visual disturbance

Related Factors

Ineffective airway clearance; ineffective breathing pattern; pain

At Risk Population

Premature infants

Associated Conditions

Alveolar-capillary membrane changes; asthma; general anesthesia; heart diseases; ventilation-perfusion imbalance

Client Outcomes

Client Will (Specify Time Frame)

- Demonstrate improved ventilation and adequate oxygenation as evidenced by blood gas levels within normal parameters for that client
- Maintain clear lung fields and remain free of signs of respiratory distress
- Verbalize understanding of oxygen supplementation and other therapeutic interventions

G

Nursing Interventions

- Monitor respiratory rate, depth, and ease of respiration. Watch for use of accessory muscles and nasal flaring.
- Auscultate breath sounds every 1 to 2 hours. The presence of crackles and wheezes may alert the nurse to airway obstruction, which may lead to or exacerbate existing hypoxia.
- The nurse should consider respiratory rate, work of breathing, and lung sounds along with PaO_2 values, arterial oxygen saturation (SaO_2), oxygen saturation continuously using pulse oximetry (SpO_2), patient tidal volume, and minute ventilation. Presence of dyspnea, asynchronous chest and abdominal movements, accessory muscles, and agitation indicate potential oxygenation problems (Barton, Vanderspank-Wright, & Shea, 2016).
- Monitor the client's behavior and mental status for the onset of restlessness, agitation, confusion, and (in the late stages) extreme lethargy.

▲ Monitor oxygen saturation continuously using pulse oximetry (SpO_2) (Lee, 2017). Note blood gas results as available.

- Monitor venous oxygen saturation to determine an index of oxygen balance to reflect between oxygen delivery and oxygen consumption (Dirks, 2017).
- Measurements of oxygenation supply in the macrocirculation include those made upstream from the tissue level. The parameters measured are arterial partial pressure of oxygen (PaO_2), arterial oxygen content (CaO_2), arterial oxygen saturation (SaO_2) determined on the basis of ABG analysis and pulse oximetry (SpO_2), and ratio of PaO_2 to fraction of inspired oxygen (FiO_2) or the PF ratio. Measurements of oxygenation or oxygen extraction or consumption in the macrocirculation made downstream from tissues include tissue oxygen consumption, mixed venous oxygen saturation (SVO_2) or

central venous oxygen saturation ($ScVO_2$), and blood levels of lactate (Siela & Kidd, 2017).

- Observe for cyanosis of the skin, and especially note color of the tongue and oral mucous membranes.
- Position the client in a semirecumbent position with the head of the bed at a 30- to 45-degree angle to decrease the aspiration of gastric, oral, and nasal secretions (Grap, 2009; Siela, 2010; American Association of Critical Care Nurses, 2016, 2017; Vollman, Dickinson, & Powers, 2017; Vollman, Sole, & Quinn, 2017).
- If the client has unilateral lung disease, position with head of bed at 30 to 45 degrees with "good lung down" in a side-lying position and affected lung up (Barton, Vanderspank-Wright, & Shea, 2016).
- ▲ If the client is acutely dyspneic, consider having the client lean forward over a bedside table, resting elbows on the table if tolerated.
- Help the client deep breathe and perform controlled coughing. Have the client inhale deeply, hold the breath for several seconds, and cough two or three times with the mouth open while tightening the upper abdominal muscles as tolerated. If the client has excessive fluid in the respiratory system, see the interventions for Ineffective **Airway** clearance.
- ▲ Monitor the effects of sedation and analgesics on the client's respiratory pattern; use judiciously (Barton, Vanderspank-Wright, & Shea, 2016).
- Schedule nursing care to provide rest and minimize fatigue.
- ▲ Administer humidified oxygen through an appropriate device (e.g., nasal cannula or Venturi mask per the healthcare provider's order); aim for an oxygen (O_2) saturation level of 90% or above. Oxygen should be titrated to target an SpO_2 of 94% to 98%, except with carbon monoxide poisoning (100% oxygen), acute respiratory distress syndrome (ARDS) (88%–95%), those at risk for hypercapnia (88%–92%), and premature infants (88%–94%) (Blakeman, 2013). Watch for onset of hypoventilation as evidenced by increased somnolence.
- Once oxygen is started, ABGs should be checked 30 to 60 minutes later to ensure satisfactory oxygenation without CO_2 retention or acidosis (GOLD, 2017).

- • Assess nutritional status including serum albumin level and body mass index (BMI).
- ▲ Assist the client to eat small meals frequently and use dietary supplements as necessary. Engage dietary in evaluating and creating an optimal nutrition plan. For some clients, drinking 30 mL of a supplement every hour while awake can be helpful.
- • If the client is severely debilitated from chronic respiratory disease, consider the use of a wheeled walker to help in ambulation.
- ▲ Watch for signs of psychological distress including anxiety, agitation, and insomnia.
- ▲ Refer the COPD client to a pulmonary rehabilitation program.

G

Critical Care

- ▲ Assess and monitor oxygen indices such as the PF ratio (FiO_2:PO_2), venous oxygen saturation/oxygen consumption (SVO_2 or $ScVO_2$) (Headley & Giuliano, 2011; Dirks, 2017; Siela & Kidd, 2017; Lough, 2018).
- ▲ Turn the client every 2 hours. Monitor mixed venous oxygen saturation closely after turning. If it drops below 10% or fails to return to baseline promptly, turn the client back into the supine position and evaluate oxygen status. If the client does not tolerate turning, consider use of a kinetic bed that rotates the client from side to side in a turn of at least 40 degrees (St. Clair & MacDermott, 2017).
- ▲ If the client has ARDS with difficulty maintaining oxygenation, then consider positioning the client prone with the upper thorax and pelvis supported. Monitor oxygen saturation and turn the client back to supine position if desaturation occurs. A PaO_2 lower than 150 mm Hg measured on at least 5 cm H_2O positive end-expiratory pressure (PEEP) is a recommended threshold for the application of proning (Gattinoni et al., 2013). Note: If the client becomes ventilator dependent, see the care plan for Impaired spontaneous **Ventilation.**
- ▲ High levels of PEEP likely improve oxygenation and gas exchange (Suzumura et al., 2014; Barton, Vanderspank-Wright, & Shea, 2016).

Geriatric

- ▲ Use central nervous system depressants and other sedating agents carefully to avoid decreasing respiration effort (rate and depth of breathing).

▲ Maintain appropriate levels of supplemental oxygen therapy for clients with impaired gas exchange and hypoxemia (GOLD, 2017).

Home Care

- Work with the client to determine what strategies are most helpful during times of dyspnea. Educate and empower the client to self-manage the disease associated with impaired gas exchange.
- Collaborate with healthcare providers regarding long-term oxygen administration for chronic respiratory failure clients with severe resting hypoxemia. Administer long-term oxygen therapy greater than 15 hours daily for PO_2 less than 55 or SaO_2 at or below 88% (GOLD, 2017).
- Assess the home environment for irritants that impair gas exchange. Help the client adjust the home environment as necessary (e.g., install an air filter to decrease the level of dust).

▲ Refer the client to occupational therapy as necessary to assist the client in adapting to the home and environment and in energy conservation (GOLD, 2017).

- Assist the client with identifying and avoiding situations that exacerbate impairment of gas exchange (e.g., stress-related situations, exposure to pollution of any kind, proximity to noxious gas fumes such as chlorine bleach).
- Refer to GOLD guidelines for management of home care and indications of hospital admission criteria (GOLD, 2017).
- Instruct the client to keep the home temperature above 68°F (20°C) and to avoid cold weather.
- Instruct the client to limit exposure to persons with respiratory infections.
- Instruct the family in the complications of the disease and the importance of maintaining the medical regimen, including when to call a healthcare provider.

▲ Refer the client for home health aide services as necessary for assistance with activities of daily living.

- When respiratory procedures are implemented, explain equipment and procedures to family members and provide needed emotional support.
- When electrically based equipment for respiratory support is implemented, evaluate home environment for electrical safety, proper

grounding, and so on. Ensure that notification is sent to the local utility company, the emergency medical team, and police and fire departments.

- ▲ Assess family role changes and coping ability. Refer the client to medical social services as appropriate for assistance in adjusting to chronic illness.
- • Support the family of the client with chronic illness.

Client/Family Teaching and Discharge Planning

- • Teach the client how to perform pursed-lip breathing and inspiratory muscle training, and how to use the tripod position. Have the client watch the pulse oximeter to note improvement in oxygenation with these breathing techniques.
- • Teach the client energy conservation techniques and the importance of alternating rest periods with activity. See nursing interventions for **Fatigue.**
- ▲ Teach the importance of not smoking. Refer to smoking cessation programs, and encourage clients who relapse to keep trying to quit. Ensure that clients receive appropriate medications to support smoking cessation from the primary healthcare provider.
- ▲ Instruct the family regarding home oxygen therapy if ordered (e.g., delivery system, liter flow, safety precautions).
- ▲ Teach the client the need to receive a yearly influenza vaccine.
- • Teach the client relaxation techniques to help reduce stress responses and panic attacks resulting from dyspnea.
- • Teach the client to use music, along with a rest period, to decrease dyspnea and anxiety (Mahler, 2014; Loscalzo, 2016).

Risk for Dysfunctional Gastrointestinal Motility

NANDA-I Definition

Susceptible to increased, decreased, ineffective, or lack of peristaltic activity within the gastrointestinal system, which may compromise health

Risk Factors

Anxiety; change in water source; eating habit change; immobility; malnutrition; sedentary lifestyle; stressors; unsanitary food preparation

At-Risk Population

Aging; ingestion of contaminated material; prematurity

Associated Condition

Decrease in gastrointestinal circulation; diabetes mellitus; enteral feedings; food intolerance; gastroesophageal reflux disease; infection; pharmaceutical agent; treatment regimen

Client Outcomes, Nursing Interventions, Client/Family Teaching and Discharge Planning

Refer to care plan for Dysfunctional **Gastrointestinal** motility.

Dysfunctional Gastrointestinal Motility

NANDA-I Definition

Increased, decreased, ineffective, or lack of peristaltic activity within the gastrointestinal system

Defining Characteristics

Abdominal cramping; abdominal pain; absence of flatus; acceleration of gastric emptying; bile-colored gastric residual; change in bowel sounds; diarrhea; difficulty with defecation; distended abdomen; hard; formed stool; increase in gastric residual; nausea; regurgitation; vomiting

Related Factors

Anxiety; change in water source; eating habit change; immobility; malnutrition; sedentary lifestyle; stressors; unsanitary food preparation

At-Risk Population

Aging; ingestion of contaminated material; prematurity

Associated Condition

Decrease in gastrointestinal circulation; diabetes mellitus; enteral feedings; food intolerance; gastroesophageal reflux disease; infection; pharmaceutical agent; treatment regimen

Client Outcomes

Client Will (Specify Time Frame)

- Be free of abdominal distention and pain
- Have normal bowel sounds
- Pass flatus rectally at intervals
- Defecate formed, soft stool every day to every third day
- State the presence of an appetite
- Be able to eat food without nausea and vomiting

Nursing Interventions

- Monitor for abdominal distention and presence of abdominal pain, weight loss, nausea, vomiting, obstipation, or diarrhea.
- Inspect, auscultate for bowel sounds noting characteristics and frequency; palpate and percuss the abdomen.
- Review history noting any anorexia or nausea/vomiting. Other symptoms may include relation of symptoms to meals, especially if aggravated by food, satiety, postprandial fullness/bloating, and weight loss or weight loss with severe gastroparesis.
- Monitor for fluid deficits by checking skin turgor and moisture of tongue, daily weights, input and output, and electrolyte values. Refer to care plan deficient **Fluid** volume if relevant.

▲ Monitor for nutritional deficits by keeping close track of food intake. Review laboratory studies that affirm nutritional deficits, such as decreased albumin and serum protein levels, liver profile, glucose, fecal analysis, and an electrolyte panel. Refer to care plan for imbalanced **Nutrition:** less than body requirements or Risk for **Electrolyte** imbalance as appropriate.

Slowed Gastric Motility

▲ Monitor daily laboratory studies and point of care testing blood glucose levels ensuring ordered glucose levels are performed and evaluated.

- Obtain a thorough gastrointestinal history if the client has diabetes, because he or she is at high risk for gastroparesis and gastric reflux.

▲ If client has nausea and vomiting, then provide an antiemetic and intravenous fluids as ordered. Offer or perform oral hygiene after vomiting. Refer to the care plans for **Nausea.**

▲ Evaluate medications the client is taking. Recognize that vasopressors, opioids, or anticholinergic medications can cause gastric slowing (Magidson & Martinez, 2016).

▲ Review laboratory and other diagnostic tools, including complete blood count, amylase, and thyroid-stimulating hormone level, glucose with other metabolic studies, upper endoscopy, and gastric-emptying scintigraphy.

▲ Consider abdominal massage for relief of constipation.

- ▲ Obtain a nutritional consult, considering a small particle–size diet or diets lower or higher in liquids or solids, depending on gastric motility.
- ▲ If the client is unable to eat or retain food, consult with the registered dietitian and healthcare provider, considering further nutritional support in the form of enteral or parenteral feedings for the client with gastroparesis.
- ▲ If the client is receiving gastric enteral nutrition, see the care plan Risk for **Aspiration.**
- ▲ Administer medications that increase gastrointestinal motility as ordered (Nagarwala, Dev, & Markin, 2016).

Postoperative Ileus

- • Observe for complications of delayed intestinal motility. Symptoms include vague abdominal pain and distention, nausea, vomiting, anorexia, sometimes bloating, and tympany to percussion. Clients may or may not pass flatus and some stool (Van Bree et al., 2014).
- ▲ Recommend chewing gum for the abdominal surgery client who is experiencing an ileus, is not at risk for aspiration, and has normal dentition.
- • Help the client out of bed to walk at least two times per day. Assist client to sit in a rocking chair to rock back and forth.
- ▲ If postoperative ileus is associated with opioid pain medication, ensure opioids are decreased or ideally discontinued. Use nonsteroidal antiinflammatory drugs for pain as feasible and if not contraindicated (Cagir, 2016).
- ▲ Note serum electrolyte levels, especially potassium and magnesium.

Increased Gastrointestinal Motility

- ▲ Observe for complications of gastric surgeries such as dumping syndrome.
- • Watch for nausea, vomiting, bloating, cramping, diarrhea, dizziness, and fatigue.
- • Monitor for low blood sugar, weakness, sweating, and dizziness 1 to 3 hours after eating because this is when late rapid gastric emptying may occur. Late rapid gastric emptying is associated with low blood sugar (Schattner & Grossman, 2016).
- ▲ Order a nutritional consult to discuss diet changes. The diet may vary depending on the kind of surgery causing dumping syndrome.

G

- ▲ Give intravenous fluids as ordered for the client complaining of diarrhea with weakness and dizziness. Monitor electrolyte panel and acid-base balance.
  - ❍ Offer bathroom, commode, or bedpan assistance, depending on frequency, amount of diarrhea, and condition of client.
  - ❍ Monitor rectal area for decreased skin integrity, and apply barrier creams as needed to protect and treat skin.
  - ❍ Consider a bowel management system for bed-bound patients with frequent loose stools. This will protect the perineal skin and minimize spread of infection.
  - • Refer to the care plans for the nursing diagnoses of Deficient **Fluid** volume, **Nausea,** Impaired **Skin** integrity, and **Diarrhea** as relevant.

Pediatric

- • Assess infants and children with suspected delayed gastric emptying for fullness and vomiting. Babies and children with delayed gastric emptying take longer to get hungry again and throw up undigested or partially digested food several hours after feeding (Westfal & Goldstein, 2017).
- ▲ Observe for nutritional and fluid deficits with assessment of skin turgor, mucous membranes, fontanels, furrows of the tongue, electrolyte panel, fluid status, input and output, and daily weights (Islam, 2015).
- ▲ Recommend gentle massage for preterm infants as appropriate.

Geriatric

- • Closely monitor diet and medication use/side effects because they affect the gastrointestinal system. Watch for constipation.
- ▲ Watch for symptoms of dysphagia, gastroesophageal reflux disease, dyspepsia, irritable bowel syndrome, maldigestion, and reduced absorption of nutrients.

Client/Family Teaching and Discharge Planning

- • Teach the client and caregivers about medications, reinforcing side effects as they relate to gastrointestinal function.
- • Teach client and caregivers to report signs and symptoms that may indicate further complications including increased abdominal girth, projectile vomiting, and unrelieved acute cramping pain (bowel obstruction).
- • Review signs and symptoms of dehydration with client and caregivers.

Risk for Unstable Blood Glucose Level

NANDA-I Definition

Susceptible to variation in serum levels of glucose from the normal range, which may compromise health

Risk Factors

Excessive stress; excessive weight gain; excessive weight loss; inadequate adherence to treatment regimen; inadequate blood glucose self-monitoring; inadequate diabetes self-management; inadequate dietary intake; inadequate knowledge of disease management; inadequate knowledge of modifiable factors; ineffective medication self-management; sedentary lifestyle

G

At-Risk Population

Individuals experiencing rapid growth period; individuals in intensive care units; individuals of African descent; individuals with altered mental status; individuals with compromised physical health status; individuals with delayed cognitive development; individuals with family history of diabetes mellitus; individuals with history of autoimmune disorders; individuals with history of gestational diabetes; individuals with history of hypoglycemia; individuals with history of pre-pregnancy overweight; low birth weight infants; Native American individuals; pregnant women >22 years of age; premature infants; women with hormonal shifts indicative of normal life stage changes

Associated Condition

Cardiogenic shock; diabetes mellitus; infections; pancreatic diseases; pharmaceutical preparations; polycystic ovary syndrome; pre-eclampsia; pregnancy-induced hypertension; surgical procedures

Client Outcomes

Client Will (Specify Time Frame)

- For most adults, maintain the following glucose targets (American Diabetes Association [ADA], 2017, S52); consult primary care provider for client-specific goals:
  - A1C less than 7% (normal level <5.7%)
  - Preprandial blood glucose between 80 and 130 mg/dL
  - Peak postprandial (1–2 hours after beginning of meal) glucose below 180 mg/dL
- For children and adolescents with type 1 diabetes, maintain the following glucose targets (ADA, 2017, S107):

- A1C less than 7.5%; a goal of less than 7% is appropriate if it can be achieved without excessive hypoglycemia
- Maintain blood glucose for children and adolescents as follows (ADA, 2017, S107):
  - Preprandial between 90 and 130 mg/dL
  - Bedtime/overnight between 90 and 150 mg/dL
- In pregnant women, maintain blood glucose as follows (ADA, 2017, S116):
  - Preprandial ≤95 mg/dL
  - One-hour postprandial level at or below 140 mg/dL
  - Two-hour postprandial at or below 120 mg/dL
- In pregnant mothers with preexisting type 1 or 2 diabetes blood glucose as follows (ADA, 2017, S115):
  - Fasting ≤95 mg/dL
  - One-hour postprandial ≤140 mg/dL
  - Two-hour postprandial glucose at ≤120 mg/dL
- In older adults, maintain blood glucose values as follows (ADA, 2017, S101):
  - Healthy older adults: preprandial blood glucose 90 to 130 mg/dL; bedtime 90 to 150 mg/dL
  - Older adults with complex coexisting chronic illness: preprandial blood glucose 90 to 150 mg/dL; bedtime 100 to 180 mg/dL
  - Older adult end-stage chronic illness or moderate to severe cognitive impairment: preprandial blood glucose 100 to 180 mg/dL; bedtime 110 to 200 mg/dL
- Maintain blood glucose in critically ill hospitalized clients between 140 and 180 mg/dL (ADA, 2017, S121)

Nursing Interventions

▲ Monitor blood glucose in hospitalized patients who are eating, before meals; who are not eating, every 4 to 6 hours; and who are receiving intravenous (IV) insulin, every 30 minutes to 2 hours.

▲ In patients receiving multiple-dose insulin (MDI) or insulin pump therapy, obtain blood glucose before meals and snacks, at bedtime, occasionally after meals, before exercise or critical tasks such as driving, if low blood glucose is suspected, and after treatment for low blood glucose until normoglycemic.

▲ Consider continuous glucose monitoring (CGM) in clients with type 1 diabetes on intensive insulin regimens.

▲ Evaluate A1C level for glucose control over previous 3 months.

- ▲ Consider monitoring 2 hours after the start of meals in individuals who have premeal glucose values within target but have A1C values above target.
- • Monitor for signs and symptoms of hypoglycemia, such as shakiness, dizziness, sweating, hunger, headache, pallor, behavior changes, confusion, or seizures.
- • If the client is experiencing signs and symptoms of hypoglycemia, test glucose; if the result is below 70 mg/dL, administer 15 to 20 g glucose. Pure glucose is the preferred treatment, but any form of carbohydrate that contains glucose will suffice (a cup of fruit juice or regular [not diet] soda, one cup of milk, a small piece of fruit, or three to four glucose tablets). Avoid treating with foods that contain fat. Repeat test in 15 minutes and repeat treatment if indicated. Once blood glucose returns to normal, the individual should consume a meal or snack to prevent recurrence of hypoglycemia.
- ▲ Clients who experience asymptomatic hypoglycemia should raise their glucose targets to avoid hypoglycemia for several weeks.
- • Avoid carbohydrate foods that are also high in protein to prevent or treat hypoglycemia.
- • Monitor for signs and symptoms of hyperglycemia, such as increased thirst or urination, or high blood or urine glucose levels.
- ▲ Monitor fluid balance and replace fluids in clients with diabetic ketoacidosis.
- ▲ Avoid use of sliding-scale insulin alone in hospitalized patients.
- • Prime IV tubing with 20 mL of diluted insulin solution before initiating insulin drip.
- ▲ Evaluate the client's medication regimen for medications that can alter blood glucose. Some asthma medications, some antipsychotic and antidepressant agents, thiazide diuretics, and glucocorticoids, among others, can cause hyperglycemia. Aspirin and beta-blockers are among agents that can cause hypoglycemia (National Prescribing Service [NPS], 2017).
- ▲ Refer client to a dietitian for individualized medical nutrition therapy (MNT) instruction.
- ▲ Refer people with type 1 diabetes and those with type 2 diabetes who are prescribed a flexible insulin therapy program for education on how to use carbohydrate counting (and in some

G

cases fat and protein gram estimation) to determine mealtime insulin dosing.

- ▲ Refer overweight and obese clients with type 2 diabetes for diet, activity, and behavioral therapy.
- • For interventions regarding foot care, refer to the care plan Ineffective peripheral **Tissue Perfusion.**

Geriatric

- • Watch for age-related cognitive changes that can impair self-management of diabetes.
- ▲ Consider relaxing glucose targets for older adults.
- ▲ In clients with diabetes who require tube feedings, use a diabetes-specific formulation such as Glucerna or Glytrol.

Pediatric

- ▲ Treat hypoglycemia in newborn infants with 0.5 mL/kg oral (buccal) dextrose gel.
- • Teach children and adolescents (and their parents) with type 1 diabetes or on intensive insulin regimens (MDI or insulin pump therapy) to perform SMBG before meals and snacks, occasionally postprandially, at bedtime, before exercise, when they suspect low blood glucose, after treating low blood glucose until they are normoglycemic, and before critical tasks such as driving.
- • Teach parents and children that children and adolescents with type 1 and 2 diabetes should spend 60 minutes daily in moderate to vigorous aerobic activity, and at least 3 days per week in muscle/bone strengthening activity.

Home Care

- ▲ Teach family and others having close contact with the person with diabetes how to use an emergency glucagon kit (as prescribed).

Multicultural

- • Provide culturally appropriate diabetes health education.
- • Involve community health workers, peers, and lay leaders in diabetes education and support in underserved communities.

Client/Family Teaching and Discharge Planning

- • Provide "survival skills" education or review for hospitalized clients, including information about (1) identification of the healthcare provider who will provide diabetes care after discharge; (2) diagnosis of diabetes, SMBG, explanation of home blood glucose goals, and when to call provider; (3) information on consistent nutrition habits; (4) when and how to take medications including insulin administration; (5) proper use and disposal of needles and syringes if applicable, (6) definition, recognition, treatment, and prevention of hyperglycemia and hypoglycemia; and (7) sick-day management.

- • Refer clients for individual or group Diabetes Self-Management Education (DSME) and Diabetes Self-Management Support (DSMS) of at least 10 hours' duration.
- • Evaluate clients' monitoring technique initially and at regular intervals.
- • Teach patients with type 2 diabetes the importance of avoiding sedentary behavior, to move around briefly at least every 20 to 30 minutes, and to walk for 15 minutes after meals.
- • Teach clients the importance of at least 150 minutes/week of aerobic physical activity spread over at least 3 days per week.
- ▲ Discuss recommending resistance training with the client's provider.
- • Teach clients with type 1 diabetes to test for blood ketones before exercise if they have unexplained hyperglycemia (≥250 mg/dL).
- ▲ Teach clients with type 1 diabetes to check blood glucose prior to exercise. Blood glucose levels prior to exercise should ideally be between 90 and 250 mg/dL (5.0 and 13.9 mmol/L). Discuss carbohydrate use prior to exercise with physician.
- • Teach clients to use alcohol with caution.

G

Maladaptive Grieving

NANDA-I Definition

A disorder that occurs after the death of a significant other, in which the experience of distress accompanying bereavement fails to follow sociocultural expectations.

Defining Characteristics

Anxiety; decreased life role performance; depressive symptoms; diminished intimacy levels; disbelief; excessive stress; experiencing symptoms the deceased experienced; expresses anger; expresses being overwhelmed; expresses distress about the deceased person; expresses feeling detached from others; expresses feeling of emptiness; expresses feeling stunned; expresses shock; fatigue;

gastrointestinal symptoms; grief avoidance; increased morbidity; longing for the deceased person; mistrust of others; nonacceptance of a death; persistent painful memories; preoccupation with thoughts about a deceased person; rumination about deceased person; searching for a deceased person; self-blame

Related Factors

Difficulty dealing with concurrent crises; excessive emotional disturbance; high attachment anxiety; inadequate social support; low attachment avoidance

At-Risk Population

Economically disadvantaged individuals; individuals experiencing socially unacceptable loss; individuals experiencing unexpected sudden death of significant other; individuals experiencing violent death of significant other; individuals unsatisfied with death notification; individuals who witnessed uncontrolled symptoms of the deceased; individuals with history of childhood abuse; individuals with history of unresolved grieving; individuals with significant pre-death dependency on the deceased; individuals with strong emotional proximity to the deceased; individuals with unresolved conflict with the deceased; individuals without paid employment; women

Client Outcomes

Client Will (Specify Time Frame)

- Express appropriate feelings of guilt, fear, anger, or sadness
- Identify somatic distress associated with grief (e.g., anxiety, changes in appetite, insomnia, nightmares, loss of libido, decreased energy, altered activity levels)
- Seek support in dealing with grief-associated issues
- Identify personal strengths and effective coping strategies
- Function at a normal developmental level and begin to successfully and increasingly perform activities of daily living

Nursing Interventions

- Assess for signs of maladaptive grieving that include symptoms that persist at least 6 months after the death and are experienced at least daily or to a disabling degree. Symptoms include feeling emotionally numb, stunned, shocked, and that life is meaningless; dysfunctional thoughts and maladaptive behaviors; experiencing mistrust and estrangement from others; anger and bitterness over the loss; identity confusion; avoidance of the reality of the loss, or excessive proximity seeking to try to feel closer to the deceased, sometimes focused on wishes to die or suicidal statements and behavior; or difficulty moving on with life.

- ▲ Determine the client's state of grieving. Use a tool such as the Prolonged Grief Disorder (PGD) scale (Jordan & Litz, 2014), the Grief Support in Health Care Scale (Anderson et al., 2010), the Hogan Grief Reaction Checklist (Hogan, Worden, & Schmidt, 2004), and the Beck Depression Inventory.
- ▲ Determine whether the client is experiencing depression, suicidal tendencies, or other emotional disorders. Refer the client for counseling or therapy as appropriate.
- • Educate the client and his or her support systems that grief resolution is not a sequential process and that the positive outcome of grief resolution is the integration of the deceased into the ongoing life of the griever.
- ▲ Assess caregivers, particularly younger caregivers, for pessimistic thinking and additional stressful life events. Refer for appropriate support.
- • See the interventions and rationales in the care plans for Chronic **Sorrow.**

Pediatric/Parent

- ▲ Refer grieving children and parents to a program to help facilitate grieving if desired, especially if the death was traumatic.
- • Encourage grieving parents to take part in activities that are supportive, such as faith-based activities.
- • Encourage grieving parents to seek mental health services as needed.
- • Help the adolescent determine sources of support and how to use them effectively. If the client is an adolescent exposed to a peer's suicide, watch for symptoms of traumatic grief and post-traumatic stress disorder, which include numbness, preoccupation with the deceased, functional impairment, and poor adjustment to the loss.

Geriatric

- • Assess for deterioration in bereaved older adults' self-care.
- • Those who have lived with older adults with dementia and experienced significant feelings of loss before the loved one's death may be at risk for more intense feelings of grief after the death of the client with dementia.

G

- Monitor the older client for maladaptive grieving manifesting in physical and mental health problems.

Multicultural

- Assess for the influence of cultural beliefs, norms, and values on the client's grief and mourning practices.
- Encourage discussion of the grief process.
- Identify whether the client had been notified of the health status of the deceased and was able to be present during illness and death.

Home Care

- Consider providing support via the Internet.

Risk for Maladaptive Grieving

NANDA-I Definition

Susceptible to a disorder that occurs after the death of a significant other, in which the experience of distress accompanying bereavement fails to follow sociocultural expectations, which may compromise health.

Risk Factors

Difficulty dealing with concurrent crises; excessive emotional disturbance; high attachment anxiety; inadequate social support; low attachment avoidance

At-Risk Population

Economically disadvantaged individuals; individuals experiencing socially unacceptable loss; individuals experiencing unexpected sudden death of significant other; individuals experiencing violent death of significant other; individuals unsatisfied with death notification; individuals who witnessed uncontrolled symptoms of the deceased; individuals with history of childhood abuse; individuals with history of unresolved grieving; individuals with significant pre-death dependency on the deceased; individuals with strong emotional proximity to the deceased; individuals with unresolved conflict with the deceased; individuals without paid employment; women

Client Outcomes, Nursing Interventions, Client/Family Teaching and Discharge Planning

Refer to care plan for Maladaptive **Grieving.**

Deficient Community Health

NANDA-I Definition

Presence of one or more health problems or factors that deter wellness or increase the risk of health problems experienced by an aggregate

Defining Characteristics

Health problem experienced by groups or populations; program unavailable to eliminate health problem(s) of a group or population; program unavailable to enhance wellness of a group or population; program unavailable to prevent health problem(s) of a group or population; program unavailable to reduce health problem(s) of a group or population; risk of hospitalization experienced by groups or populations; risk of physiological states experienced by groups or populations; risk of psychological states experienced by groups or populations

Related Factors

Inadequate consumer satisfaction with program; inadequate program budget; inadequate program evaluation plan; inadequate program outcome data; inadequate social support for program; insufficient access to healthcare provider; insufficient community experts; insufficient resources; program incompletely addresses health problem

Client Outcomes

Community/Adolescents/Minority Clients Will (Specify Time Frame)

- Provide programs for healthy behaviors
- Demonstrate goal setting
- Describe and comply with healthy behaviors
- Describe and demonstrate compliance with hepatitis B virus (HBV) education and testing

Nursing Interventions

Refer to care plans: Readiness for Enhanced community **Coping,** Ineffective Community **Coping,** Ineffective **Health** maintenance behaviors, Ineffective **Home** Maintenance Behaviors, Risk for other-directed **Violence**

- Assess for the presence of demographic variables that predict community mortality.
- Assess for needs related to the community's priority health concerns.
- Assess patients accessing health services for a history of military service and provide the necessary referrals and information.
- Implement community engagement techniques for collaboration with stakeholders to design, develop, and adapt relevant health interventions.
- Encourage attendance at community-based exercise programs.

- Implement community engagement techniques in conjunction with tailored interventions to address health deficiencies.
- Collaborate with other community-based programs to use the Short Message Service (SMS) to broadcast targeted health messages to reach large numbers of community members.

Pediatric

▲ Consider use of a clinical–community collaboration to address health deficiencies in underserved populations with children.

▲ Screen at-risk pediatric populations for lead exposure.

Geriatric

▲ Assess community-dwelling older individuals for cognitive impairment using the Brief Cognitive Assessment Tool–Short Form (BCAT-SF).

▲ Assess community-dwelling older individuals with the Identification of Seniors at Risk (ISAR) screening tool when they present for treatment in the emergency department.

▲ Screen community-dwelling older individuals for fall risk with the Timed Up and Go Test (TUG) or the Functional Gait Assessment (FGA).

Multicultural

- Provide culturally and linguistically appropriate risk reduction programs to individuals living in rural and border regions of the country.
- Use decision aids (DAs) (personal counseling, multimedia, and print materials) to facilitate communication between patients and healthcare providers to determine a plan for healthcare.

Home Care and Client/Family Teaching and Discharge Planning

- The previously mentioned interventions may be adapted for home care and client/family teaching.

Risk-Prone Health Behavior

NANDA-I Definition

Impaired ability to modify lifestyle and/or actions in a manner that improves the level of wellness

Defining Characteristics

Failure to achieve optimal sense of control; failure to take action that prevents health problem; minimizes health status change; nonacceptance of health status change; smoking; substance misuse

Related Factors

Inadequate comprehension; insufficient social support; low self-efficacy; negative perception of healthcare provider; negative perception of recommended healthcare strategy; social anxiety; stressors

At-Risk Population

Family history of alcoholism; economically disadvantaged

Client Outcomes

Client Will (Specify Time Frame)

- State acceptance of change in health status
- Request assistance in altering behaviors to adapt to change
- State personal goals for dealing with change in health status and means to prevent further health problems
- State experience of a period of grief that is proportional to the actual or perceived effect of the loss
- Report and/or demonstrate behavior changes mutually agreed upon with nurse as evidence of positive adaptation

Nursing Interventions

- Assess the client's perceptions of health, wellness, disability, and major barriers to health and wellness.
- Use motivational interviewing to help the client identify and change unhealthy behaviors.
- Encourage mindfulness and meditation to help the client cope with changes in health status.
- Allow the client adequate time to express feelings about the change in health status.
- Use open-ended questions to allow the client free expression (e.g., "Tell me about your last hospitalization" or "How does this time compare?").
- Help the client work through the stages of grief that occur as part of a psychological adaptation to illness or life change. Assess for signs of nonacceptance to illness or change.
- Assess the client for depression and refer for counseling or medical follow-up, as appropriate.
- Discuss the client's current goals and assist in modification as needed. Use a goal attainment scaling (GAS) approach, which is a therapeutic method that refers to the development of a written follow-up guide between the client and the nurse and is used for monitoring client progress.

- ▲ Encourage participation in appropriate wellness programs associated with health changes.
- • Give the client positive feedback for accomplishments, no matter how small. Support the client and family and promote their strengths and coping skills.
- ▲ Promote use of positive spiritual influences, as appropriate.
- ▲ Refer to community resources. Provide general and contact information for ease of use.

Pediatric

- • Include social history in client assessment to help identify past abuse and traumatic experiences.
- • Encourage parents to process and express grief, uncertainty, and discouragement after learning about their child's diagnosis, prognosis, and treatments. Provide parents with resources and tools to help further their understanding of the illness.
- • Provide parents of critically ill children with individualized coping resources.
- • Use distraction with children undergoing procedures or treatment with unpleasant side effects.

Geriatric

- ▲ Assess for signs of depression resulting from illness-associated changes and make appropriate referrals.
- • Support activities that promote a sense of purpose for older adults.
- • Encourage social support.

Multicultural

- • Assess for the influence of cultural beliefs, norms, and values on the client's ability to modify health behavior.
- • Assess the role of fatalism on the client's ability to modify health behavior. Fatalistic perspectives, which involve the belief that you cannot control your own fate, may influence health behaviors in some cultures.
- • Encourage spirituality as a source of support for coping.
- • Negotiate with the client regarding the aspects of health behavior that will need to be modified.
- • Acknowledge client's identified gender and sexual orientation and refer client and family members to support networks that have experience with lesbian, gay, bisexual, or transgender (LGBT) issues, as appropriate.

Home Care

- The previously mentioned interventions may be adapted for home care use.
- Take the client's perspective into consideration and use a holistic approach in assessing and responding to client planning for the future.
- Assist the client/family to adapt to his or her diagnosis and to live with their disease.
- Ensure that evaluations of the client's ability to perform activities of daily living are age appropriate and consider existing, as well as new, diagnoses.
- Refer to care plan for **Powerlessness.**

Client/Family Teaching and Discharge Planning

- Assess family/caregivers for coping and teaching/learning styles.
- Foster communication between the client/family and medical staff.
- Educate and prepare families regarding the appearance and function of the client and the environment before initial exposure.
- Teach a client and his or her family relaxation techniques (controlled breathing, guided imagery) and help them practice.
- Allow the client to proceed at his or her own pace in learning; provide time for return demonstrations (e.g., self-injection of insulin). Tailor teaching and learning materials as appropriate for client and caregiver literacy level.

Ineffective Health Self-Management

NANDA-I Definition

Unsatisfactory management of symptoms, treatment regimen, physical, psychosocial, and spiritual consequences and lifestyle changes inherent in living with a chronic condition.

Defining Characteristics

Exacerbation of disease signs; exacerbation of disease symptoms; exhibits disease sequelae; expresses dissatisfaction with quality of life; failure to attend appointments with health care provider; failure to include treatment regimen into daily living; failure to take action that reduces risk factor; inattentive to disease signs; inattentive to disease symptoms; ineffective choices in daily living for meeting health goal

Related Factors

Competing demands; competing lifestyle preferences; conflict between cultural beliefs and health practices; conflict between health behaviors and social norms; conflict between spiritual beliefs and treatment regimen; decreased perceived quality of life; depressive symptoms; difficulty accessing community resources; difficulty managing complex treatment regimen; difficulty navigating complex health care systems; difficulty with decision-making; inadequate commitment to a plan of action; inadequate health literacy; inadequate knowledge of treatment regimen; inadequate number of cues to action; inadequate role models; inadequate social support; individuals with limited decision-making experience; limited ability to perform aspects of treatment regimen; low self efficacy; negative feelings toward treatment regimen; neurobehavioral manifestations; nonacceptance of condition; perceived barrier to treatment regimen; perceived social stigma associated with condition; substance misuse; unrealistic perception of seriousness of condition; unrealistic perception of susceptibility to sequelae; unrealistic perception of treatment benefit

At-Risk Population

Children; economically disadvantaged individuals; individuals experiencing adverse reactions to medications; individuals with caregiving responsibilities; individuals with history of ineffective health self-management; individuals with low educational level; older adults

Associated Conditions

Asymptomatic disease; developmental disabilities; high acuity illness; neurocognitive disorders; polypharmacy; significant comorbidity

Client Outcomes

Client Will (Specify Time Frame)

- Describe daily food and fluid intake that meets therapeutic goals
- Describe activity/exercise patterns that meet therapeutic goals
- Describe scheduling of medications that meets therapeutic goals
- Verbalize ability to manage therapeutic regimens
- Collaborate with health professionals to decide on a therapeutic regimen that is congruent with health goals and lifestyle

Nursing Interventions

Note: This diagnosis does not have the same meaning as the diagnosis **Noncompliance.** This diagnosis is made with the client, so if the client does not agree with the diagnosis, it should not be made. The emphasis is on helping the client direct his or her own life and health, not on the client's compliance with the provider's instructions.

▲ Establish a collaborative partnership with the client for purposes of meeting health-related goals.

- Explore the client's perception of their illness experience and identify uncertainties and needs through open-ended questions.
- Assist the client to enhance self-efficacy or confidence in his or her own ability to manage the illness.
- Review factors of the health belief model (HBM) (individual perceptions of seriousness and susceptibility, demographic and other modifying factors, and perceived benefits and barriers) with the client.
- Help the client identify and modify barriers to effective self-management.
- Help the client self-manage his or her own health through education about strategies for changing habits such as overeating, sedentary lifestyle, and smoking.
- Develop a contract with the client to maintain motivation for changes in behavior.
- Use focus groups to evaluate the implementation of self-management programs.
- Refer to the care plan ineffective Family **Health** self-management.

Geriatric

- Identify the reasons for behaviors that are not therapeutic, and discuss alternatives.

Multicultural

- Assess the influence of cultural beliefs, norms, and values on the individual's perceptions of the therapeutic regimen.
- Provide health information that is consistent with the health literacy of clients.
- Assess for barriers that may interfere with client follow-up of treatment recommendations.
- Use electronic monitoring and dosing to improve management of medications.
- Validate the client's feelings regarding the ability to manage his or her own care and the impact on lifestyle.

Home Care

- Prepare and instruct clients and family members in the use of a medication box. Set up an appropriate schedule for filling the medication box, and post medication times and doses in an accessible area (e.g., attached by a magnet to the refrigerator).

- Refer to healthcare professionals for questions and self-care management.

Client/Family Teaching and Discharge Planning

- Identify the client and/or family's current knowledge and adjust teaching accordingly. Teach the client and family about all aspects of the therapeutic regimen, providing as much knowledge as the client and family will accept, in a culturally congruent manner.
- Teach ways to adjust activities of daily living (ADLs) for inclusion in therapeutic regimens.
- Teach safety in taking medications.

Readiness for Enhanced Health Self-Management

NANDA-I Definition

A pattern of satisfactory management of symptoms, treatment regimen, physical, psychosocial, and spiritual consequences and lifestyle changes inherent in living with a chronic condition, which can be strengthened.

Defining Characteristics

Expresses desire to enhance acceptance of the condition; expresses desire to enhance choices of daily living for meeting health goals; expresses desire to enhance commitment to follow-up care; expresses desire to enhance decision making; expresses desire to enhance inclusion of treatment regimen into daily living; expresses desire to enhance management of risk factors; expresses desire to enhance management of signs; expresses desire to enhance management of symptoms; expresses desire to enhance recognition of disease signs; expresses desire to enhance recognition of disease symptoms; expresses desire to enhance satisfaction with quality of life

Client Outcomes

Client Will (Specify Time Frame)

- Describe integration of therapeutic regimen into daily living
- Demonstrate continued commitment to integration of therapeutic regimen into daily living routines

Nursing Interventions

▲ Acknowledge the expertise that the client and family bring to health management.

- Review factors that contribute to the likelihood of health promotion and health protection. Use Pender's Health Promotion Model and

Becker's Health Belief Model to identify contributing factors (Khodaveisi et al., 2017).
- Further develop and reinforce contributing factors that might change with ongoing management of the therapeutic regimen (e.g., knowledge, self-efficacy, self-esteem, and perceived benefits).
- Review the client's strengths in the management of the therapeutic regimen.
- Collaborate with the client to identify strategies to maintain strengths and develop additional strengths as indicated.
- Identify contributing factors that may need to be improved now or in the future.
- Help the client maintain existing support and seek additional supports as needed.

Geriatric
- Facilitate the client and family to obtain health insurance and drug payment plans whenever needed and possible.

Multicultural
- Assess client's cultural perspectives on health management.
- Assess health literacy in clients of diverse backgrounds.
- Validate the client's feelings regarding the ability to manage his or her own care and the impact on current lifestyle.
- Facilitate the client and family to obtain financial assistance in the form of health insurance and drug payment plans whenever needed and possible.
- Use electronic monitoring to improve medication adherence.

Community Teaching
- Review therapeutic regimens and their optimal integration with daily living routines.
- Teach disease processes and therapeutic regimens to clients and peer supporters for management of disease processes.

Ineffective Family Health Self-Management

NANDA-I Definition
Unsatisfactory management of symptoms, treatment regimen, physical, psychosocial and spiritual consequences and lifestyle changes inherent in living with one or more family members' chronic condition.

Defining Characteristics

Caregiver strain; decrease in attention to illness in one or more family members; depressive symptoms of caregiver; exacerbation of disease signs of one or more family members; exacerbation of disease symptoms of one or more family members; failure to take action to reduce risk factor in one or more family members; ineffective choices in daily living for meeting health goal of family unit; one or more family members report dissatisfaction with quality of life

Related Factors

Cognitive dysfunction of one or more caregivers; competing demands on family unit; competing lifestyle preferences within family unit; conflict between health behaviors and social norms; conflict between spiritual beliefs and treatment regimen; difficulty accessing community resources; difficulty dealing with role changes associated with condition; difficulty managing complex treatment regimen; difficulty navigating complex health care systems; difficulty with decision-making; family conflict; inadequate commitment to a plan of action; inadequate health literacy of caregiver; inadequate knowledge of treatment regimen; inadequate number of cues to action; inadequate social support; ineffective communication skills; ineffective coping skills; limited ability to perform aspects of treatment regimen; low self efficacy; negative feelings toward treatment regimen; nonacceptance of condition; perceived barrier to treatment regimen; perceived social stigma associated with condition; substance misuse; unrealistic perception of seriousness of condition; unrealistic perception of susceptibility to sequelae; unrealistic perception of treatment benefit; unsupportive family relations

At-Risk Population

Economically disadvantaged families; families with member experiencing delayed diagnosis; families with members experiencing low educational level; families with members who have limited decision-making experience; families with premature infant

Associated Conditions

Chronic disease; mental disorders; neurocognitive disorders; terminal illness

Client Outcomes

Client Will (Specify Time Frame)

- Make adjustments in usual activities (e.g., diet, activity, stress management) to incorporate therapeutic regimens of its members
- Reduce illness symptoms of family members
- Desire to manage therapeutic regimens of its members
- Describe a decrease in the difficulties of managing therapeutic regimens
- Describe actions to reduce risk factors

Nursing Interventions

- Base family interventions on knowledge of the family, family context, family dynamics, family structure, and family function.
- Use a family approach when helping an individual with a health problem that requires therapeutic management.
- Review with family members the congruence and incongruence of family behaviors and health-related goals.
- Acknowledge the challenge of integrating therapeutic regimens with family behaviors.
- Review the symptoms of specific illnesses and work with the family toward development of greater self-efficacy in relation to these symptoms.
- Support family decisions to adjust therapeutic regimens as indicated.
- Advocate for the family in negotiating therapeutic regimens with health providers.
- Help the family mobilize social supports.
- Help family members modify perceptions as indicated.
- Use one or more theories of family dynamics to describe, explain, or predict family behaviors (e.g., theories of Bowen, Satir, and Minuchin).

▲ Collaborate with expert nurses or other consultants regarding strategies for working with families.

- Coaching methods can be used to help families improve their health.

Pediatric

- Support kangaroo care for infants at risk at birth. Keep infants in an upright position in skin-to-skin contact until they no longer tolerate it.

Geriatric

- Recommend that clients use the "Ask Me 3" program when communicating with their health providers (What is my main problem? What do I need to do? Why is it important for me to do this?).

Multicultural

- Acknowledge racial and ethnic differences at the onset of care.
- Ensure that all strategies for working with the family are congruent with the culture of the family.
- Facilitate modeling and role playing for the family regarding healthy ways to communicate and interact.
- Use the nursing intervention of cultural brokerage to help families deal with the healthcare system.

Client/Family Teaching and Discharge Planning

- Teach about all aspects of therapeutic regimens. Provide as much knowledge as family members will accept, adjust instruction to account for what the family already knows, and directions provide information in a culturally congruent manner.
- Teach ways to adjust family behaviors to include therapeutic regimens, such as safety in taking medications and teaching family members to act as self-advocates with health providers who prescribe therapeutic regimens.

H

Ineffective Health Maintenance Behaviors

NANDA-I Definition

Management of health knowledge, attitudes, and practices underlying health actions that is unsatisfactory for maintaining or improving well-being, or preventing illness and injury.

Defining Characteristics

Failure to take action that prevents health problem; failure to take action that reduces risk factor; inadequate commitment to a plan of action; inadequate health literacy; inadequate interest in improving health; inadequate knowledge about basic health practices; ineffective choices in daily living for meeting health goal; pattern of lack of health-seeking behavior

Related Factors

Competing demands; competing lifestyle preferences; conflict between cultural beliefs and health practices; conflict between health behaviors and social norms; conflicts between spiritual beliefs and health practices; depressive symptoms; difficulty accessing community resources; difficulty navigating complex health care systems; difficulty with decision-making; inadequate health resources; inadequate social support; inadequate trust in health care professional; individuals with limited decisionmaking experience; ineffective communication skills; ineffective coping strategies; ineffective family coping; low self efficacy; maladaptive grieving; neurobehavioral manifestations; perceived prejudice; perceived victimization; spiritual distress

At-Risk Population

Economically disadvantaged individuals; individuals from families with ineffective family coping; individuals with history of violence; men; older adults; young adults

Associated Conditions

Chronic disease; developmental disabilities; mental disorders

Client Outcomes

Client Will (Specify Time Frame)

- Discuss fear of or blocks to implementing health regimen
- Follow mutually agreed-on healthcare maintenance plan
- Meet goals for healthcare maintenance

Nursing Interventions

- Assess the client's feelings, values, and reasons for not following the prescribed plan of care. See Related Factors.
- Assess for family patterns, economic issues, and spiritual and cultural patterns that influence compliance with a given medical regimen.
- Involve the client in shared decision-making regarding health maintenance.
- Show genuine interest in the client's individual needs.
- Assist the client in finding methods to reduce stress.
- Help the client determine how to manage complex medication schedules (e.g., HIV/AIDS regimens or polypharmacy).
- Identify complementary healing modalities such as herbal remedies, acupuncture, healing touch, yoga, or cultural shamans that the client uses in addition to or instead of the prescribed allopathic regimen along with the client's perception of the complementary healing modalities.
- ▲ Refer the client to appropriate medical and social services as needed, providing adequate information on details about the service, including scheduling.
- Identify support groups related to the disease process.
- Use social media such as text messaging to remind clients of scheduled appointments.
- Use telehealth interventions to facilitate self-care.

Geriatric

- Assess the client's perception of health and health maintenance.
- Assist client to identify both life- and health-related goals.
- Provide information that supports informed decision-making.
- Discuss realistic goal setting for changes in health maintenance with the client and support person.
- Educate the client about the symptoms of life-threatening illness, such as myocardial infarction (MI), and the need for timeliness in seeking care.

Multicultural

- Assess influence of cultural beliefs, norms, and values on the client's ability to modify health behavior.
- Assess the effect of fatalism on the client's ability to modify health behavior.
- Clarify culturally related health beliefs and practices.
- Provide culturally appropriate education and healthcare services.

Home Care

- The interventions described previously may be adapted for home care use.
- ▲ Provide nurse-led case management.
- Provide a health promotion focus for the client with disabilities, with the goals of reducing secondary conditions (e.g., obesity, hypertension, pressure sores), maintaining functional independence, providing opportunities for leisure and enjoyment, and enhancing overall quality of life.
- Provide support and individual training for caregivers before the client is discharged from the hospital.
- Assist the client to develop confidence in the ability to manage the health condition.

Client/Family Teaching and Discharge Planning

- Provide the family with credible sources in which information can be obtained from social media. (Most libraries have Internet access with printing capabilities.)
- ▲ Develop collaborative multidisciplinary partnerships.
- Tailor both the information provided and the method of delivery of information to the specific client and/or family.
- Explain nonthreatening qualities before introducing more anxiety-producing information regarding possible side effects of the disease or medical regimen.

Ineffective Home Maintenance Behaviors

NANDA-I Definition

An unsatisfactory pattern of knowledge and activities for the safe upkeep of one's residence.

Defining Characteristics

Cluttered environment; difficulty maintaining a comfortable environment; failure to request assistance with home maintenance; home task-related anxiety; home task-related stress; impaired ability to regulate finances; negative affect toward home maintenance; neglected laundry; pattern of hygiene-related diseases; trash accumulation; unsafe cooking equipment; unsanitary environment

Related Factors

Competing demands; depressive symptoms; difficulty with decision-making; environmental constraints; impaired physical mobility; impaired postural balance; inadequate knowledge of home maintenance; inadequate knowledge of social resources; inadequate organizing skills; inadequate role models; inadequate social support; insufficient physical endurance; neurobehavioral manifestations; powerlessness; psychological distress

At-Risk Population

Economically disadvantaged individuals; individuals living alone; older adults

Associated Conditions

Depression; mental disorders; neoplasms; neurocognitive disorders; sensation disorders; vascular diseases

Client Outcomes

Client Will (Specify Time Frame)

- Maintain a healthy home environment
- Use community resources to assist with home care needs
- Maintain a safe home environment

Nursing Interventions

- • Assess the concerns of family members, especially the primary caregiver, about home care for a long time.
- • Provide home safety education and safety equipment when possible.
- ▲ Consider a predischarge home assessment referral to determine the need for accessibility and safety-related environmental changes.
- • Use an assessment tool to identify environmental safety hazards in the home.
- • Establish an individualized plan of care for improved home maintenance with the client and family based on the client's needs and the caregiver's capabilities.
- • Set up a system of relief for the main caregiver in the home and a plan for sharing household duties and/or outside assistance.
- ▲ Provide a multidisciplinary approach to target the home environment and the client's ability to function in the home.
- • Assess the quality of relationships among family members.

Geriatric

- All of the previously mentioned interventions are applicable for the geriatric population.
- Assess injury prevention knowledge and practices of the client and caregivers and provide information as appropriate.
- Assess functional ability to manage safely after hospital discharge.
- Explore community resources to assist with home maintenance (e.g., senior centers, Department of Aging, hospital case managers, friends and relatives, the Internet, or church parish nurse).
- Provide education related to home modification.
- Focus on the interaction between the older client and the technology, assisting the client to be an active participant in choices of and uses for technology.
- See the care plans for Risk for **Injury** and Risk for Adult **Falls.**

Multicultural

- Acknowledge the stresses unique to racial/ethnic communities.

Home Care

- The previously mentioned interventions incorporate these resources.
- See care plans **Contamination** and Risk for **Contamination.**

Client/Family Teaching and Discharge Planning

- Identify support groups within the community to assist families in the caregiver role.
- Provide counseling and support for clients and for caregivers of clients. Focus teaching on environmental hazards identified in the nursing assessment. Areas may include, but are not limited to, the following:
    - **Home Safety.** Identify the need for and use of common safety measures in the home.
    - **Food Safety.** Instruct client to avoid microbial foodborne illness by storing and cooking food at the proper temperature; regularly washing hands, food contact surfaces, and fruits and vegetables; and monitoring expiration dates.
- Teach clients to assess their homes for potential environmental health hazards in the home, including risks related to structure, moisture/mold, fire, pets, electrical, ventilation, pests, and lifestyle.
- See care plans **Contamination,** Risk for **Contamination,** Risk for Adult **Falls,** Risk for **Infection,** and Risk for **Injury.**

Readiness for Enhanced Hope

NANDA-I Definition

A pattern of expectations and desires for mobilizing energy to achieve positive outcomes, or avoid a potentially threatening or negative situation, which can be strengthened.

Defining Characteristics

Expresses desire to enhance ability to set achievable goals; expresses desire to enhance belief in possibilities; expresses desire to enhance congruency of expectations with goal; expresses desire to enhance deep inner strength; expresses desire to enhance giving and receiving of care/love; expresses desire to enhance initiative; expresses desire to enhance involvement with self-care; expresses desire to enhance positive outlook on life; expresses desire to enhance problem-solving to meet goal; expresses desire to enhance sense of meaning in life; expresses desire to enhance spirituality

Client Outcomes

Client Will (Specify Time Frame)

- Describe values, expectations, and meanings
- Set achievable goals that are consistent with values
- Design strategies to achieve goals
- Express belief in possibilities

Nursing Interventions

- Spend one-on-one time with the client. Use empathy; try to understand what the client is saying and communicate this understanding to the client to create a nonjudgmental, trusting environment to develop therapeutic relationships with the client.
- Assist clients to identify sources of gratitude in their lives using a future-oriented focus.
- Assist families to identify sources of gratitude in their lives.
- Screen the client for hope using a valid and reliable instrument as indicated.
- Focus on the positive aspects of hope.
- Assist the client to develop positive expectations outcomes and recognize the pathways to achieve the positive outcomes.
- Explore the meanings, functions, objects, sources, and nature of hope with patients as relates to their current situation.
- Teach individuals how to become aware of attention that is focused on unwanted aspects of life and how to redirect attention toward things that feel more wanted or desired by using a future-directed approach.

- Review the client's strengths and resources in conjunction with the client.
- Assist the client to consider alternatives and set long- and short-term goals that are important to him or her.
- Encourage engagement in positive and pleasant events.
- Facilitate sources of the client's resilience.
- Implement social supports and reintegration programs for postdeployment soldiers and veterans in a timely fashion.
- Encourage the client to adopt active coping strategies.
- Identify spiritual beliefs and practices.

Home Care

- The previously mentioned interventions may be adapted for home care use.

Client/Family Teaching and Discharge Planning

- Teach alternative coping strategies such as physical activity.
- ▲ Refer the client to self-help groups.
- Use a family-centered approach to provide information regarding the client's condition, treatment plan, and progress.
- Offer emotional support, active listening, and coping assistance to client families.

Hopelessness

NANDA-I Definition

The feeling that one will not experience positive emotions, or an improvement in one's condition.

Defining Characteristics

Anorexia; avoidance behaviors; decreased affective display; decreased initiative; decreased response to stimuli; decreased verbalization; depressive symptoms; expresses despondency; expresses diminished hope; expresses feeling of uncertain future; expresses inadequate motivation for the future; expresses negative expectations about self; expresses negative expectations about the future; expresses sense of incompetency in meeting goals; inadequate involvement with self-care; overestimates the likelihood of unfortunate events; passivity; reports altered sleep-wake cycle; suicidal behaviors; unable to imagine life in the future; underestimates the occurrence of positive events

Related Factors

Chronic stress; fear; inadequate social support; loss of belief in spiritual power; loss of belief in transcendent values; low self efficacy; prolonged immobility; social isolation; unaddressed violence; uncontrolled severe disease symptoms

At-Risk Population

Adolescents; displaced individuals; economically disadvantaged individuals; individuals experiencing infertility; individuals experiencing significant loss; individuals with history of attempted suicide; individuals with history of being abandoned; older adults; unemployed individuals

H

Associated Condition

Critical illness; depression; deterioration in physiological condition; feeding and eating disorders; mental disorders; neoplasms; terminal illness

Client Outcomes

Client Will (Specify Time Frame)

- Verbalize feelings
- Participate in care
- Make positive statements (e.g., "I can" or "I will try")
- Set goals
- Make eye contact, focus on speaker
- Maintain appropriate appetite for age and physical health
- Sleep appropriate length of time for age and physical health
- Express concern for another
- Initiate activity

Nursing Interventions

▲ Assess for, monitor, and document the potential for suicide. (Refer the client for appropriate treatment if a potential for suicide is identified.) Refer to the care plan risk for **Suicidal Behavior** for specific interventions.

▲ Assess and monitor potential for depression. (Refer the client for appropriate treatment if depression is identified.)

▲ Assess for hopelessness with the modified Beck Hopelessness Scale.

- Assess and monitor family caregivers for symptoms of hopelessness.
- Assess for pain and respond with appropriate measures for pain relief.
- Assist the adolescent client to develop positive expectations.
- Assist the client to explore the meaning of his or her life, satisfaction with his or her life, and life goals.
- Encourage adolescent clients to get 9 to 10 hours of sleep nightly.

- Assist the client in looking at alternatives and setting long- and short-term goals that are important to him or her.
- Explore the meanings, functions, objects, sources, and nature of hope with patients as relates to their current situation.
- Spend one-on-one time with the client. Use empathy; try to understand what the client is saying and communicate this understanding to the client to create a nonjudgmental trusting environment to develop therapeutic relationships with the client.
- Teach alternative coping strategies such as physical activity.
- Use a future-directed approach that teaches individuals how to become aware of attention that is focused on unwanted aspects of life and how to redirect attention toward things that feel more wanted or desired.
- Review the client's strengths and resources in conjunction with the client.
- Encourage the client to adopt active coping strategies.
- Offer emotional support, active listening, and coping assistance to client families.
- Implement social supports and reintegration programs for postdeployment soldiers and veterans in a timely fashion.
- For additional interventions, see the care plans for Readiness for enhanced **Hope, Spiritual** distress, Readiness for enhanced **Spiritual** well-being, and Disturbed **Sleep** pattern.

Geriatric

- Previous interventions may be adapted for geriatric clients.

▲ If depression is suspected, confer with the primary healthcare provider regarding referral for mental health services.

- Take threats of self-harm or suicide seriously and intervene as needed.
- Encourage engagement in positive and pleasant events.

Multicultural

- Assess for the influence of cultural beliefs, norms, and values on the client's feelings of hopelessness.
- Assess for the effect of fatalism on the client's expression of hopelessness.
- Use caution when highlighting health disparities of multicultural populations through public health campaigns and media broadcasts.
- Encourage spirituality as a source of support for hopelessness.

Home Care

- Previously mentioned interventions may be adapted for home care use.
- Use in-person problem-solving therapy (PST) to address depressive symptoms and hopelessness.

Client/Family Teaching and Discharge Planning

- • Provide information regarding the client's condition, treatment plan, and progress.
- ▲ Refer the client to self-help groups.

Risk for Compromised Human Dignity

NANDA-I Definition

Susceptible for perceived loss of respect and honor, which may compromise health

Risk Factors

Cultural incongruence; dehumanizing treatment; disclosure of confidential information; exposure of the body; humiliation; insufficient comprehension of health information; intrusion by clinician; invasion of privacy; limited decision-making experience; loss of control over body function; stigmatization

Client-Based Outcome

Client/Caregiver Will (Specify Time Frame)

- Perceive that dignity is maintained throughout hospitalization/encounter
- Consistently call client by name of choice
- Maintain client's privacy

Nursing Interventions

- Be authentically present when with the client, try to limit extraneous thoughts of self or others, and concentrate on the well-being of the client.
- Enter into and stay within the other's frame of reference. Connect with the inner life world of meaning and spirit of the other. Join in a mutual search for meaning and wholeness of being and becoming to potentiate comfort measures, pain control, a sense of well-being, wholeness, or even spiritual transcendence of suffering.
- Determine the client's perspective about his or her health. Example questions include "Tell me about your health." "What is it like to be in your situation?" "Tell me how you perceive yourself in this situation." "What meaning are you giving to this situation?" "Tell me about your health priorities." "Tell me about the harmony you wish to reach."
- Determine the client's preferences for when and how nursing care is needed and follow the client's guidelines if possible.

H

- Include the client in all decision-making; if the client does not choose to be part of the decision or is no longer capable of making a decision, then use the named surrogate decision-maker.
- Maintain client's privacy at all times.
- Actively listen to what the client is saying both verbally and nonverbally.
- Encourage the client to share thoughts about spirituality as desired.
- Use interventions to instill increased hope; see the care plan for Readiness for enhanced **Hope.**
- For further interventions on spirituality, see the care plan for Readiness for enhanced **Spiritual** well-being.

Geriatric

- Always ask the client how he or she would like to be addressed. Avoid calling older clients "sweetie," "honey," "Gramps," or other terms that can be demeaning unless this is acceptable in the client's culture or requested by the client.
- Treat the older client with the utmost respect, even if delirium or dementia is present with confusion.

Multicultural

- Assess for the influence of cultural beliefs, norms, and values on the client's way of communicating, and follow the client's lead in communicating in matters of eye contact, amount of personal space, voice tones, and amount of touching. If in doubt, ask the client.

Home Care

- Most of the interventions described previously may be adapted for home care use.
- Recognize that the client with the caregiver has complete autonomy in the home.

Client/Family Teaching and Discharge Planning

- Teach family and caregivers the need for the dignity of the client to be maintained at all times. How an individual cognitively perceives and emotionally deals with the illness can depend on the person's family and social relationships and ultimately can affect the ability to heal. Note: Caring is integral to maintaining dignity.

Neonatal Hyperbilirubinemia

NANDA-I Definition

The accumulation of unconjugated bilirubin in the circulation (less than 15 ml/dl) that occurs after 24 hours of life

Defining Characteristics

Abnormal blood profile; bruised skin; yellow mucous membranes; yellow sclera; yellow-orange skin color

Related Factors

Deficient feeding pattern; delay in meconium passage; infants with inadequate nutrition

At-Risk Population

ABO incompatibility; age ≤ 7 days; American Indian ethnicity; blood type incompatibility between mother and infant; East Asian ethnicity; infant who is breastfed; infant with low birth weight; maternal diabetes mellitus; populations living at high altitudes; premature infant; previous sibling with jaundice; rhesus (Rh) incompatibility; significant bruising during birth

Associated Condition

Bacterial infection; infant with liver malfunction; infant with enzyme deficiency; internal bleeding; prenatal infection; sepsis; viral infection

Client Outcomes

Client (Infant) Will (Specify Time Frame)

- Establish effective feeding pattern (breast or bottle)
- Receive bilirubin assessment and screening within the first few days of life to identify potentially harmful levels of serum bilirubin
- Receive appropriate therapy to enhance indirect bilirubin excretion
- Receive nursing assessments to determine risk for severity of jaundice
- Maintain hydration: moist buccal membranes, four to six wet diapers in 24-hour period, weight loss no greater than 10% of birth weight
- Evacuate stool within 48 hours of birth, and pass three or four stools per 24 hours by day 4 of life

Client (Parent[s]) Will (Specify Time Frame)

- Receive information on neonatal jaundice prior to discharge from birth hospital
- Verbalize understanding of physical signs of jaundice prior to discharge
- Verbalize signs requiring immediate health practitioner notification: sleepy infant who does not awaken easily for feedings, fewer than four to six wet diapers in 24-hour period by day 4, fewer than three to four stools in 24 hours by day 4, breastfeeds fewer than eight times per day
- Demonstrate ability to operate home phototherapy unit if prescribed

Nursing Interventions

- Evaluate maternal and delivery history for risk factors for neonatal jaundice (RH compatibility [RhD], ABO, G6PD deficiency, direct Coombs).
- Perform neonatal gestational age assessment once the newborn has had an initial period of interaction with mother and father.
- Encourage breastfeeding within the first hour of the neonate's life.
- Encourage skin-to-skin mother–newborn contact shortly after delivery.
- Assess infant's skin color at birth and every 8 hours thereafter until birth hospital discharge for the appearance of jaundice.
- Encourage and assist mother with frequent breastfeeding.
- Assist parents who choose to bottle feed their neonate.
- Avoid feeding supplements such as water, dextrose water, or any other milk substitutes in breastfeeding neonate.
- Assess neonate's stooling pattern in first 48 hours of life.

▲ Collect and evaluate laboratory blood specimens as prescribed or per unit protocol.

▲ Monitor transcutaneous bilirubin level in jaundiced neonate per unit protocol.

- Perform hour-specific total serum bilirubin (TSB) risk assessment before discharge from hospital or birth center and document the results.
- Monitor newborn for signs of inadequate breast milk or formula intake: dry oral mucous membranes, fewer than four to six wet diapers per 24 hours, no stool in 24 hours, and body weight loss greater than 10%.
- Assess late preterm infant (born between 34 weeks and 36$\frac{6}{7}$ weeks' gestation) for ability to breastfeed successfully and adequate intake of breast milk.
- Assist mother with breastfeeding and assess latch-on.
- Encourage alternate methods for providing expressed breast milk if maternal health status is compromised, and assist mother with collection of breast milk via use of breast pump or hand expression.
- Encourage father's participation in newborn care by changing diapers, helping position newborn for breastfeeding, and holding newborn while mother rests.
- Weigh newborn daily.

▲ When phototherapy is ordered, place seminude infant (diaper only) under prescribed amount of phototherapy lights.

• = Independent ▲ = Collaborative

- • Protect infant's eyes from phototherapy light source with eye shields; remove eye shields periodically when infant is removed from light source for feeding and parent–infant interaction.
- • Monitor infant's hydration status, fluid intake, skin status, and body temperature while undergoing phototherapy.
- ▲ Collect and evaluate laboratory blood specimens (TSB) while infant is undergoing phototherapy.
- • Encourage continuation of breastfeeding and brief infant care activities such as changing diapers while the infant is being treated with phototherapy; phototherapy may be interrupted for breastfeeding.
- • Provide emotional support for parents of infants undergoing phototherapy.

Multicultural

- • Assess infants of Asian or American Indian ethnicity for early rising bilirubin levels, especially when breastfeeding.
- • Encourage early and exclusive breastfeeding among Asian and American Indian newborns.

Client/Family Teaching and Discharge Planning

- • Teach the breastfeeding mother and support persons about the appearance of jaundice (yellow or orange color of skin) after hospital or birth center discharge, and provide healthcare resource telephone number for parents to call for concerns related to newborn's care.
- • Teach parents the signs of inadequate milk intake: fewer than three to four stools per day by day 4, fewer than four to six wet diapers in 24 hours, and dry oral mucous membranes; additional danger signs include a sleepy baby that does not awaken for breastfeeding or appears lethargic (decreased activity level from usual newborn pattern).
- ▲ Teach parents about the importance of medical follow-up in the first several days of life for the evaluation of jaundice.
- • Teach parents about the use of phototherapy (hospital or home, as prescribed), the proper use of the phototherapy equipment; feedings; and assessment of hydration, body temperature, skin status, and urine and stool output.

Quality and Safety in Nursing

- • **Client safety:** Minimizes risk of harm to client.
- • Knowledge: Nurses continually assess newborns for risk factors associated with the development of jaundice.

- Skills: Nurses use transcutaneous and serum bilirubin measurements to determine the newborn's bilirubin risk according to the hour-specific nomogram.
- Attitudes: Nurses appreciate their role as one of promoting safety for the newborn at risk for developing jaundice.
- Knowledge: Nurses implement client-focused strategies to promote serum bilirubin reduction; these include but are not limited to placing the newborn to mother's breast in first hours of life and encouraging frequent breastfeeding of no less than 10 to 12 feedings per 24 hours.
- Skills: Nurses identify individual clinical risk factors in the neonate that place him or her at risk for jaundice.
- Attitudes: Nurses value their role as a healthcare team member to promote the safe care of the newborn at discharge from the birth center and beyond.
- Knowledge: Nurses understand use of phototherapy to reduce levels of indirect bilirubin.
- Skills: Nurses use phototherapy lights appropriately.
- Skills: Nurses assess infant for untoward effects of phototherapy.
- Attitudes: Nurses appreciate the role of phototherapy as a treatment.
- Attitudes: Nurses value their role in the promotion of safety with the use of phototherapy.
- Quality and safety education for nurses at www.qsen.org.

Risk for Neonatal Hyperbilirubinemia

NANDA-I Definition

Susceptible to the accumulation of unconjugated bilirubin in the circulation (less than 15 ml/dl) that occurs after 24 hours of life which may compromise health

Risk Factors

Deficient feeding pattern; delay in meconium passage; infants with inadequate nutrition

At-Risk Population

ABO incompatibility; age ≤ 7 days; American Indian ethnicity; blood type incompatibility between mother and infant; East Asian ethnicity; infant who is breastfed; infant with low birth weight; maternal diabetes mellitus; populations living at high altitudes; premature infant; previous sibling with jaundice; rhesus (Rh) incompatibility; significant bruising during birth

Associated Condition

Bacterial infection, infant with liver malfunction; infant with enzyme deficiency; internal bleeding; prenatal infection; sepsis; viral infection

Client Outcomes

- Neonatal total serum bilirubin (TSB) will be monitored and there will be no undetected TSB values in the high-risk (95th percentile or greater) or high-intermediate risk (75th–94th percentile) zones (as determined by the hour-specific nomogram)
- Newborn will receive appropriate therapies to enhance bilirubin excretion
- Newborn will remain free of undetected signs of acute bilirubin neurotoxicity
- Establish effective feeding pattern (breast or bottle)
- Receive bilirubin assessment and screening within the first few days of life to detect increasing levels of serum bilirubin
- Receive nursing assessments to determine risk for severity of jaundice prior to discharge from birth hospital
- Maintain hydration: moist buccal membranes, four to six wet diapers in a 24-hour period, weight loss no greater than 10% of birth weight
- Evacuate stool within 48 hours of birth, and pass three to four stools per 24 hours by day 4 of life

Nursing Interventions

- Identify clinical risk factors that place the infant at greater risk for development of neonatal jaundice: exclusive breastfeeding, isoimmune or hemolytic disease, preterm birth 38⁶⁄₇ weeks' gestation or less), weight loss of 10% or more from birth weight, maternal diabetes, maternal obesity, previous sibling with jaundice, East Asian ethnicity, and significant bruising or cephalhematoma.
- Measure transcutaneous bilirubin (TcB) of all newborns in the first 24 to 48 hours of life, using a noninvasive transcutaneous bilirubinometer. Plot TcB on a nomogram standardized for the appropriate patient population; determine newborn's risk of subsequent significant hyperbilirubinemia.

Refer to care plan for Neonatal **Hyperbilirubinemia** for additional interventions for multicultural and discharge planning.

Client/Family Teaching and Discharge Planning

▲ Teach parents about the importance of medical follow-up in the first several days of life for the evaluation of jaundice, especially in the late preterm infant.

Refer to care plan for Neonatal **Hyperbilirubinemia** for additional interventions.

Quality and Safety in Nursing

Refer to care plan for Neonatal **hyperbilirubinemia** for additional interventions.

Hyperthermia

NANDA-I Definition

Core body temperature above the normal diurnal range due to failure of thermoregulation

Defining Characteristics

Abnormal posturing; apnea; coma; flushed skin; hypotension; infant does not maintain suck; irritability; lethargy; seizure; skin warm to touch; stupor; tachycardia; tachypnea; vasodilation

Related Factors

Dehydration; inappropriate clothing; increase in metabolic rate; vigorous activity

At-Risk Population

Exposure to high environmental temperature

Associated Condition

Decrease in sweat response; illness; ischemia; pharmaceutical agent; sepsis; trauma

Client Outcomes

Client Will (Specify Time Frame)

- Maintain core body temperature within adaptive levels (less than 104°F, 40°C)
- Remain free of complications of malignant hyperthermia
- Remain free of complication of neuroleptic malignant syndrome
- Remain free of dehydration
- Remain free from infection
- Verbalize signs and symptoms of heat stroke and actions to prevent heat stroke
- Verbalize personal risks for malignant hyperthermia and neuroleptic malignant syndrome to be reported during health history reviews to all healthcare professionals, including pharmacists

Nursing Interventions

Temperature Measurement

- Recognize that hyperthermia is a rise in body temperature above 40°C (104°F) that is not regulated by the hypothalamus, resulting in an uncontrolled increase in body temperature exceeding the body's ability to lose heat. It is a medical emergency (Leon & Bouchama, 2015; Gaudio & Grissom, 2016).
- Continually measure a client's core temperature with a distal esophageal probe or obtain near core body temperature measurements with a rectal or bladder temperature probe and verify with a second method.
- Use the same site and method (device) for temperature measurement for a given client so that temperature trends are assessed accurately; record site of temperature measurement.

▲ Work with the healthcare provider to help determine the cause of the temperature increase (hyperthermia), which will often help direct appropriate treatment.

- Refer to care plan for Ineffective **Thermoregulation** for interventions managing fever (pyrexia).

Heat Stroke

- Recognize that heat stroke may be separated into two categories: classic and exertional.
- Watch for risk factors for classic heat stroke, which include (Leon & Bouchama, 2015; Gaudio & Grissom, 2016):
  - Medications, especially diuretics, anticholinergic agents, beta-blockers, anti-Parkinson's medications, antidepressants, and antihistamines
  - Alcoholism
  - Mental illness
  - Obesity
  - Heart disease
- Risk factors of exertional heat stroke include (Gaudio & Grissom, 2016; Lipman et al., 2013):
  - Preexisting illness
  - Drug use (e.g., alcohol, amphetamines, ecstasy)
  - Wearing protective clothing (uniforms and athletic gear) that limits heat dissipation
- Recognize signs and symptoms of hyperthermia: core body temperature greater than 40°C (104°F), exercise-associated muscle

cramps, tachycardia, tachypnea, orthostatic dizziness, weakness, vomiting, headache, confusion, delirium, seizures, coma, acute kidney injury (rhabdomyolysis), and hot dry skin (classic heat stroke) (Pryor et al., 2013; Gaudio & Grissom, 2016).

- • Recognize that antipyretic agents are of little use in treatment of hyperthermia.
- ▲ Assess fluid loss and facilitate oral intake or administer intravenous fluids as ordered to accomplish fluid replacement and support the cardiovascular system.
- ▲ Recognize use of alpha-adrenergic agents should be avoided if possible.
- • Remove clothing and immerse young and healthy clients who have suffered exertional heat stroke in a cold water bath ensuring the head does not go underwater, or continuously douse the client with cold water.
- • For clients with classic heat stroke, remove clothes and spray or douse the skin with water and provide continual airflow over the body with a fan.
- ▲ Recognize adjunctive cooling measures include administering cold (4°C) intravenous fluids, water-circulating hydrogel-coated pads placed over the chest and legs, ice packs over the entire body, intravascular cooling catheter, and cooling blankets.
- ▲ Continuously monitor the effects of cooling measures, stop cooling interventions once the body temperature is less than 39°C; benzodiazepines may be administered to control shivering.
- ▲ Continually assess the client's neurologic and other organ function, especially kidney function (i.e., signs of rhabdomyolysis), for signs of injury from hyperthermia.

Malignant Hyperthermia

- ▲ If the client has just received general anesthesia, especially halothane, sevoflurane, desflurane, enflurane, isoflurane, or succinylcholine, recognize that the hyperthermia may be caused by malignant hyperthermia and requires immediate treatment to prevent death.
- • Monitor core temperature for all clients receiving general anesthetic agents for longer than 30 minutes.
- • Recognize that signs and symptoms of malignant hyperthermia typically occur suddenly after exposure to the anesthetic agent and include rapid rise in core body temperature, hypercarbia (increase in end tidal carbon dioxide), muscle rigidity, masseter muscle spasm,

dysrhythmias, tachycardia, tachypnea, rhabdomyolysis, acute kidney injury, and elevated serum calcium and potassium, progressing to disseminated intravascular coagulation and cardiac arrest (Rosenberg et al., 2015; SCJSA, 2017).

- ▲ If the client has malignant hyperthermia, begin treatment as ordered, including cessation of the anesthetic agent and intravenous administration of dantrolene sodium, STAT, along with cooling measures, hyperventilation with 100% oxygen, antidysrhythmics, and continued support of the cardiovascular system.
- ▲ Recognize that dysrhythmias must not be treated with calcium channel blockers (e.g., verapamil) when the client has malignant hyperthermia.
- • Provide client and family education when malignant hyperthermia occurs because it is an inherited muscle disorder.

Neuroleptic Malignant Syndrome

- ▲ Recognize that neuroleptic malignant syndrome is a rare condition associated with clients who are taking typical and atypical antipsychotic agents or after abrupt discontinuation of dopaminergic agonist agents used for Parkinson's disorder (Paden, Franjic, & Halcomb, 2013; Pileggi & Cook, 2016).
- • Watch for signs and symptoms that can range from mild to severe and include a sudden change in mental status, rapid rise in body temperature, muscle rigidity, tachycardia, tachypnea, elevated or labile blood pressure, diaphoresis, rhabdomyolysis, and acute kidney injury (Paden, Franjic, & Halcomb, 2013; Pileggi & Cook, 2016).
- ▲ Begin treatment when diagnosed, including cessation of the neuroleptic or dopamine antagonist agent or resumption of dopamine agonist agent that may have been abruptly discontinued; order administration of dantrolene, bromocriptine, amantadine, or benzodiazepine; and continue support of the cardiovascular, pulmonary, and renal systems (Paden, Franjic, & Halcomb, 2013; Pileggi & Cook, 2016).
- • A client health history that reports extrapyramidal reaction to any medication should be further explored for risk of neuroleptic malignant syndrome because this syndrome can occur at any time during a client's treatment with typical and atypical antipsychotic agents (Paden, Franjic, & Halcomb, 2013; Pileggi & Cook, 2016).
- • Recognize that clients receiving rapid dose escalation of antipsychotic agents (e.g., haloperidol) intramuscularly for acute

treatment of delirium may be at increased risk for neuroleptic malignant syndrome (Paden, Franjic, & Halcomb, 2013; Pileggi & Cook, 2016).

Pediatric

- • Assess risk factors of malignant hyperthermia, including a personal or family history of anesthesia-related complications or death or a history of muscle disorders.
- ▲ Administer dantrolene, provide oxygen and assist with ventilation, monitor heart rate and rhythm, and treat electrolyte and acid-base disorders (i.e., metabolic acidosis) as ordered if malignant hyperthermia is present.

H

Geriatric

- • Help the client seek medical attention immediately if elevated core temperature is present. To diagnose the hyperthermia, assess for possible precipitating factors, including changes in medication, environmental changes, and recent medical interventions or infectious exposures.
- • In hot weather, encourage the client to wear lightweight cotton clothing (Leon & Bouchama, 2015).
- • Provide education on the importance of drinking eight glasses of fluid per day (within their cardiac and renal reserves) regardless of whether they are thirsty and wearing appropriate clothing for the environmental temperature; assess for the need for and presence of fans or air conditioning.
- • In hot weather, monitor the older client for signs of heat stroke such as rising temperature, orthostatic blood pressure drop, weakness, restlessness, mental status changes, faintness, thirst, nausea, and vomiting. If signs are present, move the client to a cool place, have the client lie down, give sips of water, check orthostatic blood pressure, spray with lukewarm water, cool with a fan, and seek medical assistance immediately.
- • During warm weather, help the client obtain a fan or an air conditioner to increase evaporation, as needed. Help the older client locate a cool environment to which they can go for safety in hot weather.
- • Take the temperature of the older client in hot weather.

Home Care

- • Some of the interventions described previously may be adapted for home care use.

- Determine whether the client or family has a functioning thermometer, and know how to use it. Refer to the previous interventions on taking a temperature.
- Help the client and caregivers prevent and monitor for heat stroke/hyperthermia during times of high outdoor temperatures.
- To prevent heat-related injury in athletes, laborers, and military personnel, instruct them to acclimate gradually to the higher temperatures, increase fluid intake, wear vapor permeable clothing, and take frequent rests (Leon & Bouchama, 2015; CDC, 2017).
- In the event of temperature elevation above the adaptive range, institute measures to decrease temperature (e.g., get the client out of the sun and into a cool place, remove excess clothing, have the client drink fluids, spray the client with lukewarm water, fan with cool air, initiate emergency transport).

Client/Family Teaching and Discharge Planning

▲ Instruct to increase fluids to prevent heat-induced hyperthermia and dehydration in the presence of fever.

- Teach the client to stay in a cooler environment during periods of excessive outdoor heat or humidity. If the client does go out, instruct him or her to avoid vigorous physical activity; wear lightweight, loose-fitting clothing; and wear a hat to minimize sun exposure.

Hypothermia

NANDA-I Definition

Core body temperature below the normal diurnal range in individuals > 28 days of life

Defining Characteristics

Acrocyanosis; bradycardia; cyanotic nail beds; decreased blood glucose level; decreased ventilation; hypertension; hypoglycemia; hypoxia; increased metabolic rate; increased oxygen consumption; peripheral vasoconstriction; piloerection; shivering; skin cool to touch; slow capillary refill; tachycardia

Related Factors

Alcohol consumption; excessive conductive heat transfer; excessive convective heat transfer; excessive evaporative heat transfer; excessive radiative heat transfer; inactivity; inadequate caregiver knowledge of hypothermia prevention; inadequate clothing; low environmental temperature; malnutrition

At-Risk Population

Economically disadvantaged individuals; individuals at extremes of age; individuals at extremes of weight

Associated Condition

Damage to hypothalamus; decreased metabolic rate; pharmaceutical preparations; radiotherapy; trauma

Client Outcomes

Client Will (Specify Time Frame)

- Maintain body temperature within normal range
- Identify risk factors of hypothermia
- State measures to prevent hypothermia
- Identify symptoms of hypothermia and actions to take when hypothermia is present
- If hypothermia is medically induced, client/family will state goals for hypothermia treatment

Nursing Interventions

Temperature Measurement

- Recognize hypothermia as a drop in core body temperature below 35°C (95°F) (Paal et al., 2016; Zafren, 2017).
- Measure and record the client's temperature hourly, or, if the client's temperature is less than 35°C (95°F), continuously.
- Select a core or a near core measurement site based on the clinical situation and ability to obtain an accurate measurement; verify the temperature reading with a second monitoring device as needed.
- Use the same site and method (device) for a given client so that temperature trends are accurately assessed.
- See the care plan for Ineffective **Thermoregulation** as appropriate.

Accidental Hypothermia

- Recognize that there are three types of accidental hypothermia (environmental causes):
  - Acute hypothermia, also called immersion hypothermia, often from sudden exposure to cold through immersion in cold water or snow
  - Exhaustion hypothermia, caused by exposure to cold in association with lack of food and exhaustion
  - Chronic hypothermia that occurs over days or weeks and primarily affects older adults (Petrone, 2014)
- Remove the client from the cause of the hypothermic episode (e.g., cold environment, cold or wet clothing), bring into a warm environment, cover the client with warm blankets, and apply a covering to the head and neck to conserve body heat.

- Keep the moderately and severely hypothermic client horizontal and handle gently during movements.
- Monitor the client for signs of hypothermia: shivering, slurred speech, confusion, clumsy movements, fatigue progressing to a further decrease in level of consciousness, bradycardia, hypoventilation, hypotension, ventricular fibrillation, and asystole (Rischall & Rowland-Fisher, 2016; Zafren, 2017). Hypothermic patients have decreased oxygen needs and generally do not need supplemental oxygen (Zafren & Giesbrecht, 2014).
- Monitor the client's vital signs every hour and as appropriate, noting changes associated with hypothermia, such as increased pulse rate, respiratory rate, and blood pressure, as well as diuresis with mild hypothermia, progressing to a decreased pulse rate, respiratory rate and blood pressure, and oliguria with moderate to severe hypothermia.

▲ Attach electrodes and a cardiac monitor and monitor for dysrhythmias.

▲ Recognize that clients with a core temperature less than 30°C are at a higher risk for cardiac arrest; if the client arrests:
  - Check the pulse for up to 1 minute because the pulse may be slow and weak.
  - Provide chest compressions and ventilations at the same rate as for a normothermic client.
  - Limit defibrillations to one attempt at maximal power for clients with ventricular fibrillation or pulseless ventricular tachycardia until the client's core temperature is at least 30°C.
  - Medications may be withheld until the client has a core temperature greater than 30°C; double the interval between doses once the temperature is above 30°C; resume normal doses of medications once the temperature reaches 35°C.
  - Recognize prolonged cardiopulmonary resuscitation may be necessary as the client is rewarmed.

▲ Monitor for signs of coagulopathy (e.g., oozing of blood from any open areas or from intravascular catheter sites or mucous membranes) and note the results of clotting studies as available.

- For mild hypothermia (core temperature of 32.2°C to 35°C [90°F–95°F]), rewarm client passively:
  - Set room temperature to 21°C to 24°C (70°F–75°F).

H

- ○ Keep the client dry; remove any damp or wet clothing.
- ○ Layer clothing and blankets and cover the client's head.
- ○ Offer warm fluids, particularly beverages high in carbohydrates for clients who are shivering and able to safely swallow; avoid alcohol or caffeine (Zafren & Giesbrecht, 2014; Zafren, 2017).

• For mild hypothermia, allow the client to rewarm at his or her own pace as heat is generated through the normal metabolism; warm fluids help reduce further heat loss, and carbohydrates help fuel metabolic processes (Rischall & Rowland-Fisher, 2016; Zafren, 2017).

▲ For moderate hypothermia (core temperature 28°C–32.1°C [82.4°F–90°F]) or any client with a decreased level of consciousness, use active external rewarming methods, not exceeding an increase of more than 0.5°C to 1°C (1.8°F) per hour.

• Methods to rewarm the client include the following (Paal et al., 2016; Zafren, 2017):
  - ○ Forced-air warming blankets
  - ○ Circulation of warm water through external pads
  - ○ Heated and humidified oxygen (42°C–46°C) through the ventilator circuit as ordered
  - ○ Warmed (40°C–42°C) intravenous (IV) fluids and blood products using a commercial IV fluid warmer
  - ○ Radiant heat sources

▲ For severe hypothermia (core temperature below 28°C [82.4°F]), use active core rewarming techniques as ordered (Paal et al., 2016; Rischall & Rowland-Fisher, 2016):
  - ○ Hemodialysis
  - ○ Intravascular temperature management catheter
  - ○ Body cavity (thorax, peritoneal, stomach, and bladder) lavage with warmed fluid
  - ○ Recognize that warming by extracorporeal life support (ECLS) using venoarterial extracorporeal membrane oxygenation (ECMO) or cardiopulmonary bypass is essential for clients experiencing hemodynamic instability or hypothermic cardiac arrest

• Rewarm clients slowly, generally at a rate of 0.5°C to 1°C every hour.

• Measure the blood pressure frequently when rewarming and monitor for hypotension.

▲ Administer isotonic IV fluids warmed to 40°C–42°C as prescribed.

• Place a barrier between the patient and the heating blanket and monitor the client's skin.

- Determine the factors leading to the hypothermic episode, particularly if the client fails to rewarm, and treat the underlying condition; see Related Factors.
- ▲ Request a social service referral to help the client obtain the heat, shelter, and food needed to maintain body temperature.
- ▲ Encourage proper nutrition and hydration.

Targeted Temperature Hypothermia

- Recognize that targeted temperature management, also called therapeutic hypothermia, is the active lowering of the client's body temperature, in a controlled manner, to preserve neurological function after a cardiac arrest; targeted temperature management may also be considered for clients who have refractory intracranial hypertension.
- Recognize that controlled cooling of clients should be considered for all unconscious survivors of in-hospital or out-of-hospital cardiac arrest with an initial shockable (ventricular fibrillation or pulseless ventricular tachycardia) or nonshockable (asystole or pulseless electrical activity) rhythm; achieve and maintain a constant target temperature between 32°C and 36°C for at least 24 hours.
- Monitor core or near core temperatures continuously using two methods of temperature monitoring.
- Recognize that cooling may be achieved noninvasively, using fluid-filled cooling pads, or invasively, with an intravascular cooling catheter.
- Monitor for signs of infection and implement measures to prevent hospital-acquired infections.
- Obtain vital signs hourly (or via continuous monitoring) to include continuous electrocardiogram monitoring, and observe for signs of hypotension, bradycardia, and dysrhythmias. Mechanical ventilation is required to protect the client's airway and breathing during treatment.
- ▲ Observe for shivering and implement skin counterwarming with blankets; administer sedatives, opioids, neuromuscular blocking agents, buspirone, acetaminophen, or magnesium sulfate as prescribed.
- ▲ Closely inspect the skin before and throughout the cooling intervention and implement frequent turning and other pressure reduction interventions as indicated.
- ▲ Monitor and treat serum electrolytes (e.g., potassium, magnesium, calcium, phosphorus) and serum glucose closely during targeted

hypothermia and during rewarming of the client; electrolytes will fluctuate as the client is rewarmed.

- ▲ Monitor blood cell counts and observe for signs and symptoms of coagulopathy during targeted hypothermia treatment.
- • Rewarming should occur in a controlled manner, with a rise in body temperature of 0.25°C to 0.5°C per hour and targeted goal of normothermia, 37°C for 36 hours.
- ▲ Neurological and cognitive function should be assessed during targeted temperature treatment and after rewarming.

Pediatric

- • Recognize that pediatric clients have a decreased ability to adapt to temperature extremes; take the following actions to maintain body temperature in the infant/child:
  - ❍ Keep the head covered.
  - ❍ Use blankets to keep the client warm.
  - ❍ Keep the client covered during procedures, transport, and diagnostic testing.
  - ❍ Keep the room temperature at 22.2°C (72°F).
- • For the preterm or low-birth-weight newborn, set the room temperature to 25°C (77°F) before the delivery; cover the infant's head with a wool or polyethylene cap; and use specially designed bags, skin-to-skin care, transwarmer mattresses, radiant warmers, and thermal blankets to keep the infant warm.
- • Avoid bathing neonates for at least 6 hours after birth or until physiological stability is achieved; avoid removing the vernix caseosa and allow it to wear off with normal activity and handling; grossly contaminated vernix caseosa may be gently removed.
- • Targeted hypothermia to 34°C for 72 hours may be implemented in the treatment of neonates with hypoxic-ischemic encephalopathy (HIE).
- • Measure the temperature of the neonate undergoing therapeutic hypothermia for HIE with a rectal or nasopharyngeal probe.

Geriatric

- • Normal aging often includes changes in touch-related sensations, making it harder to differentiate cool and cold.
- • Recognize that older adults can develop hypothermia even from exposure to mildly cold temperatures of 60°F to 65°F (15.5°C–18.3°C).
  - ❍ Set the room temperature to 68°C to 70°C (20°C–21.1°C).

- Instruct client to wear warm clothes as appropriate (long underwear, socks, slippers, and a cap or hat) and to use a blanket to keep shoulders and legs warm while indoors.
- Instruct client to dress in layers and wear a hat, scarf, and gloves or mittens when going outside during cold weather.
- Instruct client to maintain adequate calorie intake.

• Assess neurological signs frequently, watching for confusion and decreased level of consciousness.

Home Care

• Hypothermia is not a symptom that appears in the normal course of home care, but when it occurs it is a clinical emergency, and the client/family should access emergency medical services immediately.

• Some of the interventions described earlier may be adapted for home care use.

• Before a medical crisis occurs, confirm that the client or family has a thermometer that registers accurately and the client or family can read it.

• Instruct the client or family to take the temperature when the client displays cyanosis, pallor, or shivering.

▲ Monitor temperature every hour, as noted previously; if the temperature of the client begins dropping below the normal range, apply layers of clothing or blankets, or adjust environmental heat to the comfort level, being careful to not overheat the client.

▲ If temperature continues to drop, activate the emergency system and notify a healthcare provider.

▲ If the client is in hospice care or is terminally ill, follow advance directives, client wishes, and the healthcare provider's orders; keep the client free of pain.

Client/Family Teaching and Discharge Planning

• Teach the client and family signs of hypothermia and the method of taking the temperature (age appropriate).

• Teach the client methods to prevent hypothermia: wearing adequate clothing, including a hat and mittens; heating the environment to a minimum of 20°C (68°F); and ingesting adequate food and fluid.

• Teach clients who engage in cold weather outdoor activities the importance of appropriate clothing, survival skills, and emergency planning.

▲ Teach the client and family about medications such as sedatives, opioids, and anxiolytics that predispose the client to hypothermia (as appropriate).

Risk for Hypothermia

NANDA-I Definition

Susceptible to a failure of thermoregulation that may result in a core body temperature below the normal diurnal range, in individuals > 28 days of life which may compromise health

Risk Factors

Alcohol consumption; excessive conductive heat transfer; excessive convective heat transfer; excessive evaporative heat transfer; excessive radiative heat transfer; inactivity; inadequate caregiver knowledge of hypothermia prevention; inadequate clothing; low environmental temperature; malnutrition

At-Risk Population

Economically disadvantaged individuals; individuals at extremes of age; individuals at extremes of weight

Associated Condition

Damage to hypothalamus; decreased metabolic rate; pharmaceutical preparations; radiotherapy; trauma

Client Outcomes, Nursing Interventions, Client/Family Teaching and Discharge Planning

Refer to care plan for **Hypothermia**

Risk for Perioperative Hypothermia

NANDA-I Definition

Susceptible to an inadvertent drop in core body temperature below 36°C/ 96.8°F occurring one hour before to 24 hours after surgery, which may compromise health

Risk Factors

Anxiety; body mass index below normal range for age and gender; environmental temperature < 21 °C / 69.8 °F; inadequate availability of appropriate warming equipment; wound area uncovered

At-Risk Population

Individuals aged ≥ 60 years; individuals in environment with laminar air flow; individuals receiving anesthesia for a period > 2 hours; individuals undergoing long induction time; individuals undergoing open surgery; individuals undergoing surgical procedure > 2 hours; individuals with American Society of Anesthesiologists (ASA) Physical Status classification score > 1; individuals with high Model for End-Stage Liver Disease

(MELD) score; individuals with increased intraoperative blood loss; individuals with intraoperative diastolic arterial blood pressure < 60 mmHg; individuals with intraoperative systolic blood pressure < 140 mmHg; individuals with low body surface area; neonates < 37 weeks gestational age; women

Associated Condition

Acute hepatic failure; anemia; burns; cardiovascular complications; chronic renal impairment; combined regional and general anesthesia; neurological disorder; pharmaceutical preparations; trauma

H

Client Outcomes

Client Will (Specify Time Frame)

- Maintain body temperature within normal range
- Identify risk factors of hypothermia
- State measures to prevent hypothermia
- Identify symptoms of hypothermia and actions to take when hypothermia is present
- Client will be free of surgical site infection

Nursing Interventions

Temperature Measurement

- Recognize perioperative hypothermia as a drop in core body temperature below 36°C (96.8°F) (Campbell et al., 2015; Centers for Disease Control and Prevention [CDC], 2018).
- Measure the client's temperature frequently, at least every 15 minutes, while the patient is undergoing general anesthesia and with changes in client condition (e.g., chills, change in mental status); if more than mild hypothermia is present (temperature lower than 36°C/96.85°F), use a continuous temperature-monitoring device. Two modes of temperature monitoring may be indicated. Continuous temperature monitoring using an indwelling method of temperature measurement is usually indicated to monitor effectiveness of treating body alterations in core body temperature.
- Use the same site and method (device) for temperature measurement for a given client so that temperature trends are assessed accurately, and record site of temperature measurement.
- Bladder temperature may be used because an indwelling urinary catheter is often inserted in the management of hypothermia to monitor diuresis.

Unintentional Perioperative Hypothermia

- Keep the client warm throughout the perioperative period (preoperative, intraoperatively, and postoperatively) to prevent unintentional perioperative hypothermia.
- Factors that increase the risk of perioperative hypothermia include anesthetic agents, ambient room air temperature, intravenous (IV) fluid infusion, cavity solution irrigation, blood product administration, duration and type of surgical procedure, anemia, extremes of age, neurological disorders, cachexia, and preexisting conditions (e.g., peripheral vascular disease, endocrine disease, pregnancy, burns, open wounds) (Billeter et al., 2014; American Society of PeriAnesthesia Nurses [ASPAN], 2015).
- Closely monitoring and preventing unintentional perioperative hypothermia is necessary to prevent adverse patient outcomes.
- Several interventions should be implemented to prevent unintentional perioperative hypothermia:
  - Use warming booties perioperatively
  - Use warming blankets over and under the client perioperatively
  - Use warming blankets under the client on the operating table
  - Use of reflective blankets
  - Adjust environmental room controls to maintain ambient room temperature between 68°F and 77°F
  - Use humidified heated breathing circuit
  - Use warmed forced-air blankets preoperatively, during surgery, and in the postanesthesia care unit
  - Use circulating-water mattress
  - Use warmed IV fluids and irrigation solutions
  - Designate responsibility and accountability for thermoregulation
- Using warmed IV fluids and irrigation solutions during the operative period may assist with reducing the client's risk of unintentional perioperative hypothermia.
- Active warming interventions include the use of warm blankets and forced-air warming devices.
- A heated humidified breathing circuit can be used intraoperatively to decrease hypothermia.
- Watch the client for signs of hypothermia: shivering, slurred speech, confusion, clumsy movements, fatigue, and dehydration. Shivering

increases oxygen consumption by about 40%. As hypothermia progresses, the skin becomes pale, muscles are tense, fatigue and weakness progress, breathing is decreased, and pulmonary congestion is present, compromising oxygenation. Pulses are decreased and blood pressure and heart rate decrease, progressing to lethal arrhythmias (e.g., ventricular fibrillation) (Danzl, 2012; Petrone, 2014; Torossian et al., 2016).

- ▲ Administer oxygen as ordered. Oxygenation is hampered by the change in the oxyhemoglobin curve caused by hypothermia (Danzl, 2012).
- ▲ Attach electrodes and a cardiac monitor. Watch for dysrhythmias. With hypothermia, the client is prone to dysrhythmias because of the cold myocardium; dysrhythmias may include atrial fibrillation, ventricular fibrillation, or asystole (Danzl, 2012; Petrone, 2014).
- ▲ Monitor for signs of coagulopathy (e.g., oozing of blood from any open areas or from intravascular catheter sites or mucous membranes). Also note results of clotting studies as available. Coagulopathy is a common occurrence during hypothermia (Petrone, 2014; Soreide, 2014; ASPAN, 2015).
- ▲ Monitor for signs of surgical site infection (e.g., increased incisional pain, drainage, poor healing, poor incision approximation). Unintentional perioperative hypothermia has been associated with increased risk of surgical site infections (IHI, 2012a; ASPAN, 2015; CDC, 2018).
- • See care plan for Ineffective **Thermoregulation** and **Hypothermia** as appropriate.

Pediatric

- • Interventions implemented in the care of adult clients are similar when providing care to pediatric clients to prevent hypothermia.

Home Care

- ▲ Hypothermia is not a symptom that appears in the normal course of postoperative home care. If the client continues to complain of chills or feeling cold after discharge home from a surgical procedure, provide the client with warm blankets, and if the client is allowed to drink, provide warm fluids by mouth.

- ▲ Monitor temperature every hour, as noted previously. If the temperature of the client begins dropping below the normal range, apply layers of clothing or blankets, or adjust environmental heat to the comfort level. Do not overheat. Contact a healthcare provider. Passive rewarming is the only method of rewarming that is appropriate for home care under normal circumstances.
- ▲ If temperature continues to drop, activate the emergency system and notify a healthcare provider. Hypothermia is a clinically acute condition that cannot be managed safely in the home.

Client/Family Teaching and Discharge Planning

- • Teach the client/family signs of hypothermia and the method of taking the temperature (age appropriate).
- ▲ Teach the client and family about medications such as sedatives, opioids, and anxiolytics that predispose the client to hypothermia (as appropriate). If the client has had hypothermia in the past, using alternative medications is an option if there is no contraindication (Danzl, 2012).

Disturbed Personal Identity

NANDA-I Definition

Inability to maintain an integrated and complete perception of self

Defining Characteristics

Alteration in body image; confusion about cultural values; confusion about goals; confusion about ideological values; delusional description of self; feeling of emptiness; feeling of strangeness; fluctuating feelings about self; gender confusion; inability to distinguish between internal and external stimuli; inconsistent behavior; ineffective coping strategies; ineffective relationships; ineffective role performance

Related Factors

Alteration in social role; cult indoctrination; cultural incongruence; discrimination; dysfunctional family processes; low self-esteem; manic states; perceived prejudice; stages of growth

At-Risk Population

Developmental transition; situational crisis; exposure to toxic chemical

Associated Condition

Dissociative identity disorder; organic brain disorder; pharmaceutical agent; psychiatric disorder

Client Outcomes

Client Will (Specify Time Frame)

- Demonstrate new purposes for life
- Show interests in surroundings
- Perform self-care and self-control activities appropriate for age
- Acknowledge personal strengths
- Engage in interpersonal relationships

Nursing Interventions

- • Assess and support family strengths of commitment, appreciation, and affection toward each other; positive communication; time together; a sense of spiritual well-being; and the ability to cope with stress and crisis.
- ▲ Assess for suicidal ideation and make appropriate referral for clients dealing with diversity or mental or chronic somatic illness.
- ▲ Assess clients with mood disorders and make appropriate referrals for treatment.
- ▲ Assess and make appropriate referrals for clients with physical or mental disabilities.
- ▲ Assess clients for substance abuse and make appropriate referrals.
- • Use empathetic communication and encourage the client and family to verbalize fears, express emotions, and set goals.
- • Be present for clients physically or by telephone.
- • Encourage expression of positive thoughts and emotions.
- • Help clients with serious and chronic conditions to maintain social support networks or assist in building new ones.
- ▲ Refer women facing diagnostic and curative breast cancer surgery for psychosocial support.
- • Refer for CBT.
- ▲ Refer clients with borderline personality disorder (BPD) and dual-diagnosed BPD and substance-dependent female clients for dialectical behavior therapy (DBT) and psychoanalytical-orientated day-hospital therapy.
- ▲ Refer to the care plans for Readiness for enhanced **Communication** and Readiness for enhanced **Spiritual** well-being.

Pediatric

- • Encourage adolescents to promote positive self-esteem, to enhance coping, and to prevent behavioral and psychological problems.

- Evaluate and refer children and adolescents for eating disorder prevention programs to include medical care, nutritional intervention, and mental health treatment and care coordination.
- Use computer-mediated support groups to enhance identity formation.

Geriatric

- Evaluate the effectiveness of nursing interventions used to promote positive self-identify in older adults.
- Encourage clients to discuss their "life histories." Life history–based interventions and self-esteem and life satisfaction questionnaires may be used to reinforce personal identity and foster hope.
- ▲ Refer the older client to self-help support groups.
- ▲ Refer the client with Alzheimer's disease who is terminally ill to hospice.

Multicultural

- Assess an individual's sociocultural background in teaching self-management and self-regulation as a means of supporting hope and coping.
- Decrease discrimination to promote positive ethnic identity.
- Refer to care plan for Ineffective **Coping.**

Home Care

- The interventions described previously may be adapted for home care use.
- Provide an Internet-based health coach to encourage self-management for clients with chronic conditions such as depression, impaired mobility, and chronic pain. Use computer-mediated support groups to enhance identify formation.
- ▲ Refer the client to mutual health support groups. Participating in mutual health support groups leads to enhanced coping by improving psychological and social functioning.
- ▲ Refer cancer clients and their spouses to family programs that include family-based interventions for communication, hope, coping, uncertainty, and symptom management.
- Refer combat veterans and service members directly involved in combat, as well as those providing support to combatants, including nurses, for mental health services.

Client/Family Teaching and Discharge Planning

- Teach the client about available community resources (e.g., therapists, ministers, counselors, self-help groups, family education groups).
- Teach coping skills to family caregivers of cancer clients.
- Refer to Ineffective **Coping** for additional references.

Risk for Disturbed Personal Identity

NANDA-I Definition

Susceptible to the inability to maintain an integrated and complete perception of self, which may compromise health

Risk Factors

Alteration in social role; cult indoctrination; cultural incongruence; discrimination; dysfunctional family processes; low self-esteem; manic states; perceived prejudice; stages of growth

At-Risk Population

Developmental transition; exposure to toxic chemical; situational crisis

Associated Condition

Dissociative identity disorder; organic brain disorder; pharmaceutical agent; psychiatric disorder

Client Outcomes, Nursing Interventions, Client/Family Teaching and Discharge Planning

Refer to care plan for Disturbed personal **Identity**

Risk for Complicated Immigration Transition

NANDA-I Definition

Susceptibility to experiencing negative feelings (loneliness, fear, anxiety) in response to unsatisfactory consequences and cultural barriers to one's immigration transition, which may compromise health

Related Factors

Available work below educational preparation; cultural barriers in host country; unsanitary housing; insufficient knowledge about the process to access resources in the host country; insufficient social support in host country; language barriers in host country; multiple non-related persons within household; overcrowded housing; overt discrimination; parent–child conflicts related to enculturation in the host country; abusive landlord

At-Risk Population

Forced migration; hazardous work conditions with inadequate training; illegal status in host country; labor exploitation; precarious economic situation; separation from family in home country; separation from friends in home country; unfulfilled expectations of immigration

Client Outcomes

Client Will (Specify Time Frame)

- Participate in community activities
- State satisfaction with social relationships, living arrangements, and social integration
- State satisfaction with health status and access to healthcare
- Demonstrate actions that are congruent with expressed feelings and thoughts
- State sense of belonging
- Accept strengths and limitations of new environment

Nursing Interventions

- Understand immigrants' personal perspectives/stories about their health maintenance and illness management.
- Focus on providing holistic (physical, emotional, psychological, social, and spiritual) care while caring for immigrants. When appropriate, integrate use of spirituality and connection with ethnic faith institutions.
- Acknowledge the reciprocal relationship of immigrant and his and her cultural context.
- Identify immigrant's sociocultural context, particularly to identify his or her unique perspectives with respect to cultural assimilation and cultural distinctiveness and whether or not he or she considers there is a possibility of combining both perspectives.
- Consider exploring the following factors in planning and providing care to immigrants: (1) premigration factors; (2) migration experience; (3) reception into new environment and trauma; (4) language/communication; (5) symptom expression; (6) changes in gender roles and intergenerational issues, economic stress, and marginalization; (7) resilience; and (8) multiplicity of identity need.
- Ensure that immigrants' cultural identities, rights, and needs are respected in the delivery of healthcare.
- Assist immigrants in their transition toward health and a perception of well-being.
- Be aware of the benefits and risks of involving an interpreter in providing care to immigrants.

Pediatric

- Explore current barriers and facilitators that are faced by children of immigrants to assimilate into the immigrated country's educational system.

- Invest effort in understanding the unique experiences of immigrant children, their health insurance status, and access to care.
- Explore the actual or perceived discrimination experienced by immigrant youth.
- Healthcare providers and school personnel need to encourage involvement of immigrant parents in their children's school-based activities.
- Identify the dynamics between immigrant children and their parents, including intergenerational conflict.
- Encourage children to verbalize their understanding of being separated from their parent(s) or loved ones because of migration.
- Explore acculturation process–related stress, social support, and ethnic identity of youth.
- Focus on assisting adolescent immigrants in their transition to developing bicultural competencies.

Geriatric

Note: All interventions are relevant and appropriate for geriatric immigrants.

Multicultural

Note: All interventions are relevant and appropriate for geriatric immigrants.

Home Care

- Encourage family members of immigrants to engage in home care tasks. Cultures with collective societal values are strongly expected to participate in the meeting of home care tasks for the elderly and needy.
- Educate and encourage immigrants' family members to use available home care–specific support services as needed.

Ineffective Impulse control

NANDA-I Definition

A pattern of performing rapid, unplanned reactions to internal or external stimuli without regard for the negative consequences of these reactions to the impulsive individual or to others

Defining Characteristics

Acting without thinking; asking personal questions despite the discomfort of others; gambling addiction; inability to save money or regulate finances; inappropriate sharing of personal details; irritability; overly familiar with strangers; sensation seeking; sexual promiscuity; temper outbursts; violent behavior

Related Factors

Hopelessness; mood disorder; smoking; substance misuse

Associated Condition

Alteration in cognitive functioning; alteration in development; organic brain disorder; personality disorder

Client Outcomes

Client Will (Specify Time Frame)

- Be free from harm
- Cooperate with behavioral modification plan
- Verbalize adaptive ways to cope with stress by means other than impulsive behaviors
- Delay gratification and use adaptive coping strategies in response to stress
- Verbalize understanding that behavior is unacceptable
- Accept responsibility for own behavior

Nursing Interventions

- Refer to mental health treatment for cognitive behavioral therapy (CBT).
- Assess the circumstances that led the client to seek help for their impulse control disorder.
- Assess individuals with impulsive behaviors for exposure to trauma and referral for mental health evaluation.
- Implement motivational interviewing for clients with impulse control disorders.
- Teach client mindfulness meditation techniques. Mindfulness meditation includes observing experiences in the present moment, describing those experiences without judgments or evaluations, and participating fully in one's current context.
- Refer to self-help groups such as Gambler's Anonymous.
- Use a brief intervention model to screen and provide information and referral to services for clients that may experience at-risk gambling.
- Teach clients to use urge surfing techniques when impulses or urges are triggered.
- Teach client to use cue avoidance techniques to reduce impulsive behaviors.
- Implement strategies to engage a high-level construal mindset by asking "why" abstaining from the targeted behavior will benefit the client.

Pediatric

- Assess children for environmental lead exposure.
- Assess the risk-taking and impulsive behaviors of the peer group.
- Refer to mental health treatment for CBT.

Geriatric

- Assess for impulsive symptoms and maintain increased surveillance of the client whenever the use of dopamine agonists has been initiated.
- Implement fall risk screening and precautions for geriatric clients with inattention and impulse control symptoms.
- Monitor caregivers for evidence of caregiver burden.

Client/Family Teaching and Discharge Planning

- Families should be encouraged to use practical measures to manage behavior such as limiting access to credit cards and restricting and monitoring internet access gambling and casino websites, checking medication compliance, reporting behavior typical of impulse control disorders (ICDs), and transferring control of financial affairs to a partner or other family members.

Disability-Associated Urinary Incontinence

NANDA-I Definition

Involuntary loss of urine not associated with any pathology or problem related to the urinary system.

Defining Characteristics

Adaptive behaviors to avoid others' recognition of urinary incontinence; mapping routes to public bathrooms prior to leaving home; time required to reach toilet is too long after sensation of urge; use of techniques to prevent urination; voiding prior to reaching toilet

Related Factors

Avoidance of non-hygienic toilet use; caregiver inappropriately implements bladder training techniques; difficulty finding the bathroom; difficulty obtaining timely assistance to bathroom; embarrassment regarding toilet use in social situations; environmental constraints that interfere with continence; habitually suppresses urge to urinate; impaired physical mobility; impaired postural balance; inadequate motivation to maintain continence; increased fluid intake; neurobehavioral manifestations; pelvic floor disorders

At Risk Population

Children; older adults

Associated Conditions

Heart diseases; impaired coordination; impaired hand dexterity; intellectual disability; neuromuscular diseases; osteoarticular diseases; pharmaceutical preparations; psychological disorder; vision disorders

Client Outcomes

Client Will (Specify Time Frame)

- Eliminate or reduce incontinent episodes
- Eliminate or overcome environmental barriers to toileting
- Use adaptive equipment to reduce or eliminate incontinence related to impaired mobility or dexterity
- Use portable urinary collection devices or urine containment devices when access to the toilet is not feasible

Nursing Interventions

- Introduce yourself to the client and anyone accompanying him or her and inform them of your role.
- Gain consent to provide care before proceeding further with the assessment. In clients unable to give consent, discuss permission with relevant healthcare professionals and/or family members.
- Wash hands using a recognized technique.
- Assess usual pattern of bladder management and establish the extent of the problem to include a detailed and accurate assessment of the client.
- Evaluate the client's Bladder Habits:
  - Episodes of incontinence during the day and night
  - Alleviating and aggravating factors
  - Current management strategies to include containing/collection devices, restriction of fluid intake, and avoidance of fluid/food groups that cause bladder irritation
- Complete a Lifestyle and Risk Assessment: Toilet facility access and ability to use including:
  - Distance of the toilet from the bed, chair, and living quarters
  - Characteristics of the bed, including presence of side rails and distance of the bed from the floor
  - Characteristics of the pathway to the toilet, including barriers such as stairs, loose rugs on the floor, and inadequate lighting
  - Characteristics of the bathroom, including patterns of use, lighting, height of the toilet from the floor, the presence of

handrails to assist transfers to the toilet, and breadth of the door and its accessibility for a wheelchair, walker, or other assistive device

- Assess the client's physical and mental abilities:
  - Ability to rise from chair and bed, transfer to the toilet, and ambulate, and the need for physical assistive devices such as a cane, walker, or wheelchair.
  - Ability to manipulate buttons, hooks, snaps, loop and pile closures, and zippers as needed to remove clothing.
  - Functional and cognitive status assessment should be done using a tool such as the Mini Mental Status Examination for the older client with functional incontinence.
  - Daily fluid intake included amount of types of fluids drank.
  - Risk of falls caused by dizziness, impaired vision, and hearing.
  - Functional ability decline secondary to comorbidities (cerebral vascular incidents, amputation).
- Discuss quality-of-life issues relating to socialization and family events. A comprehensive assessment enables the problem to be identified, generating a baseline of information from which to accurately diagnose and plan treatment and care (Reid, 2014).
- Review the client's past medical history:
  - Obstetrical/gynecological/urological history and surgeries
  - Relevant comorbidities such as cardiac, respiratory, renal, or neurological
  - Recurrent urinary tract infections
- Teach the client, the client's care providers, or the family to complete a bladder diary. Each 24-hour period should be subdivided into 1- to 2-hour periods and include number of urinations occurring in the toilet, actual episodes of incontinence and amount of urine leaked, reasons for episode of incontinence, type and amount of liquid intake, number of bowel movements, and incontinence pads or other products used.
- Consult with the healthcare provider and complete a medication review relating to side effects and contraindications.
- Ensure that an appropriate, safe urinary receptacle such as a three-in-one commode, female or male handheld urinal, no-spill urinal, or containment device when toileting access is limited by immobility or environmental barriers is available to assist the client

with elimination needs while other interventions are being implemented.

- ▲ Refer to occupational therapy for help in obtaining assistive devices and adapting the home for optimal toilet accessibility.
- • Provide advice to clients relating to loose-fitting clothing with stretch waistbands rather than buttoned or zippered waist; minimize buttons, snaps, and multilayered clothing; and substitute a loop-and-pile closure or other easily loosened systems such as Velcro for buttons, hooks, and zippers in existing clothing.
- • Work with the client on retraining the bladder by regular timed toileting regimens (every 2 hours). For the older client in the home or a long-term care facility who has functional incontinence and dementia:
  - Determine the frequency of current urination using an alarm system or check-and-change device.
  - Record urinary elimination and incontinent patterns in a bladder log to use as a baseline for assessment and evaluation of treatment efficacy.
  - Begin a prompted toileting program based on the results of this program; toileting frequency may vary from every 1.5 to 2 hours to every 4 hours.
  - Provide positive reinforcement.
- • Monitor older clients in a long-term care facility, acute care facility, or home for dehydration.
- • Inspect the perineal and perianal skin for evidence of incontinence-associated dermatitis, including inflammation, vesicles in skin exposed to urinary leakage, and especially skinfolds or denudation of the skin, particularly when incontinence is managed by absorptive pads or containment briefs.
- • Begin a preventive skin care regimen for all clients with urinary incontinence and treat clients with incontinence-associated dermatitis or related skin damage.
- • Advise the client about the advantages of using disposable or reusable insert pads, pad-pant systems, or replacement briefs specifically designed for urinary incontinence as indicated for short-term/long-term use, including social events.
- • Consider the use of an indwelling catheter for continuous drainage in the client who is both homebound and bedbound and is

receiving palliative or end of life care (requires a healthcare provider's order).
- When an indwelling urinary catheter is in place, follow prescribed maintenance protocols for managing the catheter, taping and replacing the catheter, the drainage bag, and care of perineal skin and urethral meatus. Teach infection control measures adapted to the home care setting.
- Assist the client in adapting to the catheter. Encourage discussion of the client's response to the catheter.
- Provide client with comprehensive written information about bladder care.
- Document all care and advice given in a factual and comprehensive manner.

Stress Urinary Incontinence

NANDA-I Definition

Involuntary loss of urine with activities that increase intra-abdominal pressure, which is not associated with urgency to void.

Defining Characteristics

Involuntary loss of urine in the absence of detrusor contraction; involuntary loss of urine in the absence of overdistended bladder; involuntary loss of urine upon coughing; involuntary loss of urine upon effort; involuntary loss of urine upon laughing; involuntary loss of urine upon physical exertion; involuntary loss of urine upon sneezing

Related Factors

Overweight; pelvic floor disorders; pelvic organ prolapse

At Risk Population

Individuals who perform high-intensity physical exercise; multiparous women; pregnant women; women experiencing menopause; women giving birth vaginally

Associated Conditions

Damaged pelvic floor muscles; degenerative changes in pelvic floor muscles; intrinsic urethral sphincter deficiency; nervous system diseases; prostatectomy; urethral sphincter injury

Client Outcomes

Client Will (Specify Time Frame)

- Report fewer stress incontinence episodes and/or a decrease in the severity of urine loss

- Experience reduction in frequency of urinary incontinence episodes as recorded on voiding diary (bladder log)
- Identify containment devices that assist in management of stress incontinence

Nursing Interventions

- Introduce yourself to the client and anyone accompanying him or her and inform them of your role.
- Gain consent to provide care before proceeding further with the assessment. In clients unable to give consent, discuss permission with relevant healthcare professionals and/or family members.
- Wash hands using a recognized technique.
- Assess usual pattern of bladder management to understand the extent of the problem and establish pattern of bladder management.
    - Review the client's past medical history to identify possible risk factors for stress incontinence (i.e., pregnancy, parity, large babies, forceps or breech deliveries, obesity, chronic cough, physical activity, previous urinary tract or gynecological surgery, smoking history).
    - Review the client's medication list (e.g., diuretics, lithium, adrenergic blockers, diabetes medications) to see what may exacerbate the client's urinary urgency.
- Review the client's bladder habits:
    - Onset and duration of urinary leakage
    - Related lower urinary tract symptoms, including voiding frequency (day/night) and urgency, severity (small, moderate, large amounts) of urinary leakage
    - Factors provoking urine loss (diuretics, bladder irritants, alcohol), focusing on the differential diagnosis of stress, urge or mixed stress, and urge urinary symptoms; consider using a symptom questionnaire that elicits relevant lower urinary tract symptoms and provides differentiation between stress and urge incontinence symptoms
- Stress urinary incontinence is more common in young and middle-aged women, is characterized by incontinence in small amounts (drops, spurts), no nocturia or incontinence at night, and incontinence without sensation of urine loss (Strothers & Friedman, 2011).

- Assess for mixed urinary incontinence (a combination of stress and urge incontinence) by asking the client:
  - Can you delay urination for a 2-hour movie or car ride?
  - How often do you wake/arise at night to urinate?
  - When you have the urge to urinate, can you reach the toilet without leaking?
- Complete a lifestyle assessment to understand the effect of stress urinary incontinence on an individual's lifestyle. Inquire about incontinence pad use and change in daily, social, or recreational activities, as well as emotional impact.
- Inspect the perineal skin for evidence of incontinence-associated dermatitis, including inflammation, vesicles in skin exposed to urinary leakage, and especially skinfolds or denudation of the skin, particularly when incontinence is managed by absorptive pads or containment briefs.

▲ Refer client for specific testing to confirm etiology of incontinence etiology and diagnosis. If trained to do so, perform the cough stress test, and request 24-hour pad test (if appropriate) and urodynamic studies (to include urine speed and flow, postvoid residual measurement, leak point pressure, and pressure flow study).

- Establish with the client the current use of containment devices; evaluate the devices for their ability to adequately contain urine loss, protect clothing, and control odor. Assist the client in identifying containment devices specifically designed to contain urinary leakage.
- Teach the client to complete a bladder diary by recording voiding frequency, the frequency and degree of urinary incontinence episodes, association with urgency (a sudden and strong desire to urinate that is difficult to defer), fluid intake, and pad usage over a 3- to 7-day period. An electronic voiding diary may be kept whenever feasible.

▲ With the client and in close consultation with the healthcare provider, review treatment options, including behavioral management; drug therapy; use of a pessary, vaginal device, or urethral insert; and surgery. Outline the potential benefits, efficacy, and side effects of each treatment option.

- Teach the client undergoing pelvic floor muscle training to identify, contract, and relax the pelvic floor muscles without contracting distal muscle groups (e.g., abdominal muscles or gluteus muscles) using verbal feedback based on vaginal or anal palpation, biofeedback, or electrical stimulation and the assistance of an incontinence specialist or healthcare provider as necessary.
- Incorporate principles of exercise physiology into a pelvic muscle training program using the following strategies:
    - Begin a graded exercise program, usually starting with 5 to 10 repetitions and advancing gradually to no more than 35 to 50 repetitions every day or every other day based on baseline and ongoing evaluation of maximal strength and endurance.
    - Continue exercise sessions over a period of 3 to 6 months.
    - Integrate muscle training into activities of daily living.
    - Assess progress every 2 weeks during the first month and every 4 to 6 weeks thereafter.
- Implement a bladder training program with the client. Assist the client in completing a bladder diary over a period of a minimum of 3 days or up to 7 days.
    - Review the results of the diary with the client, determining typical voiding frequency and establishing goals for voiding frequency.
    - Using baseline voiding frequency, as determined by the diary, teach the client to urinate by the clock when awake, typically every 30 to 120 minutes.
    - Encourage adherence to the program with timing devices, as well as verbal encouragement and support, and address individual reasons for schedule interruption.
    - Gradually increase the time between urinations to the negotiated goal. Time intervals between voiding are typically increased in increments of 15 to 30 minutes for clients with a baseline frequency of less than every 60 minutes and increments of 25 to 30 minutes for clients with a baseline frequency of more than every 60 minutes.
- Combining pelvic floor muscle training with bladder training is more effective than bladder training alone in the short term for treating stress urinary incontinence (Kaya et al., 2015).

- ▲ Teach the client to self-administer duloxetine and imipramine as ordered by the consulting healthcare provider, and to monitor for adverse side effects.
- ▲ Teach the client to self-administer topical (vaginal) estrogens as directed, and to monitor for adverse side effects.
- • Refer the female client with stress urinary incontinence and pelvic organ prolapse who wishes to use a pessary to manage stress incontinence to a nurse specialist or gynecologist with expertise in the placement and maintenance of these devices.
- • Discuss potentially reversible or controllable risk factors, such as weight loss, with the client with stress incontinence, and assist the client to formulate a strategy to eliminate these conditions.
- • Provide information about support resources such as the National Association for Continence, The Simon Foundation for Continence, or the Total Control Program.
- • Refer the client with persistent stress incontinence to a continence service, healthcare provider, or nurse who specializes in the management of this condition.
- • Teach the client to ensure good hydration. Total daily fluid intake should be approximately 2.7 L/day for women and 3.7 L/day for men.
- • Provide client with comprehensive written information about bladder care.
- • Encourage a program of self-care management. Addressing self-care activities through exercise, diet, fluid intake, and protective devices helps the client exercise control over incontinence and may reduce the substantial care provider burden affecting a significant proportion of spouse, partner, or familial care providers.
- • Assist the family with arranging care in a way that allows the client to participate in family or favorite activities without embarrassment. Elicit discussion of the client's concerns about the social or emotional burden of incontinence.
- • Document all care and advice given in a factual and comprehensive manner. Good record keeping is an integral part of nursing practice and is essential to the provision of safe and effective care (St. Aubyn and Andrews, 2015).

Urge Urinary Incontinence

NANDA-I Definition

Involuntary loss of urine in combination with or following a strong sensation or urgency to void.

Defining Characteristics

Decreased bladder capacity; feeling of urgency with triggered stimulus; increased urinary frequency; involuntary loss of urine before reaching toilet; involuntary loss of urine with bladder contractions; involuntary loss of urine with bladder spasms; involuntary loss of varying volumes of urine between voids, with urgency; nocturia

Related Factors

Alcohol consumption; anxiety; caffeine consumption; carbonated beverage consumption; fecal impaction; ineffective toileting habits; involuntary sphincter relaxation; overweight; pelvic floor disorders; pelvic organ prolapse

At Risk Population

Individuals exposed to abuse; individuals with history of urinary urgency during childhood; older adults; women; women experiencing menopause

Associated Conditions

Atrophic vaginitis; bladder outlet obstruction; depression; diabetes mellitus; nervous system diseases; nervous system trauma; overactive pelvic floor; pharmaceutical preparations; treatment regimen; urologic diseases

Client Outcomes

Client Will (Specify Time Frame)

- Report relief from urge urinary incontinence or a decrease in the frequency of incontinent episodes
- Identify containment devices that assist in the management of urge urinary incontinence

Nursing Interventions

- Introduce yourself to the client and anyone accompanying him or her and inform them of your role.
- Gain consent to perform care before proceeding further with the assessment.
- Wash hands using a recognized technique.
- Assess the usual pattern of bladder management and establish the pattern of bladder management and extent of the problem. Refer to Disability-associated urinary **Incontinence** care plan.
- Assess bladder habits and quality-of-life issues:

  - Diurnal frequency (voiding more than once every 2 hours while awake)
  - Urgency, daytime frequency, and nocturia
  - Involuntary leakage and leakage accompanied by or preceded by urgency
  - Amount of urine loss, moderate or large volume
  - Severity of symptoms
  - Alleviating and aggravating factors
  - Effect on quality of life
- ▲ Urge urinary incontinence occurs when involuntary leakage of urine is accompanied by or immediately preceded by urgency; overactive bladder is characterized by the storage symptoms of urgency with or without incontinence and is usually accompanied by frequency and nocturia (Abrams et al., 2010).
- • Ask specific questions relating to urge presentation:
  - Can you delay urination for a 2-hour movie or car ride?
  - How often do you wake at night to urinate?
  - When you have the urge to urinate, can you reach the toilet without leaking?
- ▲ In close consultation with a healthcare practitioner or advanced practice nurse, consider administering a symptom questionnaire that elicits relevant lower urinary tract symptoms and differentiates stress and urge incontinence symptoms.
- • Assess the severity of incontinence and the effect on the individual's lifestyle; inquire about incontinence pad use and change in daily, social, or recreational activities, and emotional impact.
- ▲ Perform a focused physical assessment, in close consultation with a healthcare practitioner or advanced practice nurse including:
  - Bladder palpation after voiding to check for retention
  - Bladder scanning for postvoid residual
  - Inspection of the perineal skin
  - Vaginal examination to determine hypoestrogenic changes in the mucosa (may contribute to urge incontinence)
  - Pelvic examination to determine the presence, location, and severity of vaginal wall prolapse, and reproduction of stress urinary incontinence with the cough test
  - ▲ Anal tone and constipation should be assessed.

- • Inspect the perineal and perianal skin for evidence of incontinence-associated dermatitis, including inflammation, vesicles in skin exposed to urinary leakage, and especially skinfolds or denudation of the skin, particularly when incontinence is managed by absorptive pads or containment briefs.
- • Teach the client to complete a bladder diary by recording voiding frequency, the frequency and degree of urinary incontinence episodes, their association with urgency (a sudden and strong desire to urinate that is difficult to defer), fluid intake, and pad usage over a 3- to 7-day period. An electronic voiding diary may be kept whenever feasible. In addition to these parameters, the client may be asked to record voided volume and fluid intake.
- • Review all medications the client is receiving, paying particular attention to sedatives, opioid analgesics, diuretics, antidepressants, psychotropic drugs, and cholinergics. Consult the healthcare practitioner or nurse practitioner about altering or eliminating these medications if they are suspected of affecting incontinence.
- • Assess the client for urinary retention (see the care plan for **Urinary Retention**).
- • Assess the client for functional limitations (environmental barriers, limited mobility or dexterity, and impaired cognitive function). Clients with impaired dexterity or weakness may benefit from clothing that has been modified or is without buttons and zippers (Leaver, 2017). Refer to the care plan for Disability-associated urinary **Incontinence.**
- • Consult the healthcare practitioner concerning diabetic management or pharmacotherapy for urinary tract infection when indicated. In specific cases, urgency and an increased risk of urge incontinence may be related to bacteriuria or urinary tract infection (Gupta & Trautner, 2011).
- ▲ Assess for signs and symptoms of atrophic vaginal changes in the perimenopausal or postmenopausal woman, including vaginal dryness, tenderness to touch, mucosal dryness, friability, and discomfort with gentle palpation. Specifically query the woman with atrophic vaginitis concerning associated lower urinary tract symptoms (usually voiding frequency, urgency, and dysuria). Refer the woman with atrophic vaginal changes and bothersome lower urinary tract symptoms to a gynecologist, urologist, or women's health nurse practitioner for further evaluation and management.

Pelvic Floor Training Program

- Pelvic floor muscle training is effective in the treatment of stress, urge, and mixed urinary incontinence; participation in a supervised program for at least 3 months may yield improved outcomes (Dumoulin, Hay-Smith, & Mac Habbe-Seguin, 2014).
- Teach the client undergoing pelvic floor muscle training to identify, contract, and relax the pelvic floor muscles without contracting distal muscle groups (e.g., abdominal muscles or gluteus muscles) using verbal feedback based on vaginal or anal palpation, biofeedback, or electrical stimulation, using the assistance of an incontinence specialist or healthcare provider as necessary.
- Incorporate principles of exercise physiology into a pelvic muscle training program using the following strategies:
  - Begin a graded exercise program, usually starting with 5 to 10 repetitions and advancing gradually to no more than 35 to 50 repetitions every day or every other day based on baseline and ongoing evaluation of maximal strength and endurance.
  - Continue exercise sessions over a period of 3 to 6 months.
  - Integrate muscle training into activities of daily living.
  - Assess progress every 2 weeks during the first month and every 4 to 6 weeks thereafter.

Bladder Training Program

- Assist the client in completing a voiding diary over a period of a minimum of 3 days or up to 7 days.
- Review the results with the client, determining typical voiding frequency and establishing goals for voiding frequency based on the longest time interval between voids that is comfortable for the client.
- Using baseline voiding frequency, as determined by the diary, teach the client to void first thing in the morning, every time the predetermined voiding interval passes, and before going to bed at night.
- Encourage adherence to the program with timing devices and verbal encouragement and support, and address individual reasons for schedule interruption.
- Teach distraction and urge suppression techniques (see later discussion) to control urgency while the client postpones urination.
- Gradually increase the time between urinations to the negotiated goal. Time intervals between voiding are typically increased in

increments of 15 to 30 minutes for clients with a baseline frequency of less than every 60 minutes and increments of 25 to 30 minutes for clients with a baseline frequency of more than every 60 minutes. The voiding interval should be increased by 15 to 30 minutes each week (based on the client's tolerance) until a voiding interval of 3 to 4 hours is achieved. Use a bladder diary to monitor progress.

- Review with the client the types of beverages consumed, focusing on the intake of caffeine, which is associated with a transient effect on lower urinary tract symptoms. Advise all clients to reduce or eliminate intake of caffeinated beverages or over-the-counter medications of dietary aids containing caffeine. Identify and counsel the client to eliminate other bladder irritants that may exacerbate incontinence, such as smoking, carbonated beverages, citrus, sugar substitutes, and tomato products.
- Review with the client the volume of fluids consumed; fluids may be reduced with caution to alleviate urinary frequency, especially in the evening after 6 p.m. or 3 to 4 hours before bedtime to reduce nocturia.
- Teach the client methods to avoid constipation, such as increasing dietary fiber, moderately increasing fluid intake, exercising, and establishing a routine defecation schedule.
  - Refer to **Constipation** care plans

Urge Suppression

- Teach the client the following techniques:
  - When a strong or precipitous urge to urinate is perceived, teach the client to avoid running to the toilet.
  - Pause, sit down, and relax the entire body.
  - Perform repeated, rapid pelvic muscle contractions until the urge is relieved.
  - Use distraction: count backward from 100 by sevens; recite a poem; write a letter; balance a checkbook; do handwork such as knitting; and take five deep breaths, focusing on breathing.
  - Relief is followed by micturition within 5 to 15 minutes, using nonhurried movements when locating a toilet and voiding.
  - Use urge suppression strategies on waking during the night. If the urge subsides, the client should be encouraged to go back to sleep. If after a minute or two the urge does not subside, clients should be instructed to get up to void to avoid sleep interruption.

- Teach the client to self administer antimuscarinic (anticholinergic) drugs as directed. Teach dosage side effects and administration of the medication and the importance of combining pharmacotherapy with scheduled voiding, adequate fluid intake, restriction of bladder irritants, and urge suppression techniques.
- Assist the client in selecting, obtaining, and applying a containment device for urine loss as indicated.
- Provide the client with information about incontinence support groups such as the National Association for Continence and the Simon Foundation for Continence. A helpful website titled Total Control (http://www.totalcontrolprogram.com/Pelvic+Health/Bladder+Health) can be accessed to give support and information to women with incontinence.
- Assess the functional and cognitive status of all clients with urge incontinence; use interventions to improve mobility.
- Refer client for occupational therapy for help in obtaining assistive devices and adapting the home for optimal toilet accessibility.
- Encourage the client to develop an action plan for self-care management of incontinence.
- Provide client with comprehensive written information about bladder care.
- Document all care and advice given in a factual and comprehensive manner.

Risk for Urge Urinary Incontinence

NANDA-I Definition

Susceptible to involuntary passage of urine occurring soon after a strong sensation or urgency to void, which may compromise health

Risk Factors

Alcohol consumption; anxiety; caffeine consumption; carbonated beverage consumption; fecal impaction; ineffective toileting habits; involuntary sphincter relaxation; overweight; pelvic floor disorders; pelvic organ prolapse

At Risk Population

Individuals exposed to abuse; individuals with history of urinary urgency during childhood; older adults; women; women experiencing menopause

Associated Conditions

Atrophic vaginitis; bladder outlet obstruction; depression; diabetes mellitus; nervous system diseases; nervous system trauma; overactive pelvic floor; pharmaceutical preparations; treatment regimen; urologic diseases

Client Outcomes, Nursing Interventions, Client/Family Teaching and Discharge Planning

Refer to care plan for Urge urinary **Incontinence**

Impaired Bowel Continence

NANDA-I Definition

Inability to hold stool, to sense the presence of stool in the rectum, to relax and store stool when having a bowel movement is not convenient.

Defining Characteristics

Abdominal discomfort; bowel urgency; fecal staining; impaired ability to expel formed stool despite recognition of rectal fullness; inability to delay defecation; inability to hold flatus; inability to reach toilet in time; inattentive to urge to defecate; silent leakage of stool during activities

Related Factors

Avoidance of non-hygienic toilet use; constipation; dependency for toileting; diarrhea; difficulty finding the bathroom; difficulty obtaining timely assistance to bathroom; embarrassment regarding toilet use in social situations; environmental constraints that interfere with continence; generalized decline in muscle tone; impaired physical mobility; impaired postural balance; inadequate dietary habits; inadequate motivation to maintain continence; incomplete emptying of bowel; laxative misuse; stressors

At Risk Population

Older adults; women giving birth vaginally; women giving birth with obstetrical extraction

Associated Conditions

Anal trauma; congenital abnormalities of the digestive system; diabetes mellitus; neurocognitive disorders; neurological diseases; physical inactivity; prostatic diseases; rectum trauma; spinal cord injuries; stroke

Client Outcomes

Client Will (Specify Time Frame)

- Have regular, complete evacuation of fecal contents from the rectal vault (pattern may vary from every day to every 3 days)
- Have regulation of stool consistency (soft, formed stools)
- Reduce or eliminate frequency of incontinent episodes
- Exhibit intact skin in the perianal/perineal area

- Demonstrate the ability to isolate, contract, and relax pelvic muscles (when incontinence related to sphincter incompetence or high-tone pelvic floor dysfunction)
- Increase pelvic muscle strength (when incontinence related to sphincter incompetence)
- Identify triggers that precipitate change in bowel continence

Nursing Interventions

- • In a private setting, directly question client about the presence of fecal incontinence. If the client reports altered bowel elimination patterns, problems with bowel control, or "uncontrollable diarrhea," complete a focused nursing history including previous and present bowel elimination routines, dietary history, frequency and volume of uncontrolled stool loss, and aggravating and alleviating factors.
- • Recognize that risk factors for fecal incontinence include older individuals, female sex, impaired mobility, cognitive impairment, obesity, individuals who have undergone pelvic surgery, diabetes, and structural or functional impairment of bowel function (Ditah et al., 2014; Willson et al., 2014, Young et al., 2017).
- • Recognize that additional risk factors for impaired bowel continence in hospitalized clients include antibiotic therapy, medications, enteral feeding, indwelling urinary catheter placement, immobility, inability to communicate elimination needs, acute disease processes and procedures (e.g., cancer, abdominal surgery), sedation, and mechanical ventilation (Chang & Huang, 2013; Gorina et al., 2014; Eman & Lohrmann, 2015).
- ▲ Conduct a health history assessment that includes a review of current bowel patterns/habits to include constipation and use of laxatives; diarrhea; pelvic floor injury with childbirth; acute trauma to organs, muscles, or nerves involved in defecation; gastrointestinal inflammatory disorders; functional disability; and medications (Kaiser et al., 2014; Whitehead, Palsson, & Simren, 2016).
- ▲ Closely inspect the perineal skin and skinfolds for evidence of skin breakdown in clients with incontinence.
- ▲ Use a validated tool that focuses on bowel elimination patterns to help provide a more clear understanding of the client's individual challenges and perceptions of symptoms associated with fecal incontinence (Gillibrand, 2012; Jelovsek et al., 2014).
- ▲ Complete a focused physical assessment, including inspection of perineal skin, pelvic muscle strength assessment, digital examination

of the rectum for the presence of impaction and anal sphincter strength, and evaluation of functional status (mobility, dexterity, and visual acuity).

- Complete an assessment of cognitive function; explore for a history of dementia, delirium, or acute confusion (Bliss et al., 2015; Drennan, Greenwood, & Cole, 2014).
- Document patterns of stool elimination and incontinent episodes through a bowel record, including frequency of bowel movements, stool consistency, frequency and severity of incontinent episodes, precipitating factors, and dietary and fluid intake.
- Assess stool consistency and its influence on risk for stool loss.
- Identify conditions contributing to or causing fecal incontinence.
- Improve access to toileting:
  - Identify usual toileting patterns and plan opportunities for toileting accordingly.
  - Provide assistance with toileting for clients with limited access or impaired functional status (mobility, dexterity, and access).
  - Institute a prompted toileting program for persons with impaired cognitive status.
  - Provide adequate privacy for toileting.
  - Respond promptly to requests for assistance with toileting.
- Review the client's nutritional history and evaluate methods to normalize stool consistency with dietary adjustments (e.g., avoiding high-fat content foods) and use of fiber along with assessing for use of caffeine, lactose, and sugar replacements (International Foundation for Functional Gastrointestinal Disorders [IFFGD], 2017).
- Encourage the client to keep a nutrition log to track foods that irritate the bowel (Paquette et al., 2017).
- For hospitalized clients with tube feeding–associated fecal incontinence, involve the nutrition specialist to evaluate the formula composition, osmolality, and fiber content.
- For the client with intermittent episodes of fecal incontinence related to acute changes in stool consistency, begin a bowel reeducation program consisting of the following:
  - Cleansing the bowel of impacted stool if indicated
  - Normalizing stool consistency by adequate intake of fluids (30 mL/kg of body weight per day) and dietary or supplemental fiber

  - ❍ Establishing a regular routine of fecal elimination based on established patterns of bowel elimination (patterns established before onset of incontinence)
- ▲ Implement a scheduled stimulation defecation program for persons with neurological conditions causing fecal incontinence:
  - ❍ Cleanse the bowel of impacted fecal material before beginning the program.
  - ❍ Implement strategies to normalize stool consistency, including adequate intake of fluid and fiber and avoidance of foods associated with diarrhea.
  - ❍ Determine a regular schedule for bowel elimination (typically every day or every other day) based on prior patterns of bowel elimination.
  - ❍ Provide a stimulus before assisting the client to a position on the toilet; digital stimulation, a stimulating suppository, "mini-enema," or pulsed evacuation enema may be used for stimulation.
- ▲ Begin a reeducation or pelvic floor muscle exercise program for the person with sphincter incompetence or high-tone pelvic floor muscle dysfunction of the pelvic muscles, or refer persons with fecal incontinence related to sphincter dysfunction to a nurse specialist or other therapist with clinical expertise in these techniques of care.
- ▲ Consider a sacral nerve stimulation program in clients with urgency to defecate and fecal incontinence related to weakened sphincter muscles or sphincter defect.
- • Institute a structured skin care regimen that incorporates three essential steps: cleanse, moisturize, and protect:
  - ❍ Select a cleanser with a pH range comparable to that of normal skin (usually labeled "pH balanced").
  - ❍ Moisturize with an emollient to replace lipids removed with cleansing and protect with a skin. Products containing petrolatum, dimethicone, or zinc oxide base or a no-sting skin barrier should be used.
  - ❍ Routine incontinence care should include daily perineal skin cleansing and after each episode of incontinence.
  - ❍ When feasible, select a product that combines two or all three of these processes into a single step. Ensure that products are available at the bedside when caring for a client with total incontinence in an inpatient facility.

▲ Use of absorptive pads or adult containment briefs that are applied next to the client's skin increases the risk of IAD. Absorbent underpads that wick moisture away from skin may be used with immobile clients.

▲ Consult the provider if a fungal infection is suspected. An antifungal cream or powder beneath a protective ointment may be indicated (Willson et al., 2014; Coyer, Gardner, & Doubrovsky, 2017).

• Assist the client to select and apply a containment device for occasional episodes of fecal incontinence. A fecal containment device will prevent soiling of clothing and reduce odors in the client with uncontrolled stool loss.

• In the client with frequent episodes of fecal incontinence and limited mobility, monitor the sacrum and perineal area for pressure ulcerations.

• With acutely ill clients, anticipate and evaluate the cause of acute diarrhea. Anticipate diarrhea associated with treatment or specific interventions (e.g., medications, initiation of tube feedings).

▲ Consult a provider about insertion of a bowel management system (BMS) in the critically ill client when conservative measures have failed and fecal incontinence is excessive and/or produces perianal skin injury or IAD.

Geriatric

• Evaluate all older clients for established or acute fecal incontinence when the older client enters the acute or long-term care facility, and intervene as indicated.

• Determine the client's cognitive level using a screening tool such as the Mini-Mental State Exam (MMSE), Montreal Cognitive Assessment (MoCA), the Confusion Assessment Method (CAM), or Mini-Cog.
  - Teach nursing colleagues, nonprofessional care providers, family, and clients the importance of providing toileting opportunities and adequate privacy for the client in an acute or long-term care facility.

Home Care

• The preceding interventions may be adapted for home care use.

• Assess and teach a bowel management program to support continence. Address timing, diet, fluids, and actions taken independently to deal with impaired bowel continence.

- Instruct the caregiver to provide clothing that is nonrestrictive, can be manipulated easily for toileting, and can be changed with ease.
- Evaluate self-care strategies of community-dwelling older adults, strengthen adaptive behaviors, and counsel older adults about altering strategies that compromise general health.
- Assist the family in arranging care in a way that allows the client to participate in family or favorite activities without embarrassment.
- ▲ If the client is limited to bed (or bed and chair), provide a commode or bedpan that can be easily accessed. Involve occupational and physical therapy services as indicated to promote safe transfers.
- ▲ If the client is frequently incontinent, refer for home health aide services to assist with hygiene and skin care.
- ▲ Refer the family to support services to assist with in-home management of fecal incontinence as indicated.

Note: Refer to nursing diagnoses **Diarrhea** and **Constipation** for detailed management of these related conditions.

Disorganized Infant behavior

NANDA-I Definition

Disintegration of the physiological and neurobehavioral systems of functioning

Defining Characteristics

Attention-Interaction System

Impaired response to sensory stimuli

Motor System

Alteration in primitive reflexes; exaggerated startle response; fidgeting; finger splaying; fisting; hands to face; hyperextension of extremities; impaired motor tone; tremor; twitching; uncoordinated movement

Physiological

Abnormal skin color; arrhythmia; bradycardia; feeding intolerance; oxygen desaturation; tachycardia; time-out signals

Regulatory Problems

Inability to inhibit startle reflex; irritability

State-Organization System

Active-awake; diffuse alpha electroencephalogram (EEG) activity with eyes closed; irritable crying; quiet-awake; state oscillation

Related Factors

Caregiver cue misreading; environmental overstimulation; feeding intolerance; inadequate physical environment; infant malnutrition; insufficient caregiver knowledge of behavioral cues; insufficient containment within environment; insufficient environmental sensory stimulation; pain; sensory deprivation; sensory overstimulation

At-Risk Population

Low postconceptual age; prematurity; prenatal exposure to teratogen

Associated Condition

Congenital disorder; genetic disorder; infant illness; immature neurological functioning; impaired infant motor functioning; invasive procedure; infant oral impairment

Client Outcomes

Client Will (Specify Time Frame)

Infant/Child

- Display physiological/autonomic stability: cardiopulmonary, digestive functioning
- Display signs of organized motor system (Wyngarden, DeWys, & Padnos, 1999)
- Display signs of organized state system: ability to achieve and maintain a state, and transition smoothly between states (Wyngarden, DeWys, & Padnos, 1999)
- Demonstrate progress toward effective self-regulation (Wyngarden, DeWys, & Padnos, 1999)
- Demonstrate progress toward or ability to maintain calm attention
- Demonstrate progress or ability to engage in positive interactions
- Demonstrate ability to respond to sensory information (visual, auditory, tactile) in an adaptive way

Parent/Significant Other

- Recognize infant/child behaviors as a complex communication system that expresses specific needs and wants (e.g., hunger, pain, stress, desire to engage or disengage)
- Educate parents/caregivers to recognize infant's avenues of neurobehavioral communication: autonomic/physiological, motor, state, attention/interaction
- Recognize how infants respond to environmental sensory input through stress/avoidance and approach/engagement behaviors
- Recognize and support infant's self-regulatory, coping behaviors used to regain or maintain homeostasis

- Teach parents to "tune in" to their own interactive style and how that affects their infant's behavior
- Teach parents ways to adapt their interactive style in response to infant's style of communication appropriate for developmental stage and gestational age (DeWys, 2017)
- Identify appropriate positioning and handling techniques that will enhance normal motor development (Wyngarden, DeWys, & Padnos, 1999)
- Promote infant/child's attention capabilities that support visual and auditory development (Wyngarden, DeWys, & Padnos, 1999)
- Engage parents in pleasurable parent–infant interactions that encourage bonding and attachment (Wyngarden, DeWys, & Padnos, 1999)
- Structure and modify the environment in response to infant/child's behavior and personal needs; personalize their bed space (Wyngarden, DeWys, & Padnos, 1999)
- Identify available community resources that provide early intervention services, emotional support, community health nursing, and parenting classes (Wyngarden, DeWys, & Padnos, 1999)
- Communicate the infant's medical, nursing, and developmental needs to the family in a culturally sensitive and appropriate way that is understandable (DeWys, 2017)

Nursing Interventions

- Sensitive nursing care must be implemented at the infant's admission to the neonatal intensive care unit (NICU), continued stay, and continue past discharge as the family adjusts to transitioning home and into the community.
- Recognize the neurobehavior systems through which infants communicate organized and/or disorganized/stress behaviors within the subsystems of functioning (i.e., physiological/autonomic, motor, states, attention/interactional, self-regulatory).
- Recognize and educate parents to recognize the behavior cues infants use to communicate stress/avoidance and approach/engagement.
- Provide high-quality individualized developmental care for low-birth-weight preterm infants in a family-centered care environment that promotes normal neurological, physical, and emotional developmental and prevents disabilities.
- Identify and manage pain using appropriate pain management techniques during invasive procedures (e.g., tube insertion, heel sticks, intravenous lines).

- Provide care that supports development state organization, such as the ability to achieve and maintain quiet sleep and awake states and transition smoothly between states.
- Encourage parents to speak slowly and/or sing to their babies during visits.
- Provide infants several opportunities for nonnutritive sucking (NNS).
- Provide parents opportunities to experience physical closeness through loving touch, massage, cuddling, and skin-to-skin (kangaroo care), which enhances parent–infant attachment
- Provide an environment that helps infants learn to self-regulate by encouraging self-calming behaviors (e.g., curing up, sucking fingers/fists).
- Parental engagement and early interactions in the NICU set the foundation for parent–infant attachment and social relationships.
- Support effective and pleasurable feeding practices, such as breast, bottle, or combination, as essential for healthy nutrition/calories, for mother-baby bonding and attachment, and for setting the foundation for successful feeding/eating patterns.
- Provide infants with positive sensory experiences (i.e., visual, auditory, tactile, olfactory, vestibular, proprioceptive) to enhance development of sensory pathways and avoid overstimulation of sensory systems.
- Incorporate parents as coparticipants of infant care by communicating daily progress of their infants' condition.
- Provide social support to parents including all members of the family.

Multicultural

- Identify cultural beliefs, norms, and values of family's perceptions of infant/child behavior.
- Recognize and support positive mother–infant interactive behaviors and be sensitive to cultural and ethnic backgrounds.

Client/Family Teaching and Discharge Planning

▲ Provide information or refer to community-based follow-up programs for preterm/at-risk infants and their families.

- Educate parents on safe "back-to-sleep" practice before NICU discharge.
- Educate and demonstrate to parents prior to NICU discharge a variety of development positions and handling that encourages free

body movement, hand-to-mouth and eye-hand coordination, visual scanning, and auditory localizing, and to avoid overuse of infant swings/carriers/bouncy seats.

Home Care

- NICU discharge is a vulnerable time for parents, and nurses have a key role in increasing parents' confidence by listening to fears, answering questions, and giving time to practice new skills before discharge.
- Encourage parents to use home visitation whenever possible because it enhances neonatal progress and parental support.
- Encourage families to teach extended family and support persons to recognize and respond appropriately to the infant's behavioral cues; supportive help may be most appreciated doing physical tasks.
- Provide education on positioning and handling that supports optimal infant growth and development.
- Home visitors to need to recognize maternal depression resulting from the NICU experience.
- Provide families with information about community resources, developmental follow-up services, parent-to-parent support programs, and request primary healthcare providers to follow developmental progress with parent friendly developmental questionnaires.

Readiness for Enhanced Organized Infant Behavior

NANDA-I Definition

An integrated pattern of modulation of the physiological and neurobehavioral systems of functioning, which can be strengthened

Defining Characteristics

Parent expresses desire to enhance cue recognition; parent expresses desire to enhance environmental conditions; parent expresses desire to enhance recognition of infant's self-regulatory behaviors

Client Outcomes, Nursing Interventions, Client/Family Teaching and Discharge Planning

Refer to care plans for Disorganized **Infant** behavior and Risk for disorganized **Infant** behavior

Risk for Disorganized Infant Behavior

NANDA-I Definition

Susceptible to disintegration in the pattern of modulation of the physiological and neurobehavioral systems of functioning, which may compromise health

Risk Factors

Caregiver cue misreading; environmental overstimulation; feeding intolerance; inadequate physical environment; infant malnutrition; insufficient caregiver knowledge of behavioral cues; insufficient containment within environment; insufficient environmental sensory stimulation; pain; sensory deprivation; sensory overstimulation

At-Risk Population

Low postconceptual age; prematurity; prenatal exposure to teratogen

Associated Condition

Congenital disorder; genetic disorder; infant illness; immature neurological functioning; impaired infant motor functioning; invasive procedure; infant oral impairment

Client Outcomes, Nursing Interventions, Client/Family Teaching and Discharge Planning

Refer to Disorganized **Infant** behavior

Risk for Infection

NANDA-I Definition

Susceptible to invasion and multiplication of pathogenic organisms, which may compromise health

Risk Factors

Difficulty managing long-term invasive devices; difficulty managing wound care; dysfunctional gastrointestinal motility; exclusive formula feeding; impaired skin integrity; inadequate access to individual protective equipment; inadequate adherence to public health recommendations; inadequate environmental hygiene; inadequate health literacy; inadequate hygiene; inadequate knowledge to avoid exposure to pathogens; inadequate oral hygiene habits; inadequate vaccination; malnutrition; mixed breastfeeding; obesity; smoking; stasis of body fluid

At-Risk Population

Economically disadvantaged individuals; individuals exposed to disease outbreak; individuals exposed to increased environmental pathogens; individuals with low level of education; infants who are not breastfed

Associated Condition

Alteration in pH of secretion; anemia; chronic illness; decrease in ciliary action; immunosuppression; invasive procedure; leukopenia; premature rupture of amniotic membrane; prolonged rupture of amniotic membrane; suppressed inflammatory response

Client Outcomes

Client Will (Specify Time Frame)

- Remain free from symptoms of infection during contact with healthcare providers
- State symptoms of infection before initiating a healthcare–related procedure
- Demonstrate appropriate care of infection-prone sites within 48 hours of instruction
- Maintain white blood cell count and differential within normal limits within 48 hours of treatment initiation
- Demonstrate appropriate hygienic measures such as handwashing, oral care, and perineal care within 24 hours of instruction

Nursing Interventions

- Implement targeted surveillance for methicillin-resistant *Staphylococcus aureus* (MRSA) (screen clients at risk for MRSA on admission) and other multidrug-resistant organisms (MDROs).
- Obtain a travel history from clients presenting to the healthcare site (e.g., emergency department, clinic).
- Observe and report as redness, warmth, discharge, and increased body temperature.
- Assess temperature of neutropenic clients; report a single temperature of greater than 100.5°F.
- Oral, rectal, tympanic, temporal artery, or axillary thermometers may be used to assess temperature in adults and infants.

▲ Note and report laboratory values (e.g., white blood cell count and differential, serum protein, serum albumin, cultures).

- Assess skin for color, moisture, texture, and turgor (elasticity). Keep accurate, ongoing documentation of changes.
- Carefully wash and pat dry skin, including skinfold areas. Use hydration and moisturization on all at-risk surfaces.
- Refer to care plan for Risk for impaired **Skin** integrity.

▲ Monitor client's vitamin D level.

- Refer to care plan Readiness for enhanced **Nutrition** for additional interventions.

- Use strategies to prevent healthcare–acquired pneumonia, assess lung sounds and sputum color and characteristics, provide daily oral care with chlorhexidine, use sterile technique when suctioning, suction secretions above tracheal tube before suctioning, drain accumulated condensation in ventilator tubing into a fluid trap or other collection device before repositioning the client, assess patency and placement of nasogastric tubes, and elevate the client's head to 30 degrees or higher to prevent gastric reflux of organisms in the lung (Peyrani, 2014).
- Encourage fluid intake.
- Use appropriate hand hygiene (i.e., handwashing or use of alcohol-based hand rubs).
- When using an alcohol-based hand rub, apply an ample amount of product to the palm of one hand and rub hands together, covering all surfaces of hands and fingers, until hands are dry. Note that the volume needed to reduce the number of bacteria on hands varies by product.
- Follow standard precautions and wear gloves during any contact with blood, mucous membranes, nonintact skin, or any body substance except sweat. Use goggles and gowns when appropriate. Standard precautions apply to all clients. You must assume all clients are carrying blood-borne pathogens (CDC, 2007).
- Implement respiratory hygiene/cough etiquette.
- Follow transmission-based precautions for airborne-, droplet-, and contact-transmitted microorganisms:
  - **Airborne:** Isolate the client in a room with monitored negative air pressure, with the room door closed and the client remaining in the room. Always wear appropriate respiratory protection when you enter the room. Limit the movement and transport of the client from the room to essential purposes only. Have the client wear a surgical mask during transport.
  - **Droplet:** Keep the client in a private room, if possible. If not possible, maintain a spatial separation of 3 feet from other beds or visitors. The door may remain open. Wear a surgical mask when you must come within 3 feet of the client. Some hospitals may choose to implement a mask requirement for droplet precautions for anyone entering the room. Limit transport to essential purposes and have the client wear a mask, if possible.

- **Contact:** Place the client in a private room, if possible, or with someone (cohorting) who has an active infection from the same microorganism. Wear clean, nonsterile gloves when entering the room. When providing care, change gloves after contact with any infective material such as wound drainage. Remove the gloves and clean your hands before leaving the room and take care not to touch any potentially infectious items or surfaces on the way out. Wear a gown if you anticipate your clothing may have substantial contact with the client or other potentially infectious items. Remove the gown before leaving the room. Limit transport of the client to essential purposes and take care that the client does not contact other environmental surfaces along the way. Dedicate the use of noncritical client care equipment to a single client.

▲ Use alternatives to indwelling catheters whenever possible (external catheters, incontinence pads, and bladder control techniques).

• If a urinary catheter is necessary, follow catheter management practices. All indwelling catheters should be connected to a sterile, closed drainage system (i.e., not broken), except for good clinical reasons. Cleanse the perineum and meatus twice daily using soap and water.

• Use evidence-based practices and educate personnel in care of peripheral catheters: use aseptic technique for insertion and care, label insertion sites and all tubing with date and time of insertion, inspect every 8 hours for signs of infection, record, and report.

• Use sterile technique wherever there is a loss of skin integrity.

• Ensure the client's appropriate hygienic care with handwashing; bathing; oral care; and hair, nail, and perineal care performed by either the nurse or the client.

• Recommend responsible use of antibiotics; use antibiotics sparingly.

Pediatric

Note: Many of the preceding interventions are appropriate for the pediatric client.

• Follow meticulous hand hygiene when working with children.

• Cluster nursing procedures to decrease number of contacts with infants, allowing time for appropriate hand hygiene.

• Avoid the prophylactic use of topical cream in premature infants.

- Encourage early enteral feeding with human milk.
- ▲ Monitor recurrent antibiotic use in children.
- Instruct parents on appropriate indicators for medical visits and the risks associated with overuse of antibiotics.

Geriatric

- ▲ Suspect pneumonia when the client has symptoms of lethargy or confusion. Assess response to treatment, especially antibiotic therapy.
- Most clients develop healthcare–associated pneumonia (HCAP) by either aspirating contaminated substances or inhaling airborne particles. Refer to care plan for Risk for **Aspiration.**
- Observe and report if the client has a low-grade fever or new onset of confusion.
- Recommend that the geriatric client receive an annual influenza immunization and one-time pneumococcal vaccine.
- Recognize that chronically ill geriatric clients have an increased susceptibility to *C. difficile* infection; practice meticulous hand hygiene and monitor antibiotic response to antibiotics.

Home Care

- Adapt the previously mentioned interventions for home care as needed.
- Assess and treat wounds in the home.
- Review standards for surveillance of infections in home care.
- Maintain infection prevention policies.
- Refer for nutritional evaluation; implement dietary changes to support recovery and maintain health.

Client/Family Teaching and Discharge Planning

- Teach the client risk factors contributing to surgical wound infection.
- Teach the client and family the importance of hand hygiene in preventing postoperative infections.
- ▲ Encourage high-risk persons, including healthcare workers, to get vaccinated (CDC, 2011c).
- ▲ Influenza: Teach symptoms of influenza and the importance of vaccination for influenza.

Risk for Surgical Site Infection

NANDA-I Definition

Susceptible to invasion of pathogenic organisms at surgical site, which may compromise health

Risk Factors

Alcoholism; obesity; smoking

At-Risk Population

Cold temperature of operating room; excessive number of personnel present during the surgical procedure; increased environmental exposure to pathogens; suboptimal American Society of Anesthesiologists (ASA) physical health status score; surgical wound contamination.

Associated Condition

Comorbidity, diabetes mellitus; duration of surgery; hypertension; immunosuppression; inadequate antibiotic prophylaxis; ineffective antibiotic prophylaxis; infections at other surgical sites; invasive procedure; post-traumatic osteoarthritis; Rheumatoid arthritis; type of anesthesia; type of surgical procedure; use of implants and/or prostheses

Client Outcomes

Client Will (Specify Time Frame)

- Remain free from symptoms of surgical site infections (SSIs)
- Identify personal risk factors associated with increased SSI risk
- Modify personal behaviors that increase SSI risk
- Demonstrate appropriate hygienic practices to reduce infection risk such as handwashing

Nursing Interventions

▲ The number of surgical procedures performed in the United States continues to rise, and surgical clients often have comorbidities that increase the complexity. It is estimated that approximately half of SSIs are deemed preventable using evidence based strategies (World Health Organization [WHO], 2017). SSIs are a complication of surgical care and are associated with significant morbidity, mortality, and cost (Preas, O'Hara, & Thom et al., 2017).

▲ Optimizing the client's medical condition prior to surgery and eliminating or even diminishing modifiable risk factors for infection can lower the risk of SSIs (Hutzler & Williams, 2017). The American College of Surgeons (ACS) identifies additional modifiable risk factors as poor glycemic control and diabetic status, dyspnea, alcohol and smoking history, preoperative albumin level (<3.5 mg/dL), total bilirubin >1.0 mg/dL, obesity, and immunosuppression (Ban et al., 2016).

▲ SSI prevention, known as surgical care bundles, are evidence-based interventions that, when implemented together, can reduce the risk of infection. There are different surgical care bundles for specific high-risk surgical procedures: for example, colorectal surgery bundle, pediatric spinal surgery bundle, total joint arthroplasty surgery bundle, and cardiothoracic surgery bundle.

▲ SSIs can occur because of either client-related (endogenous) or procedure-related (exogenous) risk factors. Risk factors are further stratified into preoperative, intraoperative, and postoperative risk.

• Endogenous client-related risk factors

Compromised host defenses

• Age: Extremes of ages and advanced age increase client risk.

• Wound: A wound classification scoring system is used to identify the degree of surgical site skin integrity at the time of surgery. Assess and document skin integrity during the preoperative period to identify classification of surgical site.

• Smoking: The nicotine in tobacco products results in microvascular vasoconstriction, in addition to tissue hypoxia, which can contribute to the development of SSI (Smith & Dahlen, 2013).

▲ Assess client's smoking status and offer smoking cessation information to the receptive client. Seek nicotine patch order for client use during hospital admission.

▲ Educate the client on smoking risks using the Fact Sheet on Health Effects of Cigarette Smoking (CDC, 2017).

• Nutrition status: Assess the client's nutrition status. Preoperative risk factors include albumin <3.5 mg/dL or total bilirubin >1.0 mg/dL (Ban et al., 2016). Malnutrition leads to less competent immune response and increased risk of acquiring infections (Singh, Singla, & Chaudhary, 2014).

• Immunocompromised/immunosuppression: Clients who are immunocompromised or who have immunosuppression are at increased risk of developing infection because of their weakened immune system and inability to mount a defense against pathogenic organisms. Clients who may be immunocompromised or immunosuppressed are clients receiving cancer treatment, organ transplant recipients, clients taking steroids, and clients with HIV.

• Review the client's medical history and current medications. Medications that compromise the client's immune response may increase the risk of SSI.

• Diabetes mellitus: Monitor blood glucose levels with the goal to maintain normoglycemia in the perioperative period. Educate the client of the increased risk for SSI with episodes of hyperglycemia.

When available, coordinate referral to a diabetic educator as part of the discharge education.

- Preexisting infection: Be aware of all preoperative laboratory work, positive cultures, and actions taken to treat the infection (i.e., was the client started on oral antibiotics).
- Obesity: Obesity is defined as a body mass index (BMI) >30 kg/m^2. Obese clients are at a significant risk factor for SSI, more surgical blood loss, and experience a longer operation time.

Procedure-Related Risk Factors—Exogenous

Extended procedure time

- ❍ Estimated blood loss greater than 1 L requiring blood transfusion increases the risk of SSI
- ❍ Suboptimal timing of prophylactic antibiotic places the client at increased risk of SSI.
- ❍ Preoperative infections place the client at increased risk of SSI prior to elective surgery.

- Preoperative interventions: Establish a protocol for procedure-specific preoperative testing to detect medical conditions that increase the risk of SSI. The protocol should focus on nutritional counseling, smoking cessation, preadmission infections, and reconciling mediations with adjustments prior to surgery as indicated (Anderson et al., 2017).
  - ❍ Identify high-risk clients: Clients at high risk for developing SSIs have diabetics, history of transplant, are receiving chemotherapy, are immunosuppressed and immunocompromised, are elderly, have poor dentition, are obese, and are malnourished. Clients having a high-risk procedure with an extended surgical procedure time (i.e., cardiac surgery, joint replacement, major abdominal surgery) are at increased risk of SSI.
  - ❍ Maintain glycemic control for both diabetic and nondiabetic clients.
  - ❍ Staphylococcus aureus (SA) is the most common pathogen causing SSIs. Colonization with SA, primarily in the nares, occurs in roughly one in four persons and increases the risk of SSI by 2-to 14-fold. Perform SA intranasal decolonization by using cotton-tipped applicators to apply a 2% mupirocin ointment in each nostril for up to 5 days prior to surgery, when appropriate and according to evidence-based guidelines (Bratzler et al., 2013).

- Provide education on preoperative bathing with soap (antimicrobial or nonantimicrobial) or an antiseptic agent on at least the night before and morning of the day of surgical intervention.
- Address preexisting dental and nutritional status.
- Prepare the surgical site using an alcohol-based antiseptic agent unless contraindicated to reduce SSI risk.
- Proper hair removal: When hair removal at the operative site is necessary, removal should be done using clippers.

- If possible, educate the client preoperatively on the risk of shaving the surgical site, or the area near in which the surgical incision will be, because of the risk for microscopic cuts and abrasions. These cuts and abrasions increase the risk of developing an SSI. For example, for breast surgery, instruct the client not to shave underarms because the underarm is potentially in close proximity to the surgical site. Another example is instructing the client having a total knee replacement not to shave the leg involved in the surgery.
- Intraoperative interventions:
  - Maintain glycemic control.
  - Maintain normothermia (temperature of 35.5°C [95.9°F] or above) during the perioperative period in surgical clients who have an anesthesia duration of at least 60 minutes (Anderson et al., 2014). WHO defines hypothermia as a core temperature <36°C (WHO, 2016).
  - Provide supplemental oxygenation, during surgery for intubated clients and in the immediate postoperative period for 2 to 6 hours via a nonrebreathing mask for procedures performed under general anesthesia to ensure a Hgb saturation of >95% is maintained. **EB:** Studies have found that perioperative hyperoxygenation led to a 25% decrease in SSIs (Anderson et al., 2014; WHO, 2016).
- Postoperative interventions:
  - Discharge instructions: Teach the client postoperative self-care after discharge. Provide written instructions that include information on how and when to contact the provider, date and time for the scheduled follow-up visit, and signs and symptoms of infection.
  - Wound care: Wound care instructions will be based on the type of surgical wound closure.

- Nutrition follow up. For the malnourished and obese clients, provide written dietary instructions by the registered dietician, if appropriate. Encourage a diet that supports wound healing (high protein) and glycemic control. If appropriate, provide written information on community nutrition support group options and contact information.
- Bathing/showering instructions: Review instructions with client and family on timing to shower and if/when the client can take a bath. Explain to the client that taking a bath is generally discouraged, at a minimum, for the first week after surgery. Submerging a fresh surgical wound in warm bath water and allowing it to soak is not advised because this provides an environment that potentially exposes the surgical wound to pathogenic organisms, increasing the risk for surgical wound infection.
- Physical therapy (PT): For clients prescribed PT after discharge, review options to access services, provide contact phone numbers to call and schedule therapy, and review options for transportation to PT appointments (e.g., spouse, family, friend, senior center transport, cab, Uber, Lyft, etc.). Work with the discharge coordinator for client assistance with transport options as needed.
- Medications: Review discharge medication prescription(s). Provide written instructions on medication(s) ordered, how often to take them, and side effects of the prescribed medication(s). Reinforce with client and family that client should not be driving if taking prescription narcotic medications. Review with client and family pain relief expectations, explaining that 100% postoperative pain relief is not realistic, but adequate pain relief should allow the client to function, to ambulate, and to perform activities of daily living (ADLs) with minimal pain.

Pediatric

SSI prevention measures deemed effective in adults are also indicated in the pediatric surgical population (Berríos-Torres et al., 2017).

Geriatric

- The most common cause of postoperative complication in the frail elderly is delirium (Ersan & Schwer, 2015).
- For the frail, elder client who lived independently in a private home prior to surgical procedure, work with the discharge coordinator to assess appropriate client placement in the immediate postoperative

period. Explore independent living, acute rehabilitation facility, or skilled nursing facility.

- For the cognitively impaired client being discharged back to independent living (private home or home with a family member), identify a key contact person who will participate in discharge education. Assess for any need of community services (food assistance, meal prep, transport, home healthcare, etc.) at time of discharge.
- Nutritional deficiencies can be common in elderly clients.
- As part of the discharge process, ask the client how they will be obtaining groceries: Will they be cooking? Will they need assistance with meal prep? Do they have someone (friend or family member) who can come into the home to assist with cooking? Does the client need to have a food service (i.e., Meals on Wheels) set up for the immediate postdischarge period?

Multicultural

- Consider race and ethnicity as a key factor when developing the client's plan of care.
- In the case of a language barrier, use a qualified interpreter rather than family members, unless as a last resort, to communicate with the non–English-speaking client. The use of family members to translate healthcare–specific information may risk patient privacy issues and interpretation bias. Nurses must be attentive to nonverbal cues, such as effective listening, attentive body language, and use of eye contact.
- Cultural nonverbal communication may also include values of modesty, touch, silence, and provider gender (Douglas et al., 2014). Identify the need for an interpreter at time of admission and schedule an interpreter to be available, either by phone or in person, for discussions with providers and for education sessions.
- Identify and accommodate the client that prefers same-gender providers. Effective communication may be affected in the client assigned opposite-gender caregivers, which may negatively affect recovery.

Home Care

- Previously listed interventions appropriately pertain to the home care.
- Coordinate with discharge planner, as necessary, for assessment of the client's home care situation that suggests potential safety and mobility concerns.

- Clients discharged back to independent living with new use of walker, crutches, wheelchair, oxygen, and so forth, should have egress access evaluated, and bathing/showering options and potential need for grab bars.

Risk for Injury

NANDA-I Definition

Susceptible to physical damage due to environmental conditions interacting with the individual's adaptive and defensive resources, which may compromise health

Risk Factors

Compromised nutritional source; exposure to pathogen; exposure to toxic chemical; immunization level within community; insufficient knowledge of modifiable factors; malnutrition; nosocomial agent; physical barrier; unsafe mode of transport

At-Risk Population

Extremes of age; impaired primary defense mechanisms

Associated Condition

Abnormal blood profile; alteration in cognitive functioning; alteration in psychomotor functioning; alteration in sensation; autoimmune dysfunction; biochemical dysfunction; effector dysfunction; immune dysfunction; sensory integration dysfunction; tissue hypoxia

Client Outcomes

Client Will (Specify Time Frame)

- Remain free of injuries
- Explain methods to prevent injuries
- Demonstrate behaviors that decrease the risk for injury

Nursing Interventions

Prevent iatrogenic harm to the hospitalized client by following the National Patient Safety goals.

- Accuracy of Client Identification:
  - Use at least two methods (e.g., client's name and medical record number or birth date) to identify the client on initial entrance to a client's room and before administering medications, blood products, treatments, or procedures.
  - Before beginning any invasive or surgical procedure, have a final verification to confirm the correct client, the correct procedure,

and the correct site for the procedure using active communication techniques.
  - Label containers used for blood and other specimens in the presence of the client.
- Effectiveness of Communication Among Care Staff:
  - Verbal or telephone orders should be written and then read back for verification to the individual giving the order. Avoid verbal or telephone orders whenever possible.
  - Standardize use of abbreviations, acronyms, symbols, and dose designations that are used in the institution.
  - Ensure that critical test results and values are recorded and reported in a timely manner.
  - Use a standardized approach of "handing off" communications, including opportunities to ask and answer questions.
  - Use only approved abbreviations.
  - Staff should always wear hospital nametags.
- Medication Safety:
  - Standardize and limit the number of drug concentrations used by the institution (e.g., concentrations of medications such as morphine in client-controlled analgesia pumps).
  - Label all medications and medication containers (e.g., syringes, medication cups, or other solutions on or off the surgical field).
  - Identify all of the client's current medications on admission to a healthcare facility, and ensure that all healthcare staff has access to the information.
  - Ensure that accurate medicine information is sent with the client throughout their care.
  - Reconcile all medication at admission and discharge, and provide list to the client.
  - Improve the effectiveness of alarm systems in the clinical area.
  - Standardize a list of medications that look alike or sound alike. This list needs to be updated yearly.
  - Identify and take extra care with clients who are on anticoagulants.
- Infection Control:
  - Reduce the risk of infections by following Centers for Disease Control and Prevention (CDC, 2017) hand hygiene guidelines.

- Document clearly when clients obtain injuries or die of infectious disease.
- Use proven guidelines to prevent infections that are difficult to treat.
- Use proven guidelines to prevent infection of the blood from central lines.
- Use safe practices to treat the surgical site of the client.
- Use proven guidelines to prevent catheter-associated urinary tract infections.

- Fall Prevention:
  - Evaluate all clients for fall risk daily and take appropriate actions to prevent falls.
- Client Involvement in Care:
  - Educate the client and family on how to recognize and report concerns about safety issues.
- Identify Clients with Safety Risks:
  - Identify which clients are at risk for harming themselves.
- Identify Clients Who Are Susceptible to Changes in Health Status:
  - Educate staff on how to recognize changes in client condition, how to respond quickly, and how to alert specially trained staff to intervene if needed.
  - Prevent errors in surgery by following established protocols. Update protocols yearly.
  - Standardize steps to educate staff so documents for surgery are ready before surgery.
  - Educate staff to mark the body part scheduled for surgery and engage the client in this process as well.
- See care plan for Risk for **Adult Falls.**
- Avoid use of physical and chemical restraints, if at all possible. Restraint free is now the standard of care for hospitals and long-term care facilities. Obtain a healthcare provider's order if restraints are necessary.
- Consider providing individualized music of the client's choice if a client is agitated.
- Review drug profile for potential side effects and interactions that may increase risk of injury.
- Provide a safe environment:
  - Use one-fourth– to one-half–length side rails only, and maintain bed in a low position. Ensure that wheels are locked on bed and commode. Keep dim light in room at night.

  - ❍ Remove all possible hazards in environment such as razors, medications, room clutter, wet floors, and matches.
- • Place an "at risk for injury" client in a room that is near the nurse's station.
  - ❍ If the client has a new onset of confusion (delirium), refer to the care plan for Acute **Confusion.** If the client has chronic confusion, see the care plan for Chronic **Confusion.**
- • Involve family in helping provide a culture of safety.
- • Refer the client for physical therapy for strengthening as needed.
- ▲ Use nonphysical forms of behavior management for the agitated psychotic client.

Pediatric

- • Teach parents the need for close supervision of young children playing near water.
- • If the child has an underlying medical problem that puts him or her at risk for drowning, it is recommended that the child be given showers, not tub baths. No unsupervised swimming is ever allowed.
- • Assess the client's socioeconomic status, because financial hardship may correlate with increased rates of injury.
- • Never leave young children unsupervised around cooking or open flames.
- • Teach parents and children the need to maintain safety for the exercising child, including wearing helmets when biking.
- • Encourage parents to insist on safety precautions in all phases of participation sports involving children.
- • Provide parents of children with traumatic brain injury with written instruction and emergency phone numbers. Ensure that instructions are understood before the child is discharged from a healthcare setting. Instruct parents to observe for the following symptoms: nausea, mild headache, dizziness, irritability, lethargy, poor concentration, loss of appetite, and insomnia.
- • Teach both parents and children the need for gun safety; refer to hunting safety courses.
- • Educate parents regarding proper car safety seat use.

Geriatric

- • Encourage the client to wear glasses and hearing aids and to use walking aids, including nonslip footwear when ambulating.

- Assess for orthostatic hypotension when getting up, teach methods to decrease dizziness, such as rising slowly, remaining seated several minutes before standing, flexing feet upward several times while sitting, sitting down immediately if feeling dizzy, and trying to have someone present when standing.
- Discourage driving at night.

Multicultural

- Acknowledge racial/ethnic differences at the onset of care.
- Evaluate the influence of culture on the client's perceptions of risk for injury.
- Evaluate whether exposure to community violence is a contributor to a client's risk for injury.
- Use culturally relevant injury prevention programs when possible. Validate the client's feelings and concerns related to environmental risks.

Home Care and Client/Family Teaching and Discharge Planning

- See Risk for **Trauma** for interventions and rationales.

Risk for Corneal Injury

NANDA-I Definition

Susceptible to infection or inflammatory lesion in the corneal tissue that can affect superficial or deep layers, which may compromise health

Risk Factors

Exposure of the eyeball; insufficient knowledge of modifiable factors

At-Risk Population

Prolonged hospitalization

Associated Condition

Blinking < five times per minute; Glasgow Coma Scale score < 6; intubation; mechanical ventilation; oxygen therapy; periorbital edema; pharmaceutical agent; tracheostomy

Client Outcomes

Client Will (Specify Time Frame)

- Demonstrate relaxed facial expressions and grimacing reduction
- Remain as independent as possible
- Remain free of physical harm resulting from vision injury risk
- Demonstrate improvement in visual acuity

Nursing Interventions

Emergency Department Visits or Primary Care Office Visit

- ▲ Perform a standard ophthalmic exam or examine eye with a slit lamp using fluorescein stain to optimize visualization of the abrasion injury if available.
- • Attempt visual acuity measuring using the Snellen eye chart (corrected with glasses).
- • Ensure immunization status is current, namely tetanus-diphtheria-pertussis status (every 10 years).
- • Teach the client that fingernail-induced corneal abrasions are one of the most common eye injuries and are at risk for complications (Lin & Gardiner, 2014).
- • Provide analgesia as needed. Clients with all but the most minor abrasions usually require a strong oral narcotic analgesic initially (Verma & Khan, 2014).
- • Injuries that penetrate the cornea are more serious. The outcome depends on the specific injury. Corneal abrasions usually heal quickly and without vision concerns. Even after the original injury is healed, however, the surface of the cornea is sometimes not as smooth as before.

Hospitalization

- • Traumatic corneal abrasions are very common ophthalmic injuries accounting for 6% of emergency department visits and 65% trauma related of which 24% were corneal abrasions (Wakai et al., 2017).
- • Perioperative corneal abrasions typically heal within 72 hours. Risk factors include advanced age; prominent eyes (proptosis, exophthalmos), ocular surface abnormalities (dry eye, recurrent erosion syndrome), surgery greater than 60 to 90 minutes, prone/lateral and Trendelenburg positions, head and neck in the operative field, intraoperative hypotension, and preoperative anemia. Potential sources of corneal injury in the surgical patient are after induction (laryngoscope, name badge, watch band), before incision (surgical preparation, gauze/sponges/drapes), during the procedure (instruments, chemical solutions, heat sources, pressure on globe, eye shields), and awakening/recovery (oxygen face mask, fingernails) (Segal et al., 2014; Malafa et al., 2016).
- ▲ All surgical patients should have eyelids secured in the closed position immediately after induction. A strip of tape is generally sufficient; however, in high-risk cases with Trendelenburg position patients may

benefit from use of transparent bioocclusive dressing, which can span the entire lid and provide strong uniform closure, minimizing tear evaporation and acting as a barrier to trauma (Malafa et al., 2016).

- Ocular lubricants support surface moisture, but studies comparing different types of lubricants fail to demonstrate differences in efficacy. However, preservative-free methylcellulose-based ointments are preferred because they are retained in the eye longer than aqueous solutions. Paraffin-based (petroleum) ointments disrupt tear film stability, carrying a higher risk of eye irritation, and are flammable (Malafa, 2016).
- Assess for corneal abrasion and eye dryness, which are common problems in clients in the intensive care unit. Eye dryness is the main risk factor for the development of corneal abrasions.

Client/Family Teaching and Discharge Planning

▲ First-aid principles should be reinforced in the event of an eye injury. Clients should not attempt to remove any object in the eye; reserve this for the provider. A referral to an ophthalmologist may be required (Jacobs, 2017).

- Teach clients to use caution when using household cleaners. Many household products contain strong acids, alkalis, or other chemicals. Drain and oven cleaners are particularly dangerous, and can lead to blindness if not used correctly (Vorvick, 2014).
- If chemical exposure has occurred, flush the eye immediately with clean water for 10 minutes. Seek prompt healthcare attention.
- Wear safety goggles at all times when using hand or power tools or chemicals, during high-impact sports, or in other situations when eye injury is more likely.
- Wear sunglasses that screen ultraviolet light when outdoors, even in winter.
- Pain is usually improved within 3 days. If pain becomes intolerable, an analgesic may be prescribed short term. Seek medical attention if pain is not resolving.
- Driving should be restricted for safety until client's visual acuity is evaluated.

Risk for Occupational Injury

NANDA-I Definition

Susceptible to sustain a work-related accident or illness, which may compromise health

Risk Factors

Individual

Excessive stress; improper or use of personal protective equipment; inadequate role performance; inadequate time management; ineffective coping strategies; insufficient knowledge; misinterpretation of information; psychological distress; unsafe acts of overconfidence; unsafe acts of unhealthy negative habits

Environmental

Distraction from social relationships; exposure to biological agents; exposure to chemical agents; exposure to extremes of temperature; exposure to noise; exposure to radiation; exposure to teratogenic agents; exposure to vibration; inadequate physical environment; labor relationships; lack of personal protective equipment; night shift work rotating to day shift work; occupational burnout; physical workload; shift work

Client Outcomes

Client Will (Specify Time Frame)

- Attend and participate in all required health and safety training activities
- Demonstrate safe and healthy work behaviors to reduce the risk of occupational injuries and illnesses
- Comply with the organization's health and safety policies and procedures
- Inspect all equipment and tools before use
- Report to management any work hazards, such as facility, tools, and equipment that needs to be repaired
- Demonstrate healthy personal habits, such as healthy nutritional choices, regular exercise, smoking cessation, and effective sleep patterns

Nursing Interventions

- Interventions to reduce the risks of occupational injury focus on providing resources for safe work and education to the individual to know safety rules and procedures. Occupational safety requires the individual to engage in safe acts, proper use of equipment to include personal protective equipment (PPE), cognitive focus during work, and self-identification of stressors that may adversely impact the individual's personal safety during work.
- Environmental risks that need to be addressed to ensure a safe work environment focus on elements such as excessive noise, poorly maintained equipment or lack of PPE, uneven or poorly designed work spaces, inadequate lighting, and lack of safety training.

- Alternating shift work or night shift work provides an additional risk related to reduced strength and chronic fatigue.
- Assist the client in reduction of personal and work stress and distractions to increase coping skills, improve interpersonal relationships, and increase personal job performance and satisfaction. Emphasize paying attention to work activities and environment in hazardous and normal work situations.
- The stress in the work environment negatively affects the intention of employees to perform better in their jobs.
- Maintaining good interpersonal relationships and communications with management and coworkers can be achieved by leaders who encourage high-quality relationships among employees in the workplace. Strong interpersonal relationships assist in developing trust, respect, and a willingness to share information, resources, and perspectives (Phillips, Rothbard, & Dumas, 2009).
- Cognitive distractions tend to decrease productivity and increase the number of errors workers make (Ratwani, Trafton, & Myers, 2006).
- Visual deprivation occurs when pedestrians elect to look at the cell phone screen, reducing the available skills necessary to see features in the walking environment.
- Assist in the integration of personal health behaviors that promote total worker health and safety for the employee, which translates to a more productive worker generating better-quality products, resulting in less occupational injuries and illnesses for the workers.
- A community-based study found that gender, young age, regular psychotropic drug use, and diseases influence the occupational injuries. Smokers, overweight subjects, and excess alcohol use also had increased risk for occupational injury.
- Sleep is an active process enabling the body to restore and regenerate. Adequate sleep is essential to health and cognitive function. It is critical for cell repair, immune system health, and regulation of hormones, and it critically aids in learning, memory, and emotion.
- Maintaining good sleep hygiene promotes alertness and results in decreased occupational injuries and illnesses. However, good sleep hygiene may be difficult in employees without consistent sleep patterns.
- Sensory deprivation, also called environmental isolation, occurs when the use of cell phones and other electronics results in limited hearing and peripheral vision.

- Fatigue has been associated with negative safety outcomes. Poor-quality or decreased sleep has been associated with obesity (higher body mass index [BMI]), and higher BMI rates are related to increased injury risk. Sleep is an active process; the body undergoes restoration and regeneration. According to Judd (2017), adequate sleep is essential to health and cognitive function. Sleep is critical for cell repair, a healthy immune system, and hormonal regulation, and aids in the process of learning, memory, and emotion. Inadequate sleep can lead to multiple chronic health and mental conditions over time. The occupational health nurse can be instrumental in screening for two of the most common sleep disorders, insomnia and obstructive sleep apnea, by asking workers key questions and using simple screening tools to prevent the negative effects of sleep disorders on quality of life and increase in work-related injuries (Judd, 2017).
- When the Occupational Safety and Health Administration (OSHA) professionals understand potential interruptions and adopt a task-design–oriented approach founded in ergonomics and human factors principles and methods, they can focus on aspects of the work environment that can be observed, measured, and controlled.
- Provide medical screening, surveillance, and postexposure testing for symptomatic employees to identify and provide the focus on the exposure to control effects that can lead to illness and injury.
- Although compliance with health and safety policies and procedures must be encouraged and enforced, when the employee becomes ill or injured, the occupational health nurse must provide assessment and treatment.
- Many workers have comorbidities (e.g., hypertension, diabetes, hyperlipidemia, asthma), some of which are related to lifestyle choices or the environment.
- Implementing programs that assist overweight and obese workers to increase both strengthening and cardiovascular exercise can result in weight loss and also reduce employees' risk of injury and chronic diseases and improve their mobility and quality of life. Health coaching is the use of evidence-based skillful conversation, clinical strategies, and interventions to actively and safely engage clients in health behavior change to better self-manage their health, health risk(s), and acute or chronic health conditions, resulting in optimal wellness, improved health outcomes, lowered health risk, and decreased healthcare costs (Huffman, 2016).

- Encourage early reporting of signs and symptoms related to health hazard exposures to provide early recognition and treatment, which is aimed at reducing disability, pain, and workers' compensation costs; absence; and retraining and replacement workers.
- Case management to ensure appropriate referrals and communication is necessary to achieve safe work environment goals and include follow-up assessment to ensure that the worker is not further injured or ill by the accommodated work situation.
- OSHA requires a mechanism that identifies to whom the employees report injuries and illnesses and that they are encouraged to do so as early as possible. One of OSHA's strategies is to be proactive and reduce injuries and illnesses by implementing a reporting system that would develop and communicate a simple procedure for workers to report any injuries, illnesses, incidents (including near misses/close calls), hazards, or safety and health concerns without fear of retaliation. This also includes an option for reporting hazards or concerns anonymously.
- Occupational back pain is a multifactorial condition commonly encountered in the workforce. It is very costly for the healthcare system and industry but can be prevented or limited in its severity.
- Enforce compliance with organizational and regulatory health and safety policies and procedures, demonstrating at least adequate training and the proper use of appropriate tools, equipment, and PPE to reduce risk of injury and illness and ensure that the client receives appropriate training and education on occupational tasks and equipment.
- Ensure workers have access to and wear PPE to reduce noise exposure. Engineering and administrative controls should be considered before the use of PPE.
- A critical component in safety risk management is to adequately identify hazards and mitigate its associated risk using safety program elements (Yorio and Wachter, 2014).
- Employees are at risk when exposed to welding fumes, dust, or chemicals. Continued exposure to these substances can place employees at risk for permanent lung changes.
- Noise in healthcare varies according to the type of facility and patient care rendered. Mechanical noise from equipment (i.e., from alarms, monitors) can be disruptive to concentration, especially if it is loud and unexpected; patient vocalization depending on the cause (i.e., from pain, fear, disorientation) and amount, volume, and length of time can be considered another

type of stressor. Published studies indicate that noise levels in hospitals, particularly in intensive care units (ICUs), are greater those recommended by OSHA and have been measured at 90 dB-A, the Action level of the OSHA Noise Standard. Staff exposed to excessive noise experience anxiety and stress and can cause other psychological effects associated with annoyance. The Joint Commission on Accreditation of Healthcare Organizations has identified noise as a potential risk factor for medical and nursing errors, stating that ambient sound should not exceed the level that would prohibit clinicians from clearly understanding each other, so that nurses are not at risk of error when the noise level is 40 dB-A or greater.

- Ensure that infection prevention and control policies and procedures are enforced. Blood-borne pathogen risks are inherent when providing nursing care in healthcare facilities of for injured or ill employees, and appropriate measures must be taken to avoid contact with and spread of infectious organisms.
- Ensure appropriate protection is initiated when workers are exposed to those considered contagious through airborne exposure. Respiratory protection is required when airborne or droplet exposure to disease agents is suspected. Appropriate selection, training, and fit-testing is required before use of respirators is allowed.
- Provide resources to assist with smoking/vaping cessation. According to the American Lung Association (2018), smoking is the leading cause of preventable death in the United States, causing over 438,000 deaths per year, and worsening preexisting conditions including cardiovascular disease. Cigars have many of the same health risks as cigarettes, including causing certain cancers. Marijuana smoke contains many of the same toxins, irritants, and carcinogens as tobacco smoke. Smokeless tobacco products are a known cause of cancer and are not a safe alternative to cigarettes. Secondhand smoke is a serious health hazard for people of all ages, causing more than 41,000 deaths each year (American Lung Association, 2018). Electronic cigarettes are a new tobacco product, and the potential health consequences and safety of these products are unknown. The process of using an e-cigarette is called "vaping" rather than smoking. The US Food and Drug Administration (FDA) describes an e-cigarette as a battery-operated device that turns nicotine, formaldehyde, flavorings (diacetyl that causes popcorn

lung), and other chemicals into a vapor that can be inhaled (WebMD, 2018).

- Provide interdisciplinary collaboration to reduce occupational risks to health and safety. According to Wachs (2005), teamwork is beneficial to American business and industry because of its strength through diversity when a variety of interdisciplinary health and safety professionals offer solutions to complex problems. Teamwork among occupational health and safety professionals, management, and employees is vital to solving complex problems cost-effectively. No single discipline can meet all the needs of workers and the workplace (Wachs, 2005). OSHA has identified that an effective occupational safety and health program involves many components and recommended practices.
- Maintain a drug-free workplace through the identification of abuse of prescription and illegal drugs, which includes any substance that inhibits the mental, emotional, and physical functioning of the worker.
- Provide accurate and legal documentation for medical and exposure records with adverse health effects from health and safety exposures, maintaining confidentiality of personal medical issues. Legal requirements for documentation ensure correct communication of all aspects of the injury or illness and protects the nurse in case of litigation.
- Documentation communicates information about the employee and confirms that care was provided using the NANDA nursing diagnoses, the NIC, and the NOC as the basis for documentation.
- OSHA documentation specifics include medical, exposure, and training records that must be retained for a period of time, usually at least 30 years. The documentation provides a history of the employee's exposure to hazards, assessment and treatment received, and any worksite hazard abatements or reduction to exposures, and any outcomes of exposure and treatments (OSHA, 2011).
- The Health Insurance Portability and Accountability Act (HIPAA) and Privacy Rule provide the right of privacy to the client, and this extends to all forms of documentation related to the client.

Considerations for nursing practice include the following:

- Identify high-risk work areas and processes for developing occupational injuries and illnesses through (1) auditing of injury and illness reports and insurance claims and (2) conducting periodic walkthroughs of the workplace for unsafe acts and conditions.

- Encourage employee compliance with safety policies and procedures to reduce the opportunity for (1) slips, trips, and falls; (2) breaks in skin integrity through chemical exposure, mechanical means (trauma, friction, pressure), physical exposure (heat, cold, radiation), and exposure to biological elements (viruses, bacteria, fungi); (3) musculoskeletal injuries; and (4) misuse of equipment and tools.
- Ensure appropriate training through medical, exposure, and training records and notify management to correct when necessary.
- Ensure employee availability and understanding of accurate and current Safety Data Sheets for all personnel.
- Encourage early reporting of signs and symptoms related to health and safety hazard exposures.
- Provide appropriate primary, secondary, and tertiary prevention strategies to ensure the health and safety of the workforce.
- For adverse effects of workplace exposures, counsel employees, notify management, and follow OSHA standards (and other regulatory requirements) and company policies and procedures to reduce exposure and reverse the adverse effects to workers.
- Promote and assist employees in integrating personal health behaviors that lead to total worker health and safety, such as not smoking or using vapes; exercise; weight loss; stress reduction; hypertension reduction; drug and alcohol-controlled use; and managing personal health issues, such as blood sugar levels.
- Monitor employees for an adverse health status through medical surveillance and physical assessment examinations required for workplace exposures, such as chemicals, noise, ergonomic issues, pulmonary stressors, and radiation.
- Provide employee counseling specific to employee, health status, and work processes.
- Encourage compliance with health and safety policies and procedures that reduces opportunity exposure to health hazards from inhalation; ingestion; or skin absorption from chemical, biological agent, or radiological exposure.
- Encourage early reporting of signs and symptoms related to health hazard exposures.
- Provide postexposure testing for symptomatic employees or per specific organizational policies and procedures.
- Provide interdisciplinary collaboration to reduce occupational risks to health and safety.

- Provide appropriate medical referrals as needed.
- Provide accurate and legal documentation for medical and exposure records with adverse health effects from health and safety exposures.
- Maintain confidentiality of personal medical issues.

Geriatric

- Consider the physiological changes in the aging population.
- Although older clients may experience less occupational injuries and illnesses, the aging workforce may take longer to heal injuries and return to work and normal functioning.

Multicultural

- Address differences in cultures that affect attitudes toward healthcare professionals and treatment modalities.
- According to the Centers for Disease Control and Prevention (CDC) (2018), young workers have high rates of job-related injury. These injuries are often the result of the many hazards present in the places they typically work, such as sharp knives and slippery floors in restaurants. Limited or no prior work experience and a lack of safety training also contribute to high injury rates. Middle and high school workers may be at increased risk for injury because they may not have the strength or cognitive ability needed to perform certain job duties.
- The US workforce is becoming more diverse (National Center for Public Policy Research, 2005). Baby Boomers are remaining in the workforce past traditional retirement age because their health is better and they need or want additional income (Bureau of Labor Statistics, 2008). Physical changes occur with the aging workforce that need to be addressed, such as decreased visual acuity that requires increased lighting, decreased hearing from presbycusis, difficulty with balance, and increase in healing time from musculoskeletal injuries.
- The size of the minority workforce is growing, and more women are entering the workforce (Thompson and Wachs, 2012). There is greater diversity in the workplace, and people from different backgrounds and cultures are working alongside each other, often speaking different languages with different educational and literacy backgrounds.
- Depending on the setting, comprehensive healthcare, including, for example, smoking cessation and early diagnosis and treatment of depression, could be provided to this high-risk population using culturally sensitive outreach and motivational interviewing strategies.

- As women continue to earn significantly less than their male counterparts, they may believe that they need to work harder to prove themselves to earn the promotions and higher pay scales.
- The Americans with Disabilities Act (ADA) requires that public buildings be designed to accommodate wheelchairs and other accommodations and that jobs be modified if accommodation is reasonable, so more challenged individuals gain access to buildings and jobs (see https://www.ada.gov/ada_req_ta.htm [ADA]).

Risk for Urinary Tract Injury

NANDA-I Definition

Susceptible to damage of the urinary tract structures from use of catheters, which may compromise health

Risk Factors

Confusion; inadequate caregiver knowledge regarding urinary catheter care; inadequate knowledge regarding urinary catheter care; neurobehavioral manifestations; obesity

At-Risk Population

Extremes of age

Associated Condition

Anatomical variation in the pelvic organs; condition preventing ability to secure catheter; detrusor sphincter dyssynergia; latex allergy; long-term use of urinary catheter; medullary injury; prostatic hyperplasia; repetitive catheterizations; retention balloon inflated to ≥30 mL; use of large-caliber urinary catheter

Client Outcomes

Client Will (Specify Time Frame)

- Remain free of urinary tract injury
- State absence of pain with catheter care and during urination
- Experience unobstructed urination after removal of catheter
- Identify interventions to prevent catheter-associated urinary tract infection (CAUTI)
- Maintain adequate urine volume (0.5–1.0 ml/kg per hour for adult); urine without odor; urine clear
- Maintain adequate fluid intake considering client age and comorbidities

Nursing Interventions

- • Monitor urinary elimination, including frequency, consistency, odor, volume, and color, as appropriate.
- • Teach the client and caregiver signs and symptoms of urinary tract infection and CAUTI.
- • Assess for appropriate use of an indwelling urinary catheter. Insert urinary catheters only when indicated and leave in only as long as clinically necessary.
- ▲ To prevent injury, educate the client and family and/or caregiver regarding the use of an indwelling urinary catheter (Lo et al., 2014; Scott et al., 2014).
- • Assess clinical indication for urinary catheter daily.
- • To avoid catheterizations, evaluate alternative strategies for managing urine output for the client.
- • If an indwelling urinary catheter is determined to be clinically indicated in the care of a client, proper selection of the right catheter, technique during insertion, and evidence-based care management are needed to reduce infection and injury to the urinary tract structures.
  - ❍ Perform hand hygiene and use Standard Precautions before and after insertion of the urinary catheter and any time the catheter, catheter site, or collection system is accessed (Yokoe et al., 2014; CDC, 2017).
  - ❍ Ensure that only properly trained personnel familiar with appropriate catheter care techniques are used for inserting and maintaining the catheter (Yokoe et al., 2014; CDC, 2017).
- • Selecting the smallest catheter size (e.g., smaller than 18 French) reduces irritation and inflammation of the urethra and reduces infection risk (Yokoe et al., 2014; CDC, 2017).
- • Insert the catheter using aseptic technique in the acute care setting. Wash hands and use sterile technique when opening the catheterization kit and cleansing the urethral meatus and perineal area with an antiseptic solution. Insert the catheter using a no-touch technique (Yokoe et al., 2014; CDC, 2017). In the nonacute care setting, nonsterile technique may be used for intermittent catheterization (CDC, 2017).
- • Provide routine hygiene care; once a urinary catheter is placed, optimal management includes care of the urethral meatus according to "routine hygiene" (e.g., daily cleansing of the meatal surface during bathing

with soap and water and as needed, e.g., following a bowel movement) (Yokoe et al., 2014; CDC, 2017). Do not clean the periurethral area with antiseptics while the catheter is in place (CDC, 2017).

- Secure the catheter after placement to reduce friction and pain from movement (Clarke et al., 2013; Yokoe et al., 2014).
  - Disruptions in aseptic technique, disconnection, or leakage require the catheter and collection system to be replaced using aseptic technique and sterile equipment (Yokoe et al., 2014; CDC, 2017).
  - Maintain unobstructed urine flow; maintain the catheter and collecting tube below the level of the bladder and free of kinks. Do not rest the collection bag on the floor.
- Establish workflow protocols to routinely empty the drainage bag frequently and before transport to reduce urine reflux and opportunities for infection.
- Change urinary catheters and drainage systems based on clinical indications such as infection, obstruction, or when the drainage system is not adequately maintained.
- Monitor the client with an indwelling urinary catheter for increased temperature (>38°C), suprapubic pain, frequency, urgency, and flank pain; monitor the skin around the catheter for redness, drainage, or swelling.
- Consider an ultrasound scanner for clients who require intermittent catheterization to assess urine volume and reduce unnecessary catheter insertion (CDC, 2017).

▲ Implement systemwide quality improvement programs to include the following interventions to decrease CAUTI:
  - Establish healthcare provider alerts or reminders for all clients with catheters regarding the need for continued catheterization.
  - Provide performance feedback and education to personnel responsible for catheter care (CDC 2017; Yokoe et al., 2014).
  - Establish evidence-based "bladder bundles" as part of a multimodal approach to preventing CAUTI. "Bladder bundles" may include educational interventions aimed at healthcare providers for appropriate use of urinary catheters, use of appropriately trained personnel to insert and care for the catheter, catheter restriction and removal protocols, and the use of bladder ultrasound to assess urine volume (Lo et al., 2014; Meddings et al., 2014).

Home Care and Client/Family Teaching and Discharge Planning

- Teach the client and family discharged with an indwelling urinary catheter to perform intermittent catheterization and insertion and care of the urinary catheter and collection bag using the interventions listed previously.
- Ensure client has adequate supplies at home for catheter insertion and care.
- Teach the client and family to contact the healthcare provider regarding symptoms of CAUTI including increased temperature (>38°C), suprapubic pain, frequency, urgency, and flank pain; no drainage of urine in the collection bag; and foul-smelling, cloudy, or bloody urine (Medline Plus, 2017).
- Teach the client and family methods to keep the urinary tract healthy. Refer to Client/Family Teaching in the care plan for Readiness for enhanced **Urinary** elimination.

Insomnia

NANDA-I Definition

Inability to initiate or maintain sleep, which impairs functioning

Defining Characteristics

Altered affect; altered attention; altered mood; early awakening; expresses dissatisfaction with quality of life; expresses dissatisfaction with sleep; expresses forgetfulness; expresses need for frequent naps during the day; impaired health status; increased absenteeism; increased accidents; insufficient physical endurance; nonrestorative sleep-wake cycle

Related Factors

Anxiety; average daily physical activity is less than recommended for age and gender; caffeine consumption; caregiver role strain; consumption of sugar-sweetened beverages; depressive symptoms; discomfort; dysfunctional sleep beliefs; environmental disturbances; fear; frequent naps during the day; inadequate sleep hygiene; lifestyle incongruent with normal circadian rhythms; low psychological resilience; obesity; stressors; substance misuse; use of interactive electronic devices

At Risk Population

Adolescents; economically disadvantaged individuals; grieving individuals; individuals undergoing changes in marital status; night shift workers; older adults; pregnant women in third trimester; rotating shift workers; women

Associated Condition

Chronic disease; hormonal change; pharmaceutical preparations

Client Outcomes

Client Will (Specify Time Frame)

- Verbalize plan to implement sleep-promoting routines
- Fall asleep with less difficulty a minimum of four nights out of seven
- Wake up less frequently during night a minimum of four nights out of seven
- Sleep a minimum of 6 hours most nights and more if needed to meet next stated outcome
- Awaken refreshed and not be fatigued during day most of the time

Nursing Interventions

- Obtain a sleep history including amount of time needed to initiate sleep, duration of any awakenings after sleep onset, total nighttime sleep amounts, and dissatisfaction with daytime energy levels and alertness.
- From the history, assess client's current ability to initiate and maintain sleep and the short-term versus chronic nature of inability to initiate and maintain sleep.

For short-term insomnia:

- For clients historically able to initiate and maintain sleep but unable to do so in the current situation, (1) minimize sleep disruptions (see Nursing Interventions for Disturbed **Sleep** pattern) and (2) promote sleep hygiene practices (see Nursing Interventions for Readiness for enhanced **Sleep**.)
- Also attend to the following factors often associated with short-term insomnia:
  - Assess pain medication use and, when feasible, advocate for pain medications that promote rather than interfere with sleep. (See Nursing Interventions for Acute **Pain** and Chronic **Pain.**)
  - Assess level of tension and encourage use of relaxation techniques as needed.
  - Assess level of distress and use therapeutic communication to increase comfort. (See further Nursing Interventions for Readiness for Enhanced **Comfort**).
  - Assess for signs of overactive bladder.

For chronic insomnia:

▲ Rule out/address any disorders and syndromes associated with chronic insomnia, e.g., addiction to alcohol or other psychoactive substances, anxiety and depressive disorders, chronic pain syndrome, restless leg syndrome, or other sleep disorders.

- Encourage practices that calm the mind and body prior to bedtime.
  - Introduce music into bedtime routines if client finds music relaxing.
  - Teach progressive muscle relaxation as a way to relax at bedtime.
  - Support client's meditation or prayer practices as part of bedtime rituals if client finds them relaxing.
- Encourage use of the following stimulus control strategies in addition to relaxation and sleep hygiene interventions recommended for short-term insomnia: (1) if feasible, have client arise from bed to participate in calming activities whenever anxious about failure to fall asleep; (2) if not feasible for client to get out of bed when unable to sleep, encourage sitting up in bed to engage in calming activities or simply resting in bed without attempting to fall asleep; (3) avoid a focus on what time it is and subsequent worry about amount of sleep time lost to sleeplessness; and (4) distract from sleeplessness with a focus on positive aspects of life.
- Consider use of foot baths.
- Be aware that clients diagnosed with chronic insomnia may have a low pain threshold.
- For clients whose chronic inability to initiate and maintain sleep has led to sleep deprivation, see Nursing Interventions and Rationales for **Sleep** deprivation.

▲ For clients with unremitting chronic insomnia, refer to a nurse practitioner trained in cognitive behavioral therapies for insomnia (CBT-I).

▲ Assist clients diagnosed with chronic insomnia who have been treated with CBT-I to limit use of sleeping agents and to select intermittent nights for sleeping pill use if complete discontinuance of sleeping pills is not feasible.

- Supplement other interventions with teaching about sleep and sleep promotion. (See further Nursing Interventions for Readiness for enhanced **Sleep.**)

Geriatric

- Most interventions discussed previously may be used with geriatric clients. In addition, see the Geriatric section of Nursing Interventions for (1) Readiness for enhanced **Sleep** and (2) disturbed **Sleep, and Sleep** deprivation.

- Especially helpful for the elderly client is routine exercise unless contraindicated.

▲ Monitor for uncomfortable sensations in legs and involuntary leg movements during sleep.

Home Care

- Assessments and interventions discussed previously can all be adapted for use in home care.
- In addition, see the Home Care section of Nursing Interventions and *Rationales* for Readiness for enhanced **Sleep.**

Client/Family Teaching

- Teach family about normal sleep and promote adoption of behaviors that enhance it. See Nursing Interventions for Readiness for enhanced **Sleep.**
- Teach family about sleep deprivation and how to avoid it. See Nursing Interventions for **Sleep** deprivation.
- Advise family of importance of not disrupting sleep of others unnecessarily. See Nursing Interventions for Disturbed **Sleep** pattern.
- Advise family of importance of minimizing noise and light, including light from electronic devices in the sleep environment. See Nursing Interventions for disturbed **Sleep** pattern.
    - Help family members understand the difference between insomnia and externally caused sleep disruption/resultant sleep deprivation.

Deficient Knowledge

NANDA-I Definition

Absence of cognitive information related to a specific topic, or its acquisition

Defining Characteristics

Inaccurate follow-through of instruction; inaccurate performance on a test; inaccurate statements about a topic; inappropriate behavior

Related Factors

Anxiety; depressive symptoms; inadequate access to resources; inadequate awareness of resources; inadequate commitment to learning; inadequate information; inadequate interest in learning; inadequate knowledge of resources; inadequate participation in care planning; inadequate trust in health care professional; low self efficacy; misinformation; neurobehavioral manifestations

At Risk Population

Economically disadvantaged individuals; illiterate individuals; individuals with low educational level

Associated Condition

Depression; developmental disabilities; neurocognitive disorders

Client Outcomes

Client Will (Specify Time Frame)

- Explain disease state, recognize need for medications, and understand treatments
- Describe the rationale for therapy/treatment options
- Incorporate knowledge of health regimen into lifestyle
- State confidence in one's ability to manage health situation and remain in control of life
- Demonstrate how to perform health-related procedure(s) satisfactorily
- Identify resources that can be used for more information or support after discharge

Nursing Interventions

- Consider the health literacy and the readiness to learn for all clients and caregivers (e.g., mental acuity, ability to see or hear, existing pain, emotional readiness, motivation, previous knowledge).
- Focus on the nature of spoken and written communication when teaching clients and caregivers, especially those who may have health literacy needs.
- Consider the context, timing, and order of how information is presented.
- Use client-centered approaches that engage clients and caregivers as active versus passive learners.
- Reinforce learning through frequent repetition and follow-up sessions.
- Use electronic methods for delivery of information when appropriate.
- Help the client and caregivers locate appropriate postdischarge groups and resources.
- Encourage clients and caregivers to maintain and/or expand supportive social networks as self-care learning resources when appropriate.

Pediatric

- Use family-centered approaches when teaching children and adolescents.
- Guide children and adolescents to credible information about their condition.

Geriatric

- Educate all older clients on safety issues, including fall prevention and medication management.

- Use multidisciplinary teams to enhance patient education.
- Consider using teaching methods and materials appropriate for older adults, especially those with cognitive challenges.
- Assess readiness of older adults for use of technological resources.

Multicultural

- Use educational interventions that are culturally tailored to the health literacy needs of the client.
- Assess for cultural/ethnic self-care practices.
- Consider the potential influence of medical interpreters in information sharing and decision-making and of the possible difficulties for clients when using medical interpreters.
- Consider involving bilingual members of a community who are considered outside the traditional healthcare system who may assist in the teaching of community health issues.

Home Care

- All of the previously mentioned interventions are applicable to the home setting.
- Use telehealth and technology-enhanced practices as appropriate.

Readiness for Enhanced Knowledge

NANDA-I Definition

A pattern of cognitive information related to a specific topic, or its acquisition, which can be strengthened

Defining Characteristics

Expresses desire to enhance learning

Client Outcomes

Client Will (Specify Time Frame)

- Meet personal health-related goals
- Explain how to incorporate new health regimen into lifestyle
- List sources to obtain information

Nursing Interventions

- Assume a facilitator role versus authority role when engaging clients seeking health-related knowledge.
- Consider "health coaching" and motivational interviewing techniques when focusing on health-related goals, priorities, and preferences.
- Seek teachable moments for those with chronic conditions to enhance their knowledge of health promotion.

- ▲ Refer clients to lifestyle and health promotion resources delivered in the workplace or community sites outside traditional healthcare environments.
- • Refer clients to interactive and Web-based technological resources as appropriate.
- • Refer to Deficient **Knowledge** care plan.

Pediatric

- • Consider the use of mobile text messaging as a resource for delivery of health promotion information.
- • Incorporate health promotion education that reflects the unique cultural interests and values of diverse groups.
- • Involve children and especially adolescents in designing health promotion programs and teaching methods.
- • Consider settings outside traditional healthcare centers and interdisciplinary approaches for engaging children and adolescents in preventive healthcare.
- • Refer to Deficient **Knowledge** care plan.

Geriatric and Multicultural

- • Discuss healthy lifestyle changes that promote safety, health promotion, and health maintenance for older clients.
- • Consider involving bilingual members of a community who are considered outside the traditional healthcare system who may assist in the teaching of community health issues.
- • Refer to Deficient **Knowledge** care plan.

Risk for Latex Allergy Reaction

NANDA-I Definition

Susceptible to a hypersensitive reaction to natural latex rubber products or latex reactive foods, which may compromise health

Risk Factors

Inadequate knowledge about avoidance of relevant allergens; inattentive to potential environmental latex exposure; inattentive to potential exposure to latex reactive foods

At-Risk Population

Individuals frequently exposed to latex product; individuals receiving repetitive injections from rubber topped bottles; individuals with family history of atopic dermatitis; individuals with history of latex reaction; infants undergoing numerous operations beginning soon after birth

Associated Condition

Asthma; atopy; food allergy; hypersensitivity to natural latex rubber protein; multiple surgical procedures; poinsettia plant allergy; urinary bladder diseases

Client Outcomes

Client Will (Specify Time Frame)

- State risk factors for natural rubber latex (NRL) allergy
- Request latex-free environment
- Demonstrate knowledge of plan to treat NRL allergic reaction

Nursing Interventions

- Clients at high risk for NRL allergy need to be identified.
- Clients with spina bifida are a high-risk group for NRL allergy and should remain latex free from the first day of life.
- Children who require regular medical treatments at home (e.g., catheterization, home ventilation) should be assessed for NRL allergy.
- Assess for NRL allergy in clients who are exposed to "hidden" latex.
- See care plan for **Latex Allergy** response.

Home Care

- Ensure that the client has a medical plan if a response develops.
- See care plan for **Latex Allergy** response. Note client history and environmental assessment.

Client/Family Teaching and Discharge Planning

▲ A client who has had symptoms of NRL allergy or who suspects he or she is allergic to latex needs to give this information to healthcare providers.
- Provide written information about latex allergy and sensitivity.
- Healthcare workers should avoid the use of latex gloves and seek alternatives such as unpowdered gloves made from nitrile.
- Healthcare institutions should develop prevention programs and establish latex-safe areas in their facilities.
- Institute measures that reduce or completely avoid any latex exposure to clients.

Readiness for Enhanced Health Literacy

NANDA-I Definition

A pattern of using and developing a set of skills and competencies (literacy, knowledge, motivation, culture, and language) to find, comprehend, evaluate and use health information and concepts to make daily health decisions to promote and maintain health, decrease health risks, and improve overall quality of life, which can be strengthened

Defining Characteristics

Expresses desire to enhance ability to read; write; speak; and interpret numbers for every day health needs; expresses desire to enhance awareness of civic and/or government processes that impact public health; expresses desire to enhance health communication with healthcare providers; expresses desire to enhance knowledge of current determinants of health on social and physical environments; expresses desire to enhance personal healthcare decision-making; expresses desire to enhance social support for health; expresses desire to enhance understanding of customs and beliefs to make healthcare decisions; expresses desire to enhance understanding of health information to make healthcare choices; expresses desire to obtain sufficient information to navigate the healthcare system

L

Client Outcomes

Client Will (Specify Time Frame)

- Use reputable information sources
- Seek information from healthcare providers
- Communicate with healthcare provider about understanding of information provided

Nursing Interventions

- Use a standard tool to identify the level of health literacy.
- Identify and take into consideration factors affecting health literacy such as age, ethnicity, education, and cognitive function.
- Implement health literacy universal precautions: assume that all patients may have difficulty understanding health information.
- Determine readiness for increased health literacy.
- Tailor health teaching and educational materials to accommodate the needs of those with low health literacy.
- Modify health teaching and educational materials to patient preferences.
- Use empowerment to enhance health literacy and improve patient outcomes.
- Use individual or group interventions as preferred by the patient and appropriate to the topic.

Geriatric

- The above interventions may be adapted for geriatric use.
- Use simple educational materials targeted at health-promoting behaviors.

Multicultural

- Take the patient's culture into account when designing teaching and education materials.

Client/Family Teaching and Discharge Planning

- Promote shared decision-making.

L

Risk for Impaired Liver Function

NANDA-I Definition

Susceptible to a decrease in liver function, which may compromise health

Risk Factors

Substance misuse

Associated Condition

Human immunodeficiency virus (HIV) coinfection; pharmaceutical agent; viral infection

Client Outcomes

Client Will (Specify Time Frame)

- State the upper limit of the amount of acetaminophen safely taken per day
- Verbalize understanding that over-the-counter (OTC) medications may contain acetaminophen (e.g., OTC cold medicines)
- Have normal liver enzymes, serum and urinary bilirubin levels, white blood cell count, and red blood cell count
- Be free of unexplained weight loss, jaundice, pruritus, bruising, petechiae, gastrointestinal bleeding, and hemorrhage
- Be free of abdominal tenderness/pain, increased abdominal girth, and have normal-colored stool and urine
- Be able to eat frequent small meals per day without nausea and/or vomiting
- If alcohol abuse is factor, state relationship between abuse and worsening gastrointestinal and liver disease

Nursing Interventions

- ▲ Assess for signs of liver dysfunction including fatigue, nausea, jaundice of the eyes or skin, pruritus, gastrointestinal bleeding, coagulopathy, infections, increasing abdominal girth, fluid overload, shortness of breath, mental status changes, light-colored stools, dark urine, and increased serum and urinary bilirubin levels.
- ▲ Evaluate liver function tests. Standard liver panels include the serum enzymes aspartate transaminase (AST), alanine transaminase (ALT), alkaline phosphatase, and γ-glutamyl transferase; total, direct, and indirect serum bilirubin; and serum albumin.
- ▲ Discuss with the client/family preparations for other diagnostic studies, such as ultrasound, computed tomography, and magnetic resonance imaging (MRI) exams.
- ▲ Evaluate coagulation studies such as international normalized ratio, prothrombin time, and partial thromboplastin time, especially when there is bleeding of the mouth or gums.
- • Monitor for signs of hemorrhage, especially in the upper gastrointestinal tract, because it is the most frequent site.
- • Obtain a list of all medications, including OTC nonsteroidal antiinflammatory drugs, acetaminophen, herbal remedies, and dietary supplements. Review risk of drug-induced liver disease. The list includes some antibiotics, anticonvulsants, antidepressants, antiinflammatory drugs, antiplatelets, antihypertensives, calcium channel blockers, cyclosporine, lipid-lowering drugs, chemotherapy drugs, oral hypoglycemics, proton pump inhibitors, inhaled anesthetics, and tranquilizers, among others (Hamilton, Collins-Yoder, & Collins, 2016). If client is taking either OTC medications or herbals, discuss signs and symptoms of toxic hepatitis.
- ▲ For clients receiving drugs associated with liver injury, review risk factors to prevent potentially severe drug reactions.
- ▲ Determine the total amount of acetaminophen the client is taking per day. The amount of acetaminophen ingested should not exceed 3.25 g per day, or even lower in the client with chronic alcohol intake (Hamilton, Collins-Yoder, & Collins, 2016).

L

- ▲ Evaluation of acetaminophen-associated drug-induced liver injury is done by patient history of ingestion, time, and doses of the medication per weight calculation and serum level of acetaminophen.
- ▲ If the client is on statin medications, ensure that liver enzyme testing is done at intervals. Liver enzymes can become elevated from taking statin medications; it is rare but possible for statins to cause actual liver damage (Hamilton, Collins-Yoder, & Collins, 2016).
- ▲ If the client is an alcoholic, refer to a cessation program. It is essential the client stop drinking as soon as possible to allow the liver to heal. Alcoholism is associated with malnutrition, which is harmful to the liver (Fabrellas, 2017). Alcoholism is also associated with increased plasma endotoxins and disruption of the gut barrier, which cause inflammation and resultant damage to the liver (Cassard, Gerard, & Perlemuter, 2017). See care plans for Ineffective **Denial** and Dysfunctional **Family** processes.
- ▲ Provide frequent smaller meals for easier digestion. Provide diet with optimal carbohydrates, proteins, and fats. Consult with a registered dietitian to discuss best nutritional support.
- ▲ Recognize that severe malnutrition may result in acute liver failure, which is reversible with improved nutrition.
- ▲ Review medical history with the client, recognizing that obesity and type 2 diabetes, along with hypertriglyceridemia and polycystic ovarian syndrome, are major risk factors in the development of liver disease, specifically nonalcoholic fatty liver disease.
- • Encourage vaccinations for hepatitis A and B for all ages.
- • Measure abdominal girth if individual presents with abdominal distention and pain.
- • Assess for tenderness and/or pain level in the right upper quadrant. Tenderness in this area is a symptom of biliary, liver, and/or pancreatic problems.
- • Use standard precautions for handling of blood and body fluids. Review sterile techniques when giving intravenous solution and/or medications.
- ▲ Observe for signs and symptoms of mental status changes such as confusion from encephalopathy.

Pediatric/Parents

- ▲ Prescreen pregnant women for hepatitis B surface antigens. If found, recommend nursing case management during pregnancy.
- ▲ Recommend implementation of postexposure prophylaxis, including the hepatitis B virus vaccine for an infant born to a hepatitis B surface antigen–positive woman (CDC, 2016).
- • Encourage vaccinations for hepatitis A and B for all ages.
- ▲ Recognize that children can develop fatty liver disease, which can result in liver failure. Most children are asymptomatic, but others complain of malaise, fatigue, or vague recurrent abdominal pain (Marzuillo, del Guidice, & Santoro, 2014).
- ▲ During a well-baby visit, assess for signs of potential liver problems. Observe for prolonged jaundice, pale stools, and urine that is anything other than colorless. Consult with healthcare provider to order a split bilirubin as needed (CDC, 2016).

Home Care

- • Encourage rest, optimal nutrition (high carbohydrates, sufficient protein, and essential vitamins and minerals) during initial inflammatory processes of the liver.

Client/Family Teaching and Discharge Planning

- • Teach the client and family to examine all medications the client is taking, looking for acetaminophen as an ingredient, and reinforce the 3.25-g upper limit of intake of acetaminophen to protect liver function (Hamilton, Collins-Yoder, & Collins, 2016).
- • For the caregiver or client with hepatitis A, B, or C, teach the need for careful handwashing, use of gloves, and other precautions to prevent spread of any of these diseases.
- • Teach avoidance of high-risk behaviors that cause hepatitis and ways to avoid those behaviors.
- • Educate clients and their caregivers about treatment options and interventions for hepatitis. Recommend other informational support: risk factors, side effects of the different treatment options, and dietary advice.
- • Recommend psychological support if possible during education sessions.
- • Assess for adherence to antiviral therapies for the treatment of hepatitis and institute nursing interventions such as client education,

communication, and reminder tools to assist patients in medication adherence.

- For those clients with mental health problems, collaborate with outreach programs to teach signs/symptoms of hepatitis, risk factors, and factors that increase transmission.

Risk for Loneliness

NANDA-I Definition

Susceptible to experiencing discomfort associated with a desire or need for more contact with others, which may compromise health

Risk Factors

Affectional deprivation; emotional deprivation; physical isolation; social isolation

Client Outcomes

Client Will (Specify Time Frame)

- Maintain one or more meaningful relationships (growth-enhancing versus codependent or abusive in nature)
- Sustain relationships that allow self-disclosure and demonstrate a balance between emotional dependence and independence
- Participate in personally meaningful activities and interactions that are ongoing, positive, and relevant socially
- Demonstrate positive use of time alone when socialization is not possible

Nursing Interventions

- Assess the client's perception of loneliness. (Is the person alone by choice, or are there other factors that contribute to the feelings of loneliness? Is the client in one of the at-risk populations for loneliness?)
- Use active listening skills. Establish a therapeutic relationship and spend quality time with the client.
- Assess how unmet needs challenge the client. Note: See care plan for Disturbed **Body Image** if loneliness is associated with chronic illness and/or afflictions (e.g., multiple sclerosis, skin disturbance, mental illness).

▲ Assess the bereaved client for risk of suicide and make appropriate referrals as necessary.

- Assess the client who is alone for substance abuse and make appropriate referrals.
- Evaluate the client's desire for social interaction.
- Assess the client for feelings of loneliness.
- Explore ways to increase the client's support systems.
- Show respect for the client's personal attributes.

Adolescents

- Assess the client's social support system.
- Evaluate the family stability of adolescent clients.
- Evaluate peer relationships.
- Encourage relationships with peers and involvement with groups and organizations.

Geriatric

- Evaluate the client for any health deviations that may limit or decrease his or her ability to interact with others.
- Assess family caregivers of older persons with chronic conditions for depression related to loneliness.
- Identify support systems for older adults.
- When relocation is necessary for older adults, evaluate relocation stress as a contributing factor to loneliness.
- Identify risk factors for loneliness in older persons.
- Encourage support for the client when the decision to stop driving must be made.
- Provide activities that are pleasurable to the client.

Multicultural

- Refer to the care plan for **Social** isolation.

Home Care

▲ The preceding interventions may be adapted for home care use.

▲ Assess for depression with the lonely older client and make appropriate referrals.

- If the client has unexplained somatic complaints, evaluate these complaints to ensure that his or her physical needs are being met, and assess for a possible relationship between somatic complaints and loneliness.
- Evaluate alternatives to being alone.
- Refer to the care plan for **Social** isolation.

Client/Family Teaching and Discharge Planning

- Identify the type of loneliness that the client is experiencing as emotional and/or social.
- Encourage family members' involvement, if possible, in helping alleviate client's loneliness.
- Include the family, if possible, in all client-teaching activities, and give them accurate information.
- Provide appropriate education for clients and their support persons about disease transmission and treatment if applicable.
- Refer to the care plan for **Social** isolation for additional interventions.

M

Risk for Disturbed Maternal-Fetal Dyad

NANDA-I Definition

Susceptible to disruption of the symbiotic mother–fetal relationship as a result of comorbid or pregnancy-related conditions, which may compromise health

Risk Factors

Inadequate prenatal care; presence of abuse; substance misuse

Associated Condition

Alteration in glucose metabolism; compromised fetal oxygen transport; pregnancy complication; treatment regimen

Client Outcomes

Client Will (Specify Time Frame)

- Cope with discomforts of high-risk pregnancy until delivery of baby
- Demonstrate emotional attachment to fetus
- Adhere to prescribed regimens to maintain homeostasis during pregnancy

Nursing Interventions

- Standardize internal and external transport forms using the situation, background, assessment, and recommendation (SBAR) format to provide safe and efficient care of a high-risk pregnant client.

- Assess the antenatal client for fear related to high-risk pregnancy and fetal outcomes. Encourage verbalization of feelings, beliefs, and concerns about fetal well-being, maternal health, and family functioning. Include family when possible. Refer for treatment as needed.
- Assess antepartum clients for depression using a culturally competent tool that evaluates the bio-psycho-social-spiritual dimensions.
- Offer flexible visiting hours, private space for families, and nursing support for management of family stressors; provide distractors such as music, TV, and laptops with Internet access during hospitalization for high-risk pregnancy.
- Focus on the abilities of a pregnant woman with disabilities by encouraging identification of support systems, resources, and need for environmental modification.
- Assess for lack of social support system, loneliness, depression, lack of confidence, maternal powerlessness, domestic violence, and socioeconomic problems.
- Recognize patterns of physical abuse in all pregnant and postpartum women, regardless of age, race, and socioeconomic status.
- Perform accurate blood pressure readings at each client's clinic encounter.
- Provide educational materials and support for personal autonomy about genetic counseling and testing options before pregnancy with preimplantation genetic testing or during pregnancy with fetal nuchal translucency ultrasound, quadruple screen, and cystic fibrosis screening.
- Identify adherence barriers and assist with meal selections to maintain optimal nutrition and safe pregnancy weight gain (25–35 pounds; 15–25 pounds if overweight). Identify cultural beliefs and nutritional patterns. A prenatal vitamin with 400 μcg of folate should also be strongly recommended.
- Teach pregnant women diagnosed with gestational diabetes about management and treatment.
- Assess use of tobacco and, if positive for use, offer a tobacco cessation program and explain the health risks to the unborn fetus and mother.
- Assess for alcohol use and counsel women to stop drinking during pregnancy. Give appropriate referral for treatment if needed.

M

- Screen for current illicit drug use. Emphasize the risks or drug exposure to the fetus/newborn and the potential for withdrawal. Offer nonjudgmental compassionate care.
- Refer clients who self-report drug abuse or have positive toxicology screens to a comprehensive addiction program designed for the pregnant woman. Children born to addicted mothers often have poor neonatal outcomes.
- Encourage pregnant women to use digital resources, such as Text4Baby (see https://www.text4baby.org) or https://www.whattoexpect.com, to track pregnancy progress and provide education and motivation to make healthy lifestyle choices (abstinence from poor nutrition, smoking, and alcohol).

Impaired Memory

NANDA-I Definition

Persistent inability to remember or recall bits of information or skills, while maintaining the capacity to independently perform activities of daily living.

Defining Characteristics

Consistently forgets to perform a behavior at the scheduled time; difficulty acquiring a new skill; difficulty acquiring new information; difficulty recalling events; difficulty recalling factual information; difficulty recalling familiar names; difficulty recalling familiar objects; difficulty recalling familiar words; difficulty recalling if a behavior was performed; difficulty retaining a new skill; difficulty retaining new information

Related Factors

Depressive symptoms; inadequate intellectual stimulation; inadequate motivation; inadequate social support; social isolation; water-electrolyte imbalance

At Risk Population

Economically disadvantaged individuals; individuals aged ≥ 60 years; individuals with low educational level

Associated Conditions

Anemia; brain hypoxia; cognition disorders

Client Outcomes

Client Will (Specify Time Frame)

- Demonstrate use of techniques to help with memory loss
- State he or she has improved memory for everyday concerns

Nursing Interventions

- Determine whether onset of memory loss is gradual or sudden.
- Assess overall cognitive function and memory. A brief screening instrument such as the Montreal Cognitive Assessment (s-MoCA) is useful as a first level of evaluation.
- Assess risk of malnutrition, including risk for thiamine (B_1) associated with chronic alcohol abuse, cancer, bariatric surgery, and risk of vitamin D deficiency–associated history of inadequate exposure to sunlight.
- Determine the client's sleep quality and patterns. If sleep quantity and quality is insufficient, or symptoms of obstructive sleep apnea are reported, refer to the care plan for Disturbed **Sleep** pattern.
- Teach clients, including those with cognitive disorders, to use memory techniques such as concentrating and attending, repeating information, making mental associations, and placing items in strategic places so that they will not be forgotten.
- Encourage the client to participate in a multicomponent cognitive rehabilitation program that includes stress and relaxation training, physical activity, structured learning, and social interaction.
- Encourage the client to develop an aerobic exercise program.
- For clients with memory impairments associated with dementia, also see care plan for **Chronic Confusion.**

Geriatric

- Assess for signs and symptoms of depression.
- Teach older adults that they can improve their memory and learn strategies to compensate for memory loss.

▲ Refer the client for cognitive training.

Multicultural

- When using cognitive assessments that have been translated into other languages, refer to translation-specific scoring instructions and any recommended adjustment for low-levels of education.
- Assess for the influence of cultural beliefs, norms, and values on the family or caregiver's understanding of impaired memory.
- Visitation facilitation: stigma may result in social isolation, and older adults with memory impairment may need assistance to rebuild and strengthen their social network.

Home Care

- The previously mentioned interventions may be adapted for home care use.

M

- Assist clients to select and use cuing strategies or assistive technology, such as a smart watch, smart phone, pill box, calendar, alarm clock, microwave oven, whistling tea kettle, sign, or written list to cue behaviors at designated times.

Client/Family Teaching and Discharge Planning

- When teaching the client, determine what the client knows about memory techniques and then build on that knowledge.
- When teaching a skill to the client, set up a series of practice attempts that will enhance motivation. Begin with simple tasks so the client can be positively reinforced and progress to more difficult concepts.
- ▲ Refer for care coordination if family caregiver is unavailable or unable to assist.

Risk for Metabolic Syndrome

NANDA-I Definition

Susceptible to developing a cluster of symptoms that increase risk of cardiovascular disease and type 2 diabetes mellitus, which may compromise health.

Risk Factors

Absence of interest in improving health behaviors; average daily physical activity is less than recommended for age and gender; body mass index above normal range for age and gender; excessive accumulation of fat for age and gender; excessive alcohol intake; excessive stress; inadequate dietary habits; inadequate knowledge of modifiable factors; inattentive to second-hand smoke; smoking

At-Risk Population

Individuals aged > 30 years; individuals with family history of diabetes mellitus; individuals with family history of dyslipidemia; individuals with family history of hypertension; individuals with family history of metabolic syndrome; individuals with family history of obesity; individuals with family history of unstable blood pressure

Associated Conditions

– Hyperuricemia
– Insulin resistance
– Polycystic ovary syndrome

Client Outcomes

Client Will (Specify Time Frame)

- Maintain blood glucose within normal limits
- Explain actions and precautions to decrease cardiovascular risk

- Maintain waist circumference of less than 102 centimeters/40 inches in men, or less than 88 centimeters/35 inches in women
- Explain the risk factors associated with lipid disorders
- Maintain normal laboratory results, specifically high-sensitivity C-reactive protein, triglycerides, fasting blood glucose, and high-density lipoprotein (HDL) cholesterol
- Design lifestyle modifications to meet individual long-term goal of health, using effective risk control strategies
- Maintain weight within normal range for height and age
- Develop a system of self-management, for improved dietary intake and physical activity

Nursing Interventions

- Assess for risk factors associated with metabolic syndrome. Risk factors for metabolic syndrome include central obesity, dyslipidemia, insulin resistance, and increased blood pressure.
- Assess clients for elevated waist circumference measures; greater than 102 cm/40 inches or more in men, or greater than 88 cm/35 inches or more in women.
- Examine the client's skin for acanthosis nigricans, acrochordons, keratosis pilaris, hyperandrogenism, and hirsutism, which are skin diseases associated with insulin resistance and obesity.
- Assess the effect of psychosocial risk factors on cardiovascular risk.
- Assess and report abnormal laboratory results, specifically high-sensitivity C-reactive protein, triglycerides, fasting blood glucose, and HDL cholesterol.
- Screen clients who are prescribed antipsychotic medications for metabolic syndrome during routine health treatment.
- Screen clients with a family history of polycystic ovary syndrome for metabolic syndrome.
- Assist obese clients to develop a system of self-management, which may include self-monitoring of weight, body mass index (BMI), realistic goal setting, planning, and action planning for improved dietary intake and physical activity; problem-solving; and tracking dietary intake and exercise.
- Encourage strength training for the client to address modifiable risk factors of metabolic syndrome.
- Provide nutritional teaching targeted at reducing daily energy, fat intakes, sugar intakes, and increasing the frequency of eating two portions of vegetables during each meal.

M

- Encourage the client to engage in vigorous-intensity physical activity for at least 150 minutes weekly or moderate-intensity physical activity for at least 300 minutes weekly to improve cardiorespiratory fitness and influence body shape and weight.
- Counsel clients to slow the pace of their eating during meals.
- Provide teaching about reducing intake of ultra-processed foods and increasing intake of minimally processed foods.
- Encourage once or more weekly consumption of lean fish.
- Use social media for communication with clients to implement social support and share information about lifestyle modifications.
- Refer clients with Class II and III obesity and diabetes for bariatric surgery consideration.

Pediatric

- Assess adolescent clients for vitamin D deficiency with additional screening for prediabetes if deficiencies are found.
- Provide preventive interventions for obesity during early childhood. **EBN:** A meta-analysis found that overweight or obesity in early childhood was associated with a higher risk of adult metabolic syndrome compared with the controls (Kim et al., 2017).

Geriatric

Note: Many of the preceding interventions also apply.

- Encourage strength training for older women.
- Encourage Tai chi training for older adults.

Multicultural

- Use criteria in addition to overweight and obesity when screening for cardiometabolic abnormalities in racial/ethnic minority populations.
- Provide African American women with community-based prevention education targeted toward improving knowledge, reducing clinical risk profiles, adoption of heart-healthy lifestyles, reducing inflammatory burden, and decreasing cardiometabolic risk.

Home Care

- Previously discussed interventions may be adapted for home care use.

Client/Family Teaching and Discharge Planning

- Many of the preceding interventions involve teaching.
- Work with the family members regarding information on how to identify and reduce risk factors related to metabolic syndrome.

Impaired Bed Mobility

NANDA-I Definition

Limitation of independent movement from one bed position to another

Defining Characteristics

Difficulty moving between long sitting and supine positions; difficulty moving between prone and supine positions; difficulty moving between sitting and supine positions; difficulty reaching objects on the bed; difficulty repositioning self in bed; difficulty returning to the bed; difficulty rolling on the bed; difficulty sitting on edge of bed; difficulty turning from side to side

Related Factors

Decreased flexibility; environmental constraints; impaired postural balance; inadequate angle of headboard; inadequate knowledge of mobility strategies; insufficient muscle strength; obesity; pain; physical deconditioning

At Risk Population

Children; individuals experiencing prolonged bed rest; individuals in the early postoperative period; older adults

Associated Condition

Artificial respiration; critical illness; dementia; drain tubes; musculoskeletal impairment; neurodegenerative disorders; neuromuscular diseases; Parkinson's disease; pharmaceutical preparations; sedation

Client Outcomes

Client Will (Specify Time Frame)

- Demonstrate optimal independence in positioning, exercising, and performing functional activities in bed
- Demonstrate ability to direct others on how to do bed positioning, exercising, and functional activities

Nursing Interventions

▲ Recognize that components of normal bed mobility include rolling, bridging, scooting, long sitting, and sitting upright. Activity starts with the client supine, flat in bed, and promotes normal movements that are bilateral, segmental, well timed, and involve set positions such as weight bearing and trunk centering. Refer to a physical therapist (PT) for individualized instructions and mobility strategies.

- Choose therapeutic beds and positions based on client's history and risk profile.
  - Advocate for specialty beds for bedbound patients incorporating low-airloss pressure relief, shear reduction with position changes, and turn assist.

M

- ❍ Use devices such as a trapeze, friction-reducing slide sheets, mechanical lateral transfer aids, and ceiling-mounted or floor lifts to move (rather than drag) clients in bed to prevent injury to staff.
- ❍ Use special beds and equipment to move clients, such as mattress overlay, sliding/roller board, trapeze, stirrup, and pulley attached to overhead traction system (holds one leg up during pericare).

- • Place clients in free-standing or ceiling-mounted lifts with padded slings while changing bed linen.
- • All patients can benefit from a high sitting position to potentially minimize orthostatic intolerance (Khan et al., 2002).
- • Assess to determine whether positioning for one condition may negatively affect another; use critical thinking skills for risk–benefit analysis.
- • Elevate HOB to 30 to 45 degrees unless contraindicated, and elevate HOB to 90 degrees during oral intake of fluids, solids, and oral medications.
- • Raise HOB to 30 degrees for clients with acute increased intracranial pressure and brain injury.
- ▲ Consult healthcare provider for HOB elevation for acute stroke and monitor response.
- • Raise HOB as close to 45 degrees as possible for critically ill ventilated clients to prevent pneumonia (this height may place clients at higher risk for adult pressure injuries). Elevating the HOB decreases regurgitation and risk for aspiration of gastric contents.
- • Assist client with dysphagia to sit as upright as possible for oral intake, including solids, fluids, and oral medications. Refer to care plan for Impaired **Swallowing.**
- • Periodically sit client upright as tolerated in bed; dangle client, if vital signs and oxygen saturation levels remain stable.
- • To decrease risk of pressure injury, maintain HOB at lowest elevation that is medically possible and raise the foot of the bed to prevent shear-related injury. Assess the client's sacrum, ischial tuberosities, and heels at least every 2 hours.
- • Try periods of prone positioning for clients and monitor their tolerance/response.
- • Assess client's risk for falls using a valid fall risk assessment tool, such as the Morse Fall Scale (Morse, Tylko, & Dixon, 1987) and implement specific measures to mitigate identified risk factors.
- • Beds should be kept locked and in the lowest position when occupied. Specialty low beds in which mattresses are approximately

8 to 12 inches from the floor are helpful for clients at risk for falls. Cushioned mats, 2 to 3 inches thick, with beveled edges lined with reflective tape and covered by a rubberized material are also helpful.

▲ Bed rails and restraints must be prescribed by a healthcare provider.

▲ While placing all four bed rails up is considered a form of restraint and requires a healthcare provider's prescription, two and even three rails up can be a support for bed mobility.

• Place frequently used items within client's reach; demonstrate use of call bell (Hill & Fauerbach, 2014).

• Use a formalized screening tool to identify clients who are at high risk for deep venous thrombosis, e.g., obesity, cancer diagnosis, pelvic surgery, immobility, prior history of deep vein thrombosis (DVT).

▲ Assess for injury associated with thromboembolism prophylaxis and other prescribed treatment (e.g., anticoagulants, compression stockings, elastic leg wraps, sequential compression devices, feet/ankle exercises, and hydration). Refer to care plan for Ineffective peripheral **Tissue Perfusion.**

• Use a valid and reliable tool to assess a client's risk for pressure injury.

• Implement the following interventions to prevent pressure ulcers and complications of immobility:
  - Position sitting clients with special attention to the individual's anatomy, postural alignment, distribution of weight, and foot support.
  - Use static/dynamic bed surfaces and assess for "bottoming out" under susceptible bony areas (body sinks into mattress, thus the recommended 1 inch between mattress/bones is absent). Refer to care plan for Risk for impaired **Skin** integrity.
  - Use heel protection devices that completely float or offload heels (National Pressure Ulcer Advisory Panel et al., 2014).
  - Implement a 2-hour on/off schedule for heel protector boots or high-top tennis shoes with socks underneath in clients with paralyzed feet, and check condition of heels when removed.
  - Strictly maintain leg abduction in persons with a surgical hip pinning or replacement by placing an abductor splint/pillow between legs if prescribed.
  - Place bariatric beds along a corner wall, which helps keep the bed from moving during repositioning.
  - Identify/modify hospital beds with large gaps between bed rail/mattress that create an entrapment hazard. Ensure that mattresses fit the bed; install gap fillers/rail inserts, then monitor effectiveness.

- Apply elbow pads to comatose and/or restrained clients and to those who use their elbows to prop or scoot up in bed. Apply nocturnal elbow splint as prescribed if ulnar nerve palsy exists or if painful elbow with paresthesia in ulnar side of fourth/fifth fingers develops. Reassess sensation every 2 to 4 hours.
- Explain importance of exhaling versus holding one's breath (Valsalva maneuver) and straining during bed activities.
- Reassess pain level, especially before movement and/or exercising, and accept clients' pain ratings and levels they think is appropriate for comfort. Administer analgesics based on clients' pain rating. Refer to Acute **Pain** or Chronic **Pain.**

Exercise

- Test strength in bilateral grips, arms at elbow flexion and extension, bilateral arm abduction and adduction, bilateral leg or thigh raise (one at a time in bed or chair), and quadriceps and hamstring strength to extend and flex at knee to assess baseline and interval strength gains.
- Perform passive range of motion (ROM) of three repetitions, at least twice a day, to immobile joints.
- Range or move a hemiplegic arm with the shoulder slightly externally rotated (hand up).

▲ Encourage client's practice of exercises taught by therapists (muscle setting, strengthening, contraction against resistance, and weight lifting).

Bed Positioning

- Incorporate the following measures to promote normal tone and prevent complications in clients with neurological impairment:
  - ❍ Use a flat head pillow when clients are supine. Use a small pillow behind the head and/or between shoulder blades if neck extension occurs.
  - ❍ Abduct the shoulders of clients with high paraplegia or quadriplegia horizontally to 90 degrees briefly two to three times a day while client is supine.
  - ❍ Position a hemiplegic shoulder fairly close to the client's body.
- Tilt hemiplegics onto both unaffected and affected sides with the affected shoulder slightly forward (e.g., move/lift the affected shoulder, not the forearm/hand).

▲ Elevate a client's paralyzed forearms on a pillow when client is supine. Elevate edematous legs on a pillow supporting the knees to prevent hyperextension. Apply resting wrist, hand, and foot/ankle splints and pressure garments or other devices as prescribed. Range joints before applying splints. Adhere to on/off schedule as prescribed by the PT. Remove splints and compression garments or devices.

Geriatric

- Assess caregiver's strength, health history, and cognitive status to predict ability/risk for assisting bedbound clients at home. Refer to care plan for **Caregiver Role Strain.**
- Assess the client's stamina and energy level during bed activities/exercises; if limited, spread out activities and allow rest breaks.

Home Care

- ▲ Collaborate with nurse case managers, care coordinators, social workers, and physical/occupational therapists to assess home support systems and needs, and to provide for home modifications, durable medical equipment, assistive technology, and home health services.
- Encourage use of the client's own bed unless contraindicated. Raise HOB with commercial blocks or grooved-out pieces of wood under legs; set bed against walls in a corner. Emotionally, clients may benefit from sleeping in their own beds with familiar partners.
- Stress psychological/physical benefits of clients being as self-sufficient as possible with bed mobility/care even though it may be time-consuming. Allowing independence and autonomy may help prevent disuse syndromes and feelings of helplessness and low self-esteem.
- Offer emotional support and help client identify usual coping responses to help with adjustment and loss issues. The home environment may trigger the reality of lost function and disability.
- Discuss support systems available for caregivers to help them cope. Refer to care plan for **Caregiver Role Strain.**
- ▲ In the presence of medical disorders, institute case management for frail older adults to support continued independent living as much as possible or desired by the client.
- Refer to the home care interventions in the care plan for Impaired physical **Mobility.**

Client/Family Teaching and Discharge Planning

- Use various sensory modalities to teach client/caregivers correct ROM, exercises, positioning, self-care activities, and use of devices. Readiness and learning styles vary but may be enhanced with visual/auditory/tactile/cognitive stimulus as follows:
  - Provide demonstrations, sketches, instructional videos, and written directions/schedules, notes.

M

- ○ Provide verbal instructions, recorded audiotapes, timers, reading aloud written directions, and self-talk during activities.
- ○ Use motor task practice/repetition, return demonstrations, note taking, manual guidance, or staff's-hand-on-client's-hand technique.

▲ Schedule time with family/caregivers for education and practice for nursing, physical therapy, and occupational therapy. Suggest family come prepared with questions and wear comfortable, safe clothing/shoes. Practice provides opportunity for learning; repetition helps memory retention.

▲ Implement safe approaches for caregivers/home care staff and reinforce an adequate number of people and handling equipment (e.g., friction pads, slide boards, lifts) during bed mobility, exercise, toileting, and bathing to decrease risk of injury.

▲ Coordinate evaluations for bariatric equipment for home use before discharge, including a weight-rated bed, a wheelchair or mobility device (scooter), and lift device. Doorways may need to be widened, floors reinforced, and ramps added for safety.

Impaired Physical Mobility

NANDA-I Definition

Limitation in independent, purposeful physical movement of the body or of one or more extremities

Defining Characteristics

Alteration in gait; decrease in fine motor skills; decrease in gross motor skills; decrease in range of motion; decrease in reaction time; difficulty turning; discomfort; engages in substitutions for movement; exertional dyspnea; movement-induced tremor; postural instability; slowed movement; spastic movement; uncoordinated movement

Related Factors

Decreased activity tolerance; anxiety; body mass index (BMI) >75th percentile appropriate for age and gender; cultural belief regarding acceptable activity; decrease in endurance; decrease in muscle control; decrease in muscle mass; decrease in muscle strength; depression; disuse; insufficient environmental support; insufficient knowledge of value of physical activity; joint stiffness; malnutrition; pain; physical deconditioning; reluctance to initiate movement; sedentary lifestyle

Associated Condition

Alteration in bone structure integrity; alteration in cognitive functioning; alteration in metabolism; contractures; developmental delay; musculoskeletal impairment; neuromuscular impairment; pharmaceutical agent; prescribed movement restrictions; sensory-perceptual impairment

Client Outcomes

Client Will (Specify Time Frame)

- Meet mutually defined goals of increased ambulation and exercise that include individual choice, preference, and enjoyment in the exercise prescription
- Describe feeling stronger and more mobile
- Describe less fear of falling and pain with physical activity
- Demonstrate use of adaptive equipment (e.g., wheelchairs, walkers, gait belts, weighted walking vests) to increase mobility
- Increase exercise to 20 minutes per day for those who were previously sedentary (less than 150 minutes per week). Note: Light- to moderate-intensity exercise may be beneficial in deconditioned persons. In very deconditioned individuals exercise bouts of less than 10 minutes are beneficial.
- Increase pedometer step counts by 1000 steps per day every 2 weeks to reach a daily step count of at least 7000 steps per day, with a daily goal for most healthy adults of 10,000 steps per day (approximately 5 miles)
- Perform resistance exercises that involve all major muscle groups (legs, hips, back, chest, abdomen, shoulders, and arms) performed 2 or 3 days per week
- Perform flexibility exercise (stretching) for each of the major muscle-tendon groups 2 days per week for 10 to 60 seconds to improve joint range of motion (ROM); greatest gains occur with daily exercise
- Engage in neuromotor exercise 20 to 30 minutes per day, including motor skills (e.g., balance, agility, coordination, gait), proprioceptive exercise training, and multifaceted activities (e.g., Tai chi, yoga) to improve and maintain physical function and reduce falls in those at risk for falling (older persons)
- Engage in purposeful moderate-intensity cardiorespiratory (aerobic) exercise for 30 to 60 minutes per day at least 5 days per week for a total of 2 hours and 30 minutes (150 minutes) per week

Nursing Interventions

- Adults with disabilities should follow the adult guidelines. If this is not possible, they should be as physically active as their abilities allow and avoid inactivity (US Department of Health & Human Services, 2008). Use "start low and go slow" approach for intensity and duration of physical activity if client is highly deconditioned, functionally limited, or has chronic conditions affecting performance of physical tasks. When progressing client's activities, use an individualized and tailored approach based on client's tolerance and preferences (Riebe et al., 2015).

- Assess for fear of falling.
- Screen for mobility skills in the following order: (1) bed mobility; (2) dangling and supported and unsupported sitting; (3) weight-bearing for sit to stand, transfer to chair; (4) standing and walking with assistance; and (5) walking independently.
- Assess muscle strength and other factors affecting balance, mobility, and endurance. Immobility can affect tissue perfusion and increase risk of postural hypotension; shortness of breath decreases endurance and increases fear; bowel or bladder incontinence can decrease motivation to be mobile; cognitive and neuromuscular deficits, including side effects of medication, can affect balance, coordination, and movement; and pain, fear, or sick role expectations can decrease willingness to be mobile.

- Refer to care plans for Risk for Adult **Falls,** Acute **Pain,** Chronic **Pain,** Ineffective **Coping,** or **Hopelessness.**
- Increase activity tolerance with graded increases in self-care (function-focused care [FFC]), such as bathing, walking to the bathroom instead of using a bedpan/urinal, and ROM.
- Consider patient's self-reported fear of falling.

▲ Before activity, observe for and, if possible, treat pain with massage, heat pack to affected area, or medication. Ensure that the client is not oversedated.

- Obtain any assistive devices needed for activity, such as gait belt, weighted vest, walker, cane, crutches, or wheelchair, ergonomic shower chairs; ceiling and floor-based lifts; and air-assisted lateral transfer devices.
- Monitor and record the client's response to activity, such as pulse rate, blood pressure, dyspnea, skin color, subjective report. Refer to the care plan for **Decreased Activity** tolerance.

Special considerations: Immobility

- Perform passive ROM exercises at least twice a day unless contraindicated; repeat each maneuver three times.

▲ Consult with healthcare provider for a safety evaluation before beginning an exercise program; if program is approved, begin with the following exercises:

  - ❍ Active ROM exercises using both upper and lower extremities (e.g., flexing and extending at ankles, knees, hips)

- Chin-ups and pull-ups using a trapeze in bed (may be contraindicated in clients with cardiac conditions)
- Strengthening exercises such as gluteal or quadriceps sitting exercises

• Use assistive technology for mobilizing bedbound patients. Refer to **Impaired Bed Mobility.**

• Help the client achieve mobility and start walking as soon as possible if not contraindicated.

• Initiate a "no lift" policy where appropriate assistive devices are used for manual lifting. See **Impaired Bed Mobility.**

Other clinical conditions:

▲ If the client has osteoarthritis or rheumatoid arthritis, consult with a physical therapist to on ways to integrate aerobic exercise, resistance exercise, and flexibility exercise (stretching) into care.

▲ If client has had a cerebrovascular accident (CVA) with hemiparesis, consult with physical therapist on constraint-induced movement therapy, in which the functional extremity is purposely constrained and the client is forced to use the involved extremity.

• If the client does not feed or groom self, sit side by side with the client, put your hand over the client's hand, support the client's elbow with your other hand, and help the client feed self; use the same technique to help the client comb hair.

Geriatric

• Assess ability to move using valid and reliable criterion-referenced standards for fitness testing that can predict the level of capacity associated with maintaining physical independence into later years of life (e.g., Get Up and Go test).

• Help the mostly immobile client achieve mobility as soon as possible, depending on physical condition.

• Use the FFC rehabilitative philosophy of care in older adults to prevent avoidable functional decline.

• If the client is scheduled for an elective surgery that will result in admission into the intensive care unit and immobility, or recovery from a joint replacement, for example, initiate a prehabilitation program that includes warm-up, aerobic activity, strength, flexibility, neuromotor, and functional task work.

• Use gestures and nonverbal cues when helping clients move if they are anxious or have difficulty understanding and following verbal instructions.

• Recognize that wheelchairs are not a good mobility device and often serve as a mobility restraint.

- Ensure that chairs fit clients. Chair seat should be 3 inches above the height of the knee. Provide a raised toilet seat if needed.
- If the client is mainly immobile, provide opportunities for socialization and sensory stimulation (e.g., television and visits). Refer to the care plan for Deficient **Diversional** activity.
- Recognize that immobility and a lack of social support and sensory input may result in confusion or depression in older adults. Refer to nursing interventions for Acute **Confusion** or **Hopelessness** as appropriate.

Home Care

- The preceding interventions may be adapted for home care use.
- ▲ Begin discharge planning as soon as possible with a personal health navigator (e.g., nurse care coordinator or case manager) to assess need for and arrange home support systems, assistive devices, and community or home health services. Nurses are often the first healthcare providers to assess the patient on admission; this creates the opportunity for early discharge planning (McNeil, 2016).
- ▲ Assess home environment for factors that create barriers to physical mobility. Refer to occupational therapy services if needed to assist the client in restructuring home environment and daily living patterns.
- ▲ Refer to home health aide services to support the client and family through changing levels of mobility. Reinforce need to promote independence in mobility as tolerated.
- ▲ Refer to physical therapy for gait training, strengthening, and balance training. Physical therapists can provide direct interventions and assess need for assistive devices (e.g., cane, walker) (Miller, Sabol, & Pastva, 2017).
- Assess skin condition at every visit. Establish a skin care program that enhances circulation and maximizes position changes.
- Once the client is able to walk independently, suggest that the client enter an exercise program, or walk with a friend.
- Provide support to the client and family/caregivers during long-term impaired mobility. Refer to the care plan for **Caregiver Role Strain.**

Client/Family Teaching and Discharge Planning

- Consider using motivational interviewing techniques when working with both children and adult clients to increase their activity. Refer to the care plan for **Sedentary** lifestyle.
- Teach the client and caregivers processes and tools used during care to use at home to assess fall risk and promote progressive mobility. Involve them in planning for these activities at home.

Impaired Wheelchair Mobility

NANDA-I Definition

Limitation of independent operation of wheelchair within environment

Defining Characteristics

Difficulty bending forward to pick up object from the floor; difficulty folding or unfolding wheelchair; difficulty leaning forward to reach for something above head; difficulty locking brakes on manual wheelchair; difficulty maneuvering wheelchair sideways; difficulty moving wheelchair out of an elevator; difficulty navigating through hinged door; difficulty operating battery charger of power wheelchair; difficulty operating power wheelchair on a decline; difficulty operating power wheelchair on an incline; difficulty operating power wheelchair on curbs; difficulty operating power wheelchair on even surface; difficulty operating power wheelchair on uneven surface; difficulty operating wheelchair backwards; difficulty operating wheelchair forward; difficulty operating wheelchair in corners; difficulty operating wheelchair motors; difficulty operating wheelchair on a decline; difficulty operating wheelchair on an incline; difficulty operating wheelchair on curbs; difficulty operating wheelchair on even surface; difficulty operating wheelchair on stairs; difficulty operating wheelchair on uneven surface; difficulty operating wheelchair while carrying an object; difficulty performing pressure relief; difficulty performing stationary wheelie position; difficulty putting feet on the footplates of the wheelchair; difficulty rolling across side-slope while in wheelchair; difficulty selecting drive mode on power wheelchair; difficulty selecting speed on power wheelchair; difficulty shifting weight; difficulty sitting on wheelchair without losing balance; difficulty stopping wheelchair before bumping something; difficulty transferring from wheelchair; difficulty transferring to wheelchair; difficulty turning in place while on wheelie position

Related Factors

Altered mood; environmental constraints; inadequate adjustment to wheelchair size; inadequate knowledge of wheelchair use; insufficient muscle strength; insufficient physical endurance; neurobehavioral manifestations; obesity; pain; physical deconditioning; substance misuse; unaddressed inadequate vision

At Risk Population

Individuals using wheelchair for short time; individuals with history of fall from wheelchair; older adults

Associated Condition

Musculoskeletal impairment; neuromuscular diseases; vision disorders

Client Outcomes

Client Will (Specify Time Frame)

- Demonstrate independence in operating and moving a wheelchair or other wheeled device
- Demonstrate ability to direct others in operating and moving a wheelchair or other device
- Demonstrate therapeutic positioning, pressure relief, and safety principles while operating and moving a wheelchair or other wheeled device

Nursing Interventions

▲ Refer to physical and occupational therapy or wheelchair seating clinic.

▲ Recognize that support surfaces on chairs and beds redistribute pressure and should be used for at-risk clients as an adjunct to reduce risk of pressure injury (Sprigle & Sonenblum, 2011; Requejo, Furumasu, & Mulroy, 2015). Refer to care plan for Risk for Adult **Pressure Injury**.

M

- Optimize nutrition and hydration for skin and tissue health.
- Intervene to maintain continence or use absorbent underpads or diapers to help prevent skin breakdown caused by excessive moisture and macerated skin. Some wheelchair cushions have moisture-wicking characteristics.
- Assess client's sitting posture frequently and reposition for alignment. Document specific measures to allow for reproducibility.
- Implement use of friction-coated projection hand rims and leather gloves for clients to propel manual wheelchairs.
- Manually guide or explain to the client to push forward on both wheel rims to move ahead, push the right rim to turn left and vice versa, and pull backward on both wheel rims to back up.
- Recommend that clients back wheelchair into an elevator. If entering face first, instruct them to turn chairs around to face the elevator doors and controls.

▲ In conjunction with physical therapy for teaching and assessment, reinforce principle of descending a curb backward ("popping a wheelie") if balance, trunk control, strength, and timing are adequate.

- Ascend curbs in a forward position by popping a wheelie or having someone aid in tilting the chair back, place front wheels over curb, and roll chair up. If surface is muddy or sandy, ascend backward.
- During assisted wheelies, helper must hold wheelchair until all four wheels are back on the ground and client has control of wheelchair.

▲ Follow therapist's recommendations for how clients should propel manual wheelchairs to prevent upper extremity pain and joint degeneration.

- Recognize that ultra-lightweight, push rim–activated, power-assisted, or powered wheelchairs may be indicated. Striking the balance between optimum independence and preventing injury, e.g., rotator cuff injury from years of manual propulsion, is a consideration.
- ▲ Reduce floor clutter and establish safety rules for drivers of electric/power mobility devices; make referrals to physical or occupational therapy for driver reevaluations if accidents occur or client's health deteriorates.
- Request and receive client's permission before moving an unoccupied wheelchair in the room or out to hallway.
- Reinforce compensatory strategies for unilateral neglect and agnosia (e.g., visual scanning, self-talk, self-questioning as to what could be wrong) as clients propel wheelchair through doorways and around obstacles. Refer to care plan for **Unilateral Neglect.**
- Offer support to help clients cope with issues related to physical disability. Refer to care plan for Ineffective **Role performance**.
- Provide information on support group and reliable Internet resource options.
- Provide information about advocacy, accessibility, assistive technology, and issues under the Americans with Disabilities Act as Amended (2008) (Jackson, 2017).
- ▲ Make social service or wheelchair clinic referral to educate clients on financial coverage/regulations of third-party payers and HealthCare Financing Association for wheelchairs.
- Recommend that clients test-drive wheelchairs and try out cushions/postural supports with the advice of a qualified seating professional, not a vendor, before purchasing. If a specialty chair is indicated, for example, for sports or outdoor use, having clients test-drive the wheelchair is especially important.

Pediatric

- ▲ Help client/family transition from a manual to a powered wheelchair/scooter if disability is severe.

Geriatric

- Avoid using restraints on fidgeting clients who slide down in a wheelchair. Instead, assess for deformities; spinal curvatures; abnormal tone; limited joint range; discomfort from clothing, pressure, or constriction areas; social isolation, and toileting needs.
- Ensure proper seat depth/leg positioning and use custom footrests (not elevated leg rests) to prevent older adults from sliding down in wheelchairs.

- ▲ Assess for side effects of medications and potential need for dosage readjustments to increase wheelchair tolerance. Give prescribed hydration and medications to treat orthostatic hypotension. Consider leg wraps. Assist client to perform warm-up bed exercises if possible.
- • Allow client to control speed to propel wheelchair independently if possible.
- • Assess the client's ability to safely maneuver independently using a wheelchair.

Home Care

- ▲ Establish a support system for emergency and contingency care (e.g., remote monitoring, emergency call system, alert local emergency medical system).
- • Recommend the following changes to the home to accommodate the use of a wheelchair:
  - Arrange traffic patterns so they are wide enough to maneuver a wheelchair.
  - Recognize that a 5-foot turning space is necessary to maneuver wheelchairs, doorways need to have 32 to 36 inches clear width, and entrance ramps/path slope should be assessed before permanent ramps are installed, because standardized slopes may not be appropriate. Temporary ramps are cost-effective and easier to adjust (Sofka, 2011).
  - Replace door hardware with fold-back hinges, remove doorway encasements (if too narrow), remove/replace thresholds (if too high), hang wall-mounted sinks/handrails, grade floors in showers for roll-in chairs, and use nonskid/nonslip floor coverings (e.g., nonwaxed wood, linoleum, or Berber carpet).
  - Rearrange room functions, furniture, and storage so that toileting, sleeping, bathing, and preparing/eating meals can safely take place on one level of the home.
- ▲ Request physical and occupational therapy referrals to evaluate wheelchair fitting, skills, safety, and maintenance. Suggest community resources for servicing and tuning up wheelchairs and/or locating parts so clients can service their own chairs; an annual tune-up is recommended.

Client/Family Teaching and Discharge Planning

- ▲ Assess pain levels of long-term wheelchair users and make referrals to therapists or wheelchair clinics for modifications as needed.

- Instruct and have client return-demonstrate reinflation of pneumatic tires; encourage client to monitor tire pressure every 2 to 3 weeks.
- Instruct family/clients to remove large wheelchair parts (leg rests, armrests) when lifting wheelchair into car for transport; when reassembling, check that all parts are fastened securely and temperature is tepid.
- Teach the critical importance of using seatbelts and secure chair tie-downs when riding in motor vehicles in a wheelchair. Never transport a client in an unsecured wheelchair in any kind of vehicle.
- For further information, refer to care plan for Impaired **Transfer** ability.

Impaired Mood Regulation

NANDA-I Definition

A mental state characterized by shifts in mood or affect and which is comprised of a constellation of affective, cognitive, somatic, and/or physiologic manifestations varying from mild to severe

Defining Characteristics

Change in verbal behavior; disinhibition; dysphoria; excessive guilt; excessive self-awareness; excessive self-blame; flight of thoughts; hopelessness; impaired concentration; influenced self-esteem; irritability; psychomotor agitation; psychomotor retardation; sad affect; withdrawal

Related Factors

Alteration in sleep pattern; anxiety; appetite change; hypervigilance; impaired social functioning; loneliness; pain; recurrent thoughts of death; recurrent thoughts of suicide; social isolation; substance misuse; weight change

Associated Condition

Chronic illness; functional impairment; psychosis

Client Outcomes

Client Will (Specify Time Frame)

- State feelings related to changes in mood
- Eat appropriate diet for height and weight
- Follow exercise plan
- Have no attempts at self-harm
- Attention during activities

Nursing Interventions

- Provide nutritional intake for a client who is unable to feed self.
- Encourage regular physical exercise to maintain or advance to a higher level of fitness and health.
- Reduce the risk of self-inflicted harm for a client in crisis or severe depression with a planned treatment program.
- Advise the client to listen to music in a negative mood (Gold, 2013; Aalbers et al., 2017).
- Try to perceive possible suicidal thoughts on time (Sohn et al., 2017).
- Enable the patient to express his or her feelings and try to support the patient emotionally if necessary (Kim et al., 2017).
- When possible, use (aromatherapy) massage when in a negative mood (Babaee et al., 2012; Ho et al., 2017).
- Consider recommending cognitive behavior therapy (Whitten & Stanik-Huff, 2011; Cajanding, 2016; Andersen et al., 2017).
- Consider recommending psychotherapy (Szczepanska-Gieracha et al., 2013).
- Give the patient hope, for example, about regaining his or her health (Svensson, Nilsson, & Svantesson, 2016).
- If necessary, emphasize the importance of daily activity and routine (Crowe, Beaglehole, & Inder, 2016).
- Signal and treat pain on time (Husebo et al., 2014).
- Promote the self-efficacy of the patient (Madueno Caro et al., 2017).
- In case of a persistent negative mood, recommend meditation to the patient (Yuichi et al., 2015).
- The use of a doll in people with dementia can contribute to a better mood (Shin, 2015).

Client/Network Interventions

- Provide a treatment involving the cooperation of several aid workers in neighborhood teams and providing customized treatment at the place in which the client resides.

Moral Distress

NANDA-I Definition

Response to the inability to carry out one's chosen ethical or moral decision and/or action

Defining Characteristics

Anguish about acting on one's moral choice

Related Factors

Conflict among decision-makers; conflicting information available for ethical decision-making; conflicting information available for moral decision-making; cultural incongruence; difficulty reaching end-of-life decisions; difficulty reaching treatment decision; time constraint for decision-making

At-Risk Population

Loss of autonomy; physical distance of decision-maker

Client Outcomes

Client Will (Specify Time Frame)

- Be able to act in accordance with values, goals, and beliefs
- Regain confidence in the ability to make decisions and/or act in accord with values, goals, and beliefs
- Express satisfaction with the ability to make decisions consistent with values, goals, and beliefs
- Have choices respected

M

Nursing Interventions

- Assess if moral distress is present and its relationship to intrinsic or extrinsic factors.
- Affirm the distress, commitment "to take care of yourself," and your obligations. Validate feelings and perceptions with others.
- Implement strategies to change situations causing moral distress.
- Assess sources and severity of distress.
- Give voice/recognition to moral distress and express concerns about constraints to supportive individuals.
- Engage in healthy problem-solving
- Identify/use a support system.
- Investigate whether the emotional touchpoint method (significant moments when patients were effected physically or emotionally by care) interviews of patients (N = 31) met appropriate ethical standards when used for evaluating care. The study results demonstrated that the touchpoint method was ethical and valuable in evaluating patient care.

Pediatric

- Consider the developmental age of children when evaluating decisions and conflict.

Multicultural

- Acknowledge and understand cultural differences that may influence a client's moral choices.

Geriatric and Home Care

- Previous interventions may be adapted for geriatric or home care use.

Risk for Dry Mouth

NANDA-I Definition

Susceptible to discomfort or damage to the oral mucosa due to reduced quantity or quality of saliva to moisten the mucosa, which may compromise health

Risk Factors

Dehydration; depression; excessive stress; excitement; smoking

Associated Condition

Chemotherapy; fluid restriction; inability to feed orally; oxygen therapy; pharmaceutical agent; pregnancy; radiation therapy to the head and neck; systematic disease

Client Outcomes

Client Will (Specify Time Frame)

- Maintain intact, moist oral mucous membranes that are free of ulceration, inflammation, infection, and debris
- Demonstrate measures to maintain or regain oral health
- Demonstrate oral hygiene knowledge and skills to maintain moisture within the mouth
- Be free of halitosis and oral discomfort
- State tolerable to no changes in taste sensation (dysgeusia)

Nursing Interventions

- Perform a comprehensive extraoral and intraoral examination for associated conditions and risk factors that reduce quantity or quality of saliva and patient complaints of oral dryness and difficulty speaking, eating, or swallowing.
- Assess for symptoms of dry mouth.
- Inspection and palpation of major salivary glands and lymph nodes for masses, enlargement, tenderness, purulent discharge, or absence of salivary pooling/secretions are components of a comprehensive head and neck examination to differentiate between salivary and nonsalivary causes of dry mouth (ADA, 2015).
- Inspect nasal turbinates for enlargement, swelling, polyps, and nasal flow because nasal blockages increase mouth breathing, which may exacerbate oral dryness symptoms.
- Assess patient for oral candidiasis, dental caries, and gingival recession (ADA, 2015).
- Assess patient for dental caries and gingival recession because clinical signs of hyposalivation also include increased incidence of

tooth decay at the gingival margin and nonspecific gingival inflammation (Plemons, Al-Hashimi, & Marek, 2014; ADA, 2015).

- Assess patient for difficulty chewing, swallowing (dysphagia), or speaking.
- Assess patient for mouth breathing caused by functional impairment of the upper airway and/or presence of nasal, endotracheal, or orogastric tubes that may prevent mouth closure or irritate oral mucosa, which may contribute to an increase in dry mouth symptoms experienced by clients.
- Assess patient hydration status.
- Assess fluid status because dehydration will also affect salivary flow (Plemons, Al-Hashimi, & Marek, 2014).
- ▲ Dry mouth, mouth dryness, or oral dryness (xerostomia) is a dryness of the oral cavity resulting from insufficient or complete lack of saliva secretion. Although dry mouth is a common symptom of salivary gland hyposecretion, there is a distinction between dryness caused by malfunction of the salivary glands and patient's subjective report of oral dryness despite normal salivary gland function (Tanasiewicz, Hildebrandt, & Obersztyn, 2016).
- ▲ The client may require a dental referral to evaluate salivary flow rate as a tool to monitor dry mouth symptoms (Plemons, Al-Hashimi, & Marek, 2014; ADA, 2015).
- ▲ Consider use of oral screening, patient self-report tool, and/or subjective questioning regarding dry mouth symptoms to assess client oral health and to predict need for dental intervention and degree of salivary hypofunction.
- ▲ Use client self-report to measure symptoms of dry mouth.
- Ask the client about symptoms of hyposalivation.
- ▲ Review client medication usage for dry mouth as a side effect of medication. If symptoms are present, consult with provider, or refer client to see a dentist or specialist.
- ▲ Administer pilocarpine and cevimeline as prescribed because these medications are considered first-line therapy in Sjögren's syndrome and head and neck cancer clients with radiotherapy-induced dry mouth and hyposalivation.
- ▲ ADA council on scientific affairs report identifies that pilocarpine and cevimeline have US Food and Drug Administration approval for treating dry mouth caused by Sjögren's syndrome or radiation therapy (ADA, 2015).

- ▲ Administer amifostine as prescribed to reduce the incidence of acute and late xerostomia for clients treated with standard fractionated radiation and gland-sparing radiation technique to the head and neck.
- • Teach clients about conditions that can exacerbate dry mouth symptoms, including:
  - ❍ Avoiding low-humidity environments
  - ❍ Avoidance of oral irritants: acidic fluids such as carbonated beverages and juices, caffeine, alcohol, tobacco
  - ❍ Avoidance of salty, spicy, acidic, or high-sucrose content foods.
  - ❍ Avoidance of dry, hard, and sticky foods
  - ❍ Refer patient to smoking and/or alcohol cessation program
- • Teach the client good oral hygiene:
  - ❍ Twice-daily toothbrushing with regular topical fluoride toothpaste.
  - ❍ Use of soft bristle toothbrush.
  - ❍ Daily use of dental floss or another interdental cleaner.
  - ❍ Daily use of alcohol-free mouth rinse.
  - ❍ Recommend use of prescription-strength fluoride toothpastes for severe salivary hypofunction.
- • Provide instruction regarding cleaning and assist with care of dental prosthesis as needed. Daily cleansing of dental prosthetic is accepted standard of care to maintain and promote oral health and dentition (ADA, 2015).
- ▲ Provide instruction on candidiasis prevention and control. Administer antifungal topical treatments as prescribed using available suspensions, pastilles, and lozenges for uncomplicated oral candidiasis. Systemic antifungal agents may be prescribed for complicated candidiasis mucosal infection (Mercadante et al., 2017).
- ▲ Soak partial or complete dental prosthesis overnight in 0.2% chlorhexidine HCL.
- ▲ Recommend professional dental oral examination every 3 to 6 months. Recommend professional teeth cleaning at least every 6 months.
- • Discuss selection and use of salivary substitutes with patient and healthcare provider to assist in maintaining mouth moisture.
- • Teach the client that any topical product that is acidic or contains sugar, or noted as sugarless with high fructose, should be avoided.

- Encourage the client to try several products, based on client preference, to find a suitable saliva substitute. Clients reported that use of saliva substitutes may be more helpful before sleep because of diurnal variation on reduction in salivary flow at night. It is also suggested that patients mix and match salivary agents based on their daily schedules or activities such as eating or public speaking (Baer et al., 2017).
- Lubricate lips every 2 hours, while awake, and as needed. Apply moisturizer (e.g., lanolin) to dry lips every 2 hours, as needed to assist with dryness.
- Teach patients preventative measures to reduce oral dryness:
  - Maintain adequate oral hydration by sipping water regularly and/or sucking on ice chips (AAOM, 2016).
  - While eating, drink fluids carefully.
  - Maintain oral intake log.
  - Rinse with normal saline or clean water as a part of daily oral care to prevent dry mouth, or sodium bicarbonate solution (1 teaspoon salt and 1 teaspoon baking soda to 1 L of water).
- Encourage the client to use sugar-free gum or sugar-free candy to promote salivary flow.
- Encourage the client to use saline nasal sprays to maintain open nasal passages.
- The client may find the use of a humidifier during sleep at night helpful in reducing symptoms.

▲ Discuss with the client the use of acupuncture, electrical nerve stimulation, and powered versus manual toothbrushes to assist in maintaining mouth moisture.

▲ Encourage the client to discuss use of emerging preventative treatments with the healthcare provider such as gene therapy, tissue engineering, stem cell therapy, and growth factors for etiologies associated with dry mouth.

▲ Discuss use of Bethanechol HCL saliva stimulant in head and neck cancer patients with radiotherapy-induced dry mouth and hyposalivation with the client and healthcare provider.

Geriatric

- Recognize that symptoms of dry mouth are more common in menopausal women and geriatric patients.
- Age-associated increase of systemic disease and subsequent disease treatment is the primary cause of dry mouth.

- Older adults are at risk of xerostomia from a variety of etiologies.
- Review client medication list routinely.

Multicultural and Home Care Considerations

- The previously mentioned nursing interventions and client teaching may be adapted for multicultural and home care considerations. See Care Plan on Impaired Oral **Mucous Membrane Integrity.**

Nausea

NANDA-I Definition

A subjective, phenomenon of an unpleasant feeling in the back of the throat and stomach, which may or may not result in vomiting

Defining Characteristics

Aversion toward food; gagging sensation; increase in salivation; increase in swallowing; sour taste

Related Factors

Anxiety; exposure to toxin; fear; noxious environmental stimuli; noxious taste; unpleasant visual stimuli

Associated Condition

Biochemical dysfunction; esophageal disease; gastric distention; gastro-intestinal irritation; increase in intracranial pressure (ICP); intra-abdominal tumors; labyrinthitis; liver capsule stretch; localized tumor; Ménière's disease; meningitis; motion sickness; pancreatic disease; pregnancy; psychological disorder; splenetic capsule stretch; treatment regimen

Client Outcomes

Client Will (Specify Time Frame)

- State relief of nausea
- Explain methods clients can use to decrease nausea and vomiting (N&V)

Nursing Interventions

▲ Determine cause or risk for N&V (e.g., medication effects, infectious causes [viral and bacterial gastroenteritis], disorders of the gut and peritoneum [mechanical obstruction, motility disorders, or other intraabdominal causes], central nervous system causes [including anxiety], endocrine and metabolic causes [including pregnancy], postoperative-related status).

▲ Evaluate and document the client's history of N&V, with attention to onset, duration, timing, volume of emesis, frequency of pattern, setting, associated factors, aggravating factors, and past medical and social histories.

- • Document each episode of nausea and/or vomiting separately and the effectiveness of interventions. Consider an assessment tool for consistency of evaluation.
- • Identify and eliminate contributing causative factors. This may include eliminating unpleasant odors or medications that may be contributing to nausea.
- ▲ Implement appropriate dietary measures such as nothing by mouth (NPO) status as appropriate; small, frequent meals; and low-fat meals. It may be helpful to avoid foods that are spicy, fatty, or highly salty. Reverting to previous practices when ill in the past and consuming "comfort foods" may also be helpful at this time.
- ▲ Recognize and implement interventions and monitor complications associated with N&V. This may include administration of intravenous fluids and electrolytes.
- ▲ Administer appropriate antiemetics, according to emetic cause, by most effective route, considering the side effects of the medication, with attention to and coverage for the time frames in which the nausea is anticipated.
- • Consider nonpharmacological interventions such as acupressure, acupuncture, music therapy, distraction, and slow, deliberate movements.
- • Provide oral care after the client vomits. Oral care helps remove the taste and smell of vomitus, reducing the stimulus for further vomiting.

Nausea in Pregnancy

- • Early recognition and conservative measures are recommended to successfully manage nausea in pregnancy, and to prevent progression to hyperemesis gravidarum. Dietary and lifestyle modifications should be implemented before pharmacological interventions. Avoidance of any aversive odors or foods is recommended. Eating multiple small meals per day is also recommended to have some food in the stomach at all times, avoiding hypoglycemia and gastric overdistention. Foods with higher protein (before bedtime) and carbohydrate and lower fat content are helpful (between meals and before getting out of bed early in the morning). Drinking smaller volumes of liquids at multiple times throughout the day is recommended.

- ▲ Because of the high incidence of coexisting gastroesophageal reflux disease (GERD), it is important to assess and manage these symptoms of heartburn, belching, and indigestion.
- ▲ It is well established that *Helicobacter pylori* infection is associated with hyperemesis gravidarum.
- ▲ Coexisting psychosocial factors may also influence the severity of N&V with pregnancy. Symptoms of anxiety and depression can occur in early pregnancy, especially when N&V is severe and can make the treatment of the N&V more challenging and even ineffective.
- ▲ The American College of Obstetricians and Gynecologists (ACOG) currently recommends converting the prenatal vitamin to folic acid only if nausea persists. Pharmacological options include a combination of oral pyridoxine hydrochloride (vitamin B_6, 10–25 mg) and doxylamine succinate (antihistamine 12.5 mg) to be used three to four times a day as first-line treatment for N&V of pregnancy after failure of pyridoxine alone. This combination agent of pyridoxine and doxylamine (Diclegis) is the only US Food and Drug Administration pregnancy Category A approved therapy for N&V of pregnancy. There are, however, several pharmacological treatments outlined by the ACOG.
- ▲ Nonpharmacological interventions that are recommended include P6 acupressure with wrist bands and ginger capsules, 250 mg four times a day.

Nausea After Surgery

- ▲ Evaluate for risk factors for postoperative N&V (PONV).
- ▲ Reduction of risk factors associated with PONV is beneficial for both adults and children.
- ▲ Medicate the client prophylactically for nausea as ordered, throughout the period of risk.
- ▲ Alleviate postoperative pain using ordered analgesic agents (refer to care plan for Acute **Pain**). Pain is known to be a factor in the development of PONV (Bruderer et al., 2017).
- • Consider the use of nonpharmacological techniques, such as P6 acupoint stimulation, as an adjunct for controlling PONV, which has been shown to be effective in reducing PONV by 30%. Acupoint pressure is noninvasive, inexpensive, and has no side effects; thus it is part of a combined approach with antiemetic medication.

- Include client education on the management of PONV for all outpatients and discuss key assessment criteria (Odom-Forren et al., 2014).

Nausea After Chemotherapy

- Perform risk assessment before chemotherapy administration. Risk factors include female gender, younger age, history of low alcohol consumption, history of morning sickness during pregnancy, anxiety, previous history of chemotherapy, client expectancy of nausea, and emetic potential of the regimen.
- ▲ Initiate antiemetic strategy prophylactically or when N&V occurs in accordance with evidence-based guidelines.
- ▲ Drug classes that are recommended for practice include the serotonin receptor antagonists, the NK-1 receptor antagonists, and cannabinoids.
- ▲ Consider the use of the following integrative therapies that are likely to be effective in reducing N&V: hypnosis with anticipatory N&V, and progressive muscle relaxation and guided imagery with antiemetics.
- Consider managing client expectations about CINV.

Geriatric

- There are no specific guidelines that address the prophylaxis of CINV specifically in older adults. Risk still needs to be assessed, although many older clients are often treated with less emetic chemotherapy. Chemotherapy, however, can cause increased toxicity caused by age-related decreases in organ function, comorbidities, and drug-drug interactions secondary to polypharmacy. Additionally, adherence may be an issue because of cognitive decline, impaired senses, and economic issues.

Pediatric

- Interventions for CINV should be implemented before and after chemotherapy.
- Relatively few systematic reviews exist examining the antiemetic medications used for CINV in children. It appears that 5-HT3 antagonists, with palonosetron preferred, combined with dexamethasone and aprepitant (in children 6 months of age or older) are recommended in children receiving highly emetogenic chemotherapy (Dupuis et al., 2017; Patel et al., 2017).
- Integrative therapies for control of nausea in children with cancer have not yet been studied as adequately as they have with adults.

Some integrative therapies with potential include cognitive distraction, hypnosis, and acupressure (Momani & Berry, 2017).

Home Care

- • Previously mentioned interventions may be adapted for home care use.
- ▲ In hospice care clients, N&V is common, and can considerably affect quality of life. Assessment is relevant in the management of N&V, and should include history, physical exam, and evaluation of reversible causes.
- • Assist the client and family with identifying and avoiding irritants in the home that exacerbate nausea (e.g., strong odors from food, plants, perfume, and room deodorizers). All medications except antiemetics should be given after meals to minimize the risk of nausea.

Client/Family Teaching and Discharge Planning

- • Teach the client techniques to use before and after chemotherapy, including antiemetics/medication management schedules and dietary approaches, such as eating smaller meals, avoiding spicy and fatty foods, and avoiding an empty stomach before chemotherapy (Irwin & Johnson, 2014).

N

Neonatal Abstinence Syndrome

NANDA-I Definition

A constellation of withdrawal symptoms observed in newborns as a result of in-utero exposure to addicting substances, or as a consequence of postnatal pharmacological pain management

Defining Characteristics

Diarrhea (00013); disorganized infant behavior (00116); disturbed sleep pattern (00198); impaired comfort (00214); ineffective infant suck-swallow response (00295); neurobehavioral stress; risk for aspiration (00039); risk for imbalanced body temperature (00005); risk for impaired attachment (00058); risk for impaired skin integrity (00047); risk for injury (00035)

Related Factors

To be developed

At-Risk Population

Iatrogenic substance exposure for pain control following a critical illness or surgery; in-utero substance exposure secondary to material substance use

Client Outcomes

Client will (Specify Time Frame)

- Tolerate small frequent formula feedings or frequent breast feedings
- Maintain weight and readjust feedings frequency as necessary for appropriate growth
- Provide calorie-dense formula, which is appropriate for weight gain
- Maintain proper hydration with elastic skin turgor and moist mucus membranes
- Maintain adequate nutrition that will promote adequate growth
- Preserve skin integrity in perianal area

Nursing Interventions

- Provide supportive nonpharmacological care with formula feeding as prescribed.
- Encourage breastfeeding for nutrition and nonpharmacological supportive care.
- Use nursing skills to provide supportive nonpharmacological care.
- Use vibrotactile stimulation (VS) as a nonpharmacological supportive care option.
- Practice supportive nursing interventions with an understanding of the levels of evidence.
- Provide pharmacological treatment as indicated for symptoms.
- Use of nonpharmacological and complementary therapy to comfort infants and provide relief of symptoms.
- Use of rooming-in and promotion of maternal–infant bonding for mother infant dyad.
- Provide compassionate care, free of judgment, to substance abusing mothers.

Pediatric

- When available, consider professional, supportive programs for infants with a history of NAS.

Multicultural

- Specific rural areas are high risk for NAS.

Home Care

- Consider alternative models of care for treatment for infants with NAS.

Readiness for Enhanced Nutrition

NANDA-I Definition

A pattern of nutrient intake that can be strengthened

N

Defining Characteristics

Expresses desire to enhance nutrition

Client Outcomes

Client Will (Specify Time Frame)

- Explain how to eat according to the US Dietary Guidelines
- Design dietary modifications to meet individual long-term goal of health, using principles of variety, balance, and moderation
- Maintain weight within normal range for height and age

Nursing Interventions

- Assess the meaning and importance of food in the client's life.
- Assess client readiness to determine whether he or she is ready to discuss enhanced nutrition and/or would like nutrition information.
- Use a motivational interviewing technique when working with clients to promote healthy eating and improved nutrition.
- Counsel the client to measure regularly consumed foods periodically. Help the client learn usual portion sizes. Measuring food alerts the client to normal portion sizes. Estimating amounts can be extremely inaccurate.
- Assist the client to develop a system of self-management, which may include self-monitoring of weight and BMI; realistic goal setting, planning, and action planning for improved dietary intake and physical activity; problem-solving; and tracking dietary intake and exercise.
- Document the client's height and weight and teach the significance of his or her BMI in relationship to current nutritional health. Use a chart or a website such as http://www.cdc.gov/healthyweight/assessing/bmi/index.html (Centers for Disease Control and Prevention [CDC], 2015).
- Encourage the client to engage in vigorous-intensity physical activity for at least 150 minutes weekly or moderate-intensity physical activity for at least 300 minutes weekly.
- Recommend that the client avoid eating in fast-food restaurants.
- Assist the client to reframe slips in nutrition or physical activity behavior as lapses that are a single event and not a full return to previous unhealthy behaviors. Relapse prevention strategies include managing lapses in healthy behavior, identifying high-risk situations for relapses, self-monitoring, providing social support, enhancing skills for coping, and increasing self-efficacy for avoiding relapse.

- Assist clients to engage their social support systems either digitally or face to face in ways that facilitate healthy eating and physical activity behavior change.
- Assist the client to implement informal and formal mindfulness-based interventions (MBIs). Informal MBIs include mindful eating, increasing awareness of hunger and satiety cues, taste satisfaction, and decreasing impulsive tendencies to overeat when experiencing negative emotions. Meditation practice is a formal MBI.
- Assist the client to develop stimulus control techniques designed to reduce environmental cues associated with eating behaviors. Specifically clients should be taught to limit the presence of high-calorie/high-fat foods in the home; to reduce the visibility of unhealthy food choices in the home; to limit where and when they eat; to avoid distractions like reading, using the computer, or watching television when eating; and to eat more slowly.
- Encourage 7.5 to 8.5 hours of sleep nightly.
- Recommend that clients use dietary supplements such as vitamins and minerals after consulting with their primary healthcare provider.
- Incorporate the following recommendations from the Academy of Nutrition and Dietetics: Interventions for the Treatment of Overweight and Obesity in Adults (Raynor & Champagne, 2016):
  - Assess food and nutrition-related history; anthropometric measures; biochemical data, medical tests, and procedures; nutrition-focused physical findings; and client history.
  - Assess the energy intake and nutrient content of the diet.
  - Use height and weight to calculate BMI, and waist circumference to determine risk of cardiovascular disease (CVD), type 2 diabetes, and all-cause mortality.
  - Use a measured resting metabolic rate (RMR) to determine energy needs.
  - Set a realistic weight-loss goal, such as one of the following: up to 2 pounds per week, up to 10% of baseline body weight, or a total of 3% to 5% of baseline weight if cardiovascular risk factors (hypertension, hyperlipidemia, and hyperglycemia) are present.
  - To achieve weight loss, use an individualized diet, including patient preferences and health status, to achieve and maintain

N

nutrient adequacy and reduce caloric intake, based on one of the following caloric reduction strategies: 1200 to 1500 kcal/day for women and 1500 to 1800 kcal/day for men, with an energy deficit of approximately 500 kcal/day or 750 kcal/day.

Pediatric

- Offer obese or overweight adolescents healthy methods for weight loss.
- Offer families of obese or overweight children prejudice-free, individually accepting, and supportive interventions to address weight loss.
- Recommend that families eat together for at least one meal per day.
- Recommend involving the family in planning meals and food preparation. Children can learn about nutrition as they help plan and make meals.
- Assist parents at being good role models of healthy eating.
- Recommend that the family try new foods, either a new food or recipe every week (Fulkerson et al., 2018).

Geriatric

- Determine the risks and benefits of weight loss in the older client. A BMI greater than 30 in the older client suggests a moderate weight loss approach.
- Observe for social, psychological, and economic factors that influence diet quality.

Multicultural

- Tailor nutritional interventions to be consistent with cultural beliefs, norms, and values.
- Offer tailored lifestyle counseling via the telephone.
- Integrate weight loss and weight maintenance interventions with church faith-based concepts for cultural congruence with African American clients.

Client/Family Teaching and Discharge Planning

- The majority of the preceding interventions involve teaching.
- Work with the family members regarding information on how to support and promote enhanced nutritional choices and healthy intakes.

Imbalanced Nutrition: Less Than Body Requirements

NANDA-I Definition

Intake of nutrients insufficient to meet metabolic needs

Defining Characteristics

Abdominal cramping; abdominal pain; body weight below ideal weight for age and gender; capillary fragility; constipation; delayed wound healing; diarrhea; excessive hair loss; food intake less than recommended daily allowance (RDA); hyperactive bowel sounds; hypoglycemia; inadequate head circumference growth for age and gender; inadequate height increase for age and gender; lethargy; muscle hypotonia; neonatal weight gain < 30g per day; pale mucous membranes; weight loss with adequate food intake

Related Factors

Altered taste perception; depressive symptoms; difficulty swallowing; food aversion; inaccurate information; inadequate food supply; inadequate interest in food; inadequate knowledge of nutrient requirements; injured buccal cavity; insufficient breast milk production; interrupted breastfeeding; misperception about ability to ingest food; satiety immediately upon ingesting food; sore buccal cavity; weakened muscles required for swallowing; weakened muscles required for mastication

At-Risk population

Competitive athletes; displaced individuals; economically disadvantaged individuals; individuals with low educational level; premature infants

Associated Condition

Body dysmorphic disorders; digestive system diseases; immunosuppression; Kwashiorkor; malabsorption syndromes; mental disorders; neoplasms; neurocognitive disorders; parasitic disorders

Client Outcomes

Client Will (Specify Time Frame)

- Progressively gain weight toward desired goal
- Weigh within normal range for height and age
- Recognize factors contributing to being underweight
- Identify nutritional requirements
- Consume adequate nourishment
- Be free of signs of malnutrition

Nursing Interventions

- Conduct a nutrition screen on all clients within 24 hours of admission and refer to a dietitian as deemed necessary.

- The screening tool should be based on the client population and the validity and reliability of the screening tool. The Malnutrition Universal Screening Tool (MUST), for example, is considered a quick easy-to-use tool to assess body mass index (BMI), unintentional weight loss, acuity of illness, and nutritional intake.
- Recognize the importance of rescreening and monitoring oral intake in hospitalized individuals to help facilitate the early identification and prevention of nutritional decline.
- Recognize the characteristics that classify individuals as malnourished and refer to a dietitian for a complex nutritional assessment and intervention.
- Recognize clients who are likely to experience malnutrition in the context of social or environmental circumstances, characterized by pure chronic starvation and anorexia nervosa without the presence of an inflammatory process (White, Guenter, & Gordon, 2012).
  - Chronic disease–related malnutrition: those with organ failure, pancreatic cancer, rheumatoid arthritis, sarcopenic obesity
  - Acute disease or injury-related malnutrition: those with major infection, burns, trauma, closed-head injuries accompanied by a marked inflammatory response (White, Guenter, & Gordon, 2012)

▲ Note laboratory values cautiously; decrease in albumin and prealbumin may be indicators of the inflammatory response that often accompanies acute malnutrition, but it should not be used to diagnose malnutrition. Other potential indicators of inflammatory response include C-reactive protein, white blood cell count, and blood glucose values.

- Weigh the client daily in acute care and weekly to monthly in extended care at the same time (usually before breakfast) with same amount of clothing.
- Observe for potential barriers to eating such as willingness, ability, and appetite.

Note: If the client is unable to feed self, refer to Nursing Interventions for Feeding **Self-Care** deficit. If the client has difficulty swallowing, refer to Nursing Interventions for Impaired **Swallowing.** If the client is receiving tube feedings, refer to the Nursing Interventions for Risk for **Aspiration.**

- Advocate for the implementation of a feeding protocol, if not already in place, to avoid unnecessary and/or prolonged nothing by mouth (mouth)/clear liquid diet (NPO/CLD) status in hospitalized clients.

- For the client with anorexia nervosa, consider offering high-calorie foods and snacks often.
- For the client who is able to eat but has a decreased appetite, try the following activities:
  - Offer oral nutritional supplements (ONS) early after admission and continue to encourage intake of ONS throughout the hospital stay.
  - Avoid interruptions during mealtimes and offer companionship; meals should be eaten in a calm and peaceful environment.
  - Allow for access to meals or snacks during "off times" if the client is not available at time of meal delivery, monitor food and ONS intake, and communicate with dietitian/healthcare provider.
  - If the client lacks endurance, schedule rest periods before meals, and open packages and cut up food for the client.
- Vitamin D deficiency has been shown to be associated with greater risk of falls and fractures in older people. For the client with fracture caused by a fall, consider the need for vitamin D supplementation.
- For the client who has had a stroke, repeat nutritional screenings weekly and provide timely interventions for those at risk or who may already be malnourished.
- Recognize the importance of offering high-protein foods and beverages to most hospitalized individuals (use caution with those with compromised renal/liver function).
- Monitor state of oral cavity (gums, tongue, mucosa, and teeth). Provide good oral hygiene before each meal.

▲ Administer antiemetics and pain medications as ordered and needed before meals.

- If client is nauseated, remove cover of food tray before bringing it into the client's room. The sudden, concentrated food odors that come when the cover is removed in front of the client can trigger nausea.
- Work with the client to develop a plan for increased activity. Immobility leads to negative nitrogen balance, which fosters anorexia.

Critical Care

- Recognize the need to begin enteral feeding within 24 to 48 hours of admission to the critical care environment, once the client is free of hemodynamic compromise, if the client is unable to eat.
- Recognize that it is important to administer feedings to the client and that frequently checking for gastric residual and fasting clients for procedures can be a limiting factor to adequate nutrition in the tube-fed client.

N

Pediatric

- ▲ Use a nutritional screening tool designed for nurses such as the Subjective Global Nutrition Assessment (SGNA), and if the child's malnutrition is identified as moderate or severe, refer to a dietitian.
- • Watch for symptoms of malnutrition in the child including short stature; thin arms and legs; poor condition of skin and hair; visible vertebrae and rib cage; wasted buttocks; wasted facial appearance; lethargy; and in extreme cases, edema.
- • Weigh and measure the length (height) of the child and use a growth chart to help determine growth pattern, which reflects nutrition.
- ▲ Refer to a healthcare provider and a dietitian a child who is underweight for any reason.
- • Work with the child and parent to develop an appropriate weight gain plan.
- • Recognize that a large percentage of girls and teenagers are dieting, which can result in nutritional problems.

Geriatric

- • Screen for malnutrition in older clients.
- • Screen for dysphagia in all older clients.
- • Recognize that geriatric clients with moderate or severe cognition impairment have a significant risk for developing malnutrition.
- ▲ Interpret laboratory findings cautiously. Watch the color of urine for an indication of fluid balance; darker urine demonstrates dehydration. Low axillary moisture could indicate mild to moderate dehydration.
- • Consider using dining assistants and trained nonnursing staff, to provide feeding assistance care in extended care facilities to ensure adequate time for feeding clients as needed.
- • Consider offering healthy snacks such as yogurt, which is a good source of protein, calcium, zinc, B vitamins, and probiotics.
- • Encourage high-protein foods for the older client, unless medically contraindicated by organ failure.
- • Encourage physical activity throughout the day as tolerated.
- • Recognize the implications of malnutrition on client strength and mobility.
- • Monitor for onset of depression.
- • Consider offering nutritional supplement drinks served in a glass rather than with a straw inserted directly into the container.
- • Advise families that enteral nutrition may not be indicated for clients with dementia. For strategies for feeding clients with

dementia, please refer to the ESPEN Guidelines on nutrition in dementia (Volkert et al., 2015). Note: If the client is unable to feed self, refer to Nursing Interventions and *Rationales* for Feeding **Self-Care** deficit. If client has impaired physical function, malnutrition, depression, or cognitive impairment, refer to care plan for **Frail Elderly** syndrome.

- Emphasize the importance of good oral care in the older client.
- Consult the dietitian if the client has pressure ulcers.

Home Care

- The preceding interventions may be adapted for home care use.
- Screen for malnutrition using the MUST, which is easy and simple. Recognize that the client may also use MUST as a self-screening tool in the home setting.
- Monitor food intake. Instruct the client in the intake of small frequent meals of foods with increased calories and protein.
- Assess the client's willingness and ability to eat.
- Consider social factors that may interfere with nutrition (e.g., lack of transportation, inadequate income, lack of social support).
- Continue to encourage intake of oral nutritional support to help optimize oral intake.
- ▲ Recognize that the client on home parenteral nutrition requires regularly scheduled lab work for electrolyte monitoring, increased risk of catheter-related complication, parenteral nutrition–associated liver disease (PNALD), and metabolic bone disease.

Client/Family Teaching and Discharge Planning

- Help the client/family identify the area to change that will make the greatest contribution to improved nutrition.
- Build on the strengths in the client/family's food habits. Adapt changes to their current practices.
- Select appropriate teaching aids for the client/family's background.
- Implement instructional follow-up to answer the client/family's questions.
- Recommend that clients discuss with their primary healthcare provider before taking any supplements such as vitamins and minerals.
- Suggest community resources, such as Meals on Wheels and community centers as suitable food sources.
- Teach the client and family how to manage tube feedings or parenteral therapy at home as needed.

N

Impaired Oral Mucous Membrane Integrity

NANDA-I Definition

Injury to the lips, soft tissue, buccal cavity, and/or oropharynx

Defining Characteristics

Bad taste in mouth; bleeding; cheilitis; coated tongue; decrease in taste sensation; desquamation; difficulty eating; difficulty speaking; enlarged tonsils; exposure to pathogen; geographic tongue; gingival hyperplasia; gingival pallor; gingival pocketing deeper than 4 mm; gingival recession; halitosis; hyperemia; impaired ability to swallow; macroplasia; mucosal denudation; oral discomfort; oral edema; oral fissure; oral lesion; oral mucosal pallor; oral nodule; oral pain; oral papule; oral ulcer; oral vesicles; presence of mass; purulent oral–nasal drainage; purulent oral–nasal exudates; smooth atrophic tongue; spongy patches in mouth; stomatitis; white patches in mouth; white plaque in mouth; white; curdlike oral exudate; xerostomia

Related Factors

Alcohol consumption; barrier to dental care; barrier to oral self-care; chemical injury agent; decrease in salivation; dehydration; depression; inadequate nutrition; inadequate oral hygiene; insufficient knowledge of oral hygiene; malnutrition; mouth breathing; smoking; stressors

At-Risk Population

Economically disadvantaged

Associated Condition

Allergy; alteration in cognitive functioning; autoimmune disease; autosomal disorder; behavioral disorder; chemotherapy; cleft lip; cleft palate; decrease in hormone level in women; decrease in platelets; immunodeficiency; immunosuppression; infection; loss of oral support structure; mechanical factor; nil per os (NPO) > 24 hours; oral trauma; radiation therapy; Sjögren's syndrome; surgical procedure; trauma; treatment regimen

Client Outcomes

Client Will (Specify Time Frame)

- Maintain intact, moist oral mucous membranes that are free of ulceration, inflammation, infection, and debris
- Demonstrate measures to maintain or regain intact oral mucous membranes
- Demonstrate oral hygiene knowledge and skills

Nursing Interventions

- ▲ Inspect the oral cavity/teeth/gingiva at least once daily and note any discoloration; presence of debris; amount of plaque buildup; presence of lesions such as white lesions or patches, edema, or bleeding; and intactness of teeth. Refer to a dentist or periodontist as appropriate.
- • If the client is free of bleeding disorders and able to swallow, encourage toothbrushing with a soft toothbrush using fluoride-containing toothpaste at least two times per day.
- • Recommend the use of a power, rotation-oscillation toothbrush for removal of dental plaque and prevention of gingivitis.
- • Use foam sticks to moisten the oral mucous membranes, clean out debris, and swab out the mouth of the edentulous client. **Do not use foam sticks to clean the teeth** unless the platelet count is very low and the client is prone to bleeding gums. Foam sticks are useful for cleansing the oral cavity of a client who is edentulous.
- • If the client does not have a bleeding disorder, encourage the client to floss once per day or use an interdental cleaner.
- • Use an antimicrobial mouthwash as ordered or tap water or saline only for a mouth rinse. Do not use commercial mouthwashes containing alcohol or hydrogen peroxide. Also, do not use lemon-glycerin swabs.
- • Provide oral hygiene if the client is unable to care for himself or herself. The nursing diagnosis Bathing **Self-Care** deficit is then applicable.
- • If the client is unable to brush own teeth, follow this procedure:
  - ○ Position the client sitting upright or on side.
  - ○ Use a soft-bristle toothbrush.
  - ○ Use fluoride toothpaste and tap water or saline as a solution.
  - ○ Brush teeth in an up-and-down manner.
  - ○ Suction as needed.
- • Monitor the client's nutritional and fluid status to determine whether it is adequate. Refer to the care plan for Deficient **Fluid** volume or Imbalanced **Nutrition:** less than body requirements if applicable.
- • Encourage fluid intake of up to 3000 mL/day if not contraindicated by the client's medical condition.

O

- ▲ Determine the client's usual method of oral care and address any concerns regarding oral hygiene. If the client has a dry mouth (xerostomia):
  - ❍ Recognize that more than 50 classes of medications may cause xerostomia, which is often exacerbated by polypharmacy. When feasible, medications can be discontinued or replaced to increase the client's comfort (Villa et al., 2015).
  - ❍ Provide saliva substitutes as ordered.
  - ❍ Suggest the client chew sugarless gum or sugarless sour candy to promote salivary flow.
  - ❍ Examine the oral cavity for signs of caries, dental plaque, infection, mucositis ulceration, and oral candidiasis.
- • Recommend that the client decrease or preferably stop intake of soft drinks. Sugar-containing soft drinks can cause cavities, and the low pH of the drink can cause erosion in teeth (ADA, 2017a).
- • If client has halitosis, review good oral care with the client, including brushing teeth, using floss, and brushing the tongue. Halitosis can be a beginning sign of gingivitis and can be eradicated by a good program of dental hygiene (ADA, 2017b).
- • Instruct the client with halitosis to clean the tongue when performing oral hygiene; brush tongue with tongue scraper or toothbrush and follow with a mouth rinse. **EB:** A meta-analysis found that tongue cleaning in addition to toothbrushing was effective for short-term control of halitosis (Kuo et al., 2013; ADA 2017b).
- ▲ Assess the client for underlying medical condition that may be causing halitosis.
- • Keep the lips well lubricated using a water-based or aloe-based lip balm.

Client Receiving Chemotherapy/Radiation

- • Ensure that the client receives a comprehensive oral examination before initiation of chemotherapy or radiation, with aggressive preventive dental care given as needed (Radvansky, Pace, & Siddiqui, 2013; Maria, Eliopoulos, & Muanza, 2017).
- • Provide both verbal and written instruction about the need for and method of providing frequent oral care to the client before radiation therapy or chemotherapy. Assess the condition of the oral cavity daily in the client receiving radiation or chemotherapy (Radvansky, Pace, & Siddiqui, 2013).

- For measurement of presence or severity of mucositis, use the Oral Mucositis Assessment Scale (OMAS).
- Use a protocol to prevent/treat mucositis that includes the following:
  - Use a soft toothbrush that is replaced on a regular basis; brush teeth at least two times a day and for at least 90 seconds.
  - Continue to floss teeth daily.
  - Use a bland, alcohol-free rinse to remove debris and moisten the oral cavity. Rinse the mouth often (every 2 hours while awake) if the client has mouth sores.
  - Avoid tobacco, alcohol, and irritating foods (hot, rough, acidic, or spicy).
  - Use a valid and reliable pain assessment tool and treatment of pain as needed.
- Help the client use a mouth rinse of normal saline or salt and soda every 1 to 2 hours for prevention and treatment of stomatitis. A typical mixture is 1 teaspoon of salt or sodium bicarbonate per pint of water. Clients are directed to take a tablespoon of the rinse and swish it in the mouth for 30 seconds, then expectorate.

▲ If the mouth is severely inflamed and it is painful to swallow, contact the healthcare provider for a topical anesthetic or analgesic order. Modification of oral intake (e.g., soft or liquid diet) may also be necessary to prevent friction trauma.

- If the client's platelet count is lower than 50,000/mm^3 or the client has a bleeding disorder, use a specially made toothbrush designed for sensitive or diseased tissue, or a toothette that is not soaked in glycerin or flavorings; if the client cannot tolerate a toothbrush or a toothette, a piece of gauze wrapped around a finger can be used to remove plaque and debris (Radvansky, Pace, & Siddiqui, 2013).

Critical Care—Client on a Ventilator

- Use a soft toothbrush to brush teeth to clean the client's teeth at least every 12 hours; use suction to remove secretions. Provide oral moisturizer to oral mucosa and lips every 4 hours. Recognize that good oral care is paramount in the prevention of ventilator-associated events (VAE) and ventilator-associated pneumonia (VAP).

▲ Apply chlorhexidine gluconate mouthwash or gel in the oral cavity after performing tooth brushing, which may reduce the risk of the client developing VAE and VAP.

O

Geriatric

- Determine the functional ability of the client to provide his or her own oral care. Refer to Bathing **Self-Care** deficit.
- Provide appropriate oral care to older adults with a self-care deficit, brushing the teeth after breakfast and in the evening.
- If the client has dementia or delirium and exhibits care-resistant behavior, such as fighting, biting, or refusing care, then use the following method:
  - ❍ Ensure client is in a quiet environment such as own bathroom, sitting or standing at the sink to prime memory for appropriate actions.
  - ❍ Approach the client at eye level within his or her range of vision.
  - ❍ Approach with a smile and begin conversation with a touch of the hand and gradually move up.
  - ❍ Use mirror–mirror technique, standing behind the client, and brush and floss teeth.
  - ❍ Use respectful adult speech, not "elder speak" (sing-song voice, or diminutive terms such as "dearie" or "honey").
  - ❍ Promote self-care in which client brushes own teeth if possible.
  - ❍ Use distractors when needed: talking, reminiscing, singing.
- Carefully observe the oral cavity and lips for abnormal lesions such as white or red patches, masses, ulcerations with an indurated margin, or a raised granular lesion.
- Ensure that dentures are removed and cleaned regularly, preferably after every meal and before bedtime.

Home Care

- The interventions described previously may be adapted for home care use.
- Instruct the client in ways to soothe the oral cavity (e.g., cool beverages, popsicles, viscous lidocaine).

▲ If necessary, refer for home health aide services to support the family in oral care and observation of the oral cavity.

Client/Family Teaching and Discharge Planning

- Teach the client how to inspect the oral cavity and monitor for signs and symptoms of infection or complications, and when to call the healthcare provider (Radvansky, Pace, & Siddiqui, 2013; Eilers et al., 2014).

- Recommend the client not smoke, use chewing tobacco, or drink excessive amounts of alcohol.
- Teach the client and family, if necessary, how to perform appropriate mouth care. Use the motivational interviewing technique.

Risk for impaired Oral Mucous Membrane

NANDA-I Definition

Susceptible to injury to the lips, soft tissues, buccal cavity, and/or oropharynx, which may compromise health

Risk Factors

Alcohol consumption; barriers to dental care; barrier to oral self-care; chemical injury agent; decrease in salivation; dehydration; depression; inadequate nutrition; inadequate oral hygiene; insufficient knowledge of oral hygiene; malnutrition; mouth breathing; smoking; stressors

At-Risk Population

Economically disadvantaged

Associated Condition

Allergy; alteration in cognitive functioning; autoimmune disease; autosomal disorder; behavioral disorder; chemotherapy; cleft lip; cleft palate; decrease in hormone level in women; decrease in platelets; immunodeficiency; immunosuppression; infection; loss of oral support structure; mechanical factor; nil per os (NPO) > 24 hours; oral trauma; radiation therapy; surgical procedure; Sjögren's syndrome; trauma; treatment regimen

Client Outcomes, Nursing Interventions, Client/Family Teaching

Refer to care plan for Impaired **Oral Mucous Membrane**

Obesity

NANDA-I Definition

A condition in which an individual accumulates excessive fat for age and gender that exceeds overweight

Defining Characteristics

ADULT: Body mass index (BMI) >30 kg/m^2; CHILD <2 years: term not used with children at this age; CHILD 2 to 18 years: Body mass index (BMI) >95th percentile or 30 kg/m^2 for age and gender

Related Factors

Average daily physical activity is less than recommended for gender and age; consumption of sugar-sweetened beverages; disordered eating behaviors; disordered eating perceptions; energy expenditure below energy intake based on standard assessment; excessive alcohol consumption; fear regarding lack of food supply; frequent snacking; high frequency of eating restaurant or fried food; low dietary calcium intake in children; portion sizes larger than recommended; sedentary behavior occurring for ≥2 hours/day; shortened sleep time; sleep disorder; solid foods as major food source at <5 months of age

At-Risk Population

Economically disadvantaged; formula- or mixed-fed infants; heritability of interrelated factors; high disinhibition and restraint eating behavior score; maternal diabetes mellitus; maternal smoking; overweight in infancy; paternal obesity; premature pubarche; rapid weight gain during childhood; rapid weight gain during infancy; including the first week; first 4 months; and first year

Associated Condition

Genetic disorder

Client Outcomes

Client Will (Specify Time Frame)

- Explain how to eat according to the US Dietary Guidelines
- Design dietary modifications to meet individual long-term goal of health, using principles of variety, balance, and moderation
- Maintain weight within normal range for height and age

Nursing Interventions

- Assess the meaning and importance of food in the client's life.
- Assess client readiness to determine whether the client is ready to discuss weight loss and/or would like weight loss information.
- Use a motivational interviewing technique when working with clients to promote healthy eating and weight loss.
- Counsel the client to measure regularly consumed foods periodically. Help the client learn usual portion sizes. Measuring food alerts the client to normal portion sizes. Estimating amounts can be extremely inaccurate.
- Assist the client to develop a system of self-management, which may include self-monitoring of weight and BMI; realistic goal setting, planning, and action planning for improved dietary intake and physical activity; problem-solving; and tracking dietary intake and exercise.

- Document the client's height and weight and teach the significance of his or her BMI in relationship to current health. Use a chart or a website such as http://www.cdc.gov/healthyweight/assessing/bmi/index.html (Centers for Disease Control and Prevention [CDC], 2015).
- Encourage the client to engage in vigorous-intensity physical activity for at least 150 minutes weekly or moderate-intensity physical activity for at least 300 minutes weekly.
- Recommend that the client avoid eating in fast-food restaurants.
- Assist the client to reframe slips in weight loss or physical activity behavior as lapses that are a single event and not a full return to previous unhealthy behaviors. Relapse prevention strategies include managing lapses in healthy behavior, identifying high risk situations for relapses, self-monitoring, providing social support, enhancing skills for coping, and increasing self-efficacy for avoiding relapse.
- Assist clients to engage their social support systems either digitally or face to face in ways that facilitate weight loss, healthy eating, and physical activity behavior change. **EB:** Significant others, family, friends, and coworkers can facilitate or hinder weight loss success (Romo, 2018).
- Assist the client to reframe the goal from a focus on outcome (weight loss) to a focus on process (eating behaviors) for weight loss.
- Assist the client to implement informal and formal mindfulness-based interventions (MBIs). Informal MBIs include mindful eating, increasing awareness of hunger and satiety cues, taste satisfaction, and decreasing impulsive tendencies to overeat when experiencing negative emotions. Meditation practice is a formal MBI. **EB:** Results of a research review suggested that a combination of formal and informal MBIs are effective in reducing weight and improving obesity-related eating behaviors among individuals with overweight and obesity (Carrière et al., 2018).
- Assist the client to develop stimulus control techniques designed to reduce environmental cues associated with eating behaviors. Specifically clients should be taught to limit the presence of high-calorie/high-fat foods in the home; to reduce the visibility of unhealthy food choices in the home; to limit where and when they eat; to avoid distractions like reading, using the computer, or watching television when eating; and to eat more slowly.

O

- Encourage 7.5 to 8.5 hours of sleep nightly.
- Refer the client to a weight-loss–related therapy group.
- Incorporate the following recommendations from the Academy of Nutrition and Dietetics: Interventions for the Treatment of Overweight and Obesity in Adults (Raynor & Champagne, 2016):
  - Assess food- and nutrition-related history; anthropometric measures; biochemical data, medical tests, and procedures; nutrition-focused physical findings; and client history.
  - Assess the energy intake and nutrient content of the diet.
  - Use height and weight to calculate BMI, and waist circumference to determine risk of cardiovascular disease (CVD), type 2 diabetes, and all-cause mortality.
  - Use a measured resting metabolic rate (RMR) to determine energy needs.
  - Set a realistic weight loss goal such as one of the following: up to 2 pounds per week, up to 10% of baseline body weight, or a total of 3% to 5% of baseline weight if cardiovascular risk factors (hypertension, hyperlipidemia, and hyperglycemia) are present.
  - To achieve weight loss, use an individualized diet, including patient preferences and health status, to achieve and maintain nutrient adequacy and reduce caloric intake, based on one of the following caloric reduction strategies: 1200 to 1500 kcal/day for women and 1500 to 1800 kcal/day for men, with an energy deficit of approximately 500 kcal/day or 750 kcal/day.

Pediatric

- Offer obese or overweight adolescents healthy methods for weight loss.
- Offer families of obese or overweight children prejudice-free, individually accepting, and supportive interventions to address weight loss.
- Recommend that families eat together for at least one meal per day.
- Recommend involving the family in planning meals and food preparation. Children can learn about nutrition as they help plan and make meals.
- Assist parents at being good role models of healthy eating.
- Recommend that the family try new foods, either a new food or recipe every week.

Geriatric

- Determine the risks and benefits of weight loss in the older client. A BMI greater than 30 in the older client suggests a moderate weight loss approach.
- Observe for social, psychological, and economic factors that influence diet quality.

Multicultural

- Tailor nutritional interventions to be consistent with cultural beliefs, norms, and values.
- Offer tailored lifestyle counseling via the telephone.
- Integrate weight loss and weight maintenance interventions with church faith-based concepts for cultural congruence with African American clients.

Client/Family Teaching and Discharge Planning

- The majority of the preceding interventions involve teaching.
- Work with the family members regarding information on how to support and promote weight loss and healthy intakes.

Overweight

NANDA-I Definition

A condition in which an individual accumulates abnormal or excessive fat for age and gender

Defining Characteristics

ADULT: Body mass index (BMI) >25 kg/m^2; CHILD <2 years: Weight-for-length >95th percentile; CHILD 2–18 years: Body mass index (BMI) >85th percentile or 25 kg/m^2 but <95th percentile or 30 kg/m^2 for age and gender

Related Factors

Average daily physical activity is less than recommended for gender and age; consumption of sugar-sweetened beverages; disordered eating behaviors disordered eating perceptions; energy expenditure below energy intake based on standard assessment; excessive alcohol consumption; fear regarding lack of food supply; frequent snacking; high frequency of restaurant or fried food; insufficient knowledge of modifiable factors; low dietary calcium intake in children; portion sizes larger than recommended; sedentary behavior occurring for >2 hours/day; shortened sleep time; sleep disorder; solid foods as major food source of <5 months of age

Associated Condition

Genetic Disorder

At-Risk Population

ADULT: Body mass index (BMI) approaching 25 kg/m^2; CHILD <2 years: Weight-for-length approaching 95th percentile; CHILD 2–18 years: Body mass index (BMI) approaching 85th percentile or 25 kg/m^2; children who are crossing body mass index (BMI) percentiles upward; children with high body mass index (BMI) percentiles; economically disadvantaged; formula-fed or mixed-fed infants; heritability of interrelated factors; high disinhibition and restraint eating behavior score; maternal diabetes mellitus; maternal smoking; obesity in childhood; paternal obesity; premature pubarche; rapid weight gain during childhood; rapid weight gain during infancy; including the first week; first 4 months; and first year

Nursing Interventions

- Assess the meaning and importance of food in the client's life.
- Assess client readiness to determine whether the client is ready to discuss weight loss and/or would like weight-loss information.
- Use a motivational interviewing technique when working with clients to promote healthy eating and weight loss.
- Counsel the client to measure regularly consumed foods periodically. Help the client learn usual portion sizes. Measuring food alerts the client to normal portion sizes. Estimating amounts can be extremely inaccurate.
- Assist the client to develop a system of self-management, which may include self-monitoring of weight and BMI; realistic goal setting, planning, and action planning for improved dietary intake and physical activity; problem-solving; and tracking dietary intake and exercise.
- Document the client's height and weight and teach the significance of his or her BMI in relationship to current health. Use a chart or a website such as http://www.cdc.gov/healthyweight/assessing/bmi/index.html (Centers for Disease Control and Prevention [CDC], 2015).
- Encourage the client to engage in vigorous-intensity physical activity for at least 150 minutes weekly or moderate-intensity physical activity for at least 300 minutes weekly.
- Recommend the client avoid eating in fast-food restaurants.
- Assist the client to reframe slips in weight loss or physical activity behavior as lapses that are a single event and not a full return to previous unhealthy behaviors. Relapse prevention strategies include managing lapses in healthy behavior, identifying high-risk situations

for relapses, self-monitoring, providing social support, enhancing skills for coping, and increasing self-efficacy for avoiding relapse.

- Assist clients to engage their social support systems either digitally or face to face in ways that facilitate weight loss, healthy eating, and physical activity behavior change.
- Assist the client to reframe the goal from a focus on outcome (weight loss) to a focus on process (eating behaviors) for weight loss.
- Assist the client to implement informal and formal mindfulness-based interventions (MBIs). Informal MBIs include mindful eating, increasing awareness of hunger and satiety cues, taste satisfaction, and decreasing impulsive tendencies to overeat when experiencing negative emotions. Meditation practice is a formal MBI.
- Assist the client to develop stimulus control techniques designed to reduce environmental cues associated with eating behaviors. Specifically clients should be taught to limit the presence of high-calorie/high-fat foods in the home; to reduce the visibility of unhealthy food choices in the home; to limit where and when they eat; to avoid distractions like reading, using the computer, or watching television when eating; and to eat more slowly.
- Encourage 7.5 to 8.5 hours of sleep nightly.
- Refer the client to a weight-loss–related therapy group.
- Recommend that clients use dietary supplements such as vitamins and minerals after consulting with their primary healthcare provider.
- Incorporate the following recommendations from the Academy of Nutrition and Dietetics: Interventions for the Treatment of Overweight and Obesity in Adults (Raynor & Champagne, 2016):
    - Assess food- and nutrition-related history; anthropometric measures; biochemical data, medical tests, and procedures; nutrition-focused physical findings; and client history.
    - Assess the energy intake and nutrient content of the diet.
    - Use height and weight to calculate BMI, and waist circumference to determine risk of cardiovascular disease (CVD), type 2 diabetes, and all-cause mortality.
    - Use a measured resting metabolic rate (RMR) to determine energy needs.

- Set a realistic weight loss goal such as one of the following: up to 2 pounds per week, up to 10% of baseline body weight, or a total of 3% to 5% of baseline weight if cardiovascular risk factors (hypertension, hyperlipidemia, and hyperglycemia) are present.
- To achieve weight loss, use an individualized diet, including patient preferences and health status, to achieve and maintain nutrient adequacy and reduce caloric intake, based on one of the following caloric reduction strategies: 1200 kcal to 1500 kcal/day for women and 1500 to 1800 kcal/day for men, and energy deficit of approximately 500 kcal/day or 750 kcal/day.

Pediatric

- Offer obese or overweight adolescents healthy methods for weight loss.
- Offer families of obese or overweight children prejudice-free, individually accepting, and supportive interventions to address weight loss.
- Recommend that families eat together for at least one meal per day.
- Recommend involving the family in planning meals and food preparation. Children can learn about nutrition as they help plan and make meals.
- Assist parents at being good role models of healthy eating.
- Recommend that the family try new foods, either a new food or recipe every week.

Geriatric

- Determine the risks and benefits of weight loss in the older client. A BMI greater than 30 in the older client suggests a moderate weight loss approach.
- Observe for social, psychological, and economic factors that influence diet quality.

Multicultural

- Tailor nutritional interventions to be consistent with cultural beliefs, norms, and values.
- Offer tailored lifestyle counseling via the telephone.
- Integrate weight loss and weight maintenance interventions with church faith-based concepts for cultural congruence with African American clients.

Client/Family Teaching and Discharge Planning

- The majority of the preceding interventions involve teaching.
- Work with the family members regarding information on how to support and promote weight loss and healthy intakes.

Risk for Overweight*

NANDA-I Definition

Susceptible to excessive fat accumulation for age and gender, which may compromise health

Risk Factors

Average daily physical activity is less than recommended for gender and age; consumption of sugar-sweetened beverages; disordered eating behaviors; disordered eating perceptions; energy expenditure below energy intake based on standard assessment; excessive alcohol consumption; fear regarding lack of food supply; frequent snacking; high frequency of eating restaurant or fried food; insufficient knowledge of modifiable factors; low dietary calcium intake in children; portion sizes larger than recommended; sedentary behavior occurring for >2 hours/day; shortened sleep time; sleep disorder; solid foods as major food source at <5 months of age

At-Risk Population

ADULT: Body mass index (BMI) approaching 25 kg/m^2; CHILD < 2 years: Weight-for-length approaching 95th percentile; CHILD: 2–18 years: Body mass index (BMI) approaching 85th percentile; or 25 kg/m^2; children who are crossing body mass index (BMI) percentiles upward; children with high BMI percentiles; economically disadvantaged; formula- or mixed-fed infants; heritability of interrelated factors; high disinhibition and restraint eating behavior score; maternal diabetes mellitus; maternal smoking; obesity in childhood; parental obesity; premature pubarche; rapid weight gain during childhood; rapid weight gain during infancy; including the first week; first 4 months; and the first year

Associated Condition

Genetic disorder

*Previously Risk for imbalanced Nutrition: more than body requirements

Nursing Interventions

- Assess the meaning and importance of food in the client's life.
- Assess client readiness to determine whether the client is ready to discuss weight loss and/or would like weight loss information.
- Use a motivational interviewing technique when working with clients to promote healthy eating and weight loss.
- Counsel the client to measure regularly consumed foods periodically. Help the client learn usual portion sizes. Measuring food alerts the client to normal portion sizes. Estimating amounts can be extremely inaccurate.
- Assist the client to develop a system of self-management, which may include self-monitoring of weight and BMI; realistic goal setting, planning, and action planning for improved dietary intake and physical activity; problem-solving; and tracking dietary intake and exercise.
- Document the client's height and weight and teach significance of his or her BMI in relationship to current health. Use a chart or a website such as http://www.cdc.gov/healthyweight/assessing/bmi/index.html (Centers for Disease Control and Prevention [CDC], 2015).
- Encourage the client to engage in vigorous-intensity physical activity for at least 150 minutes weekly or moderate-intensity physical activity for at least 300 minutes weekly.
- Recommend that the client avoid eating in fast-food restaurants.
- Assist the client to reframe slips in weight loss or physical activity behavior as lapses that are a single event and not a full return to previous unhealthy behaviors. Relapse prevention strategies include managing lapses in healthy behavior, identifying high-risk situations for relapses, self-monitoring, providing social support, enhancing skills for coping, and increasing self-efficacy for avoiding relapse.
- Assist clients to engage their social support systems either digitally or face to face in ways that facilitate weight loss, healthy eating, and physical activity behavior change.
- Assist the client to reframe the goal from a focus on outcome (weight loss) to a focus on process (eating behaviors) for weight loss.
- Assist the client to implement informal and formal mindfulness-based interventions (MBIs). Informal MBIs include mindful

eating, increasing awareness of hunger and satiety cues, taste satisfaction, and decreasing impulsive tendencies to overeat when experiencing negative emotions. Meditation practice is a formal MBI.

- • Assist the client to develop stimulus control techniques designed to reduce environmental cues associated with eating behaviors. Specifically, clients should be taught to limit the presence of high-calorie/high-fat foods in the home; to reduce the visibility of unhealthy food choices in the home; to limit where and when they eat; to avoid distractions like reading, using the computer, or watching television when eating; and to eat more slowly.
- • Encourage 7.5 to 8.5 hours of sleep nightly.
- • Refer the client to a weight-loss–related therapy group.
- • Recommend that clients use dietary supplements such as vitamins and minerals after consulting with their primary healthcare provider.
- • Incorporate the following recommendations from the Academy of Nutrition and Dietetics: Interventions for the Treatment of Overweight and Obesity in Adults (Raynor & Champagne, 2016):
    - ❍ Assess food- and nutrition-related history; anthropometric measures; biochemical data, medical tests, and procedures; nutrition-focused physical findings; and client history.
    - ❍ Assess the energy intake and nutrient content of the diet.
    - ❍ Use height and weight to calculate BMI, and waist circumference to determine risk of cardiovascular disease (CVD), type 2 diabetes, and all-cause mortality.
    - ❍ Use a measured resting metabolic rate (RMR) to determine energy needs.
    - ❍ Set a realistic weight loss goal such as one of the following: up to 2 pounds per week, up to 10% of baseline body weight, or a total of 3% to 5% of baseline weight if cardiovascular risk factors (hypertension, hyperlipidemia, and hyperglycemia) are present.
    - ❍ To achieve weight loss, use an individualized diet, including patient preferences and health status, to achieve and maintain nutrient adequacy and reduce caloric intake, based on one

O

of the following caloric reduction strategies: 1200 to 1500 kcal/day for women and 1500 to 1800 kcal/day for men and energy deficit of approximately 500 kcal/day or 750 kcal/day.

Pediatric

- Offer obese or overweight adolescents healthy methods for weight loss.
- Offer families of obese or overweight children prejudice-free, individually accepting, and supportive interventions to address weight loss.
- Recommend that families eat together for at least one meal per day.
- Recommend involving the family in planning meals and food preparation. Children can learn about nutrition as they help plan and make meals.
- Assist parents at being good role models of healthy eating.
- Recommend that the family try new foods, either a new food or recipe every week.

Geriatric

- Determine the risks and benefits of weight loss in the older client. A BMI greater than 30 in the older client suggests a moderate weight loss approach.
- Observe for social, psychological, and economic factors that influence diet quality.

Multicultural

- Tailor nutritional interventions to be consistent with cultural beliefs, norms, and values.
- Offer tailored lifestyle counseling via the telephone.
- Integrate weight loss and weight maintenance interventions with church faith-based concepts for cultural congruence with African American clients.

Client/Family Teaching and Discharge Planning

- The majority of the preceding interventions involve teaching.
- Work with the family members regarding information on how to support and promote weight loss and healthy intakes.

Acute Pain

NANDA-I Definition

Unpleasant sensory and emotional experience associated with actual or potential tissue damage, or described in terms of such damage (International Association for the Study of Pain); sudden or slow onset of any intensity from mild to severe with an anticipated or predictable end, and with a duration of less than 3 months

Defining Characteristics

Appetite change; change in physiological parameter; diaphoresis; distraction behavior; evidence of pain using standardized pain behavior checklist for those unable to communicate verbally; expressive behavior; facial expression of pain; guarding behavior; hopelessness; narrowed focus; positioning to ease pain; protective behavior; proxy report of pain behavior/activity changes; pupil dilation; self-focused; self-report of intensity using standardized pain scale; self-report of pain characteristics using standardized pain instrument

Related Factors

Biological injury agent; chemical injury agent; physical injury agent

P

Client Outcomes

Client Will (Specify Time Frame)

For the client who is able to provide a self-report

- Use a self-report pain tool to identify current pain intensity level and establish a comfort-function goal
- Report that the pain management regimen achieves comfort-function goal without side effects
- Describe nonpharmacological methods that can be used to help achieve comfort-function goal
- Perform activities of recovery or activities of daily living (ADLs) easily
- Describe how unrelieved pain will be managed
- State ability to obtain sufficient amounts of rest and sleep
- Notify member of the healthcare team promptly for pain intensity level that is consistently greater than the comfort-function goal, or occurrence of side effects

For the client who is unable to provide a self-report

- Decrease in pain-related behaviors
- Perform activities of recovery or ADLs easily as determined by client condition
- Demonstrate the absence of side effects of analgesics

- No pain-related behaviors will be evident in the client who is completely unresponsive; a reasonable outcome is to demonstrate the absence of side effects related to the prescribed pain treatment plan

Nursing Interventions

- During the initial assessment and interview, if the client is experiencing pain, or when pain first occurs, conduct and document a comprehensive pain assessment, using appropriate pain assessment tools.
- Implement or request orders to implement pain management interventions to achieve a satisfactory level of comfort. Components of this initial assessment include location, quality, onset/duration, temporal profile, intensity, aggravating and alleviating factors, and effects of pain on function and quality of life.
- Assess if the client is able to provide a self-report of pain intensity, and if so, assess pain intensity level using a valid and reliable self-report pain tool, such as the 0 to 10 numerical pain rating scale.
- Ask the client to describe prior experiences with pain, effectiveness of pain management interventions, responses to analgesic medications including occurrence of side effects, and concerns about pain and its treatment (e.g., fear about addiction, worries, anxiety) and informational needs.
- Using a self-report pain tool, ask the client to identify a comfort-function goal that will allow the client to perform necessary or desired activities easily.
- Use the Hierarchy of Pain Measures as a framework for pain assessment (Herr et al., 2011; Drew & Peltier, 2018): (1) attempt to obtain the client's self-report of pain; (2) consider the client's condition and search for possible causes of pain (e.g., presence of tissue injury, pathological conditions, exposure to procedures/interventions that are thought to result in pain); (3) observe for behaviors that may indicate pain presence (e.g., facial expressions, crying, restlessness, changes in activity); (4) evaluate physiological indicators, with the understanding that these are the least sensitive indicators of pain and may be related to conditions other than pain (e.g., shock, hypovolemia, anxiety); and (5) conduct an analgesic trial.
- Assume that pain is present if the client is unable to provide a self-report and has tissue injury, a pathological condition, or has undergone a procedure that is thought to produce pain, and conduct an analgesic trial.

- ▲ Obtain and review an accurate and complete list of medications the client is taking or has taken.
- ▲ Describe the adverse effects of unrelieved pain.
- ▲ Explain to the client the pain management approach, including pharmacological and nonpharmacological interventions, the assessment and reassessment process, potential side effects, and the importance of prompt reporting of unrelieved pain.
- ▲ Discuss the client's fears of undertreated pain, side effects, and opioid use disorder (OUD), and reassure the client that there will be regular assessment and treatment of pain, and assessment for side effects and signs of OUD.
- • Teach the client about pain and pharmacological and nonpharmacological interventions when pain is relatively well controlled.
- ▲ Regularly reassess the client for the presence of pain and response to pain management interventions, including effectiveness and the presence of adverse effects related to pain management interventions. Review the client's pain flow sheet and medication administration record to evaluate effectiveness of pain relief, previous 24-hour opioid requirements, and occurrence of side effects.
- ▲ Advocate for and manage acute pain using a multimodal, opioid-sparing approach.
- ▲ Select the route for administration of analgesics based on client condition and pain characteristics.
- ▲ Provide perineural infusions and intraspinal analgesia when appropriate and available.
- ▲ Use diverse analgesic delivery methods such as PCA to increase client's satisfaction with pain management, to lower cost, and to decrease occurrence of adverse reactions.
- ▲ Administer a nonopioid analgesic for mild to moderate pain and add an opioid analgesic if indicated for moderate to severe acute pain.
- • Avoid administering analgesics based solely on a client's pain intensity rating.
- • Administer analgesics around the clock for continuous pain (expected to be present approximately 50% of the day, such as postoperative pain) and as needed (PRN) for intermittent or breakthrough pain.

P

- Prevent pain by administering analgesia before painful procedures whenever possible (e.g., endotracheal suctioning, wound care, heel puncture, venipunctures, and peripherally inserted IV catheters).
- Perform nursing care during the peak effect of analgesics to optimize client comfort and participation in care.
- Advocate for the use of "as needed" opioid range orders to provide effective and appropriate pain relief.
- Choose analgesic and dose based on orders that reflect the client's report of pain severity and response to the previous dose in terms of pain relief, occurrence of side effects, and ability to perform the activities of recovery or ADLs.
- ▲ When converting opioids from parenteral doses to oral doses (the preferred route when the client can tolerate and absorb oral medications), use equianalgesic dosing charts and carefully monitor the client's response to the new medication route and dose.
- ▲ Clients who are receiving opioids for acute pain require frequent assessment for effectiveness of opioids and assessment for serious opioid-related adverse effects. This includes respiratory assessment (rate, rhythm, noisiness, and depth) and systematic assessment of sedation level using a sedation scale (Eksterowicz & DiMaggio, 2018).
- ▲ When opioids are included in the multimodal analgesic plan, clients need regular assessment for common side effects such as constipation, nausea, pruritus, lack of appetite, and changes in rest and sleep, and preventive measures are implemented when possible.
- Monitor frequency of bowel movements and provide the client with adequate hydration, a stool softener, and stimulant to prevent/treat opioid-related constipation.
- ▲ Support the client's use of nonpharmacological methods to supplement pharmacological analgesic approaches to help control pain, such as distraction, imagery, music therapy, simple massage, relaxation, and application of heat and cold.
- ▲ Assist client to identify resources for coping with psychological impact of pain.

Pediatric

- Assess for the presence of pain using a valid and reliable pain scale based on age, cognitive development, and the child's ability to provide a self-report.

▲ Administer prescribed analgesics using a multimodal approach to treat pain in children, infants, and neonates.
- Prevent procedural pain in neonates, infants, and children by using opioid analgesics and anesthetics, as indicated, in appropriate dosages.
- Use a topical local anesthetic treatment or other nonpharmacologic treatment before performing venipuncture in neonates, infants, and children.
- For the neonate, use oral sucrose and nonnutritional sucking (NNS) or human milk for pain of short duration such as heel stick or venipuncture. Neonates, especially preterm neonates, are more sensitive to pain than older children.
- Recognize that breastfeeding has been shown to reduce behavioral indicators of pain.
- As with adults, use nonpharmacological analgesic interventions to supplement, not replace, pharmacological interventions in pediatric clients.

Geriatric

- Refer to the Nursing Interventions and *Rationales* in the care plan for Chronic **Pain**.

Multicultural

- Refer to the Nursing Interventions and *Rationales* in the care plan for Chronic **Pain**.

Home Care

▲ Develop the treatment plan with the client and caregivers.
▲ Assess the client's full medication profile, including medications prescribed by all healthcare providers and all over-the-counter medications for drug interactions, and instruct the client to refrain from mixing medications without healthcare provider approval.
▲ Assess the client/family's knowledge of side effects and safety precautions associated with pain medications.
- If medication is administered using highly technological methods, assess the home for the necessary resources (e.g., electricity) and ensure that there will be responsible caregivers available to assist the client with administration.
- Assess the knowledge base of the client and family regarding highly technological medication administration and provide necessary education, including the procedure to follow if analgesia is unsatisfactory.

P

Client/Family Teaching and Discharge Planning

Note: To avoid the negative connotations associated with the words "drugs" and "narcotics," use the term "pain medicine" when teaching clients.

- • Discuss the various discomforts encompassed by the word "pain" and ask the client to give examples of previously experienced pain. Explain the pain assessment process and the purpose of the pain rating scale.
- • Teach the client to use the self-report pain tool to rate the intensity of past or current pain. Ask the client to set a comfort-function goal by selecting a pain level on the self-report tool that will allow performance of desired or necessary activities of recovery with relative ease (e.g., turn, cough, deep breathe, ambulate, participate in physical therapy). If the pain level is consistently above the comfort-function goal, the client should take action that decreases pain or notify a member of the healthcare team so that effective pain management interventions may be implemented promptly.
- • Provide written educational materials on various aspects of pain control to improve client understanding of pain and pain-related interventions.
- • Discuss and evaluate the client's understanding about the total plan for pharmacological and nonpharmacological treatment, including the medications prescribed and their indication, proper dosing schedule, and adverse events and what to do should they occur.
- • Teach basic principles of pain management using a variety of educational strategies, and evaluate learning.
- ▲ Reinforce the importance of taking pain medications to maintain the comfort-function goal.
- ▲ Reinforce that short-term use of opioids for acute pain relief is an appropriate part of their multimodal pain treatment plan.
- ▲ Reinforce the importance of safe storage of opioid medications out of the reach of others, and to responsibly dispose of any unused opioids.
- ▲ Demonstrate the use of appropriate nonpharmacological approaches in addition to pharmacological approaches to help control pain, such as application of heat and/or cold, distraction techniques, relaxation breathing, visualization, rocking, stroking, listening to music, and watching television.

P

Chronic Pain

NANDA-I Definition

Unpleasant sensory and emotional experience associated with actual or potential tissue damage, or described in terms of such damage (International Association for the Study of Pain); sudden or slow onset of any intensity from mild to severe, constant or recurring without an anticipated or predictable end, and with a duration of greater than 3 months

Defining Characteristics

Alteration in ability to continue previous activities; alteration in sleep pattern; anorexia; evidence of pain using standardized pain behavior checklist for those unable to communicate verbally; facial expression of pain; proxy report of pain behavior/activity changes; self-focused; self-report of intensity using standardized pain scale; self-report of pain characteristics using standardized pain instrument

Related Factors

Alteration in sleep pattern; emotional distress; fatigue; increase in body mass index; ineffective sexuality pattern; injury agent; malnutrition; nerve compression; prolonged computer use; repeated handling of heavy loads; social isolation; whole-body vibration

P

At-Risk Population

Age >50 years; female gender; history of abuse; history of genital mutilation; history of indebtedness; history of static work postures; history of substance misuse; history of vigorous exercise

Associated Condition

Chronic musculoskeletal condition; contusion; crush injury; damage to the nervous system; fracture; genetic disorder; imbalance of neurotransmitters; neuromodulators; and receptors; immune disorder; impaired metabolic functioning; ischemic condition; muscle injury; post-trauma related condition; prolonged increase in cortisol level; spinal cord injury; tumor infiltration

Client Outcomes

Client Will (Specify Time Frame)

For the client who is able to provide a self-report

- Provide a description of the pain experience including physical, social, emotional, and spiritual aspects
- Use a self-report pain tool to identify current pain level and establish a comfort-function goal
- Report that the pain management regimen achieves comfort-function goal without the occurrence of side effects

- Describe nonpharmacological methods that can be used to supplement, or enhance, pharmacological interventions and help achieve the comfort-function goal
- Perform necessary or desired activities at a pain level less than or equal to the comfort-function goal
- •Demonstrate the ability to pace activity, taking rest breaks before they are needed
- Describe how unrelieved pain will be managed
- State the ability to obtain sufficient amounts of rest and sleep
- Notify a member of the healthcare team for pain level consistently greater than the comfort-function goal or occurrence of side effect

For the client who is unable to provide a self-report

- Demonstrate decrease or resolved pain-related behaviors
- Perform desired activities as determined by client condition
- Demonstrate the absence of side effects
- No pain-related behaviors will be evident in the client who is completely unresponsive; a reasonable outcome is to demonstrate the absence of side effects related to the prescribed pain treatment plan

P

Nursing Interventions

▲ During the initial assessment and interview, if the client is experiencing pain, conduct and document a comprehensive pain assessment, using appropriate pain assessment tools.

▲ Determine the quality of the pain and whether the pain has persisted beyond the usual duration for tissue healing. **Refer to the acute Pain section for the Hierarchy of Pain Measures for assessment approach in clients who are unable to provide self-report of pain.**

▲ Perform a pain assessment using a reliable self-report pain tool.

▲ Ask the client to describe prior experiences with pain, effectiveness of pain management interventions, responses to analgesic medications including occurrence of side effects, and concerns about pain and its treatment (e.g., fear about addiction, worries, anxiety) and informational needs.

• Using a self-report tool, ask the client to identify a comfort-function goal that will allow the client to perform necessary or desired activities easily. Assess the client for the presence of acute pain (see care plan for Acute **Pain**).

▲ Assess chronic pain regularly, including the effect of chronic pain on activity; sleep; eating habits; and social conditions including relationships, finances, and employment.

- ▲ Assess the client for the presence of psychiatric conditions, including anxiety and depression.
- ▲ If opioid therapy is considered, assist the provider with aspects of an opioid risk assessment, which includes a comprehensive client interview and examination with a pain focus, mental health screening, use of an opioid risk assessment tool, examination of prescription drug monitoring program results, and urine drug screening.
- ▲ For the client who is receiving outpatient opioid therapy, at each visit, assess effect of opioids on pain status, function, goal achievement, and presence of side effects including sleep disturbance and sexual dysfunction; assessment for signs of misuse and SUD should be included, which may involve the use of random urine drug toxicology screening, pill counts, and review of prescription-monitoring database.
- • Ask the client to maintain a diary (if able) of pain ratings, timing, precipitating events, medications, and effectiveness of pain management interventions.
- ▲ Obtain and review an accurate and complete list of medications the client is taking or has taken.
- ▲ Explain to the client the pain management approach that has been ordered or revised, including therapies, medication administration, side effects, and complications.
- • Discuss the client's fears of undertreated pain, side effects, opioid use disorder (OUD), and overdose and reassure the client that there will be regular assessment and treatment of pain and assessment for side effects and signs of OUD.
- ▲ Manage chronic pain using an individualized, multimodal nonopioid or opioid-sparing approach.
- ▲ Select the route of administration of analgesics based on client condition and pain characteristics.
- ▲ When chronic pain has a neuropathic component, treat with adjuvant analgesics, such as anticonvulsants, antidepressants, and topical local anesthetics.
- ▲ Administer a nonopioid analgesic for mild to moderate chronic pain and as a component of the treatment for all levels of pain for clients with cancer pain.
- ▲ Recognize that opioid therapy may be indicated for some clients experiencing chronic pain.

P

- ▲ Administer analgesics around the clock for continuous pain and as needed (PRN) for intermittent or breakthrough pain as may be experienced by clients with cancer pain.
- ▲ Long-acting or extended-release opioids may be indicated for patients with cancer or with chronic non-cancer pain if patients require the regular use of short-acting opioids, and receive adequate relief with them.
- ▲ At regular intervals, assess inpatient clients with chronic pain for opioid-related adverse events and include frequent assessment of pain level, assessment of respiratory status (including rate, rhythm, noisiness, and depth), and systematic assessment of sedation level using a sedation scale.
- ▲ During outpatient follow-up, assess clients receiving opioids for risk factors that may increase opioid-related harm.
- ▲ Provide the client with a stool softener and stimulant to prevent/treat opioid-related constipation. Ask about other opioid-related side effects including nausea, pruritus, lack of appetite, and changes in rest and sleep.
- ▲ In addition to administering analgesics, support the client's use of nonpharmacological methods to help control pain, such as distraction, imagery, relaxation, and application of heat and cold.
- • Teach and implement nonpharmacological interventions when pain is relatively well controlled with pharmacological interventions.
- ▲ Encourage the client to plan activities around periods of greatest comfort whenever possible.
- ▲ Explore appropriate resources for management of pain on a long-term basis (e.g., hospice, pain care center).
- ▲ If the client has progressive cancer pain, assist the client and family with handling issues related to death and dying and provide access to palliative care programs and hospice services.

Pediatric

- • Assess for the presence of pain using a valid and reliable pain scale based on age, cognitive development, and the child's ability to provide a self-report.
- ▲ Manage chronic pain children, infants, and neonates with an interdisciplinary and multimodal approach.
- • Use a variety of nonpharmacological analgesic interventions to address chronic pain in pediatric clients.

Geriatric

▲ An older client's report of pain should be taken seriously and assessed and treated.
• When assessing pain, speak clearly, slowly, and loudly enough for the client to hear, ensure hearing aids and glasses are in place as appropriate; enlarge pain scales and written materials, and repeat information as needed.
• Handle the client's body gently and allow the client to move at his or her own speed.
▲ Use nonpharmacological approaches including physical therapy, exercise, or other movement-based programs as the core components to persistent pain management in the older adult.
▲ When pharmacological measures are needed to address chronic pain in the elderly, use a multimodal approach, including nonopioid analgesics for mild to moderate pain.
▲ Use opioids cautiously in the older client with moderate to severe pain.
▲ Monitor for signs of depression in older clients and refer to specialists with relevant expertise.

Multicultural

▲ Assess for pain disparities among racial and ethnic minorities.
▲ Assess for the influence of cultural beliefs, norms, and values on the client's perception and experience of pain.
▲ Use a family-centered approach to care.
▲ Use culturally relevant pain scales to assess pain in the client.

Home Care

• The interventions previously described may be adapted for home care use. Refer to the Nursing Interventions and *Rationales* in the care plan for Acute **Pain**.

Client/Family Teaching and Discharge Planning

Note: To avoid the negative connotations associated with the words "drugs" and "narcotics," use the term "pain medicine" when teaching clients.

• Discuss the various discomforts encompassed by the word "pain" and ask the client to give examples of previously experienced pain. Explain the pain assessment process and the purpose of the pain rating scale.
• Teach the client that if the pain level is consistently above the comfort-function goal, the client should take action that decreases pain or should notify a member of the healthcare team so that effective pain management interventions may be implemented promptly. (See information on teaching clients to use the pain rating scale.)

- • Provide educational materials on various aspects of pain control to improve client understanding of pain and pain-related interventions.
- • Discuss and evaluate the client's understanding about the total plan for pharmacological and nonpharmacological treatment, including the medication plan, the maintenance of a pain diary, and the use of supplies and equipment.
- • Reinforce the importance of taking pain medications to maintain the comfort-function goal.
- ▲ Reinforce that, when prescribed, opioids for pain relief are an appropriate part of their multimodal pain treatment plan.
- ▲ Reinforce the importance of safe storage of opioid medications out of the reach of others, and to responsibly dispose of any unused opioids.
- • Demonstrate the use of appropriate nonpharmacological approaches in addition to pharmacological approaches for helping control pain, such as application of heat and/or cold, distraction techniques, relaxation breathing, visualization, rocking, stroking, listening to music, and watching television. Teach these methods when pain is relatively well controlled, because pain interferes with cognition.
- ▲ Emphasize to the client the importance of participating in a structured, individualized pacing activity and taking rest breaks before they are needed.
- • Teach nonpharmacological methods when pain is relatively well controlled.

Chronic Pain Syndrome

NANDA-I Definition

Recurrent or persistent pain that has lasted at least 3 months and that significantly affects daily functioning or well-being

Defining Characteristics

Anxiety (00146); constipation (00011); disturbed sleep pattern (00198); fatigue (00093); fear (00148); impaired mood regulation (00241); impaired physical mobility (00085); insomnia (00095); social isolation (00053); stress overload (00177)

Related Factors

Body mass index above normal range for age and gender; fear of pain; fear-avoidance beliefs; inadequate knowledge of pain management behaviors; negative affect; sleep disturbances

Client Outcomes, Nursing Interventions, Client/Family Teaching and Discharge Planning

Refer to care plan for Acute **Pain** and Chronic **Pain**

Labor Pain

NANDA-I Definition

Sensory and emotional experience that varies from pleasant to unpleasant, associated with labor and childbirth

Defining Characteristics

Altered blood pressure; altered heart rate; altered muscle tension; altered neuroendocrine functioning; altered respiratory rate; altered urinary functioning; anxiety; appetite change; diaphoresis; distraction behavior; expressive behavior; facial expression of pain; narrow focus; nausea; perineal pressure; positioning to ease pain; protective behavior; pupil dilation; reports altered sleep-wake cycle; self-focused; uterine contraction; vomiting

Related Factors

Behavioral Factors

Insufficient fluid intake; supine position

Cognitive Factors

Fear of childbirth; inadequate knowledge about childbirth; inadequate preparation to deal with labor pain; low self efficacy; perception of labor pain as nonproductive; perception of labor pain as negative; perception of labor pain as threatening; perception of labor pain as unnatural; perception of pain as meaningful

Social Factors

Interference in decision-making; unsupportive companionship

Unmodified Environmental Factors

Noisy delivery room; overcrowded delivery room; turbulent environment

At Risk Population

Women experiencing emergency situation during labor; women from cultures with negative perspective of labor pain; women giving birth in a disease-based health care system; women whose mothers have a high level of education; women with history of pre-pregnancy dysmenorrhea; women with history of sexual abuse during childhood; women without supportive companion

Associated Conditions

Cervical dilation; depression; fetal expulsion; high maternal trait anxiety; prescribed mobility restriction; prolonged duration of labor

Client Outcomes

Client Will (Specify Time Frame)

- Recognize pharmacological and nonpharmacological interventions to address labor pain
- Demonstrate coping strategies to address labor pain
- Verbalize pain relief effectiveness throughout the labor process

Nursing Interventions

- Initial assessment and interview; if the client is experiencing pain, conduct and document a comprehensive pain assessment, using appropriate pain assessment tools.
- Assess pain on pain level tool such as the 0 to 10 numerical pain rating scale (NRS) if appropriate or alternatively use the Coping with Labor Algorithm (Roberts et al., 2010). Discuss with client the desire for pain management for this labor, past experiences with labor and effectiveness of pain management techniques employed at that time, concerns about pain and its treatment, and information needs (e.g., pain-coping techniques that are both analgesic and nonpharmaceutical).
- Goal is for the client to manage labor pain from admission until delivery of infant with either natural childbirth and associated pain management techniques, or pharmaceutical measures to reduce pain experience.
- Based on the client's ability to cope with labor pain, discuss with client pain management options, including pharmacological and nonpharmacological interventions.
- Based on the client's ability to cope, assess the physiological-natural process of labor, physical environment, and emotional/psychosocial dynamics (Roberts et al., 2010).
- Based on the client's ability to cope, offer intervention (either nonpharmacological or pharmacological).
- Nonpharmacological pain relief measures are low-risk and low-resource interventions (Simkin & Klein, 2017). These approaches can encompass the physical sensation of pain and the psychoemotional and spiritual components of care. By addressing all aspects of client needs (physical, emotional, and spiritual), suffering can be reduced during labor (Simkin & Klein, 2017).
  - Ambulation/rocking/swaying is a safe and effective coping measure for labor pain. This is usually a client-initiated response to labor pain; however, caregivers can encourage women to ambulate or change position to ease pain or allow clients to cope better with labor pain.

- ○ Hydrotherapy either as immersion in water or bathing can be used to promote relaxation, decrease anxiety, help client cope with pain, and possibly correct uterine contraction dystocia (Benfield et al., 2010).
- ○ TENS is a small, handheld device that transmits low-voltage electrical impulses to the skin (Simkin & Klein, 2017). The device suppresses the conduction of pain through pain fibers by using small electrical impulses (Shahoei et al., 2017).
- Pharmacological measures for pain relief are high resource and high risk; they require professional training for administration, incur cost, and have a greater risk to mother and baby (Simkin & Klein, 2017).
- Nitrous oxide is a blend of 50% nitrous oxide with 50% oxygen. The use of nitrous oxide may not alleviate pain, but it may help with satisfaction of the birth experience (American College of Nurse-Midwives [ACNM], 2010).
- IV medications for pain management are an alternative for some women who do not desire an epidural; IV medications are generally opioids. These are advantageous because they are easy to administer, are widely available, and are less invasive than neuraxial techniques of pain relief, i.e., an epidural (Grant, 2017).
- Epidural, combined spinal-epidural (CSE), and dural puncture epidural (DPE) are appropriate for laboring women when requested by the client (unless there is a contraindication).
- Account for clients' abilities to cope with labor pain regarding their psychosocial, cultural, and spiritual backgrounds. A woman's positive perceptions of how she will be able to cope with labor are associated with reduced anxiety, pain, and intervention during labor (Van der Gucht & Lewis, 2015; Simkin & Klein, 2017).

P

Impaired Parenting

NANDA-I Definition

Limitation of primary caregiver to nurture, protect, and promote optimal growth and development of the child, through a consistent, empathic exercise of authority and appropriate behavior in response to the child's needs.

Defining Characteristics

Infant or Child

Anxiety; conduct problems; delayed cognitive development; depressive symptoms; difficulty establishing healthy intimate interpersonal relations;

difficulty functioning socially; difficulty regulating emotion; extreme mood alterations; low academic performance; obesity; role reversal; somatic complaints; substance misuse

Parental Externalizing Symptoms

Hostile parenting behaviors; impulsive behaviors; intrusive behaviors; negative communication

Parental Internalizing Symptoms

Decreased engagement in parent-child relations; decreased positive temperament; decreased subjective attention quality; extreme mood swings; failure to provide safe home environment; inadequate response to infant behavioral cues; inappropriate child-care arrangements; rejects child; social alienation

Related Factors

Altered parental role; Altered parental role; decreased emotion recognition abilities; depressive symptoms; difficulty managing complex treatment regimen; dysfunctional family processes; emotional vacillation; high use of internet-connected devices; inadequate knowledge about child development; inadequate knowledge about child health maintenance; inadequate parental role model; inadequate problem-solving skills; inadequate social support; inadequate transportation; inattentive to child's needs; increased anxiety symptoms; low self efficacy; marital conflict; nonrestorative sleep-wake cycle; perceived economic strain; social isolation; substance misuse; unaddressed intimate partner violence

At-Risk Population

Infant or Child

Children experiencing prolonged separation from parent; children with difficult temperament; children with gender other than that desired by parent; children with history of hospitalization in neonatal intensive care; premature infants

Parental

Adolescents; eonomically disadvantaged individuals; homeless individuals; individuals experiencing family substance misuse; individuals experiencing situational crisis; individuals with family history of post-traumatic shock; individuals with history of being abused; individuals with history of being abusive; individuals with history of being neglected; individuals with history of exposure to violence; individuals with history of inadequate prenatal care; individuals with history of prenatal stress; individuals with low educational level; sole parents

Associated Condition

Infant or Child

Behavioral disorder; complex treatment regimen; emotional disorder; neurodevelopmental disabilities

Parental

Depression; mental disorders

Client Outcomes

Client Will (Specify Time Frame)

- Initiate appropriate measures to develop a safe, nurturing environment
- Acquire and display attentive, supportive parenting behaviors and child supervision
- Identify appropriate strategies to manage a child's inappropriate behaviors
- Identify strategies to protect child from harm and/or neglect and initiate action when indicated

Nursing Interventions

- • Use the Parenting Sense of Competence (PSOC) scale to measure parental self-efficacy.
- • Examine the characteristics of parenting style and behaviors. Consider dysfunctional child-centered and parent-centered cognitions as potentially critical correlates of abusive behavior.
- ▲ Institute abuse/neglect protection measures if evidence exists of an inability to cope with family stressors or crisis, signs of parental substance abuse are observed, or a significant level of social isolation is apparent.
- ▲ For a mother with a toddler, assess maternal depression. Make the appropriate referral.
- • Appraise the parent's resources and the availability of social support systems. Determine the single mother's particular sources of support, especially the availability of her own mother and partner. Encourage the use of healthy, strong support systems.
- • Promotion of better-quality relationships between parents and children is an effective strategy that can lead to enhanced learning. Good-quality parenting leads to improved cognitive and social skills for children.
- • Support parents' competence in appraising their infant's behavior and responses and aim supportive interventions to minimize parents' experiences of strain or stress.
- • Encourage mothers to understand and capitalize on their infant's capacity to interact, particularly in the early months of life.
- ▲ Provide programs for homeless mothers with severe mental illness who have lost physical custody of their children.
- ▲ Provide a recovery program that includes instruction in parenting skills and child development for mothers who are addicted to cocaine.

P

- Refer to Readiness for enhanced **Parenting** for additional interventions.

Multicultural

- Acknowledge that value conflicts from acculturation stresses may contribute to increased anxiety and significant conflict with children.
- Clarify parents' feelings, expectations, perceptions, and availability regarding participation in the care of their sick child.
- Carefully assess the meaning of terms used to describe health status when working with Native Americans.
- Provide support for Chinese families caring for children with disabilities.
- Facilitate modeling and role playing to help the family improve parenting skills.

Home Care

- The interventions previously described may be adapted for home care use.
- Assess parenting stress at each home visit to provide appropriate support and anticipatory guidance to families of children with a chronic disease.
- ▲ Assess the single mother's history regarding childhood and partner abuse and current status regarding depressive symptoms, abusive parenting attitudes (lack of empathy, favorable opinion of corporal punishment, parent–child role reversal, and inappropriate expectations). Refer for mental health services as indicated.

Client/Family Teaching and Discharge Planning

- Consider individual and/or group-based parenting programs for teenaged mothers.
- Consider group-based parenting programs for parents of children younger than 3 years with emotional and behavioral problems.
- Consider group-based parenting programs for parents with anxiety, depression, and/or low self-esteem.
- ▲ Refer adolescent parents for comprehensive psychoeducational parenting classes.
- Parent training is one of the most effective interventions for behavior problems in young children.
- ▲ Initiate referrals to community agencies, parent education programs, stress management training, and social support groups. Consider the use of technology and the media.
- Provide information regarding available telephone counseling services and Internet support.

Readiness for Enhanced Parenting

NANDA-I Definition

A pattern of primary caregiver to nurture, protect, and promote optimal growth and development of the child, through a consistent, empathic exercise of authority and appropriate behavior in response to the child's needs, which can be strengthened.

Defining Characteristics

Expresses desire to enhance acceptance of child; expresses desire to enhance attention quality; expresses desire to enhance child health maintenance; expresses desire to enhance childcare arrangements; expresses desire to enhance engagement with child; expresses desire to enhance home environmental safety; expresses desire to enhance mood stability; expresses desire to enhance parent-child relations; expresses desire to enhance patience; expresses desire to enhance positive communication; expresses desire to enhance positive parenting behaviors; expresses desire to enhance positive temperament; expresses desire to enhance response to infant behavioral cues

Client Outcomes

Client/Family Will (Specify Time Frame)

- Affirm desire to improve parenting skills to further support growth and development of children
- Demonstrate loving relationship with children
- Provide a safe, nurturing environment
- Assess risks in home/environment and take steps to prevent possibility of harm to children
- Meet physical, psychosocial, and spiritual needs or seek appropriate assistance

Nursing Interventions

- Use family-centered care and role modeling for holistic care of families.
- Assess parents' feelings when dealing with a child who has a chronic illness.
- Promote low-technology interventions, such as massage, multisensory interventions (maternal voice, eye-to-eye contact, and rocking), and music, to reduce maternal and infant stress and improve mother–infant relationship.
- When the person who is ill is the parent, use family-centered assessment skills to determine the effect of an adult's illness on the child, and then guide the parent through those topics that are most likely to be of concern.

- Refer to the care plan for Impaired **Parenting** for additional interventions.

Multicultural

- Assess the influence of cultural beliefs, norms, and values on the client's perception of parenting.
- Acknowledge racial and ethnic differences at the onset of care and provide appropriate health information and social support.
- Support programs for parents of young children in specific cultural communities.
- Acknowledge and praise parenting strengths noted.

Home Care

- The nursing interventions previously described should be used in the home environment with adaptations as necessary.

▲ Refer to a parenting program to facilitate learning of parenting skills.

Client/Family Teaching and Discharge Planning

- Refer to Client/Family Teaching and Discharge Planning for Impaired **Parenting** for suggestions that may be used with minor adaptations.
- Teach parents home safety: reduction of hot water temperature, proper poison storage, use of smoke alarms, and installation of safety gates for stairs.
- Teach parents and young teens conflict resolution by using a hypothetical conflict solution with and without a structured conflict resolution guide. Support self-direction of the families with minimal therapist intervention.
- Refer mothers of children with type 1 diabetes for community support in babysitting, child care, or respite.
- Teach families the importance of monitoring television viewing, social media, video gaming, and so forth to limit exposure to violence.
- See impaired **Parenting** for additional references.

Risk for Impaired Parenting

NANDA-I Definition

Primary caregiver susceptible to a limitation to nurture, protect, and promote optimal growth and development of the child, through a consistent, empathic exercise of authority and appropriate behavior in response to the child's needs

Risk Factors

Altered parental role; decreased emotion recognition abilities; depressive symptoms; difficulty managing complex treatment regimen; dysfunctional family processes; emotional vacillation; high use of internet-connected devices; inadequate knowledge about child development; inadequate knowledge about child health maintenance; inadequate parental role model; inadequate problem-solving skills; inadequate social support; inadequate transportation; inattentive to child's needs; increased anxiety symptoms; low self efficacy; marital conflict; nonrestorative sleep-wake cycle; perceived economic strain; social isolation; substance misuse; unaddressed intimate partner violence

At-Risk Population

Infant or Child

Children experiencing prolonged separation from parent; children with difficult temperament; children with gender other than that desired by parent; children with history of hospitalization in neonatal intensive care; premature infants

Parental

Adolescents; economically disadvantaged individuals; homeless individuals; individuals experiencing family substance misuse; individuals experiencing situational crisis; individuals with family history of post-traumatic shock; individuals with history of being abused; individuals with history of being abusive; individuals with history of being neglected; individuals with history of exposure to violence; individuals with history of inadequate prenatal care; individuals with history of prenatal stress; individuals with low educational level; sole parents

P

Associated Condition

Infant or Child

Behavioral disorder; complex treatment regimen; emotional disorder; neurodevelopmental disabilities

Parental

Depression; mental disorders

Client Outcomes, Nursing Interventions, Client/Family Teaching and Discharge Planning

Refer to care plans for Readiness for enhanced **Parenting** and Impaired **Parenting**

Risk for Perioperative Positioning Injury

NANDA-I Definition

Susceptible to inadvertent anatomical and physical changes as a result of posture or positioning equipment used during an invasive/surgical procedure, which may compromise health.

Risk Factors

Decreased muscle strength; dehydration; factors identified by standardized, validated screening tool; inadequate access to appropriate equipment; inadequate access to appropriate support surfaces; inadequate availability of equipment for individuals with obesity; malnutrition; obesity; prolonged non-anatomic positioning of limbs; rigid support surface

At Risk Population

Individuals at extremes of age; individuals in lateral position; individuals in lithotomy position; individuals in prone position; individuals in Trendelenburg position; individuals undergoing surgical procedure > 1 hour

Associated Condition

Diabetes mellitus; edema; emaciation; general anesthesia; immobilization; neuropathy; sensoriperceptual disturbance from anesthesia; vascular diseases

Client Outcomes

Client Will (Specify Time Frame)

- Demonstrate unchanged skin condition, with exception of the incision, throughout the perioperative experience
- Demonstrate resolution of redness of the skin at points of pressure within 30 minutes after pressure is eliminated
- Remain injury-free related to surgical positioning, including intact skin and absence of pain and/or numbness associated with surgical positioning
- Demonstrate unchanged or improved physical mobility from preoperative status
- Demonstrate unchanged or improved peripheral sensory integrity from preoperative status

P

Nursing Interventions

General Interventions for Any Surgical Client

- Assess the client's skin integrity throughout the perioperative process to avoid skin breakdown during surgical/invasive procedures.
- Recognize that surgery increases a patients risk for skin injury because of the time the patient is immobile for the procedure (Spruce, 2017).

Prevention of Pressure Injuries

- Complete a preoperative assessment to identify patient factors that will increase a patient's risk for pressure injuries. This includes physical alterations that may require additional precautions for procedure-specific positioning and to identify specific procedural positioning needs, type of anesthesia, and so on.

- Identify procedure risk factors such as length and type of surgery, potential for intraoperative hypotensive episodes, low core temperatures, and decreased mobility on postoperative day 1.
- Recognize that all surgical clients should be considered at high risk for adult pressure injury development, because pressure ulcers can develop in as little as 20 minutes in the operating room.
- Remove all patient jewelry and accessories.
- Protect the heels during surgery by elevating the heels completely.
- Use pressure-reducing devices and pressure-relieving mattresses as necessary to prevent pressure injury.
- Avoid using rolled sheets and towels as positioning devices because they tend to produce high and inconsistent pressures. Special positioning devices are available that redistribute pressure.
- Avoid covering positioning devices or placing extra blankets on top of a pressure-reducing surface.
- The nurse should demonstrate knowledge not only of the equipment but also of anatomy and the application of physiological principles to properly position the client.
- Monitor patient position and pressure being applied to the client intraoperatively by staff, equipment, and/or instruments.
- Use additional pressure-redistributing padding on all bony prominences.
- Recognize that reddened areas or areas injured by pressure should not be massaged.
- Implement measures to prevent inadvertent hypothermia.
- Many surgical clients have medical devices placed as a part of the surgical procedure. Avoid positioning the client on the medical device and perform frequent assessments of the skin under and around the device (Apold & Rydrych, 2012; NPUAP/EPUAP, 2014).

Positioning the Perioperative Client

- Ensure that linens on the operating room table are free of wrinkles.
- Lock the operating room table, cart, or bed and stabilize the mattress before transfer/positioning the client. Monitor the client while on the operating room table at all times.
- Lift rather than pull or slide the client when positioning to reduce the incidence of skin injury from shearing and/or friction.
- Ensure that appropriate numbers of personnel are present to assist in positioning the client.
- Recognize that, optimally, clients (especially those with limited range of motion/mobility) should be asked to position themselves under

the nurse's guidance before induction of anesthesia so that he or she can verify that a position of comfort has been obtained.

- Ensure that nerves are protected by positioning extremities carefully.
- Use slow and smooth movements during positioning to allow the circulatory system to readjust.
- Reassess the client after positioning and periodically during the procedure to maintain proper alignment and skin integrity.
- Frequently assess the eyes and/or monitor intraocular pressure, especially when client is in the prone, Trendelenburg, or knee-chest position.
- Position hips in proper alignment with knees flexed. Unaligned hips can cause pressure to the low back and hip joints.
- Position the arms extended on arm boards so that they do not extend beyond a 90-degree angle. The arms should be at the level of the bed and should not be allowed to hang off the bed. Do not position arms at sides unless surgically necessary.
- Protect the client's skin surfaces from injury by preventing pooling of preparative solutions, blood, irrigation, urine, and feces.
- Keep the client appropriately covered and limit traffic in the room during the procedure. Reducing unnecessary exposure provides privacy and dignity for the client during positioning and helps prevent hypothermia (Van Wicklin, 2017).
- When positioning the client prone, care should be taken to ensure the head and neck are properly positioned. In addition, 5- to 10-degree reverse Trendelenburg should be used, if possible, to reduce intraocular pressure and decrease facial edema.
- Recognize that clients positioned in the lithotomy position should be kept in this position for as short a time as possible.
- The lowest heel position should be used in the lithotomy position.
- Maintain normal body alignment.
- When applying body supports and restraint straps (safety belt), apply loosely and secure over waist or midthigh at least 2 inches above the knees, avoiding bony prominences by placing a blanket between the strap and the client.
- Assess the client's skin integrity immediately postoperatively.
- Ensure that complete, concise, accurate documentation of client assessment and use of positioning devices is in the client's medical record.

Risk for Peripheral Neurovascular Dysfunction

NANDA-I Definition

Susceptible to disruption in the circulation, sensation, and motion of an extremity, which may compromise health

Risk Factors

To be developed

Associated Condition

Burn injury; fracture; immobilization; mechanical compression; orthopedic surgery; trauma; vascular obstruction

Client Outcomes

Client Will (Specify Time Frame)

- Maintain circulation, sensation, and movement of an extremity within client's own normal limits
- Explain signs of neurovascular compromise

Nursing Interventions

- Recognize the risk factors that may result in peripheral neurovascular dysfunction.
- Assess for the early onset of compartment syndrome, and report to provider promptly. Perform neurovascular assessment as ordered or as needed based on client's condition. Use the "five Ps" of assessment as outlined in the following list.
  - Pain: Assess severity (using an appropriate pain scale), quality, radiation, and relief by medications. Pain "out of proportion" to the injury, requiring strong opiates, often described as burning, feeling deep in the muscle or structure, and elicited with passive stretching of the compartment is the most reliable sign of compartment syndrome and peripheral neurovascular dysfunction (Donaldson, Haddad & Khan, 2014).
  - Pulses: Check the pulses distal to the injury and compare with the unaffected limb. Pulselessness is a late sign of compartment syndrome (Garner et al., 2014).
  - Pallor: Check color and temperature changes below the injury site and compare with unaffected limb. Check capillary refill. A cold, pale, or bluish extremity indicates poor arterial perfusion or venous congestion. If pallor, cyanosis, mottling, or changes in temperature are present, report to provider promptly and record your assessment findings (Garner et al., 2014; Long, 2016).

P

- ❍ Paresthesia (change in sensation): Check by lightly touching the skin proximal and distal to the injury. Ask if the client has any unusual sensations such as hypersensitivity, tingling, prickling, decreased feeling, or numbness. Check nerve function (e.g., whether the client can feel a touch to the area of concern, such as the first web space of the foot [deep peroneal nerve] with tibial fracture). Paresthesia may occur as an early sign of compartment syndrome caused by ischemia of peripheral nerves (Garner et al., 2014).
- ❍ Paralysis: Ask the client to perform appropriate range-of-motion exercises in the unaffected and then the affected extremity. Loss of movement (paralysis) is a late symptom of compartment syndrome. Decreased range of motion and loss of movement can indicate impending muscle, nerve, and cellular death (Donaldson et al., 2014).
- ❍ In addition to the five Ps, assess for swelling or increase in compartment pressure by feeling the extremity; note new onset of firmness or swelling of the extremity, and a firm "wooden" feeling on deep palpation. Intercompartmental pressures may also be measured with proprietary monitoring devices. Internal pressure or external confinement or restriction can proceed to the point at which cellular exchange is diminished. Swelling and tightness of the involved compartment are indications of increased pressure. Not only are surgical or trauma clients at risk for neurovascular compromise, but they also are clients on bed rest because of changes in blood flow through the cardiovascular system (Donaldson et al., 2014).

▲ All the Ps may not be present, and they are not specific for compartment syndrome. Have a high index of suspicion for any of the Ps. Noting two or more of the Ps increases the probability of compartment syndrome. Monitor the client for compartment syndrome of the nonoperative leg and the operative leg.

• Monitor appropriate application and function of corrective device (e.g., cast, splint, traction) as needed.

• For prevention of deep vein thrombosis (DVT), nursing care of DVT, and pulmonary embolism, refer to the interventions on DVT prevention and treatment in the care plan for Ineffective peripheral **Tissue Perfusion**.

Risk for Poisoning

NANDA-I Definition

Susceptible to accidental exposure to, or ingestion of, drugs or dangerous products in sufficient doses, which may compromise health.

Risk Factors

External

Access to dangerous product; access to illicit drugs potentially contaminated by poisonous additives; access to pharmaceutical agent; occupational setting without adequate safeguards

Internal

Emotional disturbance; inadequate precautions against poisoning; insufficient knowledge of pharmacological agents; insufficient knowledge of poisoning prevention; insufficient vision

Associated Condition

Alteration in cognitive functioning

Client Outcomes

Client Will (Specify Time Frame)

- Prevent inadvertent ingestion of or exposure to toxins or poisonous substances
- Explain and undertake appropriate safety measures to prevent ingestion of or exposure to toxins or poisonous substances
- Verbalize appropriate response to apparent or suspected toxic ingestion or poisoning

P

Nursing Interventions

- • When a client comes to the hospital with possible poisoning, begin care following the airway, breathing, circulation (ABCs) and administer oxygen if needed.
- ▲ It is important for the triage nurse to call the poison control center.
- • Obtain a thorough history of what was ingested, how much, and when, and ask to look at the containers. Note the client's age, weight, medications, medical conditions, and any history of vomiting, choking, coughing, or change in mental status. Also take note of any interventions performed before seeking treatment.
- ▲ Note results of toxicology screens, arterial blood gases, blood glucose levels, and any other ordered laboratory tests.
- ▲ Initiate any ordered treatment for poisoning quickly. The poison control center will specify any treatment or medications that need to be administered.

Safety Guidelines for Medication Administration

- Prevent iatrogenic harm to the hospitalized client by following these guidelines for administering medications:
  - Use at least two methods to identify the client before administering medications or blood products, such as the client's name and medical record number or birth date. Do not use the client's room number. Use the bar code scanning system for client identification if used by your facility.
  - When taking verbal or telephone orders, the orders should be written down and read back for verification to the individual giving the order. The healthcare provider who gave the orders for the medication then needs to confirm the information that was read back.
- Standardize use of abbreviations, acronyms, symbols, and dose designations and eliminate those that are prone to cause errors. (Refer to The Joint Commission, Critical Access Hospital National Patient Safety Goals for list of abbreviations, acronyms, symbols, and dose designations that should not be used [The Joint Commission, 2014].)
  - Be aware of the medications that look/sound alike and ensure that the correct medication is ordered and administered.
  - Use the eight rights of medication administration to decrease the potential for error: right client, right medication, right reason, right dose, right frequency, right route, right site, and right time (College of Nurses of Ontario, 2014).
  - Take high-alert medications off the nursing unit, such as potassium chloride. Standardize concentrations of medications such as morphine in patient-controlled analgesia pumps.
  - Follow agency policy/procedures for medications that require a two-person check and co-signature.
  - Label all medications and medication containers or other solutions that are on or off a sterile field for a procedure. Label them when they are first taken out of the original packaging to another container. Label with medication name, strength, amount, and expiration date/time. Review the labels whenever there is a change of personnel.
  - Use only intravenous (IV) pumps that prevent free flow of IV solution when the tubing is taken out of the pump.
- Identify all the client's current medications on admission to a healthcare facility and compare the list with the current ordered

medications. Reconcile any differences in medications. Use the expertise of the pharmacy department if there is any uncertainty regarding the accuracy of the client's medications. Reconcile the list of medications if the client is transferred from one unit to another, when there is a handoff to the next provider of care, and when the client is discharged.

- Detect possible interactions and cumulative or other adverse effects among prescribed medications, self-administered over the-counter products, culturally based home treatments, herbal remedies, and foods. Medication reconciliation is an important safety issue because of the number of people taking multiple medications and involves determining what medications the person should be taking, medications they are actually taking, and resolving discrepancies (Aronson, 2017).

Pediatric

▲ Evaluate lead exposure risk and consult the healthcare provider regarding lead screening measures as indicated (public/ambulatory health).

- Provide guidance for parents and caregivers regarding age-related safety measures, including the following:
  - ❍ Store prescription and over-the-counter medications, vitamins, herbs, and alcohol in a locked cabinet far from children's reach.
  - ❍ Do not take medications in front of children (Rodgers et al., 2012).
  - ❍ Store cleaning products including things like dishwashing liquids in a high cabinet, out of children's reach.
  - ❍ Use safety latches on cabinets that contain poisonous substances.
  - ❍ Store potentially harmful substances in the original containers with safety closures intact.
  - ❍ Recognize that no container is completely childproof.
  - ❍ Do not store medications or toxic substances in food containers or near or with food products.
  - ❍ Do not leave alcoholic drinks, cosmetics, or toiletries where children can reach them.
  - ❍ Remove poisonous houseplants from the home. Teach children not to put leaves or berries in their mouths (Oerther, 2011).
  - ❍ Do not suggest that medications are candy.
  - ❍ If interrupted when using a harmful product, take it with you; children can get into it within seconds.
  - ❍ Store poisonous automotive or gardening supplies in a locked area.
  - ❍ Use extreme caution with pesticides and gardening materials close to children's play areas.

  - When visitors enter the home, place their handbags or backpacks up high where children are unable to reach them, and ask about any potential poisonous substances.
- Advise families that syrup of ipecac is no longer recommended to be kept and used in the home. Advise families that over-the-counter cough and cold suppressant medications are not recommended and are no longer considered safe for children 2 or younger (US Food and Drug Administration, 2014).
- Recognize that some children may have been exposed to methamphetamines or the components used to make methamphetamines.

Geriatric

- Caution the client and family to avoid storing medications with similar appearances close to one another (e.g., nitroglycerin ointment near toothpaste or denture creams). Remind older clients to store medications out of reach when young children come to visit. Childhood poisonings are common events that involve exposure to both prescription and nonprescription pharmaceuticals in the home, resulting in an increased number of serious outcomes (Spiller et al., 2013).
- Perform medication reconciliation in all older clients entering the healthcare system and on discharge.

Home Care

- The interventions previously described may be adapted for home care use.
- Provide the client and/or family with a poison control poster to be kept on the refrigerator or a bulletin board. Ensure that the telephone number for local poison control information is readily available and/or preprogrammed into household telephones.
- Prepour medications for a client who is at risk for ingesting too much of a given medication because of mistakes in preparation. Delegate this task to the family or caregivers if possible.
- Identify poisonous substances in the immediate surroundings of the home, such as a garage or barn, including paints and thinners, fertilizers, rodent and bug control substances, animal medications, gasoline, and oil. Label with the name, a poison warning sign, and a poison control center number. Lock out of the reach of children.
- Identify the risk of toxicity from environmental activities such as spraying trees or roadside shrubs. Contact local departments of

agriculture or transportation to obtain material safety data sheets or to prevent the activity in desired areas.

- To prevent carbon monoxide poisoning, instruct the client and family in the importance of using a carbon monoxide detector in the home and changing it every 6 months, having the home heating system serviced every year by a qualified technician, and ensuring proper installation and venting of all combustion equipment. Carbon monoxide results from fumes produced by portable generators, stoves, lanterns, gas ranges, running vehicles, or burning charcoal and wood, which can build up in enclosed or partially enclosed spaces and result in harm or death for people and animals exposed.

Multicultural

- Prompt caregivers to take action to prevent lead poisoning.
- If children live in a high-lead environment, teach the need for handwashing before each meal, annual blood testing for lead levels, and avoidance of high-lead areas.

Client/Family Teaching and Discharge Planning

- Teach parents that any substance that is absorbed by the body by a variety of means and can affect health and cause mortality is considered a poison. The increasing use of medications and home cleaning products puts children at risk for poison because of the potential for access in the home environment.

Safety Guidelines

- Counsel the client and family members regarding the following points of medication safety:
  - Avoid sharing prescriptions.
  - Always use good light when preparing medication. Do not dispense medication during the night without a light on.
  - Read the label before you open the bottle, after you remove a dose, and again before you give it.
  - Always use child-resistant caps and lock all medications away from your child or confused older adult.
  - Give the correct dose. *Never* guess.
  - Do not increase or decrease the dose without calling the healthcare provider.
  - Always follow the weight and age recommendations on the label.
  - Avoid making conversions. If the label calls for 2 teaspoons and you have a dosing cup labeled only with ounces, do not use it.

- Be sure the healthcare provider knows if you are taking more than one medication at a time.
- Never let young children take medication by themselves.
- Read and follow labeling instructions on all products; adjust dosage for age.
- Avoid excessive amounts and/or frequency of doses. ("If a little does some good, a lot should do more.")

- Data from the Nationwide Emergency Department Sample (NEDS) from 2006 to 2012 show there were 21,928 pediatric ED visits for prescription opioid poisonings. An increase in adult prescription opioid abuse contributes to unintentional ingestion of medications in children (Tadros et al., 2016).
- Advise the family to post first-aid charts and poison control center instructions in an accessible location. Poison control center telephone numbers should be posted close to each telephone and the number programmed into cell phones.
- Advise family when calling the poison control center to do the following:
  - Give as much information as possible, including your name, location, and telephone number, so that the poison control operator can call back in case you are disconnected or summon help if needed.
  - Give the name of the potential poison ingested and, if possible, the amount and time of ingestion. If the bottle or package is available, give the trade name and ingredients if they are listed.
  - Be prepared to divulge the child's height, weight, age, and medical history.
  - Describe the state of the poisoning victim. Is the victim conscious? Does he or she have any symptoms? What is the person's general appearance, skin color, respiration, breathing difficulties, mental status (alert, sleepy, unusual behavior)? Is the person vomiting? Having convulsions?
- Rapid initiation of proper treatment reduces mortality and morbidity rates. Consultation with a poison control center is necessary to assess and treat poisoned clients.
- Encourage the client and family to take first-aid and other types of safety-related programs.

▲ Initiate referrals to peer group interventions, peer counseling, and other types of substance abuse prevention/rehabilitation programs when substance abuse is identified as a risk factor.

- Teach parents and other caregivers that cough and cold medications bought over the counter are not safe for children younger than 2 unless specifically ordered by a healthcare provider. Analysis of exposures to cough/cold preparations supports the concept that poisoning exposure occurs in children with substances that they can easily access (Spilller et al., 2013).
- Teach parents that they can be a source of lead exposure for their children via contaminated work clothing from a lead-related occupation such as transportation workers or automobile repair or if they engage in certain hobbies such as stained glass or ceramics (Schnur & John, 2014). Precautions should be taken to eliminate the risk of exposure.

Post-Trauma Syndrome

NANDA-I Definition

Sustained maladaptive response to a traumatic, overwhelming event

Defining Characteristics

Aggression; alienation; alteration in concentration; alteration in mood; anger; anxiety (00146); avoidance behaviors; compulsive behavior; denial; depression; dissociative amnesia; enuresis; exaggerated startle response; fear (00148); flashbacks; gastrointestinal irritation; guilt; headache; heart palpitations; history of detachment; hopelessness (00124); horror; hypervigilance; intrusive dreams; intrusive thoughts; irritability; neurosensory irritability; nightmares; panic attacks; rage; reports feeling numb; repression; shame; substance misuse

Related Factors

Diminished ego strength; environment not conducive to needs; exaggerated sense of responsibility; insufficient social support; perceives event as traumatic; self-injurious behavior; survivor role

At-Risk Population

Destruction of one's home; displacement from home; duration of traumatic event; event outside the range of usual human experience; exposure to disaster; exposure to epidemic; exposure to event involving multiple deaths; exposure to war; history of abuse; history of being a prisoner of war; history of criminal victimization; history of torture; human service occupations; serious accident; serious injury to loved one; serious threat to loved one; serious threat to self; witnessing mutilation; witnessing violent death

Client Outcomes

Client Will (Specify Time Frame)

- Return to pretrauma level of functioning as quickly as possible
- Acknowledge traumatic event and begin to work with the trauma by talking about the experience and expressing feelings of fear, anger, anxiety, guilt, and helplessness
- Identify support systems and available resources and be able to connect with them
- Return to and strengthen coping mechanisms used in previous traumatic event
- Acknowledge event and perceive it without distortions
- Assimilate event and move forward to set and pursue life goals

Nursing Interventions

- Observe for a reaction to a traumatic event in all clients regardless of age or sex.
- After a traumatic event, assess for intrusive memories, avoidance and numbing, and hyperarousal.
- Remain with the client and provide support during periods of overwhelming emotions.
- Help the individual comprehend the trauma if possible.
- Use touch with the client's permission (e.g., a hand on the shoulder, holding a hand).
- Explore and enhance available support systems.
- Help the client regain previous sleeping and eating habits.

▲ Provide the client pain medication if he or she has physical pain.

▲ Assess the need for pharmacotherapy.

▲ Refer for appropriate psychotherapy: cognitive therapy, exposure therapy, eye movement desensitization and reprocessing (EMDR), and cognitive-behavioral therapy (CBT).

- Help the client use positive cognitive restructuring to reestablish feelings of self-worth.
- Provide the means for the client to express feelings through therapeutic drawing.
- Encourage the client to return to his or her normal routine as quickly as possible.
- Talk to and assess the client's social support after a traumatic event.

Pediatric

- Refer to nursing care plan Risk for **Post-Trauma** syndrome.

P

▲ Carefully assess children exposed to disasters and trauma. Note behavior specific to developmental age. Refer for therapy as needed.

Geriatric

- Carefully screen older adults for signs of PTSD, especially after a disaster.
- Consider using the Horwitz Impact of Event Scale, which is an appropriate instrument to measure the subjective response to stress in the older population.

▲ Monitor the client for clinical signs of depression and anxiety; refer to a healthcare provider for medication if appropriate.

- Instill hope.

Multicultural

- Assess the influence of cultural beliefs, norms, and values on the client's ability to cope with a traumatic experience.
- Acknowledge racial and ethnic differences at the onset of care.

▲ Carefully assess refugees for PTSD and refer for treatment as appropriate; encourage them to learn the language of their new residence.

- Use a family-centered approach when working with Latin, Asian, African American, and Native American clients.
- When working with Asian American clients, provide opportunities by which the family can save face.
- Incorporate cultural traditions as appropriate.

Home Care

▲ Assess family support and the response to the client's coping mechanisms. Refer the family for medical social services or other counseling as necessary.

- Assess the effect of the trauma on family and significant others and provide empathy and caring to them.

Client/Family Teaching and Discharge Planning

- Teach positive coping skills and avoidance of negative coping skills.
- Teach stress reduction methods such as deep breathing, visualization, meditation, and physical exercise. Encourage their use especially when intrusive thoughts or flashbacks occur.
- Encourage other healthy living habits
- Refer the client to peer support groups.
- Consider the use of complementary and alternative therapies.

P

Risk for Post-Trauma Syndrome

NANDA-I Definition

Susceptible to sustained maladaptive response to a traumatic, overwhelming event, which may compromise health

Risk Factors

Diminished ego strength; environment not conducive to needs; exaggerated sense of responsibility; insufficient social support; perceives event as traumatic; self-injurious behavior; survivor role

At-Risk Population

Destruction of one's home; displacement from home; duration of traumatic event; event outside the range of usual human experience; exposure to disaster; exposure to epidemic; exposure to event involving multiple deaths; exposure to war; history of abuse; history of being a prisoner of war; history of criminal victimization; history of torture; human service occupations; serious accident; serious injury to loved one; serious threat to loved one; serious threat to self; witnessing mutilation; witnessing violent death

Client Outcomes

Client Will (Specify Time Frame)

P

- Identify symptoms associated with post-traumatic stress disorder (PTSD) and seek help
- Acknowledge event and perceive it without distortions
- Identify support systems and available resources and be able to connect with them
- State that he/she is not to blame for the event

Nursing Interventions

- Assess for PTSD in a client who has chronic/critical illness, anxiety, or personality disorder; was a witness to severe injury or death; or experienced sexual molestation.
- Consider the use of a self-reported screening questionnaire.
- Assess for ongoing symptoms of post-traumatic stress such as dissociation, avoidance behavior, hypervigilance, and reexperiencing.
- Assess for past experiences with traumatic events.
- Consider screening for PTSD in a client who is a high user of medical care.

▲ Provide deployed combat veterans with previous history of low mental or physical health status before deployment with appropriate referral after deployment.

- Provide peer support to contact coworkers experiencing trauma to remind them that others in the organization are concerned about their welfare.

- Provide post-trauma debriefings. Effective post-trauma coping skills are taught, and each participant creates a plan for his or her recovery.
- Provide post-trauma counseling. Counseling sessions are extensions of debriefings and include continued discussion of the traumatic event and post-trauma consequences and the further development of coping skills.
- Consider exposure therapy for civilian trauma survivors after an assault or motor vehicle crash.

Things to Try: Critical Incident Stress Debriefing

- Instruct the client to use the following critical incident stress management techniques:

▲ Within the first 24 to 48 hours, engage in periods of appropriate physical exercise alternating with relaxation to alleviate some of the physical reactions; structure your time; keep busy; you are normal and are having normal reactions; do not label yourself as "crazy";
talk to people; talk is the most healing medicine;
be aware of numbing the pain with overuse of drugs or alcohol; you do not need to complicate the stress with a substance abuse problem; reach out; people do care; maintain as normal a schedule as possible; spend time with others; help your coworkers as much as possible by sharing feelings and checking out how they are doing; give yourself permission to feel rotten and share your feelings with others;
keep a journal; write your way through those sleepless hours; do things that feel good to you; realize that those around you are under stress; do not make any big life changes; do make as many daily decisions as possible to give yourself a feeling of control over your life (e.g., if someone asks you what you want to eat, answer the person even if you are not sure);
get plenty of rest; recurring thoughts, dreams, or flashbacks are normal; do not try to fight them because they will decrease over time and become less painful;
eat well-balanced and regular meals (even if you do not feel like it).

▲ Assess for a history of life-threatening illness such as cancer and provide appropriate counseling.

Pediatric

- Children with cancer should continue to be assessed for PTSD into adulthood.
- Provide protection for a child who has witnessed violence or who has had traumatic injuries. Help the child acknowledge the event and express grief over the event.

P

- • Assess for a medical history of anxiety disorders.
- ▲ Assess children of deployed parents for PTSD and provide appropriate referrals.
- • Consider implementation of a school-based program for children to decrease PTSD after catastrophic events.

Geriatric and Multicultural

- • Refer to the care plan for **Post-Trauma** syndrome.

Home Care

- ▲ Evaluate the client's response to a traumatic or critical event. If screening warrants, refer to a therapist for counseling/treatment.
- • Refer to the care plan for **Post-Trauma** syndrome.

Client/Family Teaching and Discharge Planning

- • Instruct family and friends to use the following critical incident stress management techniques:
- ▲ Listen carefully; spend time with the traumatized person; offer your assistance and a listening ear, even if the person has not asked for help; help the person with everyday tasks such as cleaning, cooking, caring for the family, and minding children; and give the person some private time. Do not take the individual's anger or other feelings personally, and do not tell the person that he or she is "lucky it wasn't worse." Such statements do not console traumatized people. Instead, tell the person that you are sorry such an event has occurred and you want to understand and assist him or her (National Interagency Fire Center, CISM Information Sheets, 2014).
- ▲ After exposure to trauma, teach the client and family to recognize symptoms of PTSD and seek treatment for "recurrent and intrusive distressing recollections of the traumatic event," insomnia, irritability, difficulty concentrating, and hypervigilance.
- • Provide education to explain that acute stress disorder symptoms may be common when preparing combatants for their role in deployment. Provide referrals if the symptoms persist.

Readiness for Enhanced Power

NANDA-I Definition

A pattern of participating knowingly in change for well-being, which can be strengthened.

Defining Characteristics

Expresses desire to enhance awareness of possible changes; expresses desire to enhance identification of choices that can be made for change; expresses desire to enhance independence with actions for change; expresses desire to enhance involvement in change; expresses desire to enhance knowledge for participation in change; expresses desire to enhance participation in choices for daily living; expresses desire to enhance participation in choices for health; expresses desire to enhance power

Client Outcomes

Client Will (Specify Time Frame)

- Describe power resources
- Identify realistic perceptions of control
- Develop a plan of action based on power resources
- Seek assistance as needed

Nursing Interventions

- Assess the meaning of the event to the person.
- Collaborate with and encourage the person to identify resources to put a plan into action.
- Provide support for client families to identify the balance between client care responsibilities and self-care.
- Initiate and facilitate family health conversations between the client and their family.
- Identify the client's health literacy and provide access to information.
- Help client mobilize social supports, which is a power resource.
- Refer client to an empowerment support group.

Pediatric

- Provide empowerment-based education for parents that includes a focus on caregiving knowledge, caring behaviors, self-efficacy, and indicators of the child's recovery.
- Initiate problem-solving opportunities, empowering discussions, and reflection to help families take action to manage their child's illness.

Geriatric

- Provide health education for older individuals that is tailored, interactive, structured, continuous, and incorporates motivational and encouragement techniques.

Multicultural

In addition to the preceding interventions as appropriate:

- Assess for the influence of communication patterns, cultural differences in medical consultations, and client perceptions of inequalities in care quality as contributors to client feelings of powerlessness.
- Provide support and educational interventions that are culturally tailored.

Home Care

- The preceding interventions may be adapted for home care use.

P

Powerlessness

NANDA-I Definition

A state of actual or perceived loss of control or influence over factors or events that affect one's well-being, personal life, or the society (adapted from American Psychology Association)

Defining Characteristics

Delayed recovery; depressive symptoms; expresses doubt about role performance; expresses frustration about inability to perform previous activities; expresses lack of purpose in life; expresses shame; fatigue; loss of independence; reports inadequate sense of control; social alienation

Related Factors

Anxiety; caregiver role strain; dysfunctional institutional environment; impaired physical mobility; inadequate interest in improving one's situation; inadequate interpersonal relations; inadequate knowledge to manage a situation; inadequate motivation to improve one's situation; inadequate participation in treatment regimen; inadequate social support; ineffective coping strategies; low self-esteem; pain; perceived complexity of treatment regimen; perceived social stigma; social marginalization

At-Risk Population

Economically disadvantaged individuals; individuals exposed to traumatic events

Associated Condition

Cerebrovascular Disorders; cognition disorders; critical illness; progressive illness; unpredictability of illness trajectory

Client Outcomes

Client Will (Specify Time Frame)

- State feelings of powerlessness and other feelings related to powerlessness (e.g., anger, sadness, hopelessness)
- Identify factors that are uncontrollable
- Participate in planning and implementing care; make decisions regarding care and treatment when possible
- Ask questions about care and treatment
- Verbalize hope for the future and sense of participation in planning and implementing care

Nursing Interventions

Note: Before implementation of interventions in the face of client powerlessness, nurses should examine their own philosophies of care to ensure that control issues or lack of faith in client capabilities will not bias the ability to intervene sincerely and effectively.

- Assess powerlessness with tools that are available for general and specific client groups:
  - Measure of Powerlessness for Adult Patients (De Almeida & Braga, 2006)
  - Personal Progress Scale–Revised, tested with women (Johnson, Worell, & Chandler, 2005)
  - Life Situation Questionnaire–Powerlessness subscale, tested with stroke caregivers (Larson et al., 2005)
  - Making Decisions Scale, tested in clients with mental illness (Hansson & Bjorkman, 2005)
  - Family Empowerment Scale, tested on parents of children with emotional disorders (Koren, DeChillo, & Friesen, 1992)
- Observe for factors contributing to powerlessness (e.g., immobility, hospitalization, unfavorable prognosis, lack of support system, misinformation about situation, inflexible routine, chronic illness, addiction, history of trauma, gender). Help clients channel their behaviors in an effective manner.
- Engage with clients using respectful listening and questioning to develop an awareness of clients' most important concerns.
- Provide support for client families to identify the balance between client care responsibilities and self-care.
- Use a rehabilitative behavioral learning model that assists clients to understand how the mechanisms of habit and ritual work to reinforce powerlessness in their lives.
- Refer client to an empowerment support group.
- Refer to the care plans for **Hopelessness** and **Spiritual** distress.

Pediatric

- Provided empowerment-based educational preparation for parents that includes a focus on caregiving knowledge, caring behaviors, self-efficacy, and indicators of the child's recovery.
- Initiate problem-solving opportunities, empowering discussions, and reflection to help families take action to manage their child's illness.
- Provide nursing care that shifts the focus from the illness to the child.

Geriatric

- In addition to the preceding interventions, as appropriate:
- Initiate and facilitate family health conversations between the older client and their family.

- Provide health education for older individuals that is tailored, interactive, structured, continuous, and incorporates motivational and encouragement techniques.

Multicultural

- In addition to the preceding interventions, as appropriate:
- Assess for the influence of communication patterns, cultural differences in medical consultations, and client perceptions of inequalities in care quality as contributors to client feelings of powerlessness.
- Provide support and educational interventions that are culturally tailored.

Home Care

- In addition to the preceding interventions, as appropriate:
  - Assess for denial in clients with cancer and provide support for caregivers.

Client/Family Teaching and Discharge Planning

- The preceding interventions may be adapted for home care use.

P

Risk for Powerlessness

NANDA-I Definition

Susceptible to a state of actual or perceived loss of control or influence over factors or events that affect one's well-being, personal life, or the society, which may compromise health (adapted from American Psychology Association).

Risk Factors

Anxiety; caregiver role strain; dysfunctional institutional environment; impaired physical mobility; inadequate interest in improving one's situation; inadequate interpersonal relations; inadequate knowledge to manage a situation; inadequate motivation to improve one's situation; inadequate participation in treatment regimen; inadequate social support; ineffective coping strategies; low self-esteem; pain; perceived complexity of treatment regimen; perceived social stigma; social marginalization

At-Risk Population

Economically disadvantaged individuals; individuals exposed to traumatic events

Associated Conditions

Cerebrovascular disorders; cognition disorders; critical illness; progressive illness; unpredictability of illness trajectory

Client Outcomes, Nursing Interventions, Client/Family Teaching and Discharge Planning

See the care plan for **Powerlessness**

Risk for Adult Pressure Injury

NANDA-I Definition

Adult susceptible to localized damage to the skin and/or underlying tissue, as a result of pressure, or pressure in combination with shear, which may compromise health (European Pressure Ulcer Advisory Panel, 2019).

Risk Factors

External Factors

Altered microclimate between skin and supporting surface; excessive moisture; inadequate access to appropriate equipment; inadequate access to appropriate health services; inadequate availability of equipment for individuals with obesity; inadequate caregiver knowledge of pressure injury prevention strategies; increased magnitude of mechanical; load; pressure over bony prominence; shearing forces; surface friction; sustained mechanical load; use of linen with insufficient moisture wicking property

Internal Factors

Decreased physical activity; decreased physical mobility; dehydration; dry skin; hyperthermia; inadequate adherence to incontinence treatment regimen; inadequate adherence to pressure injury prevention plan; inadequate knowledge of pressure injury prevention strategies; protein-energy malnutrition; smoking; substance misuse

Other Factors

Factors identified by standardized, validated screening tool

At-Risk Population

Individuals in aged care settings; individuals in intensive care units; individuals in palliative care settings; individuals in rehabilitation settings; individuals in transit to or between clinical care settings; individuals receiving home-based care; individuals with American Society of Anesthesiologists (ASA) Physical health status score ≥3; individuals with body mass index above normal range for age and gender; individuals with body mass index below normal range for age and gender; individuals with history of pressure injury; individuals with physical disability; older adults

Associated Conditions

Anemia; cardiovascular diseases; chronic neurological conditions; critical illness; decreased serum albumin level; decreased tissue oxygenation; decreased tissue perfusion; diabetes mellitus; edema; elevated C-reactive protein; hemodynamic instability; hip fracture; immobilization; impaired circulation; intellectual disability; medical devices; peripheral neuropathy; pharmaceutical preparations; physical trauma; prolonged duration of surgical procedure; sensation disorders; spinal cord injuries

Client Outcomes

Client Will (Specify Time Frame)

- Report any altered sensation or pain at site of tissue impairment
- Skin, without redness over bony prominences and capillary refill of less than 6 seconds over areas of redness
- Be repositioned off of bony prominences frequently if risk for pressure injuries is high (e.g., Braden scale score ≤ 18)
- Demonstrate understanding of plan to reduce pressure injury risk
- Describe measures to protect the skin

Nursing Interventions

▲ NPUAP redefined the definition of a pressure ulcer, which is now referred to as pressure injuries, during the NPUAP 2016 Staging Consensus Conference in 2016. The new definitions more accurately define alterations in tissue integrity from pressure. Classify pressure injuries (NPUAP, 2016) using national guidelines and definitions (see http://www.npuap.org/resources/educational-and-clinical-resources/npuap-pressure-injury-stages/).

- **Pressure Injury:** A pressure injury is localized damage to the skin and underlying soft tissue usually over a bony prominence or related to a medical or other device. The injury can present as intact skin or an open ulcer and may be painful. The injury occurs as a result of intense and/or prolonged pressure or pressure in combination with shear. The tolerance of soft tissue for pressure and shear may also be affected by microclimate, nutrition, perfusion, comorbidities, and condition of the soft tissue (NPUAP, 2016).
  - **Stage 1 Pressure Injury:** Nonblanchable erythema of intact skin Area of localized nonbleachable erythema that may appear differently in darkly pigmented skin, and changes in sensation, temperature, or firmness may precede visual changes. Color changes do not include purple or maroon discoloration which, is more likely to indicate deep tissue pressure injury (NPUAP, 2016).
  - **Stage 2 Pressure Injury:** Partial-thickness skin loss with exposed dermis
    Partial-thickness skin loss with exposed dermis in which the wound bed is pink/red and moist and adipose (fat) and deeper tissues are not visible. Granulation tissue, slough, and eschar are not present. A stage 2 pressure injury may also present as an intact or ruptured blister. These injuries commonly result from adverse microclimate and shear in the skin over the pelvis and shear in the heel. This stage should not be used to describe moisture-associated

skin damage (MASD) including incontinence-associated dermatitis (IAD), intertriginous dermatitis (ITD), medical adhesive–related skin injury (MARSI), or traumatic wounds (skin tears, burns, and abrasions) (NPUAP 2016).

- **Stage 3 Pressure Injury:** Full-thickness skin loss
  Full-thickness loss of skin, in which adipose is visible and granulation tissue and epibole (rolled wound edges) are often present and undermining/tunneling may occur. Slough and/or eschar may also be visible. Fascia, muscle, tendon, ligament, cartilage, and/or bone are not exposed. The depth of tissue damage varies by anatomical location, and areas of significant adiposity can develop deep wounds. If slough or eschar obscures the extent of tissue loss, then this is an unstageable pressure injury (NPUAP, 2016).
- **Stage 4 Pressure Injury:** Full-thickness skin and tissue loss
  Full-thickness skin and tissue loss with exposed or directly palpable fascia, muscle, tendon, ligament, cartilage or bone, and slough and/or eschar may be visible. Epibole, undermining, and/or tunneling often occur, and depth varies by anatomical location. If slough or eschar obscures the extent of tissue loss, then this is an unstageable pressure injury (NPUAP, 2016).
- **Deep Tissue Pressure Injury:** Persistent nonblanchable deep red, maroon, or purple discoloration
  Intact or nonintact skin with localized area of persistent nonblanchable deep red, maroon, or purple discoloration or epidermal separation revealing a dark wound bed or blood-filled blister. Pain and temperature change often precedes skin color changes. Discoloration may appear differently in darkly pigmented skin. This injury results from intense and/or prolonged pressure and shear forces at the bone–muscle interface. The wound may evolve rapidly to reveal the actual extent of tissue injury, or it may resolve without tissue loss. If necrotic tissue, subcutaneous tissue, granulation tissue, fascia, muscle, or other underlying structures are visible, then this indicates a full-thickness pressure injury (unstageable, stage 3, or stage 4). Do not use deep tissue pressure injury to describe vascular, traumatic, neuropathic, or dermatological conditions (NPUAP, 2016).
- **Unstageable Pressure Injury:** Obscured full-thickness skin and tissue loss
  Full-thickness skin and tissue loss in which the extent of tissue damage within the ulcer cannot be confirmed because it is obscured

by slough or eschar. If slough or eschar is removed, a stage 3 or stage 4 pressure injury will be revealed. Stable eschar (i.e., dry, adherent, intact without erythema or fluctuance) on the heel or ischemic limb should not be softened or removed (NPUAP, 2016).

- Routinely assess clients for risk of pressure injuries using a valid and reliable risk assessment tool (NPUAP/European Pressure Ulcer Advisory Panel [EPUAP], 2014). A validated risk assessment tool such as the Norton scale or Braden scale should be used to identify clients at risk for pressure-related skin breakdown (NPUAP/EPUAP, 2014).
- Pressure injury risk assessment should be completed on admission, daily, and after procedures or changes in the client's condition (NPUAP/EPUAP, 2014; Baranoski & Ayello, 2016).
- Inspect the skin daily, especially bony prominences and dependent areas, for pallor, redness, and breakdown. In addition to assessing pressure injury risk, client-specific interventions should be implemented to prevent tissue injury. Implement the following interventions to prevent tissue breakdown:
  - Turn and reposition all individuals at risk for pressure injury, unless contraindicated because of medical condition or medical treatments.
  - Position client properly; use pressure-reducing or pressure-relieving devices (e.g., pillows, gel or foam cushions, alternating pressure mattress, air-fluidized bed, kinetic bed) if indicated. Continue to turn and reposition the individual regardless of the support surface in use. Establish turning frequency based on the characteristics of the support surface and the individual's response (NPUAP/EPUAP, 2014).
  - Lift and move client carefully using a turn sheet and adequate assistance; keep bed linens dry and wrinkle-free.
  - Perform actions to keep client from sliding down in bed (e.g., bend knees slightly when head of bed is elevated 30 degrees or higher) to reduce the risk of skin surface abrasion and shearing. Use the 30-degree tilted side-lying position (alternately, right side, back, left side) or the prone position if the individual can tolerate this and his or her medical condition allows (NPUAP/EPUAP, 2014).
  - Select a seated posture that is acceptable for the individual and minimizes the pressures and shear exerted on the skin and soft tissues (NPUAP/EPUAP, 2014).
  - Keep client's skin clean. Thoroughly dry skin after bathing and as often as needed, paying special attention to skinfolds and

opposing skin surfaces (e.g., axillae, perineum, beneath breasts). Pat skin dry rather than rub, and use a mild soap for bathing. Apply moisturizing lotion at least once a day.
- ❍ Protect the skin from contact with urine and feces (e.g., keep perineal area clean and dry, apply a protective ointment or cream to perineal area).
- ❍ Provide and encourage adequate daily fluid intake for hydration for an individual assessed to be at risk of or with a pressure injury (NPUAP, 2016). This must be consistent with the individual's comorbid conditions and goals (NPUAP/EPUAP, 2014).
- ❍ If the individual cannot be moved or is positioned with the head of the bed elevated over 30 degrees, then place a polyurethane foam dressing on the sacrum (NPUAP, 2016). Use heel offloading device or polyurethane foam dressings on individuals at high risk for heel ulcers (NPUAP, 2016).
- ❍ Consult with nutrition/dietary specialist to evaluate client's nutritional status.
- ❍ Increase activity as allowed.

• Medical device–related pressure injuries (MDRPIs) result from the use of devices designed and applied for diagnostic or therapeutic purposes. The resultant pressure injury generally conforms to the pattern or shape of the device. The injury should be staged using the NPUAP pressure injury staging system and the etiology of the pressure injury noted to be caused by the device (NPUAP, 2016).
- ❍ The head/face/neck, heel/ankle/foot, coccyx/buttocks, abdomen, and extremities are common body regions for MDRPI.
- ❍ Common devices associated with pressure-related tissue injury include oxygen delivery and monitoring devices (e.g., face mask, nasal cannula, pulse oximetry, bilevel positive airway pressure [BiPAP] mask), feeding tubes (e.g., nasogastric, gastric, jejunal tubes), endotracheal devices (oral and/or nasal endotracheal tubes, tracheostomy tubes), urinary and bowel elimination equipment (indwelling urinary catheter, fecal containment catheter), and musculoskeletal appliances (cervical collar, splints, braces).
- ❍ Assess and evaluate the purpose and function of the medical device.
- ❍ Assess proper fit of the medical device and securement to prevent rubbing, torque, or pulling on the device and skin.
- ❍ Protect the skin below and around the device to reduce pressure.

- If tissue breakdown occurs, notify a healthcare provider or wound care specialist. See care plan for Impaired **Skin** integrity for additional interventions if a pressure ulcer occurs.

Pediatric

- Perform an age-appropriate pressure injury (NPUAP, 2016) risk assessment using a valid and reliable tool.
- Implement a comprehensive plan to reduce the client's risk of skin breakdown from pressure. Assessment should include the following:
  - Client independent activity and mobility levels
  - Body mass index and/or birth weight; lower weight may increase client risk of pressure-associated skin breakdown
  - Skin maturity
  - Adequate nutritional and hydration status
  - Perfusion and oxygenation
  - Presence of external devices
  - Duration of hospital stay
- Select an age-appropriate support surface for premature neonates and pediatric clients at high risk for pressure injuries.

P

- Document risk assessment and interventions implemented to reduce the client's risk for pressure injury (NPUAP, 2016) development.

Geriatric

- Consider the older client's cognitive status when assessing the skin and in developing a comprehensive plan of care to prevent pressure injuries (NPUAP/EPUAP, 2014; NPUAP, 2016).
- Aging skin, medications (e.g., steroids), and moisture place the older client at increased risk for pressure-associated skin breakdown.
- For older clients with continence concerns, develop and implement an individualized continence management program (NPUAP/EPUAP, 2014).

Home Care

- The interventions described previously may be adapted for home care use.
- Instruct and assist the client and caregivers in how to assess the skin for excessive pressure. Provide written instructions for actions they can implement to reduce the risk of pressure injury (NPUAP, 2016) development.
- Educate client and caregivers on proper nutrition and when to call the agency and/or healthcare provider with concerns.

▲ It may be beneficial to initiate a consultation in a case assignment with a wound, ostomy, continence nurse (or wounds specialist) to establish a comprehensive plan for pressure ulcer risk reduction for clients at high risk for skin breakdown.

Ineffective Protection

NANDA-I Definition

Decrease in the ability to guard self from internal or external threats such as illness or injury

Defining Characteristics

Altered sweating anorexia; chilling; coughing; disorientation; dyspnea; expresses itching; fatigue; impaired physical mobility; impaired tissue healing; insomnia; leukopenia; low serum hemoglobin; maladaptive stress response; neurosensory impairment; pressure injury; psychomotor agitation; thrombocytopenia; weakness

Related Factors

Depressive symptoms; difficulty managing complex treatment regimen; hopelessness; inadequate vaccination; ineffective health self-management; low self-efficacy; malnutrition; physical deconditioning; substance misuse

P

At-Risk Population

Extremes of age

Associated Condition

Blood coagulation disorders; immune system diseases; neoplasms; pharmaceutical preparations; treatment regimen

Client Outcomes

Client Will (Specify Time Frame)

- Remain free of infection while in contact during contact with healthcare
- Remain free of any evidence of new bleeding as evident by stable vital signs
- Explain precautions to take to prevent infection including hand hygiene
- Explain precautions to take to prevent bleeding including fall prevention

Nursing Interventions

- • Take temperature, pulse, and blood pressure (e.g., every 1–4 hours).
- ▲ Observe nutritional status (e.g., weight, serum protein and albumin levels, muscle mass, and usual food intake). Work with the dietitian to improve nutritional status if needed.
- • Observe the client's sleep pattern; if altered, see Nursing Interventions and *Rationales* for Disturbed **Sleep** pattern.
- • Identify stressors in the client's life. If stress is uncontrollable, see Nursing Interventions and *Rationales* for Ineffective **Coping**.

Prevention of Infection

- ▲ Monitor for and report any signs of infection (e.g., fever, chills, flushed skin, drainage, edema, redness, abnormal laboratory values, pain) and notify the healthcare provider promptly.
- • If white blood cell count is severely decreased (i.e., absolute neutrophil count of less than 1000/mm^3), initiate the following precautions:
  - ❍ Take vital signs every 2 to 4 hours.
  - ❍ Complete a head-to-toe assessment twice daily, including inspection of oral mucosa, invasive sites, wounds, urine, and stool; monitor for onset of new reports of pain.
- ▲ Avoid any invasive procedures, including catheterization, injections, or rectal or vaginal procedures unless absolutely necessary.
  - ❍ Consider warming the client before elective surgery. Normothermia is associated with low postoperative infection rates (Moucha, 2016).
- ▲ Administer granulocyte growth factor as ordered.
  - ❍ Take meticulous care of all invasive sites; use chlorhexidine gluconate for cleansing.
  - ❍ Provide frequent oral care.
  - ❍ Follow Standard Precautions, especially performing hand hygiene to prevent healthcare–associated infections.
- ▲ Refer for appropriate prophylactic antifungal treatment and avoid pathogen exposure (through air filtration, regular hand hygiene, and avoidance of plants and flowers).
  - ❍ Have the client wear a mask when leaving the room.
  - ❍ Help the client bathe daily.
  - ❍ Practice food safety; a neutropenic diet may not be necessary.
  - ❍ Ensure that the client is well nourished. Provide food with protein, and consider vitamin supplements. If appetite is suppressed, institute a dietary referral. Keep track of serum albumin levels and transferrin and prealbumin levels.
  - ❍ Help the client cough and practice deep breathing regularly. Maintain an appropriate activity level.
  - ❍ Obtain a private room for the client. Use high-energy particulate air filters if available and appropriate. Protective isolation is not recommended. Recognize that cotton cover gowns may not be effective in decreasing infection.
- ▲ Watch for signs of sepsis, including change in mental status, fever, shaking, chills, and hypotension. If present, notify the healthcare provider promptly.

P

- Refer to care plan for Risk for **Infection**.
- Refer to care plan for Readiness for enhanced **Nutrition** for additional interventions.

Pediatric

- Suggest kangaroo care (KC), frequent and exclusive or nearly exclusive breastfeeding, and early discharge from hospital for low-birth-weight infants.
- Assess postoperative fever in pediatric oncology clients promptly.
- For hand hygiene with low-birth-weight infants, use alcohol hand rub and gloves.

Geriatric

▲ If not contraindicated, promote exercise to promote improved quality of life in older adults.

- Refer to the care plan for Risk for **Infection** for more interventions related to the prevention of infection.

Prevention of Bleeding

▲ Monitor the client's risk for bleeding; evaluate results of clotting studies and platelet counts.

- Watch for hematuria, melena, hematemesis, hemoptysis, epistaxis, bleeding from mucosa, petechiae, and ecchymoses.

▲ Give medications orally or intravenously only; avoid giving intramuscularly, subcutaneously, or rectally.

- Apply pressure for a longer time than usual to invasive sites, such as venipuncture or injection sites.
- Take vital signs often; watch for changes associated with fluid volume loss. Excessive bleeding causes decreased blood pressure and increased pulse and respiratory rates (Ackley & Ladwig, 2014).
- Monitor menstrual flow if relevant; have the client use pads instead of tampons.
- Have the client use a moistened toothette or a very soft child's toothbrush instead of an adult toothbrush. Follow the dentist's recommendation for flossing and appropriate rinses to use. Control gum bleeding by applying pressure to gums with gauze pad soaked in ice water.
- Ask the client either to not shave or to use only an electric razor.

▲ To decrease risk of bleeding, avoid administering salicylates or nonsteroidal antiinflammatory drugs (NSAIDs) if possible.

Home Care

- Some of the interventions previously described may be adapted for home care use.

P

- ▲ Consider using a nurse-led patient-centered medical home (PCMH) for monitoring anticoagulant therapy.
- • For terminally ill clients, teach and institute all of the previously mentioned noninvasive precautions that maintain quality of life. Discuss with the client, family, and healthcare provider the consequences of contracting infection. Determine which precautions do not maintain quality of life and should not be used (e.g., physical assessment twice daily or multiple vital sign assessments).

Client/Family Teaching and Discharge Planning

- • Depressed immune function
  - ❍ Teach the client and family how to take a temperature. Encourage the family to take the client's temperature between 3 and 7 p.m. at least once daily. Teach precautions to use to decrease the chance of infection (e.g., avoiding uncooked fruits and vegetables, using appropriate self-care including good hand hygiene, ensuring a safe environment). Teach the client to avoid crowds and contact with persons who have infections. Teach the need for good nutrition, avoidance of stress, and adequate rest to maintain immune system function.
- • Bleeding disorder
  - ❍ Teach the client to wear a medical alert bracelet and notify all healthcare personnel of his or her bleeding disorder. Teach the client and family the signs of bleeding, precautions to take to prevent bleeding, and action to take if bleeding begins. Caution the client to avoid taking over-the-counter medications without the permission of the healthcare provider.
  - ❍ Teach the client to wear loose-fitting clothes and avoid physical activity that might cause trauma.

R

Rape-Trauma Syndrome

NANDA-I Definition

Sustained maladaptive response to a forced, violent sexual penetration against the victim's will and consent

Defining Characteristics

Aggression; agitation; alteration in sleep pattern; anger; anxiety (00146); change in relationship(s); confusion; denial; dependency; depression; disorganization; dissociative identity disorder; embarrassment; fear (00148); guilt; helplessness; history of suicide attempt; humiliation; hyperalertness; impaired decision-making; low self-esteem; mood swings; muscle spasm;

muscle tension; nightmares; paranoia; perceived vulnerability; phobias; physical trauma; powerlessness (00125); self-blame; sexual dysfunction (00059); shame; shock; substance misuse; thoughts of revenge

Related Factors

To be developed

At-Risk Population

Rape

Client Outcomes

Client Will (Specify Time Frame)

- Share feelings, concerns, and fears
- Recognize that the rape or attempt was not client's own fault
- State that, no matter what the situation, no one has the right to assault another
- Describe medical/legal treatment procedures and reasons for treatment
- Report absence of physical complications or pain
- Identify support resources and attend psychotherapy/group assistance in coping with the trauma and effects of the traumatic experience
- Function at same level as before crisis, including sexual functioning
- Recognize that it is normal for full recovery to take a minimum of 1 year

Nursing Interventions

- Escort the client to a treatment room immediately on arrival to the emergency department. Stay with (or have a trusted person stay with) the client.
- Assure the client of confidentiality.
- ▲ Provide a sexual assault response team (SART), if available, that includes a sexual assault nurse examiner (SANE), rape counseling advocate, and representative of law enforcement for best possible outcomes.
- Observe for signs of physical injury.
- Document the client's chief complaint and request an event history of the sexual assault in his or her own words.
- Encourage the client to verbalize his or her feelings.
- Make sure that the victim understands everything you are doing.
- Explain to the client that all or some of the client's clothing may be kept for evidential purposes and photographs may be taken (with consent) to document the client's injuries.
- ▲ If a law enforcement interview is permitted, provide support by staying with the client at his or her request.
- Use the sexual assault evidence collection kits that have been reviewed by the SART members and provided by your state to collect adequate and accurate evidence for analysis by a forensic laboratory.

R

- ▲ Discuss the possibility of pregnancy and sexually transmitted infections (STIs) and the treatments available.
- ▲ Encourage the client to report the sexual assault to a law enforcement agency.
- ▲ For those interested in a spiritual connection, make the appropriate recommendation.
- ▲ Stress the necessity of follow-up care with a mental health professional to recognize and intervene with problems associated with the effects of rape-trauma/sexual assault.
- • Stress the importance of awareness throughout the community of the scope and severity of the effects of sexual abuse as a means of additional healing empowerment.

Geriatric

- • Build a trusting relationship with the client.
- • All examinations should be done on older adults as they would be done on any adult client after sexual assault, with modifications for comfort if necessary.
- • Assess for mobility limitations and cognitive impairment.
- • Explain and encourage the client to report sexual abuse.
- • Observe for psychosocial distress.
- ▲ Consider arrangements for safe housing victim of abuse.

Multicultural

- ▲ Assess for the influence of cultural beliefs, norms, and values on the client's ability to cope with the trauma of the rape experience.

Home Care

- • Some of the interventions described previously may be adapted for home care use.
- • Corroborate the client's feelings of self-worth. Post-traumatic disorders were the most common consequences in women victims of violence.
- • Assist the client with realistically assessing the home setting for safety and/or selecting a safe environment in which to live.
- ▲ Ensure that the client has systems in place for long-term support.
- ▲ Design a practical discharge plan to include a safe shelter if needed, follow-up care for physical injury, and follow-up referral for psychological support.
- ▲ Assess for other client vulnerabilities, such as mental health issues or addiction, and refer the client to social agencies for implementation of a therapeutic regimen.

Client/Family Teaching and Discharge Planning

- Emphasize the client's needs for safety and to decrease the opportunities for repeat attacks. Recognize the vulnerability of the client.
- Note: PTSD has a high probability of being a psychological sequela to rape. Research demonstrated two effective treatments for the improvement of PTSD in rape victims: prolonged exposure and stress inoculation training. Prolonged exposure involves reliving the rape experience by imagining it as vividly as possible, describing it aloud in the present tense, taping this description and listening to the tape at least once daily. Stress inoculation training uses breathing exercises to diminish anxiety and instruction in coping skills, thought stopping, cognitive restructuring, self-dialog, and role playing. Research suggests that a combination of both treatments may provide the optimal effect. Furthermore, for those who reported the assault to police, lower levels of legal system success and satisfaction were linked to higher levels of perceived control over present recovery.

Ineffective Relationship

NANDA-I Definition

A pattern of mutual partnership that is insufficient to provide for each other's needs

Defining Characteristics

Delay in meeting of developmental goals appropriate for family life cycle stage; dissatisfaction with complementary relationship between partners; dissatisfaction with emotional need fulfillment between partners; dissatisfaction with idea sharing between partners; dissatisfaction with information sharing between partners; dissatisfaction with physical need fulfillment between partners; inadequate understanding of partner's compromised functioning; insufficient balance in autonomy between partners; insufficient balance in collaboration between partners; insufficient mutual respect between partners; insufficient mutual support in daily activities between partners; partner not identified as support person; unsatisfying communication with partner

Related Factors

Ineffective communication skills; stressors; substance misuse; unrealistic expectations

At-Risk Population

Developmental crisis; history of domestic violence; incarceration of one partner

Associated Condition

Alteration in cognitive functioning in one partner

Client Outcomes, Nursing Interventions, Client/Family Teaching and Discharge Planning

Refer to care plan Readiness for enhanced **Relationship**

Readiness for Enhanced Relationship

NANDA-I Definition

A pattern of mutual partnership to provide for each other's needs, which can be strengthened

Defining Characteristics

Expresses desire to enhance autonomy between partners; expresses desire to enhance collaboration between partners; expresses desire to enhance communication between partners; expresses desire to enhance emotional need fulfillment for each partner; expresses desire to enhance mutual respect between partners; expresses desire to enhance satisfaction with complementary relationship between partners; expresses desire to enhance satisfaction with emotional need fulfillment for each partner; expresses desire to enhance satisfaction with idea sharing between partners; expresses desire to enhance satisfaction with information sharing between partners; expresses desire to enhance satisfaction with physical need fulfillment for each partner; expresses desire to enhance understanding of partner's functional deficit

Client Outcomes

Family/Client Will (Specify Time Frame)

- Share thoughts and feelings with each other
- Communicate openly with each other
- Assist in performing family roles and tasks
- Provide support for each other
- Obtain appropriate assistance

Nursing Interventions

- Assess the ways in which the relationship has been altered (communication, sexuality, intimacy, etc.) from both partner's perspective.

- Assess relationship quality using the Relationship Flourishing Scale.
- Focus on helping couples maintain or develop marital closeness.
- Assist couples to identify sources of their own perceived *dyadic* empathy in the relationship.
- Assist families to identify sources of gratitude in their lives.
- Assist clients to identify sources of gratitude in their lives using a future-oriented focus.
- Encourage couples to engage in reappraisal of conflict in their relationship.
- Encourage the use of positive relational humor and humor evaluation between partners.
- Provide support resources to provide military members and their families with assistance in preparation for deployments and education about the importance of maintaining communication during deployment.
- Encourage couples to participate together in leisure activities like dance.
- Refer to care plans Readiness for enhanced **Family** processes and Readiness for enhanced family **Coping.**

Pediatric

- Encourage guidance and information on communication for parents of seriously ill children.

Geriatric

- Assess geriatric spousal caregivers for positive and negative consequences of providing medical care.
- Assess sexuality needs and support consensual sexual expression.
- Facilitate and increase opportunities for social connectedness for older individuals through the use of technology training.

Multicultural

- Provide a relationship-focused intervention to enhance communication for multicultural couples.
- Use culturally tailored cognitive behavioral techniques to promote communication, problem-solving, self-disclosure, empathic response skills, and sexual education and counseling.

Risk for Ineffective Relationship

NANDA-I Definition

Susceptible to developing a pattern that is insufficient for providing a mutual partnership to provide for each other's needs

Risk Factors

Ineffective communications skills; stressors; substance misuse; unrealistic expectations

At-Risk Population

Developmental crisis; history of domestic violence; incarceration of one partner

Associated Condition

Alteration in cognitive functioning in one partner

Client Outcomes, Nursing Interventions

Refer to care plan for Ineffective **Relationship**

Impaired Religiosity

NANDA-I Definition

Impaired ability to exercise reliance on beliefs and/or participate in rituals of a particular faith tradition.

Defining Characteristics

Desire to reconnect with previous belief pattern; desire to reconnect with previous customs; difficulty adhering to prescribed religious beliefs; difficulty adhering to prescribed religious rituals; distress about separation from faith community; questioning of religious belief patterns; questioning of religious customs

Related Factors

Anxiety; cultural barrier to practicing religion; depression; environmental barrier to practicing religion; fear of death; ineffective caregiving; ineffective coping strategies; insecurity; insufficient social support; insufficient socio-cultural interaction; insufficient transportation; pain; spiritual distress

At-Risk Population

Aging; end-stage life crisis; history of religious manipulation; hospitalization; life transition; personal crisis; spiritual crisis

Associated Condition

Illness

Client Outcomes

Client Will (Specify Time Frame)

- Express satisfaction with the ability to express religious practices
- Express satisfaction with access to religious materials and rituals
- Demonstrate balance between religious practices and healthy lifestyles
- Avoid high-risk, controlling religious relationships that inflict physical, sexual, or emotional harm and/or exploitation

Nursing Interventions

- Recognize when clients integrate religious practices in their life.
- Encourage and/or coordinate the use of and participation in usual religious rituals or practices that support coping.
- Encourage the use of prayer or meditation as appropriate.
- Promote family coping using religious practices to help cope with loss, as appropriate.
- ▲ Refer to a religious leader, professional counseling, or support group as needed.

Geriatric

- Promote established religious practices in older adults.

Multicultural

- Promote religious practices that are culturally appropriate:
  - African American
  - Korean
  - African
  - Jordanian
  - Hispanic
  - Sexual Minority Individuals (Lesbian, Gay, Bisexual, Transgendered, Queer)

R

Readiness for Enhanced Religiosity

NANDA-I Definition

A pattern of reliance on religious beliefs and/or participation in rituals of a particular faith tradition, which can be strengthened

Defining Characteristics

Expresses desire to enhance belief patterns used in the past; expresses desire to enhance connection with a religious leader; expresses desire to enhance forgiveness; expresses desire to enhance participation in religious experiences; expresses desire to enhance participation in religious practices; expresses desire to enhance religious customs used in the past; expresses desire to enhance religious options; expresses desire to enhance use of religious material

Client Outcomes, Nursing Interventions, Client/Family and Discharge Planning

See care plan for Impaired **Religiosity**

Pediatric

- Provide spiritual care for children based on developmental level. Theory: When nurses are comfortable providing spiritual care, they can implement numerous spiritual care activities and interventions to meet the spiritual needs of the child and family. After determining the child's spiritual beliefs and spiritual needs, a plan of care is developed based on the child's developmental age (Fowler, 1981, 1987; Burkhart, 2016).
    - **Parents:** Incorporate religious traditions and faith practices for parents with hospitalized and chronically ill children.
    - **School-age:** Encourage faith community involvement and religious attendance with parent(s).
    - **School Age:** Encourage children to participate in faith community health programs.
    - **Adolescents:** Encourage religious coping in the adolescent population.
    - **Adolescents:** Encourage prayer, particularly within the African American community.
    - **Adults:** Encourage centering prayer or other forms of mediation to promote mental and spiritual health.
    - **Interprofessional:** Chaplain referral when individuals engage in religious coping mechanisms. **EB:** When individuals engage in religious coping, additional religious struggles follow, which may benefit from chaplain expertise to promote spiritual well-being (Fox et al., 2016).
    - **African American:** Collaborate with faith communities to promote wellness.
    - **African American:** Incorporate faith traditions in coping with chronic disease.
    - **Latino:** Collaborate with faith communities to promote wellness.
    - **Latino:** Incorporate faith traditions among patients and families in pediatric settings.
    - **Uninsured/low income:** Explore faith community nurses to provide wellness services and care monitoring.
    - **Geriatrics:** Encourage listening to religious music.

R

Risk for Impaired Religiosity

NANDA-I Definition

Susceptible to an impaired ability to exercise reliance on religious beliefs and/or participate in rituals of a particular faith tradition, which may compromise health

Risk Factors

Insufficient transportation; pain; anxiety; depression; fear of death; ineffective caregiving; ineffective coping strategies; insecurity; insufficient social support; cultural barrier to practicing religion; environmental barrier to practicing religion; insufficient sociocultural interaction; spiritual distress

At-Risk Population

Aging; end-stage life crisis; life transition; history of religious manipulation; hospitalization; personal crisis; spiritual crisis

Associated Condition

Illness

Client Outcomes, Nursing Interventions

Refer to care plan for Impaired **Religiosity**

Relocation Stress Syndrome

NANDA-I Definition

Physiological and/or psychosocial disturbance following transfer from one environment to another

Defining Characteristics

Alienation; aloneness; alteration in sleep pattern; anger; anxiety (00146); concern about relocation; dependency; depression; fear (00148); frustration; increase in illness; increase in physical symptoms; increase in verbalization of needs; insecurity; loneliness; loss of identity; loss of self-worth; low self-esteem; pessimism; preoccupation; unwillingness to move; withdrawal

Related Factors

Ineffective coping strategies; insufficient predeparture counseling; insufficient support system; language barrier; move from one environment to another; powerlessness; significant environmental change; social isolation; unpredictability of experience

At-Risk Population

History of loss

Associated Condition

Compromised health status; deficient mental competence; impaired psychosocial functioning

Client Outcomes

Client Will (Specify Time Frame)

- Recognize and know the name of at least one staff member or new neighbor within 1 week of relocating
- Express concern about move when encouraged to do so during individual contacts within 24 hours of awareness of impending relocation
- Perform activities of daily living (ADLs) in usual manner
- Maintain previous mental and physical health status (e.g., nutrition, elimination, sleep, social interaction, physical activity) within 2 months of relocating

Nursing Interventions

- Be aware that relocation to retirement communities may be a positive change.
- Begin relocation planning as early in the decision process as possible.
- Obtain a history, including the reason for the move, the client's usual coping mechanisms, history of losses, and family support for the client.
- Identify to what extent the client can participate in the relocation decisions and advocate for this participation.
- Assess client's readiness to relocate and relocation self-efficacy.
- Consult an evidence-based practice guide for relocation.
- Assess family members' perceptions of client's ability to participate in relocation decisions. Particularly in cases of dementia, be alert to care workers' involvement in making the decision to relocate. They may need support and encouragement through the process.
- Consider the cultural and ethnic values of the client and family as much as possible when choosing roommates, foods, and other aspects of care.
- Promote clear communication between all participants in the relocation process.
- Observe the following procedures if the client is being transferred to an extended care facility or assisted living facility:
  - Facilitate the client's participation in decisions and choice of placement, and arrange a preadmission visit if possible.
  - If the client cannot visit the new facility, arrange for a visit or telephone call by a member of the staff to welcome the client and show a videotape or at least provide pictures of the new care facility.

  - Have a familiar person accompany the client to the new facility. This lessens client and family anxiety, confusion, and dissatisfaction.
  - Recommend that the caregiver write a journal of thoughts and feelings regarding the relocation of his or her loved one.
  - Continue to assess caregiver psychological distress during a 6-month period after relocation. Caregivers experience distress because of the responsibility of moving their loved one.
- Identify previous routines for ADLs. Try to maintain as much continuity with the previous schedule as possible.
- Bring in familiar items from home (e.g., pictures, clocks, afghans). Familiarity eases transition and symbolizes safeness.
- Establish the way the client would like to be addressed (Mr., Mrs., Miss, first name, or nickname).
- Thoroughly orient the client and the family to the new environment and routines; repeat directions as needed.
- Spend one-to-one time with the client. Allow the client to express feelings and convey acceptance of them; emphasize that the client's feelings are real and individual and that it is acceptable to be sad or angry about moving.
- Allocate a caring staff member to help the client adjust to the move. Assign the same staff members to the client for care if compatible with client; maintain consistency in the personnel with whom the client interacts.
- Ask the client to state one positive aspect of the new living situation each day. Helping the client focus on the positive aspects of the move can help change attitude and reframe the situation in a positive fashion.
- Ask the client to state one positive aspect of the new living situation each day.
- Monitor the client's health status and provide appropriate interventions for problems with social interaction, nutrition, sleep, new onset of infection, or elimination problems.
- If the client is being transferred within a facility, have staff members from the new unit visit the client before transfer.
- Work with the caregivers and family members helping them deal with stages of "making the best of it," "making the move," and "making it better."

R

- If a client is being transferred from the intensive care unit (ICU), have previous staff make occasional visits until the client is comfortable in the new surroundings. Ensure that the family is told relevant information.
- Watch for coping problems (e.g., withdrawal, regression, angry behavior, impaired sleeping, refusal to eat, flat affect, anxiety) and intervene immediately.
- Encourage the client to express grief for the loss of the old situation; explain that it is normal to feel sadness over change and loss.
- Assess the client's psychological needs along with physiological needs.

Encourage the client to participate in care as much as possible and make his or her own decisions when possible (e.g., placement of the bed, choice of roommate, bathing routines).

Pediatric

- Assess family history and contact information from children relocated to rescue shelters.
- Be aware that community relocation may be beneficial for children and assess community resources of new location.
- Provide support for a child and family who must relocate to be near a transplant center.
- In divorce situations, recommend alternative dispute resolution versus traditional litigated settlement.
- Assess presence of allergies before and after relocation.
- If the client is an adolescent, try to avoid a move in the middle of the school year, find a newcomers' club for the adolescent to join, and refer for counseling if needed.
- Assess adolescents' perceptions of their acceptance by peers.
- Help parents recognize that relocation stress syndrome may persist for prolonged periods (e.g., 2 years) in adolescents.
- Be aware that young people may cope with the transition by exerting control in particular domains.
- The effects of frequent relocation may not manifest immediately and may have long-term effects on physical and mental health.

Geriatric

- Monitor the need for transfer and transfer only when necessary.
- Implement discharge planning early and engage the older adult in decisions about relocation decisions.

- Use technologies, such as sensing devices, to measure average in-home gait speed (AIGS) as a predictor of fall risk.
- Implement a registered nurse (RN) care coordination model to restore older adults' health, maintain their independence, and reduce care costs.
- After the transfer, determine the client's mental status. Document and observe for any new onset of confusion. Confusion can follow relocation because of the overwhelming stress and sensory overload.
- Facilitate visits from companion animals.

Client/Family Teaching and Discharge Planning

- Teach family members and remind direct care staff about relocation stress syndrome. Encourage them to monitor for signs of the syndrome.
- Help significant others learn how to support the client in the move by setting up a schedule of visits, arranging for holidays, bringing familiar items from home, and establishing a system for contact when the client needs support.
- Assist family members and the relocating older adult to use Internet/webcam technology for interaction to supplement in-person visits.

R

Risk for Relocation Stress Syndrome

NANDA-I Definition

Susceptible to physiological and/or psychosocial disturbance following transfer from one environment to another, which may compromise health

Risk Factors

Ineffective coping strategies; insufficient predeparture counseling; insufficient support system; language barrier; move from one environment to another; powerlessness; significant environmental change; social isolation; unpredictability of experience

At-Risk Population

History of loss

Associated Condition

Compromised health status; deficient mental competence; impaired psychosocial functioning

Client Outcomes, Nursing Interventions, Client/Family Teaching and Discharge Planning

Refer to care plan for **Relocation** stress syndrome

Impaired Resilience

NANDA-I Definition

Decreased ability to recover from perceived adverse or changing situations, through a dynamic process of adaptation

Defining Characteristics

Decreased interest in academic activities; decreased interest in vocational activities; depression; guilt; impaired health status; ineffective coping strategies; ineffective integration; ineffective sense of control; low self-esteem; renewed elevation of distress; shame; social isolation

Related Factors

Community violence; disruption in family rituals; disruption in family roles; disturbance in family dynamics; dysfunctional family processes; inadequate resources; inconsistent parenting; ineffective family adaptation; insufficient impulse control; insufficient resources; insufficient social support; multiple coexisting adverse situations; perceived vulnerability; substance misuse

At-Risk Population

Chronicity of existing crisis; demographics that increase chance of maladjustment; economically disadvantaged; ethnic minority status; exposure to violence; female gender; large family size; low intellectual ability; low maternal educational level; new crisis; parental mental illness

Associated Condition

Psychological disorder

Client Outcomes

Client Will (Specify Time Frame)

- Demonstrate reduced or cessation of drug and alcohol usage
- State effective life events on feelings about self
- Seek help when necessary
- Verbalize or demonstrate cessation of abuse
- Adapt to unexpected crises or challenges
- Verbalize positive outlook on illness, family, situation, and life
- Use available resources to meet coping needs
- Identify role models
- Identify available assets and resources
- Be able to verbalize meaning of one's life

Nursing Interventions

- Encourage positive, health-seeking behaviors.
- Ensure access to biological, psychological, and spiritual resources.
- Foster communication skills through basic communication skill training.

- Foster cognitive skills in decision-making.
- Assist client in cognitive restructuring of negative thought processes.
- Facilitate supportive family environments and communication.
- Promote engagement in positive social activities.
- Assist client to identify strengths, and reinforce these.
- Help the client identify positive emotions during adverse situations.
- Build on supportive counseling and therapy.
- Identify protective factors such as assets and resources to enhance coping.
- Provide positive reinforcement and emotional support during the learning process.
- Encourage mindfulness, a conscious attention, and awareness of self.
- Educate and encourage the use of stress reduction techniques, such as guided imagery, in which the client focuses on positive images and emotions.
- Enhance knowledge and use of self-care strategies.
- Assist the client to have an optimistic worldview.

Pediatric

- The preceding interventions may be adapted for the pediatric client.
- Promote nurturing, supportive relationships with family.
- Support the seeking of opportunities to improve cognitive abilities, such as tutoring and other resources; the development of positive and supportive relations, such as family, community members, or mentors; and the improvement of general health.
- Promote the development of positive mentor relationships.

▲ Consider referral to appropriate community resources, such as faith-based communities for children who have had adverse childhood experiences.

Readiness for Enhanced Resilience

NANDA-I Definition

A pattern of ability to recover from perceived adverse or changing situations, through a dynamic process of adaption, which can be strengthened

Defining Characteristics

Expresses desire to enhance available resources; expresses desire to enhance communication skills; expresses desire to enhance environmental safety; expresses desire to enhance goal-setting; expresses desire to enhance involvement in activities; expresses desire to enhance own responsibility for action; expresses desire to enhance positive outlook; expresses desire to enhance progress toward goal; expresses desire to enhance relationships with others; expresses desire to enhance resilience; expresses desire to enhance self-esteem; expresses desire to enhance sense of control; expresses desire to enhance support system; expresses desire to enhance use of conflict management strategies; expresses desire to enhance use of coping skills; expresses desire to enhance use of resource

Client Outcomes

Client Will (Specify Time Frame)

- Adapt to adversities and challenges
- Communicate clearly and appropriately for age
- Take responsibility for own actions
- Make progress toward goals
- Use effective coping strategies
- Express emotions

Nursing Interventions

- Listen to and encourage expressions of feelings and beliefs.
- Establish a therapeutic relationship based on trust and respect.
- Assist client in rating current level of resilience.
- Facilitate supportive family environments and communication.
- Assist client to identify and reinforce strengths.
- Enhance skills associated with social and executive functioning.
- Provide positive reinforcement and emotional support during implementation of care.
- ▲ Facilitate the development of mentorship and volunteer opportunities.
- Determine how family behavior affects the client.
- Promote use of mindfulness and other stress reduction techniques.
- Establish individual/family/community goals.

Pediatric

- The preceding interventions may be adapted for the pediatric client.
- Encourage the promotion of protective factors by fostering the seeking of opportunities to improve cognitive abilities, such as tutoring and other resources; the development of positive and supportive relations such as family, community members, or mentors; and the improvement of general health.

Multicultural

- Use teaching strategies that are culturally and age appropriate.

Risk for Impaired Resilience

NANDA-I Definition

Susceptible to decreased ability to recover from perceived adverse or changing situations, through a dynamic process of adaptation, which may compromise health

Risk Factors

Community violence; disruption in family rituals; disruption in family roles; disturbance in family dynamics; dysfunctional family processes; inadequate resources; inconsistent parenting; ineffective family adaptation; insufficient impulse control; insufficient resources; insufficient social support; multiple coexisting adverse situations; perceived vulnerability; substance misuse

At-Risk Population

Chronicity of existing crisis; demographics that increase chance of maladjustment; economically disadvantaged; ethnic minority status; exposure to violence; female gender; large family size; low intellectual ability; low maternal educational level; new crisis; parental mental illness

Associated Condition

Psychological disorder

Client Outcomes

Client Will (Specify Time Frame)

- Identify available community resources
- Propose practical, constructive solutions for disputes
- Identify and access community resources for assistance
- Accept assistance with activities of daily living from family and friends
- Verbalize an enhanced sense of control
- Verbalize meaningfulness of one's life

Nursing Interventions

- Determine how family behavior affects client.
- Help identify personal rights, responsibilities, and conflicting norms.
- Encourage consideration of values underlying choices and consequences of the choice.
- Help client practice conversational and social skills.
- Assist client to prioritize values.
- Help create an accepting, nonjudgmental atmosphere.
- Help identify self-defeating thoughts.
- ▲ Refer to community resources/social services as appropriate.
- ▲ Help clarify problem areas in interpersonal relationships.

- ▲ Promote a sense of an individual's autonomy and control over choices to be made in one's environment.
- ▲ Identify and enroll high-risk families in follow-up programs.

Parental Role Conflict

NANDA-I Definition

Parental experience of role confusion and conflict in response to crisis

Defining Characteristics

Anxiety; concern about change in parental role; concern about family; disruption in caregiver routines; fear; frustration; guilt; perceived inadequacy to provide for child's needs; perceived loss of control over decisions relating to child; reluctance to participate in usual caregiver activities

Related Factors

Interruptions in family life caused by home care regimen; intimidated by invasive modalities; intimidation by restrictive modalities; parent–child separation

At-Risk Population

Change in marital status; home care of a child with special needs; living in nontraditional setting

Client Outcomes

Client Will (Specify Time Frame)

- Express feelings and perceptions regarding effects of illness, disability, and/or hospitalization on parental role
- Participate in hospital and home care as much as able given the availability of resources and support systems
- Exhibit assertiveness and responsibility in active family decision-making regarding care of the child
- Describe and select available resources to support parental management of the needs of the child and family

Nursing Interventions

- Assess and support parent's previous coping behaviors.
- Determine parent/family sources of stress, usual methods of coping, and perceptions of illness/condition. Maximize the identified strengths.
- Evaluate the family's perceived strength of its social support system, including religious beliefs. Encourage the family to use social support.

- Determine the older childbearing woman's support systems and expectations for motherhood.
- Consider the use of family-centered theory as the conceptual foundation to help guide interventions.
- Be available to accept and support parents by listening and discussing concerns.
- ▲ Maintain parental involvement in shared decision-making regarding care by using the following steps: incorporate parents' information concerning the child's typical routines, behaviors, fears, likes, and dislikes; provide clear and direct firsthand information concerning the child's condition and progress; normalize the home/hospital environment as much as possible; collaborate in care by providing choices when possible.
- Seek and support parental participation in care.
- Provide support for each parent's primary coping strategies and needs.
- ▲ Inform parents of financial resources, respite care, and home support to assist them in maintaining sufficient energy and personal resources to continue caregiving responsibilities.
- Encourage the parent to meet his or her own needs for rest, nutrition, and hygiene. Provide bed space so that the parent may stay with the sick child.
- Provide family-centered care: allow parents to touch and talk to the child, and assist in the handling of medical equipment; offer a comfortable chair, preferably a rocking chair. Provide opportunities and offer praise for successful caregiving.
- Refer parents to available telephone and/or Internet support groups.
- Involve new mother's partner or parents in clinical encounters and invite family members to discuss their expectations and parenting experiences.

Multicultural

- Acknowledge racial/ethnic differences at the onset of care.
- Assess for the influence of cultural beliefs, norms, and values on the client's perceptions of the parental role.
- Acknowledge that value conflicts arising from acculturation stresses may contribute to increased anxiety and significant conflict with the parental role.
- Promote the female parenting role by providing a treatment environment that is culturally based and woman centered.

R

- Support the client's parenting role in her usual setting via social exchange, including online support.

Home Care

- The interventions described previously may be adapted for home care use.
- Assess family adjustment prenatally and postpartum; assist new parents to renegotiate parenting roles and responsibilities with coparenting. Encourage the father to take an active role in infant care with the mother's support.

Client/Family Teaching and Discharge Planning

- Offer family-led education interventions to improve participants' knowledge about their condition and its treatment and decreasing their information needs.
- For children and their parents involved in bereavement support groups, identify the family's positive way of coping.
- ▲ Refer parents of children with behavioral problems to parenting programs.
- Involve parents in formal and/or informal social support situations, such as Internet support groups.
- Teach the client about available community resources (e.g., therapists, ministers, counselors, self-help groups).
- Encourage parents with chronic illnesses to identify areas of family conflicts and assist to integrate interventions into the family.

Ineffective Role Performance

NANDA-I Definition

A pattern of behavior and self-expression that does not match the environmental context, norms, and expectations

Defining Characteristics

Alteration in role perceptions; anxiety; change in capacity to resume role; change in other's perception of role; change in self-perception of role; change in usual patterns of responsibility; depression; discrimination; domestic violence; harassment; inappropriate developmental expectations; ineffective adaptation to change; ineffective coping strategies; ineffective role performance; insufficient confidence; insufficient external support for role enactment; insufficient knowledge of role requirements; insufficient motivation; insufficient opportunity for role enactment; insufficient self-management; insufficient skills; pessimism; powerlessness; role ambivalence;

role conflict; role confusion; role denial; role dissatisfaction; role strain; system conflict; uncertainty

Related Factors

Alteration in body image; conflict; depression; domestic violence; fatigue; inadequate role model; inappropriate linkage with the healthcare system; insufficient resources; insufficient rewards; insufficient role preparation; insufficient role socialization; insufficient support system; low self-esteem; pain; stressors; substance misuse; unrealistic role expectations

At-Risk Population

Developmental level inappropriate for role expectation; economically disadvantaged; high demands of job schedule; low educational level; young age

Associated Condition

Neurological defect; personality disorder; physical illness; psychosis

Client Outcomes

Client Will (Specify Time Frame)

- Identify realistic perception of role
- State personal strengths
- Acknowledge problems contributing to inability to perform usual role
- Accept physical limitations regarding role responsibility and consider ways to change lifestyle to accomplish goals associated with role performance
- Demonstrate knowledge of appropriate behaviors associated with new or changed role
- State knowledge of change in responsibility and new behaviors associated with new responsibility
- Verbalize acceptance of new responsibility

Nursing Interventions

- Assess the client's level of resilience and implement nursing actions that increase client resilience and sense of coherence.
- Assess the effect of uncertainty on the client's role and provide support and education.
- Assess the client's social support system.
- Assess for the presence of shame related to current health situation.
- Assess for the characteristics of role stress.
- Assess male military members for gender role stressors with the Male Gender Role Stressor Inventory (MGRSI).
- Ask the client what they need to feel prepared for the tasks and demands of their role.

▲ Refer the client to Acceptance and Commitment Therapy (ACT).

R

- Support the client's spirituality practices.
- Refer to the care plans for Readiness for enhanced family **Coping,** Readiness for enhanced **Decision-Making,** Ineffective **Home** Maintenance Behaviors, Impaired **Parenting,** Risk for **Loneliness,** Readiness for enhanced community **Coping,** Readiness for enhanced **Self-Care,** and Ineffective **Sexuality** pattern.

Pediatric

▲ Provide parents of disabled children with information about and referrals to educational and social resources available to assist their child.
- Assist new parents to adjust to changes in workload associated with childbirth. Mothers may need additional support.
- Assess mothers who present with depressive symptoms in the postpartum period for evidence of role performance distress.
- Provide parents with information about mindfulness-based interventions (MBIs) to enhance coping when the role change is associated with a critically and chronically ill child.
- Provide parents with information to increase their awareness of their child's psychological and social needs after a critical illness.

Geriatric

R

- Assess older adults' choices regarding their care and enable them to live as they wish and receive the help they want by carefully listening to their stories.
- Assess older adults for a sense of competence in their daily life.
- Provide support and practice for older adults to use technology.
- Support the client's spiritual beliefs and activities and provide appropriate spiritual support persons.
- Explore community needs after assessing the client's strengths. Encourage older adults to participate in volunteer programs.

Multicultural

- Assess for the influence of cultural beliefs, norms, values, and expectations on the individual's role.
- Assess for conflicts between the caregiver's cultural role, obligations, and competing factors, such as employment or school.
- Negotiate with the client regarding the aspects of their role that can be modified and still honor cultural beliefs.
- Identify perceived barriers to family to use support groups or other service programs to assist with role changes.
- The preceding interventions may be adapted for home care use.

Client/Family Teaching and Discharge Planning

- ▲ Refer client to comprehensive services to assist with transition needs at discharge.
- • Provide educational materials to family members on client behavior management plus caregiver stress-coping management.
- • Help the client identify resources for assistance in caring for a disabled or aging parent (e.g., adult day care, nursing home placement).

Sedentary Lifestyle

NANDA-I Definition

An acquired mode of behavior that is characterized by waking hour activities that require low energy expenditure.

Defining Characteristics

Average daily physical activity is less than recommended for gender and age; chooses a daily routine lacking in physical exercise; does not exercise during leisure time; expresses preference for low physical activity; performs majority of task in a reclining posture; performs majority of tasks in a sitting posture; physical deconditioning

Related Factors

Conflict between cultural beliefs and health practices; Decreased activity tolerance; difficulty adapting areas for physical activity; exceeds screen time recommendations for age; impaired physical mobility; inadequate interest in physical activity; inadequate knowledge of consequences of sedentarism; inadequate knowledge of health benefits associated with physical activity; inadequate motivation for physical activity; inadequate resources for physical activity; inadequate role models; inadequate social support; inadequate time management skills; inadequate training for physical exercise; low self efficacy; low self-esteem; negative affect toward physical activity; pain; parenting practices that inhibit child's physical activity; perceived physical disability; perceived safety risk

At Risk Population

Adolescents; individuals aged ≥60 years; individuals living in urban areas; individuals living with a partner; individuals with high educational level; individuals with high socioeconomic status; individuals with significant time restraints; married individuals; women

S

Client Outcomes

Client Will (Specify Time Frame)

- Engage in purposeful moderate-intensity cardiorespiratory (aerobic) exercise for 30 to 60 minutes per day on 5 or more days per week for a total of 2 hours and 30 minutes (150 minutes) per week
- Increase exercise to 20 minutes per day (less than 150 minutes per week); light- to moderate-intensity exercise may be beneficial in deconditioned persons
- Increase pedometer step counts by 1000 steps per day every 2 weeks to reach a daily step count of at least 7000 steps per day, with a daily goal for most healthy adults of 10,000 steps per day
- Perform resistance exercises that involve all major muscle groups (legs, hips, back, chest, abdomen, shoulders, and arms) performed 2 to 3 days per week
- Perform flexibility exercise (stretching) for each of the major muscle-tendon groups 2 days per week for 10 to 60 seconds to improve joint range of motion; greatest gains occur with daily exercise
- Engage in neuromotor exercise 20 to 30 minutes per day including motor skills (e.g., balance, agility, coordination, and gait), proprioceptive exercise training, and multifaceted activities (e.g., Tai chi and yoga) to improve and maintain physical function and reduce falls in those at risk for falling (older persons)

Nursing Interventions

- Observe the client for sedentary behaviors such as prolonged sitting, physical inactivity, and prolonged sleep.
- Use the Self-Efficacy for Exercise Scale (Resnick & Jenkins, 2000) and the Outcome Expectation for Exercise Scale (Resnick et al., 2001) to determine client's self-efficacy and outcome expectations toward exercise (Resnick & D'Adamo, 2011).
- Assess client with exercise preparticipation health screening prior to implementing physical activity interventions.
- Recommend the client enter an exercise program with an active person who supports exercise behavior (e.g., friend or exercise buddy).
- Recommend the client use a mobile fitness application for customizing, cueing, tracking, and analyzing an exercise program.
- Recommend participation in group physical activity programs.
- Recommend client begin performing resistance exercises for additional health benefits.
- Encourage prescriptive resistance exercise of each major muscle group (hips, thighs, legs, back, chest, shoulders, and abdomen) using a variety of exercise equipment.

- Encourage gradual progression of greater resistance, more repetitions per set, and/or increasing frequency.

Multicultural

- Assess for reasons why the client would be unable to participate in regular physical activity; address reasons and refer to resources as needed.
- Assess for their perceptions of the neighborhood they reside in.

Pediatric

- Assess the child's current activity status using the Pediatric Inactivity Triad (Faigenbaum et al., 2018).
- Children and adolescents should participate in 60 minutes (1 hour) or more of physical activity daily.
    - Aerobic: Sixty or more minutes a day should be either moderate-intensity or vigorous-intensity aerobic physical activity, and should include vigorous-intensity physical activity at least 3 days a week.
    - Muscle-strengthening: As part of daily physical activity, children and adolescents should include muscle-strengthening physical activity on at least 3 days of the week.
    - Bone-strengthening: As part of daily physical activity, children and adolescents should include bone-strengthening physical activity on at least 3 days of the week.
    - Providing activities that are age appropriate, enjoyable, and offer a variety will encourage young people to participate in physical activities (US Department of Health and Human Services, 2018).
- Assist families to develop family-based interventions to increase child physical activity.
- Encourage parents and caregivers to adhere to the following American Academy of Pediatrics guidelines for children's media use (Chassiakos et al., 2016):
    - For children younger than 18 months, avoid use of screen media other than video-chatting.
    - Parents of children 18 to 24 months of age who want to introduce digital media should choose high-quality programming and watch it with their children to help them understand what they are seeing.
    - For children ages 2 to 5 years, limit screen use to 1 hour per day of high-quality programs. Parents should co-view media with children to help them understand what they are seeing and apply it to the world around them.
    - For children ages 6 and older, place consistent limits on the time spent using media, and the types of media, and make sure media

does not take the place of adequate sleep, physical activity, and other behaviors essential to health.
  - ❍ Designate media-free times together, such as dinner or driving, and media-free locations at home, such as bedrooms.
  - ❍ Have ongoing communication about online citizenship and safety, including treating others with respect online and offline.
  - ❍ Encourage parents and caregivers to create their personalized family media plan (see https://www.healthychildren.org/English/media/Pages/default.aspx).

Geriatric

- • Use valid and reliable criterion-referenced standards for fitness testing (e.g., Senior Fitness Test) designed for older adults that can predict the level of capacity associated with maintaining physical independence into later years of life (e.g., get up and go test).
- • Recommend the client begin a regular exercise program, even if generally active.
- ▲ Refer the client to physical therapy for resistance exercise training, as able, involving all major muscle groups.
- • Implement progressive resistance training plus balance exercise for older adults as indicated.
- • Use the Function-Focused Care (FFC) rehabilitative philosophy of care with older adults in residential nursing facilities to prevent avoidable functional decline.
- • Recommend the older client practice Tai chi.
- • Prior to surgery, refer clients to a personalized prehabilitation program that includes a warm-up followed by aerobic, strength, flexibility, neuromotor, and functional task work.

Home Care

- • The preceding interventions may be adapted for home care use.
- ▲ Assess home environment for factors that create barriers to mobility. Refer to physical and occupational therapy services if needed to assist the client in restructuring home environment and daily living patterns.

Client/Family Teaching and Discharge Planning

- • Work with the client using theory-based interventions (e.g., social, cognitive, theoretical components such as self-efficacy; transtheoretical model).
- • Consider using motivational interviewing techniques when working with both children and adult clients to increase their activity.

Readiness for Enhanced Self-Care

NANDA-I Definition

A pattern of performing activities for oneself to meet health-related goals, which can be strengthened

Defining Characteristics

Expresses desire to enhance independence with health; expresses desire to enhance independence with life; expresses desire to enhance independence with personal development; expresses desire to enhance independence with well-being; expresses desire to enhance knowledge of self-care strategies; expresses desire to enhance self-care

Client Outcomes

Client Will (Specify Time Frame)

- Evaluate current levels of self-care as optimum for abilities
- Express the need or desire to continue to enhance levels of self-care
- Seek health-related information as needed
- Identify strategies to enhance self-care
- Perform appropriate interventions as needed
- Monitor level of self-care
- Evaluate the effectiveness of self-care interventions at regular intervals

Nursing Interventions

- For assessment of self-care, use a valid and reliable screening tool if available for specific characteristics of the person, such as arthritis, diabetes, stroke, heart failure (HF), or dementia.
- Support the person's awareness that enhanced self-care is an achievable, desirable, and positive life goal.
- Show respect for the person, regardless of characteristics and/or background.
- Promote trust and enhanced communication between the person and healthcare providers.
- Promote opportunities for spiritual care and growth.
- Promote social support through facilitation of family involvement.
- Provide opportunities for ongoing group support through establishment of self-help groups on the Internet.
- Help the person identify and reduce the barriers to self-care.
- Provide literacy-appropriate education for self-care activities.
- Facilitate self-efficacy by ensuring the adequacy of self-care education.
- Provide alternative mind–body therapies such as reiki, guided imagery, yoga, and self-hypnosis.
- Promote the person's hope to maintain self-care.

S

Pediatric

- Assess and evaluate a child's level of self-care and adjust strategies as needed.
- Assist families to engage in and maintain social support networks.

Multicultural

- Identify cultural beliefs, values, lifestyle practices, and problem-solving strategies when assessing the client's level of self-care.
- Recognize the effect of culture on SCBs.
- Provide culturally competent care.

Home Care

- The nursing interventions described previously may also be used in home care settings.
- Assist individuals and families to prevent exacerbations of chronic illness symptoms so rehospitalization is not necessary.
- Use educational guidelines for stroke survivors.
- Enhance individual and family coping with chronic illnesses.
- Implement a community care management program.

Client/Family Teaching and Discharge Planning

- Teach clients how to regularly assess their level of self-care.
- Instruct clients that a variety of interventions may be needed to enhance self-care.
- Help clients understand that enhanced self-care is an achievable goal.
- Empower clients.
- Teach clients about the decision-making process and self-care activities needed to manage their illness state and promote well-being.
- Continuously stress that all self-care activities must be regularly evaluated to ensure that enhanced levels of self-care can be maintained.

Bathing Self-Care Deficit

NANDA-I Definition

Inability to independently complete cleansing activities

Defining Characteristics

Impaired ability to access bathroom; impaired ability to access water; impaired ability to dry body; impaired ability to gather bathing supplies; impaired ability to regulate bath water; impaired ability to wash body

Related Factors

Anxiety; decrease in motivation; environmental barrier; pain; weakness

Associated Condition

Alteration in cognitive functioning; impaired ability to perceive body part; impaired ability to perceive spatial relationships; musculoskeletal impairment; neuromuscular impairment; perceptual disorders

Client Outcomes

Client Will (Specify Time Frame)

- Remain free of body odor and maintain intact skin
- State satisfaction with ability to use adaptive devices to bathe
- Use methods to bathe safely and effectively with minimal difficulty
- Bathe with assistance of caregiver as needed and report satisfaction and dignity maintained during bathing experience
- Bathe with assistance of caregiver as needed without exhibiting defensive (aggressive) behaviors

Nursing Interventions

- QSEN (Patient-Centered): Ask patients about their bathing preferences, which can increase patient privacy and satisfaction.
- QSEN (Safety): Warm bathing area above 25.1°C (77.18°F) while bathing, especially on cold days.
- QSEN (Safety): Use chlorhexidine-impregnated cloths rather than soap and water for daily patient bathing.
- QSEN (Safety): Consider using a prepackaged bath, especially for patients at high risk for infection (older adult, immunocompromised, invasive procedures, wounds, catheters, drains), to avoid patient exposure to multidrug-resistant pathogens from contaminated bath basins.
- QSEN (Safety): Use chlorhexidine gluconate for bath basin bathing.
- QSEN (Patient-Centered): Use patient-centered bathing interventions: plan for patient's comfort and bathing preferences, show respect in communications, critically think to solve issues that arise, and use a gentle approach.

▲ Provide pain relief measures, such as ice packs, heat, and analgesics for sore joints 45 minutes before bathing; move extremities slowly and carefully; and inform the client before movements associated with pain occur (walking; transferring to a new location; moving joints; and washing genitals, face, and between toes and under arms). Have the client wash painful areas; recognize indicators of pain and apologize for any pain caused.

- Use a comfortable padded shower chair with foot support, or adapt a chair: pad it with towels/washcloths, cover the cold back with dry towels, and cover the arms with foam pipe insulation.

S

- Ensure that bathing assistance preserves client dignity through use of privacy with a traffic-free bathing area and posted privacy signs, timeliness of personal care, and conveyance of honor and recognition of the deservedness of respect and esteem of all persons.
- For cognitively impaired clients, avoid upsetting factors associated with bathing: instead of using the terms *bath, shower,* or *wash,* use comforting words, such as *warm, relaxing,* or *massage.* Start at the client's feet and bathe upward; bathe the face last after washing hands and using a clean cloth. Use a beautician/barber or wash hair at another time to avoid water dripping in the face.
- Use towel bathing to bathe client in bed, a bath blanket, and warm towels to keep the client covered the entire time. Warm and moisten towels/washcloths and place in plastic bags to keep them warm. Use the towels to massage large areas (front, back) and one washcloth for facial areas and another one for genital areas. No rinsing or drying is needed as is commonly thought for bathing.
- **QSEN** (Patient-Centered): For shower bathing use patient-centered techniques, keep patient covered with towels and cleanse under the towels, use no-rinse products, use favorite bathing items, and use a handheld shower with adjustable spray.

▲ **QSEN** (Teamwork and Collaboration): Request referral of patient who has had a stroke to rehabilitation services.

▲ **QSEN** (Patient-Centered): Use a wrapped warm footbath for relaxation in patients with cancer.

Geriatric

- **QSEN** (Patient-Centered, Safety): Advocate for the use of the Bathing Without a Battle educational program for patients with dementia.
- **QSEN** (Patient-Centered): Provide nighttime bathing options for nursing home residents.
- Design the bathing environment for comfort: **Visual.** Reduce clutter and use partitions to hide equipment storage. Laminate and put artwork or decorative objects in bather's view, or place cue cards to bathing process (wall, ceiling, shower). Stand or sit in bather's position to experience what he or she sees. Decrease glare from tiles, white walls, and artificial lights. Use contrasting colors and soft but adequate lighting on a dimming switch for adjustment.
- Arrange the bathing environment to promote sensory comfort: **Auditory.** Reduce noise of voices and water. Do not allow traffic

into bathing room. Add fabric to absorb sound (three to four times the width of the opening for sound-absorbing folds). Play soft music.

- Design the bathing environment for comfort: **Tactile.** Use heat lamps or radiant heat panels to keep the room warm. Use powder-coated grab bars in decorative colors with nonslip grip. Provide a soft rug to stand on. Ensure that flooring is not slippery (a high coefficient of friction, ideally above 80, is desired and obtained through flooring coatings).
- Use music during shower for clients with dementia.
- Train caregivers bathing clients with dementia to avoid behaviors that can trigger assault: confrontational communication, invalidation of the resident's feelings, failure to prepare a resident for a task, initiating shower spray or touch during bathing without verbal prompts beforehand, washing the hair and face, speaking disrespectfully to the client, and hurrying the pace of the bath.
- Develop awareness of the ethics of presence during bathing to better meet clients' needs. Raholm (2012) found in a phenomenological study of nurses in elder care (*N* = 7) who discussed bathing that one must go beyond being physically present and enter into a caring relationship in which there is no indifference to the client's unique needs.
- Focus on the abilities of the client with dementia to obtain client's participation in bathing.
- **QSEN** (Patient-Centered): Use a Chinese herb formula in bath water to reduce paraplegia spasm.

Multicultural

- **QSEN** (Patient-Centered): Ask the patient for input on bathing habits and cultural bathing preferences.

Home Care

- If in a typical bathing setting for the client, assess the client's ability to bathe self via direct observation using physical performance tests for ADLs.
- **QSEN** (Safety): Turn down temperature of water heater and recommend use of a water temperature–sensing shower valve to prevent scalding.

Client/Family Teaching and Discharge Planning

- Inform clients with extremity casts or bandages of inexpensive options to protect these devices during showering such as with plastic newspaper bags or bread bags. In a case study, Naram, Makhijani, & Chao (2011) reported on the use of inexpensive or free cast and bandage protector bags.

S

Dressing Self-Care Deficit

NANDA-I Definition

Inability to independently put on or remove clothing.

Defining Characteristics

Impaired ability to choose clothing; impaired ability to fasten clothing; impaired ability to gather clothing; impaired ability to maintain appearance; impaired ability to pick up clothing; impaired ability to put clothing on lower body; impaired ability to put clothing on upper body; impaired ability to put on various items of clothing; impaired ability to remove clothing item; impaired ability to use assistive device; impaired ability to use zipper

Related Factors

Anxiety; decrease in motivation; discomfort; environmental barrier; fatigue; pain; weakness

Associated Condition

Alteration in cognitive functioning

Client Outcomes

Client Will (Specify Time Frame)

- Dress and groom self to optimal potential
- Use assistive technology to dress and groom
- Explain and use methods to enhance strengths during dressing and grooming
- Dress and groom with assistance of caregiver as needed

S

Nursing Interventions

▲ QSEN (Patient-Centered): Assess independence in dressing and bathing skills after rehabilitation to determine the need for follow-up care.

▲ QSEN (Teamwork and Collaboration): Assess functional impairment and report functional changes to healthcare provider to aid in earlier cancer diagnosis.

▲ QSEN (Teamwork and Collaboration): Refer patients after stroke to occupational therapy for ADL rehabilitation.

• **QSEN (Patient-Centered):** For clients with spinal cord injury, encourage their self-efficacy and involve them in decision-making.

• QSEN (Patient-Centered): Use adaptive dressing and grooming equipment as needed (e.g., button hooks, dressing stick, elastic shoelaces, long-handled shoehorn, reacher, sock application devices, Velcro clothing and shoes, zipper pull, long-handled brushes, soap-on-a-rope, suction holders).

• QSEN (Patient-Centered): Provide client analgesics prior to dressing as needed, sufficient time for dressing, and assist as needed.

Geriatric

- ▲ QSEN (Teamwork and Collaboration): Refer older cognitively impaired patients to physical and/or occupational therapy for functional rehabilitation with ADLs.
- • QSEN (Patient-Centered): Offer residents choices in what to wear and ensure staff is trained to do so.
- • QSEN (Patient-Centered): Allow post-stroke patients who are cognitively impaired, especially if unimanual, to practice dressing.
- • QSEN (Patient-Centered): Inform patient that a winter coat with a funnel sleeve design can be easier to put on.

Multicultural

- • Consider use of assistive technology versus personal care assistance for Native Americans.

Home Care

- • QSEN (Patient-Centered): Teach assisted living staff the philosophy and methods to increase resident participation in dressing.

Client/Family Teaching and Discharge Planning

- • QSEN (Teamwork and Collaboration): Include caregiver's perceptions of client rehabilitation needs after stroke.

S

Feeding Self-Care Deficit

NANDA-I Definition

Inability to eat independently

Defining Characteristics

Impaired ability to bring food to the mouth; impaired ability to chew food; impaired ability to get food onto utensils; impaired ability to handle utensils; impaired ability to manipulate food in mouth; impaired ability to open containers; impaired ability to pick up cup; impaired ability to prepare food; impaired ability to self-feed a complete meal; impaired ability to self-feed in an acceptable manner; impaired ability to swallow food; impaired ability to swallow sufficient amount of food; impaired ability to use assistive device

Related Factors

Anxiety; decrease in motivation; discomfort; environmental barrier; fatigue; pain; weakness

Associated Condition

Alteration in cognitive functioning; musculoskeletal impairment; neuromuscular impairment; perceptual disorders

Client Outcomes

Client Will (Specify Time Frame)

- Feed self safely and effectively
- State satisfaction with ability to use adaptive devices for feeding
- Use assistance with feeding when necessary (caregiver)

Nursing Interventions

- • QSEN (Safety): Consider assessment of patients in the intensive care unit (ICU) and stepdown patients or of patients with acute stroke for readiness of an oral diet with a 3-ounce water swallow challenge by a trained provider.
- • QSEN (Patient-Centered): Conduct repeat structured observations of patients at mealtime after a stroke to detect patients with eating difficulties to prevent possible social and functional consequences.
- ▲ QSEN (Patient-Centered): Develop an overriding guideline for assisted feeding so it is less dependent on a caregiver's own beliefs, time pressures, and organizational characteristics.
- ▲ QSEN (Patient-Centered): Prioritize assisted feeding as important in a caregiver's assignment to allow adequate dedicated time to the activity.
- ▲ QSEN (Teamwork and Collaboration): Give priority to continuity in the cooperation between the parties involved in assisted feeding for those who are completely dependent.
- • QSEN (Patient-Centered): Consult patient on the benefit or desire to use assistive devices for feeding.
- • QSEN (Safety): Presentation of feeding: provide 1 teaspoon of solid food or 10 to 15 mL of liquid at a time; wait until patient has swallowed the prior food/liquid.
- • QSEN (Safety): Ensure oral care is provided to all patients regardless of type of feeding.

Geriatric

- • QSEN (Safety): Assess for tooth loss in older patients prior to feeding.
- • QSEN (Patient-Centered): Assess the ability of patients with dementia to self-feed, and supervise the feeding of those with moderate dependency by providing verbal or physical assistance.
- • QSEN (Patient-Centered): Implement Montessori interventions for patients with dementia who have eating problems, such as playing music to signal learning session start for hand-eye coordination, scooping, pouring, and squeezing activities.

- ▲ QSEN (Patient-Centered): Reduce interruptions during mealtimes and provide additional feeding assistance for older patients, especially those with cognitive impairment.
- • QSEN (Patient-Centered): Use high-calorie oral supplements for patients with advanced dementia.
- • QSEN (Patient-Centered): Provide nutritional supplement drinks in a glass to older adults with cognitive impairment.
- • QSEN (Patient-Centered): Allow a resident an average of 42 minutes of staff time per meal and 13 minutes per between-meal snack to improve oral intake.
- • QSEN (Patient-Centered): Discuss meaningful life topics, as identified by family members, with residents with dementia during mealtimes.
- • QSEN (Patient-Centered): Encourage family visits at mealtimes for patients with dementia.
- • QSEN (Patient-Centered): Play familiar music during meals for clients with dementia.
- • Use aromatherapy with the smell of baking bread for those with dementia.
- ▲ QSEN (Teamwork and Collaboration): Provide feeding training and education programs for nursing home staff.

Multicultural

- • QSEN (Patient-Centered): For those with impaired hand function who use chopsticks, suggest adapted chopsticks.
- • QSEN (Patient-Centered): Use the simplified Chinese Edinburgh Feeding Evaluation in Dementia scale to measure feeding problems in people with dementia from Mainland China and other Chinese cultural groups.

Home Care

- • QSEN (Teamwork and Collaboration): Request referral for physical therapy and occupational therapy to assess client's ability to position and self-feed and provide client and caregiver support with feeding.

Client/Family Teaching and Discharge Planning

- • QSEN (Teamwork and Collaboration): Discuss with family caregivers, who are involved in the feeding of a family member with advanced dementia, the feeding experience to provide support to ensure that the mealtime purpose is preserved.

▲ QSEN (Patient-Centered): Educate family members that neither insertion of a feeding tube nor timing of its insertion affects client survival for those with advanced dementia who have eating problems.

Toileting Self-Care Deficit

NANDA-I Definition

Inability to independently perform tasks associated with bowel and bladder elimination

Defining Characteristics

Impaired ability to complete toilet hygiene; impaired ability to flush toilet; impaired ability to manipulate clothing for toileting; impaired ability to reach toilet; impaired ability to rise from toilet; impaired ability to sit on toilet

Related Factors

Anxiety; decrease in motivation; environmental barrier; fatigue; impaired ability to transfer; impaired mobility; pain; weakness

Associated Condition

Alteration in cognitive functioning; musculoskeletal impairment; neuromuscular impairment; perceptual disorders

Client Outcomes

S

Client Will (Specify Time Frame)

- Remain free of incontinence and impaction with no urine or stool on skin
- State satisfaction with ability to use adaptive devices for toileting
- Explain and demonstrate use of methods to be safe and independent in toileting

Nursing Interventions

- QSEN (Safety): Assess patients for fall risk using established and valid fall risk assessment tools (Morse and Heindrich) and implement fall prevention interventions for those at risk for falling or in physical restraints.
- QSEN (Patient-Centered): Assess patient's prior use of incontinence briefs and avoid use for hospitalized continent but limited mobility patient.
- QSEN (Patient-Centered): Assess patients who have had sphincter-saving surgery for self-care strategies to manage bowel symptoms to help support these strategies.

- QSEN (Safety): Make assistance call button readily available to the client and answer call light promptly.
- QSEN (Safety): Provide folding commode chairs in client bathrooms/at bedside.
- QSEN (Patient-Centered): Before use of a bedpan, discuss its use with clients.
- QSEN (Patient-Centered): Use necessary assistive toileting equipment.
- QSEN (Safety): Close toilet lid before flushing toilet and teach patient to do so.

Geriatric

- Assess residents without dementia for risk factors associated with toileting disability (such as rating health as fair or poor; living in a residence with four or less residents or that is for-profit, incontinence; physical, visual, or hearing impairment; and need for ADL or transferring assistance) to guide prevention interventions.
- QSEN (Patient-Centered): Consider use of urine alarm systems for patients with dementia.
- QSEN (Patient-Centered): Assess the patient's functional ability to manipulate clothing for toileting, and if necessary modify clothing with Velcro fasteners, elastic waists, drop-front underwear, or slacks.
- QSEN (Patient-Centered): Provide patients with dementia access to regular exercise.

Multicultural

- QSEN (Patient-Centered): Remove barriers to toileting, support patient's cultural beliefs, and preserve dignity.

Home Care

- QSEN (Patient-Centered): To design a bathroom for an older adult, consider adaptable bath fixtures/furniture and safety needs.

Client/Family Teaching and Discharge Planning

- Teach men who perform routine clean intermittent catheterization that a 40-cm intermittent catheter was found to provide ease of use, instill confidence in bladder emptying, and draining of urine into a receptacle.
- Have the family install a toilet seat of a contrasting color.
- Explain to family and caregivers of clients with dementia that toilet self-care activities decrease when self-awareness is lost.

S

Readiness for Enhanced Self-Concept

NANDA-I Definition

A pattern of perceptions or ideas about the self, which can be strengthened

Defining Characteristics

Acceptance of limitations; acceptance of strengths; actions are congruent with verbal expression; expresses confidence in abilities; expresses desire to enhance role performance; expresses desire to enhance self-concept; expresses satisfaction with body image; expresses satisfaction with personal identity; expresses satisfaction with sense of worth; expresses satisfaction with thoughts about self

Client Outcomes

Client Will (Specify Time Frame)

- State willingness to enhance self-concept
- State satisfaction with thoughts about self, sense of worthiness, role performance, body image, and personal identity
- Demonstrate actions that are congruent with expressed feelings and thoughts
- State confidence in abilities
- Accept strengths and limitations

S

Nursing Interventions

- Encourage client to express feelings through song writing.
- Refer to nutritional and exercise programs to support weight loss.
- Offer client complementary and alternative medicine (CAM) interventions like acupressure, aromatherapy, compress, and massage.
- Support homeless individuals to identify and endorse a positive self-concept.
- Support unemployed individuals to cope with identity threats and support individual identity growth.
- Support establishing community-based partnerships to address health needs.
- For clients with a history of trauma, offer a mindfulness-based intervention of hatha yoga.

Pediatric

- Consider the development of a Healthy Kids Mentoring Program that has four components: (1) relationship building, (2) self-esteem

enhancement, (3) goal setting, and (4) academic assistance (tutoring). Mentors met with students twice each week for 1 hour each session on school grounds. During each meeting, mentors devoted time to each program component.
- Facilitate healthy relationships with teachers, coaches, and other supportive adults in the adolescents' lives.
- Provide parents with information designed to promote body satisfaction, healthy eating, and weight management in early childhood.
- Promote the adoption of a recovery identity through online interactions and support groups for individuals with eating disorders.
- Provide activities to bolster physical self-concept.
- ▲ Consider wheelchair dancing for disabled adolescents.
- ▲ Provide overweight adolescents access to group-based weight control interventions.
- Provide an alternative school-based program for pregnant and parenting adolescents.

Geriatric
- Assess for depression as needed.
- Encourage clients to consider a web-based support program when they are in a caregiving situation.
- Encourage activity and a strength, mobility, balance, and endurance training program.
- Support meaning and purpose in the lives of older adults through a focus on everyday well-being and facilitation of personally treasured activities.
- Use an approach that reduces the emphasis put on ageist self-concept attributions when working with older clients.

Multicultural
- Carefully assess each client and allow families to participate in providing care that is acceptable based on the client's cultural beliefs.
- Refer to the care plans Disturbed **Body Image,** Readiness for enhanced **Coping,** Chronic low **Self-Esteem,** and Readiness for enhanced **Spiritual** well-being.

Home Care
- Previously discussed interventions may be used in the home care setting.

S

Chronic Low Self-Esteem

NANDA-I Definition

Long-standing negative perception of self-worth, self-acceptance, self-respect, competence, and attitude toward self.

Defining Characteristics

Dependent on others' opinions; depressive symptoms; excessive guilt; excessive seeking of reassurance; expresses loneliness; hopelessness; insomnia; loneliness; nonassertive behavior; overly conforming behaviors; reduced eye contact; rejects positive feedback; reports repeated failures; rumination; self-negating verbalizations; shame; suicidal ideation; underestimates ability to deal with situation

Related Factors

Decreased mindful acceptance; difficulty managing finances; disturbed body image; fatigue; fear of rejection; impaired religiosity; inadequate affection received; inadequate attachment behavior; inadequate family cohesiveness; inadequate group membership; inadequate respect from others; inadequate sense of belonging; inadequate social support; ineffective communication skills; insufficient approval from others; low self efficacy; maladaptive grieving; negative resignation; repeated negative reinforcement; spiritual incongruence; stigmatization; stressors; values incongruent with cultural norms

At-Risk Population

Economically disadvantaged individuals; individuals experiencing repeated failure; individuals exposed to traumatic situation; individuals with difficult developmental transition; individuals with history of being abandoned; individuals with history of being abused; individuals with history of being neglected; individuals with history of loss

Associated Condition

Depression; functional impairment; mental disorders; physical illness

Client Outcomes

Client Will (Specify Time Frame)

- Demonstrate improved ability to interact with others (e.g., maintains eye contact, engages in conversation, expresses thoughts/feelings)
- Verbalize increased self-acceptance through positive self-statements about self
- Identify personal strengths, accomplishments, and values
- Identify and work on small, achievable goals
- Improve independent decision-making and problem-solving skills

Nursing Interventions

- Actively listen to and respect the client.
- Assess the client's environmental and everyday stressors, including physical health concerns and the potential for abusive relationships.

- Assess existing strengths and coping abilities, and provide opportunities for their expression and recognition.
- Assess the client's self-esteem using valid and established tools like the Rosenberg Self-Esteem Scale.
- Assess the client for addictive use of social media.
- Reinforce the personal strengths and positive self-perceptions that a client identifies.
- Encourage self-affirmations by reflecting on values and strengths, in response to daily threats.
- Identify client's negative self-assessments.
- Assess individuals with low self-esteem for nonsuicidal self-injury (NSSI).
- Assess individuals with low self-esteem for symptoms of depression.
- Encourage realistic and achievable goal setting and resources and identify impediments to achievement.
- Assist client to challenge negative perceptions of self and performance.
- Encourage the client's usual religious or spiritual practices.
- Promote maintaining a level of functioning in the community and a sense of community feeling.

Pediatric

- Assess children/adolescents with chronic illness for evidence of reduced self-esteem and make needed referrals.
- Encourage mothers of premature infants to use kangaroo care for at least 30 minutes per day.
- Implement interventions that promote and maintain positive peer relations for adolescent patients.
- Encourage attendance at social support groups.
- Encourage parents to praise children in ways that are not overly positive or inflated.
- Provide parents with information designed to promote body satisfaction, healthy eating, and weight management in early childhood.
- Assess children/adolescents that express a body image of self-perceived underweight, self-perceived overweight (OW), and/or frustration with appearance for evidence of bullying.

▲ Provide bully prevention programs and include information on cyberbullying.

Geriatric

- Support client in identifying and adapting to functional changes.
- Use reminiscence therapy and productive activities.

- • Encourage older adult clients to participate in flexibility, toning, and balance exercise.
- • Encourage regular physical activity with prerecorded workouts.
- • Encourage participation in intergenerational social activities.
- • Encourage activities in which a client can support/help others.

Multicultural

- • Assess for the influence of cultural beliefs, norms, and values on the client's sense of self-esteem.
- • Assess individuals with low self-esteem for symptoms of depression.
- • Validate the client's feelings regarding ethnic or racial identity.

Home Care

- • Assess a client's immediate support system/family for relationship patterns and content of communication.
- ▲ Refer to continuous support and help from medical social services to assist the family in care of the client and support the caregiver's well-being.
- ▲ If a client is involved in counseling or self-help groups, monitor and encourage attendance. Help the client identify the value of group participation after each group encounter.

Client/Family Teaching and Discharge Planning

- ▲ Refer to community agencies for psychotherapeutic counseling.
- ▲ Refer to psychoeducational groups on stress reduction and coping skills.
- ▲ Refer to self-help support groups specific to needs.

Situational Low Self-Esteem

NANDA-I Definition

Change from positive to negative perception of self-worth, self-acceptance, self-respect, competence, and attitude toward self in response to a current situation.

Defining Characteristics

Depressive symptoms; expresses loneliness; helplessness; indecisive behavior; insomnia; loneliness; nonassertive behavior; purposelessness; rumination; self-negating verbalizations; underestimates ability to deal with situation

Related Factors

Behavior incongruent with values; decrease in environmental control; decreased mindful acceptance; difficulty accepting alteration in social role; difficulty managing finances; disturbed body image; fatigue; fear of rejection; impaired religiosity; inadequate attachment behavior; inadequate family cohesiveness; inadequate respect from others; inadequate social support;

ineffective communication skills; low self efficacy; maladaptive perfectionism; negative resignation; powerlessness; stigmatization; stressors; unrealistic self-expectations; values incongruent with cultural norms

At-Risk Population

Individuals experiencing a change in living environment; individuals experiencing alteration in body image; individuals experiencing alteration in economic status; individuals experiencing alteration in role function; individuals experiencing death of a significant other; individuals experiencing divorce; individuals experiencing new additions to the family; individuals experiencing repeated failure; individuals experiencing unplanned pregnancy; individuals with difficult developmental transition; individuals with history of being abandoned; individuals with history of being abused; individuals with history of being neglected; individuals with history of loss; individuals with history of rejection

Associated Condition

Depression; functional impairment; mental disorders; physical illness

Client Outcomes

Client Will (Specify Time Frame)

- State effect of life events on feelings about self
- State personal strengths
- Acknowledge presence of guilt and not blame self if an action was related to another person's appraisal
- Seek help when necessary
- Demonstrate self-perceptions are accurate given physical capabilities
- Demonstrate separation of self-perceptions from societal stigmas

S

Nursing Interventions

▲ Assess the client for signs and symptoms of depression and potential for suicide and/or violence. If present, immediately notify the appropriate personnel of symptoms. See care plans for **Risk for other-directed Violence** and **Risk for Suicidal Behavior.**

- Assess the client's environmental and everyday stressors, including evidence of abusive relationships.

▲ Assess the client's self-esteem using valid and established tools like the Rosenberg Self-Esteem Scale.

- Assess for unhealthy coping mechanisms, such as substance abuse, and make appropriate referrals.
- Encourage expressions of gratitude through a gratitude journal or kind acts.
- Use a cognitive approach like problem-solving education (PSE) to assist in the identification of problems and situational factors that contribute to problems and offer options for resolution.

- Mutually identify strengths, resources, and previously effective coping strategies.
- Encourage self-affirmations by reflecting on values and strengths, in response to daily threats.
- Accept client's own pace in working through grief or crisis situations.
- Encourage the client to accept their own defenses, feelings, and urges in dealing with the crisis.
- Provide information about support groups of people who have common experiences or interests.
- Teach the client mindfulness techniques to cope more effectively with strong emotional responses.
- Encourage objective appraisal of self and life events and challenge negative or perfectionist expectations of self.
- Provide psychoeducation to client and family.
- Acknowledge the presence of societal stigma. Teach management tools.
- Validate the effect of negative past experiences on self-esteem and work on corrective measures.

Geriatric and Multicultural

- See care plan for Chronic low **Self-Esteem.**

Home Care

- Establish an emergency plan and contract with the client for its use. Having an emergency plan is reassuring to the client. Establishing a contract validates the worth of the client and provides a caring link between the client and society.
- Access supplies that support a client's success at independent living.
- See care plan for Chronic low **Self-Esteem.**

Client/Family Teaching and Discharge Planning

- Assess the person's support system (family, friends, and community) and involve them if desired.
- ▲ Refer to self-help support groups specific to needs.
- ▲ Refer to appropriate community resources or crisis intervention centers.
- ▲ Refer to resources for handicap and/or disability services.
- See care plan for Chronic low **Self-Esteem.**

Risk for Chronic Low Self-Esteem

NANDA-I Definition

Susceptible to long-standing negative perception of self-worth, self-acceptance, self-respect, competence, and attitude toward self, which may compromise health.

Risk Factors

Decreased mindful acceptance; difficulty managing finances; disturbed body image; fatigue; fear of rejection; impaired religiosity; inadequate affection received; inadequate attachment behavior; inadequate family cohesiveness; inadequate group membership; inadequate respect from others; inadequate sense of belonging; inadequate social support; ineffective communication skills; insufficient approval from others; low self efficacy; maladaptive grieving; negative resignation; repeated negative reinforcement; spiritual incongruence; stigmatization; stressors; values incongruent with cultural norms

At-Risk Population

Economically disadvantaged individuals; individuals experiencing repeated failure; individuals exposed to traumatic situation; individuals with difficult developmental transition; individuals with history of being abandoned; individuals with history of being abused; individuals with history of being neglected; individuals with history of loss

Associated Condition

Depression; functional impairment; mental disorders; physical illness

Client Outcomes, Nursing Interventions

Refer to care plan for Chronic low **Self-Esteem**

Risk for Situational Low Self-Esteem

NANDA-I Definition

Susceptible to change from positive to negative perception of self-worth, self-acceptance, self-respect, competence, and attitude toward self in response to a current situation, which may compromise health.

Risk Factors

Behavior incongruent with values; decrease in environmental control; decreased mindful acceptance; difficulty accepting alteration in social role; difficulty managing finances; disturbed body image; fatigue; fear of rejection; impaired religiosity; inadequate attachment behavior; inadequate family cohesiveness; inadequate respect from others; inadequate social support; individuals experiencing repeated failure; ineffective communication skills; low self efficacy; maladaptive perfectionism; negative resignation; powerlessness; stigmatization; stressors; unrealistic self-expectations; values incongruent with cultural norms

At-Risk Population

Individuals experiencing a change in living environment; individuals experiencing alteration in body image; individuals experiencing alteration in economic status; individuals experiencing alteration in role function; individuals experiencing death of a significant other; individuals experiencing divorce; individuals experiencing new additions to the family; individuals experiencing unplanned pregnancy; individuals with difficult developmental transition; individuals with history of being abandoned; individuals with history of being abused; individuals with history of being neglected; individuals with history of loss; individuals with history of rejection

Associated Conditions

Depression; functional impairment; mental disorders; physical illness

Nursing Interventions

- Assist client to challenge negative perceptions of self and performance.
- Assess the client's self-esteem using valid and established tools like the Rosenberg Self-Esteem Scale.
- Encourage client to maintain highest level of community functioning.
- Encourage self-affirmations by reflecting on values and strengths, in response to daily threats.
- Encourage realistic and achievable goal setting and resources and identify impediments to achievement.

▲ Assess the client for symptoms of depression and anxiety. Refer to specialist as needed. Prompt and effective treatment can prevent exacerbation of symptoms or safety risks.

- See care plans for Disturbed personal **Identity,** Situational low **Self-Esteem,** and Chronic low **Self-Esteem.**

S

Pediatric

- Assess children/adolescents with chronic illness for evidence of reduced self-esteem and make needed referrals.
- Identify environmental and/or developmental factors that increase risk for low self-esteem, especially in children/adolescents, to make needed referrals.
- Encourage attendance at social support groups.
- Assess children/adolescents who are either a victim or an offender of cyberbullying for low self-esteem.

▲ Encourage a combination of extracurricular activity for adolescents in a safe, supportive, and empowering environment.

Geriatric

- Support humor as a coping mechanism.
- Support client in identifying and adapting to functional changes.
- Encourage participation in intergenerational social activities.
- Assist the client in life review and identifying positive accomplishments.
- Help client establish a peer group and structured daily activities.
- See care plans for Situational low **Self-Esteem** and Chronic low **Self-Esteem.**

Home Care

- Assess current environmental stresses and identify community resources.
- Encourage family members to acknowledge and validate the client's strengths.
- Assess the need for establishing an emergency plan.
- See care plans for Situational low **Self-Esteem** and Chronic low **Self-Esteem.**

Client/Family Teaching and Discharge Planning

- ▲ Refer the client/family to community-based self-help and support groups.
- ▲ Refer to psychoeducational groups on stress reduction and coping skills.
- ▲ Refer the client to community agencies that offer support and environmental resources. Make referrals as needed.
- • See care plans for Situational low **Self-Esteem** and Chronic low **Self-Esteem.**

Risk for Self-Mutilation

NANDA-I Definition

Susceptible to deliberate behavior causing tissue damage with the intent of causing nonfatal injury to attain relief of tension

Risk Factors

Absence of family confidant; alteration in body image; dissociation; disturbance in interpersonal relationships; eating disorder; emotional disturbance; feeling threatened with loss of significant relationship; impaired self-esteem; impulsiveness; inability to express tension verbally; ineffective communication between parent and adolescent; ineffective coping strategies; irresistible urge for self-directed violence; irresistible urge to cut self; isolation from peers; labile behavior; loss of control over problem-solving situation; low self-esteem; mounting tension that is intolerable; negative feeling; pattern of inability to plan solutions; pattern of inability to see long-term consequences; perfectionism; requires rapid stress reduction; substance misuse; use of manipulation to obtain nurturing relationship with others

At-Risk Population

Adolescence; battered child; childhood illness; childhood surgery; developmental delay; family divorce; family history of self-destructive behavior; family substance misuse; history of childhood abuse; incarceration; living in nontraditional setting; loss of significant relationship; peers who self-mutilate; sexual identity crisis; violence between parental figures

Associated Condition

Autism; borderline personality disorder; character disorder; depersonalization; psychotic disorder

Client Outcomes

Client Will (Specify Time Frame)

- Refrain from self-injury
- Identify triggers to self-mutilation
- State appropriate ways to cope with increased psychological or physiological tension
- Express feelings
- Seek help when having urges to self-mutilate
- Maintain self-control without supervision
- Use appropriate community agencies when caregivers are unable to attend to emotional needs

Nursing Interventions

Note: Before implementing interventions in the face of self-injury, nurses should examine their own knowledge base and emotional responses to incidents of self-injury to ensure that interventions will not be based on countertransference reactions.

- A nonjudgmental approach to clients is critical.
- Assess for history of self-harm behavior.
- Assess client's ability to regulate his or her own emotional states. These states may be influenced by the client's perception of his or her body or by the presence of a psychiatric disorder.
- Assess client's perception of powerlessness. Refer to the care plan for **Powerlessness.**
- Assessment data from the client and family members may have to be gathered at different times; allowing a family member or trusted friend with whom the client is comfortable to be present during the assessment may be helpful.
- Perform a thorough skin assessment at least annually and check for behavioral cues of self-harm.
- Assess for co-occurring disorders that require response, especially childhood abuse, substance abuse, and suicide attempts. Implement reporting or referral as indicated.
- Assess family dynamics and the need for family therapy and community support.
- Assess for the presence of medical disorders, mental retardation, medication effects, or disorders such as autism that may include

S

self-mutilation. Initiate referral for evaluation and treatment as appropriate.

- • Be alert to other risk factors of self-mutilation in clients with psychosis, including acute intoxication, dramatic changes in body appearance, preoccupation with religion and sexuality, and anticipated or perceived object loss.
- • Monitor the client's behavior closely by using engagement and support as elements of safety checks while avoiding intrusive overstimulation. Offer activities that will serve as a distraction.
- • Focus on understanding the function that self-harm serves for the client and on managing the client's distress.
- • Establish trust, show a caring attitude and hope for recovery, listen to client, convey safety, promote client's verbal expression, and assist in developing positive goals for the future. Assist client to identify triggers and identify prevention activities.
- ▲ Refer to mental health counseling. Multiple therapeutic modalities are available for treatment.
- ▲ Case finding and referral by school nurses for psychological or psychiatric treatment is critical. Treatment includes starting therapy and medications, increasing coping skills, facilitating decision-making, encouraging positive relationships, and fostering self-esteem.
- • Inform the client of expectations for appropriate behavior and consequences within the unit. Emphasize that the client must comply with the rules. Give positive reinforcement for compliance and minimize attention paid to disruptive behavior while setting limits.
- • Clients need to learn to recognize distress as it occurs and express it verbally rather than as a physical action against the self.
- • Assist the client to identify the motives/reasons for self-mutilation that have been perceived as positive. Self-harm serves as a defense mechanism.
- • Assist clients to identify ways to soothe themselves and generate hopefulness when faced with painful emotions.
- • Reinforce alternative ways of dealing with depression and anxiety, such as exercise, engaging in unit activities, or talking about feelings.
- • Keep the environment safe; remove all harmful objects from the area. Use of unbreakable glass is recommended for the client at risk for self-injury.
- • Anticipate trigger situations and intervene to assist the client in applying alternatives to self-mutilation.
- • If self-mutilation does occur, use a calm, nonpunitive approach. Whenever possible, assist the client to assume responsibility for

S

consequences (e.g., dress self-inflicted wound). Refer to the care plan for **Self-Mutilation.**
- • If the client is unable to control self-mutilation behavior, provide interactive supervision, not isolation.
- ▲ Refer to protective services if evidence of abuse exists.
- • Refer to the care plan for **Self-Mutilation.**

Pediatric
- • The same dynamics described previously applies to adolescents.
- • Maintaining a therapeutic relationship with teens requires explicit assurances of confidentiality, consistency of clinical routines, and a nonjudgmental communication style.
- • Encourage expression of painful experiences and provide supportive counseling.
- • Assess for the presence of an eating disorder, history of sexual abuse and/or substance abuse, or nascent psychiatric disorders. Attend to the themes that preoccupy teens with eating disorders who self-mutilate.
- • Be mindful of possible social influences on self-harm behaviors.
- • Evaluate for suicidal ideation/suicide risk. Refer to the care plan for **Suicide** for additional information.
- • Be aware that there is no complete overlap between self-mutilation and suicidal behavior. The motivation may be different (coping with difficult feelings rather than ending life), and the method is usually different.
- • Use treatment approaches detailed in nursing interventions, with modifications as appropriate for this age group.

Geriatric
- • Provide hand or back rubs and calming music when older clients experience anxiety.
- • Provide soft objects for older clients to hold and manipulate when self-mutilation occurs as a function of delirium or dementia. Apply mitts, splints, helmets, or restraints as appropriate.
- • Be aware that older adults may demonstrate self-neglect. Older adults who show self-destructive behaviors should be evaluated for dementia.

Home Care
- • Communicate degree of risk to family/caregivers; assess the family and caregiving situation for ability to protect the client and to understand the client's self-mutilative behavior. Provide family and caregivers with guidelines on how to manage self-harm behaviors in the home environment.

- • Establish an emergency plan, including when to use hotlines and 911. Develop a contract with the client and family for use of the emergency plan. Role-play access to the emergency resources with the client and caregivers.
- • Assess the home environment for harmful objects. Have family remove or lock objects as able.
- ▲ If client behaviors intensify, institute an emergency plan for mental health intervention. The degree of disturbance and the ability to manage care safely at home determine the level of services needed to protect the client.
- ▲ Refer for homemaker or psychiatric home healthcare services for respite, client reassurance, and implementation of therapeutic regimen.
- ▲ If the client is on psychotropic medications, assess client and family knowledge of medication administration and side effects.
- ▲ Evaluate the effectiveness and side effects of medications. Accurate clinical feedback improves healthcare provider's ability to prescribe an effective medical regimen specific to client needs.

Client/Family Teaching and Discharge Planning

- • Explain all relevant symptoms, procedures, treatments, and expected outcomes for self-mutilation that is illness based (e.g., borderline personality disorder, autism).
- • Assist family members to understand the complex issues of self-mutilation. Provide instruction on relevant developmental issues and on actions that parents can take to avoid media that glorify self-harm behaviors.
- • Provide written instructions for treatments and procedures for which the client will be responsible.
- • Instruct the client in coping strategies (assertiveness training, impulse control training, deep breathing, and progressive muscle relaxation).
- • Role-play responses to stressful situations (e.g., say, "Tell me how you will respond if someone ignores you").
- • Teach cognitive-behavioral activities, such as active problem-solving, reframing (reappraising the situation from a different perspective), or thought-stopping (in response to a negative thought, picture a large stop sign and replace the image with a prearranged positive alternative). Teach the client to confront his or her own negative thought patterns (or cognitive distortions), such as catastrophizing (expecting the very worst), dichotomous thinking (perceiving events

S

in only one of two opposite categories), or magnification (placing distorted emphasis on a single event).

- ▲ Provide the client and family with phone numbers of appropriate community agencies for therapy and counseling. Continuous follow-up care should be implemented; therefore the method to access this care must be given to the client.
- ▲ Give the client positive things on which to focus by referring to appropriate agencies for job-training skills or education.

Self-Mutilation

NANDA-I Definition

Deliberate self-injurious behavior causing tissue damage with the intent of causing nonfatal injury to attain relief of tension

Defining Characteristics

Abrading; biting; constricting a body part; cuts on body; hitting; ingestion of harmful substance; inhalation of harmful substance; insertion of object into body orifice; picking at wound; scratches on body; self-inflicted burn; severing of a body part

Related Factors

Absence of family confidant; alteration in body image; dissociation; disturbance in interpersonal relationships; eating disorder; emotional disorder; feeling threatened with loss of significant relationship; impaired self-esteem; impulsiveness; inability to express tension verbally; ineffective communication between parent and adolescent; ineffective coping strategies; irresistible urge for self-directed violence; irresistible urge to cut self; isolation from peers; labile behavior; loss of control over problem solving; low self-esteem; mounting tension that is intolerable; negative feeling; pattern of inability to plan solutions; pattern of inability to see long-term consequences; perfectionism; requires rapid stress reduction; substance misuse; use of manipulation to obtain nurturing relationship with others

At-Risk Population

Adolescence; battered child; childhood illness; childhood surgery; developmental delay; family divorce; family history of self-destructive behavior; family substance misuse; history of childhood abuse; history of self-directed violence; incarceration; living in nontraditional setting; peers who self-mutilate; sexual identity crisis; violence between parental figures

Associated Condition

Autism; borderline personality disorder; character disorder; depersonalization; psychotic disorder

Client Outcomes

Client Will (Specify Time Frame)

- Have injuries treated
- Refrain from further self-injury
- State appropriate ways to cope with increased psychological or physiological tension
- Express feelings
- Seek help when having urges to self-mutilate
- Maintain self-control without supervision
- Use appropriate community agencies when caregivers are unable to attend to emotional needs

Nursing Interventions

Note: Before implementing interventions in the face of self-mutilation, nurses should examine their own knowledge base and emotional responses to incidents of self-harm to ensure that interventions will not be based on countertransference reactions.

- • A nonjudgmental approach to clients is critical.
- • Consider using a measure of self-harm risk that is available for clients.
- ▲ Provide medical treatment for injuries. Use aseptic technique when caring for wounds. Care for the wounds in a matter-of-fact manner.
- • Assess for risk of suicide or other self-damaging behaviors.
- • Assess for signs of psychiatric disorders, including depression, anxiety, borderline personality disorder, dissociative disorders, eating disorders, and impulsivity.
- • Assess for the presence of hallucinations. Ask specific questions: "Do you hear voices that other people do not hear?" "Are they telling you to hurt yourself?"
- ▲ Assure the client that he or she will be safe during hallucinations, and engage supportively. Provide referrals for medication.
- ▲ Assess for the presence of medical disorders, mental retardation, medication effects, or disorders such as autism that may include self-mutilation. Initiate referral for evaluation and treatment as appropriate.
- ▲ Case finding and referral by school nurses for psychological or psychiatric treatment is critical.
- • Monitor the client's behavior closely, using engagement and support as elements of safety checks while avoiding intrusive overstimulation.
- • Focus on understanding the function that self-harm serves for the client and on managing the client's distress.

S

- Establish trust, listen to client, convey safety, and assist in developing positive goals for the future.
- Problem-solving therapy, access to emergency contacts, and long-term psychological therapy may be helpful. Although some studies suggest interventions that may be helpful, findings should be used with caution.
- ▲ Use a collaborative approach for care. A collaborative approach to care is more helpful to the client.
- Refer to the care plan for Risk for **Self-Mutilation** for additional information.

Pediatric

- Self harm is a major concern in children and adolescents, although few interventions have been adequately tested.

Home Care and Client/Family Teaching and Discharge Planning

- See the care plan for Risk for **Self-Mutilation.**

Self-Neglect

NANDA-I Definition

S

A constellation of culturally framed behaviors involving one or more self-care activities in which there is a failure to maintain a socially accepted standard of health and well-being (Gibbons, Lauder, & Ludwick, 2006)

Defining Characteristics

Insufficient environmental hygiene; insufficient personal hygiene; nonadherence to health activity

Related Factors

Deficient executive function; fear of institutionalization; inability to maintain control; lifestyle choice; stressors; substance misuse

Associated Condition

Alteration in cognitive functioning; Capgras syndrome; frontal lobe dysfunction; functional impairment; learning disability; malingering; psychiatric disorder; psychotic disorder

Client Outcomes

Client Will (Specify Time Frame)

- Reveal improvement in cognition (e.g., if reversible and treatable)
- Show improvement in mental health problems
- Show improvement in chronic medical problems
- Demonstrate improvement in functional status (e.g., basic and IADLs)

- Demonstrate adherence to health activities (e.g., medications and medical appointments)
- Exhibit improved personal hygiene
- Exhibit improved environmental hygiene
- Have fewer hospitalizations and emergency room visits
- Increase safety of client
- Increase safety of community in which client lives
- Agree to necessary personal and environmental changes that eliminate risk/endangerment to self or others (e.g., neighbors)
- Improve social networks
- Identify eligibility for public services and other benefits

Note: Because self-neglect is present along a continuum of severity and includes an array of behavioral and environmental issues, a change in a client's status must occur in such a way that balances obligation for protection and respects individual rights (e.g., autonomy and self-determination) while ensuring individual health and well-being. This is accomplished through a client–provider partnership that keeps the door open even though the client may initially decline help. Building a relationship with the client will improve trust and assist in developing an individually tailored care plan to address problems contributing to self-neglect. Interdisciplinary collaboration and teamwork, and in some instances assistance of next of kin and/or adult protective services (APS), may be needed (e.g., a state agency or local social services program).

S

Nursing Interventions

- Monitor individuals with acute or chronic mental and physical illness for defining characteristics for self-neglect.
- Assist individuals with complex mental and physical health issues to adopt positive health behaviors so that they may maintain their health status in the community.
- Assist individuals with reconnecting with family, friends, and other social networks available to them.
- Assist individuals whose self-care is failing with managing their medications regimen.
- Assist persons with self-care deficits caused by ADL or IADL impairments.
- Assess persons with failing self-care for changes in cognitive function (e.g., dementia or delirium).
- Refer persons with failing self-care to appropriate specialists (e.g., psychologist, psychiatrist, social worker) and therapists (e.g., physical therapy, occupational therapy).

- • Use behavioral modification as appropriate to bring about client changes that lead to improvement in personal hygiene, environmental hygiene, and adherence to medical regimen.
- • Monitor persons with substance abuse problems (i.e., drugs, alcohol, smoking) for adequate safety.
- ▲ Refer persons with failing self-care who are significantly impaired cognitively (e.g., executive function, dementia) or functionally and/or who are suspected victims of abuse to APS.

Geriatric

- ▲ Assess client's socioeconomic status and refer for appropriate support.
- ▲ Refer persons demonstrating a significant decline in self-care abilities (e.g., posing a threat to themselves or to their community) for formal evaluation of capacity and executive function.

Multicultural

- • Deliver healthcare that is sensitive to the culture and philosophy of individuals whose self-care appears inadequate.

Sexual Dysfunction

NANDA-I Definition

A state in which an individual experiences a change in sexual function during the sexual response phases of desire, arousal, and/or orgasm, which is viewed as unsatisfying, unrewarding, or inadequate.

Defining Characteristics

Alteration in sexual activity; alteration in sexual excitation; alteration in sexual satisfaction; change in interest toward others; change in self-interest; change in sexual role; decrease in sexual desire; perceived sexual limitation; seeking confirmation of desirability; undesired change in sexual function

Related Factors

Absence of privacy; inadequate role model; insufficient knowledge about sexual function; misinformation about sexual function; presence of abuse; psychosocial abuse; value conflict; vulnerability

At-Risk Population

Absence of significant other

Associated Condition

Alteration in body function; alteration in body structure

Client Outcomes

Client Will (Specify Time Frame)

- • Identify individual cause of sexual dysfunction

- Identify stressors that contribute to dysfunction
- Discuss alternative, satisfying, and acceptable sexual practices for self and partner
- Identify the degree of sexual interest by the client and partner
- Adapt sexual technique as needed to cope with sexual problems
- Discuss with partner concerns about body image and sex role

Nursing Interventions

- • Gather the client's sexual history, noting normal patterns of functioning and the client's vocabulary, and encouraging clients to ask questions or discuss sexual problems experienced.
- ▲ Assess duration and risk factors for sexual dysfunction and explore potential causes such as medications, medical problems, aging process, or psychosocial issues.
- ▲ Assess for history of sexual abuse.
- ▲ Assess and provide treatment for sexual dysfunction, involving the person's partner in the process, and evaluating pharmacological and nonpharmacological interventions.
- • Assess risk factors for sexual dysfunction, especially with varying sexual partners.
- • Observe for stress and anxiety as possible causes of dysfunction.
- ▲ Assess for depression as a possible cause of sexual dysfunction, and institute appropriate treatment.
- • Observe for grief-related loss (e.g., amputation, mastectomy, ostomy), because a change in body image often precedes sexual dysfunction. See care plan for Disturbed **Body Image.**
- ▲ Explore physical causes of sexual dysfunction such as diabetes, cardiovascular disease, arthritis, or BPH.
- ▲ Consider that ED may indicate the presence of cardiovascular disease, and screening and referral of men is recommended.
- • Certain chronic diseases such as cancer often have significant effects on sexual function, and both the disease process and treatment can contribute to sexual dysfunction.
- • Consider that neurological diseases can affect sexual function directly, with secondary effects caused by disability related to the illness and social and emotional effects.
- • Explore behavioral or other causes of sexual dysfunction, such as smoking, dietary factors, or obesity.
- ▲ Consider medications as a cause of sexual dysfunction.
- ▲ Refer to appropriate medical providers for consideration of medication for premature ejaculation, ED, or orgasmic problems.

- Refer to the care plan **Ineffective Sexuality Pattern** for additional interventions.

Geriatric

▲ Carefully assess the sexuality needs and sexual dysfunction of older adults and refer for counseling if needed.
- Teach about normal changes that occur with aging that may be perceived as sexual dysfunction, such as reduction in vaginal lubrication and reduction in duration and resolution of orgasm for women; for men these changes include increased time required for erection and for subsequent erections, erection without ejaculation, less firm erection, and decreased volume of seminal fluid.
- If prescribed, instruct clients with chronic pain to take pain medication before sexual activity.
- See care plan for **Ineffective Sexuality Pattern**.

Multicultural

- Evaluate culturally influenced risk factors for sexual function and dysfunction.
- Validate client feelings and emotions regarding the changes in sexual behavior by letting the client know that the nurse heard and understands what was said, promoting the nurse–client relationship.

Home Care

S
- Previously discussed interventions may be adapted for home care use.

▲ Identify specific sources of concern about sexual dysfunction and provide reassurance and instruction on appropriate expectations as indicated.

▲ Confirm that physical reasons for dysfunction have been addressed, and refer for therapy and/or support groups if appropriate.
- See care plan for Ineffective Sexuality Pattern.

Client/Family Teaching and Discharge Planning

- Provide accurate information for clients regarding interventions for sexual dysfunction.
- Teach the client and partner about condom use, for those at risk.

▲ Refer to appropriate community resources, such as a clinical specialist, family counselor, or cardiac rehabilitation, including the partner if appropriate; for complex issues, a referral to a sex counselor, urologist, gynecologist, or other specialist may be needed.

▲ Refer for medical advice when ED lasts longer than 2 months or is recurring.
- Teach the following interventions to decrease the likelihood of ED: limit or avoid the use of alcohol, stop smoking, exercise regularly,

reduce stress, get enough sleep, deal with anxiety or depression, and see a healthcare provider for regular checkups and medical screening tests.
- See care plan for Ineffective **Sexuality** pattern.

Ineffective Sexuality Pattern

NANDA-I Definition

Expressions of concern regarding own sexuality

Defining Characteristics

Alterations in relationship with significant other; alteration in sexual activity; alteration in sexual behavior; change in sexual role; difficulty with sexual activity; difficulty with sexual behavior; value conflict

Related Factors

Conflict about sexual orientation; conflict about variant preference; fear of pregnancy; fear of sexually transmitted infection; impaired relationship with a significant other; inadequate role model; insufficient knowledge about alternatives related to sexuality; skill deficit about alternatives related to sexuality; absence of privacy

At-Risk Population

Absence of significant other

Client Outcomes

Client Will (Specify Time Frame)

- State knowledge of difficulties, limitations, or changes in sexual behaviors or activities
- State knowledge of sexual anatomy and functioning
- State acceptance of altered body structure or functioning
- Describe acceptable alternative sexual practices
- Identify importance of discussing sexual issues with significant other
- Describe practice of safe sex with regard to pregnancy and avoidance of sexually transmitted infections (STIs)

Nursing Interventions

- After establishing rapport or therapeutic relationship, give the client permission to discuss issues dealing with sexuality, for example, "Have you been or are you concerned about functioning sexually because of your health status?"
- Use assessment questions and standardized instruments to assess sexual problems, where possible.

▲ Assess any risks associated with sexual activity, particularly coronary risks.

- Assess knowledge about sexual functioning and return to sexual activity after experiencing a health problem with both patients and partners.
- Encourage the client to discuss concerns with his or her partner.
- Explore attitudes about sexual intimacy and changes in sexuality patterns.
- Assess psychosocial function such as anxiety, fear, depression, and low self-esteem.
- Discuss alternative sexual expressions for altered body functioning or structure, including closeness and sexual and nonsexual touching as other forms of expression.
- Assess the client's sexual orientation and usual pattern of sexual activities, and discuss prevention of illnesses for which the client may be at increased risk (e.g., anorectal cancer), asking specific questions about sexual orientation, for example, "Do you have sexual relationships with men, women, or both?" Assess use of safer sex practices (e.g., condom use); the frequency of anal intercourse; number of sexual partners in the last year; last HIV screening/results; and use of medications, alcohol, and illicit drugs.
- Specific guidelines for sexual activity for clients who have had total hip arthroplasty (THA) include the following: sexual activity can be generally resumed 1 to 2 months after surgery, and positioning to avoid hip dislocation, e.g., a supine position ("missionary") at maximum abduction in extension, or the man and woman standing, with the woman's legs slightly bent and the man approaching the woman from behind (McFadden, 2013).
- Specific guidelines for those who have had an MI include the following: sexual activity can generally be resumed 1 week after MI unless complications are experienced, such as arrhythmias or cardiac arrest, if the client does not have cardiac symptoms during mild to moderate physical activity; begin with activities that require less exertion, such as fondling or kissing, building confidence in tolerance for sexual activity prior to sexual intercourse; engage in sexual activity in familiar surroundings with the usual partner; have a comfortable room temperature, and be well rested to minimize cardiac stress; avoid heavy meals or alcohol for 2 to 3 hours before sexual activity; and choose a position of comfort to minimize stress of the cardiac client (Steinke et al., 2013).
- Specific guidelines include that those who have had complete coronary revascularization, in addition to those mentioned with MI, including those with successful percutaneous cardiovascular

revascularization without complication, can resume sex within a few days, and those who have had standard coronary artery bypass grafting (CABG) or noncoronary open heart surgery may resume sex in 6 to 8 weeks. Incisional pain with sexual activity can be managed by premedicating with a mild pain reliever, and reassurance should be provided to the partner that sexual activity will not harm the sternum as long as direct pressure is avoided (Steinke et al., 2013).

- Specific guidelines for those with an implantable cardioverter defibrillator (ICD) include returning to sexual activity is generally safe after ICD implantation if moderate physical activity does not precipitate arrhythmias; avoid strain on the incision at the implant site; assure the client and partner that fears about being shocked during sexual activity are normal; if the ICD discharges with sexual activity, the client should stop, rest, and later notify the healthcare provider that the device fired so that a determination can be made if this was an appropriate shock or not; report any dyspnea, chest pain, or dizziness with sexual activity (Steinke et al., 2013).
- Specific guidelines for those with chronic lung disease include planning for sexual activity when energy level is highest; use of controlled breathing techniques; avoiding physical exertion prior to sexual activity; using positions that minimize shortness of breath, such as a semireclining position; engaging in sexual activity when medications are at peak effectiveness; use of an oxygen cannula, if prescribed, to provide oxygen before, during, or after sex; and use of continuous positive airway pressure (CPAP) therapy, if prescribed (Steinke, 2013b).
- Specific guidelines for those with MS include treatment of symptoms with prescribed medications, assessing changes in body image, and supportive therapies to assist with a more satisfying sexual experience, including treatment of neuropathic pain, sexual positions that are most supportive, discussing changes in sensation and stimulation with the partner, use of stretching exercise for tight muscles prior to sexual activity, and avoiding a distended bowel or bladder that may cause discomfort.
- Refer to the care plan **Sexual** dysfunction for additional interventions.

Pediatric

- Initiate discussions regarding sexual health, attitudes, and knowledge about sexual behavior, and sexual abstinence, providing information that is age-appropriate and accurate regarding sexual activity and risky sexual behaviors.

S

- Provide age-appropriate information for adolescents regarding HIV/AIDS and sexual behavior, and discuss STIs, particularly human papillomavirus, including the risks of perinatal transmission and methods to reduce risks among HIV-infected adolescents.
- Provide age-appropriate information regarding potential for sexual abuse.

Geriatric

- Carefully assess the sexuality needs of the older client and refer for counseling if needed; the ability to form satisfying social relationships and to be intimate with others, including building strong emotional intimate connections, contributes to adaptation and successful aging (Steinke, 2013b).
- ▲ Explore possible changes in sexuality related to health status, menopause, medications, and sexual risk, and make appropriate referrals.
- Allow the client to verbalize feelings regarding loss of sexual partner, and acknowledge problems such as disapproving children, lack of available partner for women, and environmental variables that make forming new relationships difficult.
- ▲ Provide a milieu that allows for discussion of sexual issues and a higher level of sexual satisfaction, including allowing couples to room together and the provision of privacy.
- See care plan for **Sexual** dysfunction.

Multicultural

- Assess for the influence of cultural beliefs, norms, and values on client's perceptions of sexual behavior.

Home Care

- Previously discussed interventions may be adapted for home care use. Also see care plan for **Sexual** dysfunction.
- Help the client and significant other identify a place and time in the home and daily living for privacy in sharing sexual or relationship activity, and, if necessary, help the client communicate the need for privacy to family members.
- Confirm that physical reasons for dysfunction have been addressed, and provide support for coping behaviors, including participation in support groups or therapy if appropriate.

Client/Family Teaching and Discharge Planning

- ▲ Refer to appropriate community agencies (e.g., certified sex counselor, Reach to Recovery, Ostomy Association, American Association of Sex Educators, Counselors, and Therapists).

▲ Sexuality education is important to all populations, whether hearing or deaf, sighted or blind, disabled or not disabled; discuss contraceptive choices as appropriate, safer sexual practices, and refer to a health professional (e.g., gynecologist, urologist, nurse practitioner).

Risk for Shock

NANDA-I Definition

Susceptible to an inadequate blood flow to the body's tissues that may lead to cellular dysfunction, which may compromise health

Risk Factors

Bleeding; deficient fluid volume; factors identified by standardized, validated screening tool; hyperthermia; hypothermia; hypoxemia; hypoxia; inadequate knowledge of bleeding management strategies; inadequate knowledge of infection management strategies; inadequate knowledge of modifiable factors; ineffective medication self-management; nonhemorrhagic fluid losses; smoking; unstable blood pressure

At Risk Population

Individuals admitted to the emergency care unit; individuals at extremes of age; individuals with history of myocardial infarction

Associated Condition

Artificial respiration; burns; chemotherapy; diabetes mellitus; embolism; heart diseases; hypersensitivity; immunosuppression; infections; lactate levels ≥ 2 mmol/L; liver diseases; medical devices; neoplasms; nervous system diseases; pancreatitis; radiotherapy; sepsis; sequential Organ Failure Assessment (SOFA) Score ≥ 3; simplified Acute Physiology Score (SAPS) III > 70; spinal cord injuries; surgical procedures; systemic inflammatory response syndrome (SIRS); trauma

Client Outcomes

Client Will (Specify Time Frame)

- Discuss precautions to prevent complications of disease
- Maintain adherence to agreed-on medication regimens
- Maintain adequate hydration
- Monitor for infection signs and symptoms
- Maintain a mean arterial pressure (MAP) above 65 mm Hg
- Maintain a heart rate between 60 and 100 with a normal rhythm
- Maintain urine output greater than 0.5 mL/kg/hr
- Maintain warm, dry skin

S

Nursing Interventions

- Review data pertaining to client risk status including age, primary diseases, immunosuppression, antibiotic use, and presence of hemodynamic alterations such as tachycardia, tachypnea, and decrease in blood pressure (BP).
- Review client's medical and surgical history, noting conditions that place the client at higher risk for shock, including trauma, myocardial infarction, pulmonary embolism, head injury, dehydration, infection, endocrine problems, certain medications, and pregnancy.
- Complete a full nursing physical examination. However, the presence of skin mottling, especially over the knees, ears, and fingers, suggests tissue hypoperfusion states often seen in shock (Contou & de Prost, 2016).
- Monitor circulatory status (e.g., BP, MAP, skin color, skin temperature, heart sounds, heart rate and rhythm, presence and quality of peripheral pulses, pulse oximetry, and end-tidal carbon dioxide monitoring [$EtCO_2$]).
- Maintain intravenous (IV) access and provide isotonic IV fluids such as 0.9% normal saline or Ringer's lactate as ordered; these fluids are commonly used in the prevention and treatment of shock.
- Monitor for inadequate tissue oxygenation (e.g., apprehension, increased anxiety, altered mental status, agitation, oliguria, cool/mottled periphery) and determinants of tissue oxygen delivery (e.g., Pao_2, SpO_2, $ScvO_2$/SvO_2, MAP, hemoglobin levels, lactate levels, CO).

▲ Maintain vital signs (BP, pulse, respirations, and temperature) and pulse oximetry within normal parameters.

▲ Administer oxygen immediately to maintain SpO_2 greater than 90%, and antibiotics and other medications as prescribed to any client presenting with symptoms of early shock.

▲ Monitor trends in noninvasive hemodynamic parameters (e.g., MAP) as appropriate.

▲ Monitor serum lactate levels and interpret them within the context of each client.

Critical Care

▲ Prepare the client for the placement of an additional IV line, central line, and/or a pulmonary artery catheter as prescribed.

▲ Monitor trends in hemodynamic parameters (e.g., central venous pressure [CVP], CO, cardiac index [CI], systemic vascular resistance [SVR], pulmonary artery pressure [PAP], and MAP) as appropriate.

S

▲ Monitor electrocardiography. Tachycardia may be present as a result of decreased fluid volume, which will be seen before a decrease in BP as a compensatory mechanism.
▲ Monitor arterial blood gases, coagulation, blood chemistries, blood glucose, cardiac enzymes, blood cultures, and hematology labs.
▲ Administer vasopressor agents as prescribed.
• If the client is in shock, refer to the following care plans: Risk for ineffective **Renal** perfusion, Risk for ineffective **Gastrointestinal** perfusion, Impaired **Gas** exchange, and Decreased **Cardiac** output.

Client/Family Teaching and Discharge Planning

▲ Teach client and family or significant others about any medications prescribed. Instruct the client to report any adverse side effects to his or her healthcare provider.
• Instruct the client and family on disease process and rationale for care.
• Instruct clients and their family members on the signs and symptoms of low BP to report to their healthcare provider (dizziness, lightheadedness, fainting, dehydration and unusual thirst, lack of concentration, blurred vision, nausea, cold, clammy, pale skin, rapid and shallow breathing, fatigue, and depression).
• Promote a culture of client safety and individual accountability.

Impaired Sitting

S

NANDA-I Definition

Limitation of ability to independently and purposefully attain and/or maintain a rest position that is supported by the buttocks and thighs, in which the torso is upright

Defining Characteristics

Impaired ability to adjust position of one or both lower limbs on uneven surface; impaired ability to attain a balanced position of the torso; impaired ability to flex or move both hips; impaired ability to flex or move both knees; impaired ability to maintain the torso in balanced position; impaired ability to stress torso with body weight

Related Factors

Insufficient endurance; insufficient energy; insufficient muscle strength; malnutrition; pain; self-imposed relief posture

Associated Condition

Alteration in cognitive functioning; impaired metabolic functioning; neurological disorder; orthopedic surgery; prescribed posture; psychological disorder; sarcopenia

Client Outcomes

Client Will (Specify Time Frame)

- Verbalize importance of being able to sit as a method to engage in activities of daily living
- Understand somatic physiology of posture control
- Choose healthcare options that enhance ability to sit
- Engage in physical conditioning exercises to enhance sitting ability
- Understand relationship of posture and emotions
- Control pain to increase ability to sit

Nursing Interventions

- Acknowledge the importance of being able to sit as a method to engage in activities of daily living.
- Understand the somatic physiology of posture control.
- Choose the musculoskeletal options that enhance ability to sit properly.
- Engage in physical conditioning exercises to enhance proper sitting ability.
- Understand the relationship of posture and emotions.
- Maintain pain levels below 3 to 4 on a 0 to 10 scale to increase ability to sit.

Pediatric

- Increase cognitive and physical functioning by promoting proper sitting ability.

Geriatric

- Increase cognitive and physical functioning by promoting prober sitting ability.

Multicultural

- Understand the importance of unimpaired sitting to different populations.

Home Care

- Encourage proper sitting posture in the home environment to promote health.

Impaired Skin Integrity

NANDA-I Definition

Altered epidermis and/or dermis

Defining Characteristics

Abscess; acute pain; altered skin color; altered turgor; bleeding; blister; desquamation; disrupted skin surface; dry skin; excoriation; foreign matter piercing skin; hematoma; localized area hot to touch; macerated skin; peeling; pruritus

Related Factors

External

Excessive moisture; excretions; humidity; hyperthermia; hypothermia; inadequate caregiver knowledge about maintaining tissue integrity; inadequate caregiver knowledge about protecting tissue integrity; inadequate use of chemical agent; pressure over bony prominence; psychomotor agitation; secretions; shearing forces; surface friction; use of linen with insufficient moisture wicking property

Internal

Body mass index above normal range for age and gender; body mass index below normal range for age and gender; decreased physical activity; decreased physical mobility; edema; inadequate adherence to incontinence treatment regimen; inadequate knowledge about maintaining tissue integrity; inadequate knowledge about protecting tissue integrity; malnutrition; psychogenic factor; self mutilation; smoking; substance misuse; water-electrolyte imbalance

At-Risk Population

Individuals at extremes of age; individuals in intensive care units; individuals in long-term care facilities; individuals in palliative care settings; individuals receiving home-based care

Associated Conditions

Altered pigmentation; anemia; cardiovascular diseases; decreased level of consciousness; decreased tissue oxygenation; decreased tissue perfusion; diabetes mellitus; hormonal change; immobilization; immunodeficiency; impaired metabolism; infections; medical devices; neoplasms; peripheral neuropathy; pharmaceutical preparations; punctures; sensation disorders

S

Client Outcomes

Client Will (Specify Time Frame)

- Regain integrity of skin surface
- Report any altered sensation or pain at site of skin impairment
- Demonstrate understanding of plan to heal skin and prevent reinjury or complications
- Describe measures to protect and heal the skin and to care for any skin lesion

Nursing Interventions

- NPUAP redefined the definition of a pressure ulcer, now referred to as pressure injuries, during the NPUAP 2016 Staging Consensus Conference. The new definitions more accurately define alterations in tissue integrity from pressure as the following: *A pressure injury is localized damage to the skin and underlying soft tissue usually over a bony prominence or related to a medical or other device. The injury can present as intact skin or an open ulcer and may be painful. The injury occurs as a result of intense and/or prolonged pressure or pressure in combination with shear. The tolerance of soft tissue for pressure and shear may also be affected by microclimate, nutrition, perfusion, comorbidities, and condition of the soft tissue* (NPUAP, 2016).

- Pressure ulcer is no longer a current clinical term; rather, pressure injury is used to describe an alteration in tissue integrity from pressure (NPUAP, 2016). Similarly, hospital-acquired pressure ulcers (HAPUs) are currently referred to as hospital-acquired pressure injury (HAPIs).
- Assess site of skin impairment and determine cause or type of wound (e.g., acute or chronic wound, burn, dermatological lesion, pressure injury, skin tear).
- Use a risk assessment tool to systematically assess client risk factors for skin breakdown caused by pressure.
- Determine the extent of the skin impairment caused by pressure using the revised classification system and definition for pressure injuries (NPUAP, 2016).
  - **Stage 1 Pressure Injury:** Non-blanchable erythema of intact skin
    Area of localized nonbleachable erythema that may appear differently in darkly pigmented skin, and changes in sensation, temperature, or firmness may precede visual changes. Color changes do not include purple or maroon discoloration, which is more likely to indicate deep tissue pressure injury (NPUAP, 2016).
  - **Stage 2 Pressure Injury:** Partial-thickness skin loss with exposed dermis
    Partial-thickness skin loss with exposed dermis in which the wound bed is pink/red and moist and adipose (fat) and deeper tissues are not visible. Granulation tissue, slough, and eschar are not present. A stage 2 pressure injury may also present as an intact or ruptured blister. These injuries commonly result from adverse microclimate and shear in the skin over the pelvis and shear in the heel. This stage should not be used to describe moisture-associated skin damage (MASD) including incontinence-associated dermatitis (IAD), intertriginous dermatitis (ITD), medical adhesive–related skin injury (MARSI), or traumatic wounds (skin tears, burns, and abrasions) (NPUAP 2016).
  - **Stage 3 Pressure Injury:** Full-thickness skin loss
    Full-thickness loss of skin, in which adipose is visible and

S

granulation tissue and epibole (rolled wound edges) are often present and undermining/tunneling may occur. Slough and/or eschar may also be visible. Fascia, muscle, tendon, ligament, cartilage, and/or bone are not exposed. The depth of tissue damage varies by anatomical location, and areas of significant adiposity can develop deep wounds. If slough or eschar obscures the extent of tissue loss this is an unstageable pressure injury (NPUAP, 2016).

- **Stage 4 Pressure Injury:** Full-thickness skin and tissue loss
  Full-thickness skin and tissue loss with exposed or directly palpable fascia, muscle, tendon, ligament, cartilage or bone, and slough and/or eschar may be visible. Epibole, undermining, and/or tunneling often occur, and depth varies by anatomical location. If slough or eschar obscures the extent of tissue loss, this is an unstageable pressure injury (NPUAP, 2016).
- **Deep Tissue Pressure Injury:** Persistent nonblanchable deep red, maroon, or purple discoloration
  Intact or nonintact skin with localized area of persistent nonblanchable deep red, maroon, or purple discoloration or epidermal separation revealing a dark wound bed or blood-filled blister. Pain and temperature change often precede skin color changes. Discoloration may appear differently in darkly pigmented skin. This injury results from intense and/or prolonged pressure and shear forces at the bone–muscle interface. The wound may evolve rapidly to reveal the actual extent of tissue injury, or it may resolve without tissue loss. If necrotic tissue, subcutaneous tissue, granulation tissue, fascia, muscle, or other underlying structures are visible, this indicates a full-thickness pressure injury (unstageable, stage 3, or stage 4). Do not use the term deep tissue pressure injury to describe vascular, traumatic, neuropathic, or dermatological conditions (NPUAP, 2016).
- **Unstageable Pressure Injury:** Obscured full-thickness skin and tissue loss
  Full-thickness skin and tissue loss in which the extent of tissue damage within the ulcer cannot be confirmed because it is obscured by slough or eschar. If slough or eschar is removed, a stage 3 or stage 4 pressure injury will be revealed. Stable eschar (i.e., dry, adherent, intact without erythema or fluctuance) on the heel or ischemic limb should not be softened or removed (NPUAP, 2016).

- ○ **Mechanical device–related pressure injury** is used to describe alterations in tissue integrity caused by pressure from mechanical devices used in the care of clients (e.g., indwelling urinary catheters, endotracheal tubes, nasogastric tubes, drains, etc.). The pressure injury typically conforms to the shape of the device (NPUAP, 2016).
- • Inspect and monitor site of skin impairment at least once a day for color changes, redness, swelling, warmth, pain, or other signs of infection. Determine whether the client is experiencing changes in sensation or pain. Closely assess high-risk areas such as bony prominences, skinfolds, the sacrum, and heels.
- • Monitor the client's skin care practices, noting type of soap or other cleansing agents used, temperature of water, and frequency of skin cleansing.
- • Consider using normal saline to clean the pressure injury or as ordered by the healthcare provider, but if necessary, tap water suitable for drinking may be used to clean the wound.
- • Maintain good skin hygiene, using mild nondetergent soap, drying gently, and lubricating with lotion or emollient to reduce the risk of dermal trauma, improve circulation, and promote comfort. Provide client education on good skin hygiene practices (Doenges, Moorhouse, & Murr, 2016).
- • Urinary and fecal incontinence can cause skin breakdown.
- • For clients with limited mobility and activity, use a risk assessment tool to systematically assess immobility and activity-related risk factors.
- • Do not position the client on site of skin impairment. If consistent with overall client management goals, reposition the client as determined by individualized tissue tolerance and overall condition. Reposition and transfer the client with care to protect against the adverse effects of external mechanical forces such as pressure, friction, and shear.
- • Evaluate for use of support surfaces (specialty mattresses, beds), chair cushions, or devices as appropriate. Maintain the head of the bed at the lowest possible degree of elevation to reduce shear and friction, and use lift devices, pillows, foam wedges, and pressure-reducing devices in the bed (Brienza et al., 2016; NPUAP/EPUAP, 2014).
- • Implement a written treatment plan for topical treatment of the site of skin impairment.
- • Select a topical treatment that will maintain a moist wound-healing environment (stage 2) that is balanced with the need to absorb exudate. Stage 1 pressure injuries may be managed by keeping the client off of

S

the area and using a protective dressing (Baranoski & Ayello, 2016).

- Avoid massaging around the site of skin impairment and over bony prominences.
- Assess the client's nutritional status. Refer for a nutritional consult and/or institute dietary supplements as necessary.
- Identify the client's phase of wound healing (inflammation, proliferation, or maturation) and stage of injury.

Home Care

- The interventions described previously may be adapted for home care use.
- Instruct and assist the client and caregivers in how to change dressings and maintain a clean environment. Provide written instructions and observe the client completing the dressing change before hospital discharge and in the home setting.
- Educate client and caregivers on proper nutrition, signs and symptoms of infection, and when to call the agency and/or healthcare provider with concerns.
- It may be beneficial to initiate a consultation in a case assignment with a wound, ostomy, continence nurse (or wounds specialist) to establish a comprehensive plan for complex wounds.

Client/Family Teaching and Discharge Planning

- Teach skin and wound assessment and ways to monitor for signs and symptoms of infection, complications, and healing. Early assessment and intervention help prevent serious problems from developing.
- Teach the client why a topical treatment has been selected.
- If consistent with overall client management goals, teach how to reposition as client condition warrants.
- Teach the client to use pillows, foam wedges, chair cushions, and pressure-redistribution devices to prevent pressure injury (Brienza et al., 2016).

Risk for Impaired Skin Integrity

NANDA-I Definition

Susceptible to alteration in epidermis and/or dermis, which may compromise health

Risk Factors

External

Excessive moisture; excretions; humidity; hyperthermia; hypothermia; inadequate caregiver knowledge about maintaining tissue integrity; inadequate caregiver knowledge about protecting tissue integrity; inadequate use of chemical agent; pressure over bony prominence; psychomotor agitation; secretions; shearing forces; surface friction; use of linen with insufficient moisture wicking property

Internal

Body mass index above normal range for age and gender; body mass index below normal range for age and gender; decreased physical activity; decreased physical mobility; edema; inadequate adherence to incontinence treatment regimen; inadequate knowledge about maintaining tissue integrity; inadequate knowledge about protecting tissue integrity; malnutrition; psychogenic factor; self mutilation; smoking; substance misuse; water-electrolyte imbalance

At-Risk Population

Individuals at extremes of age; individuals in intensive care units; individuals in long-term care facilities; individuals in palliative care settings; individuals receiving home-based care

Associated Condition

Altered pigmentation; anemia; cardiovascular diseases; decreased level of consciousness; decreased tissue oxygenation; decreased tissue perfusion; diabetes mellitus; hormonal change; immobilization; immunodeficiency; impaired metabolism; infections; medical devices; neoplasms; peripheral neuropathy; pharmaceutical preparations; punctures; sensation disorders

S

Client Outcomes

Client Will (Specify Time Frame)

- Report altered sensation or pain at risk areas as soon as noted
- Demonstrate understanding of personal risk factors for impaired skin integrity
- Verbalize a personal plan for preventing impaired skin integrity

Nursing Interventions

- The NPUAP redefined the definition of a pressure ulcer, which is now referred to as a pressure injury, during the NPUAP 2016 Staging Consensus Conference in 2016. The new definition more accurately defines alterations in tissue integrity from pressure as the following: A pressure injury is localized damage to the skin and underlying soft tissue usually over a bony prominence or related to a medical or other device. The injury can present as intact skin or an open ulcer and may be painful. The injury occurs as a result of intense and/or prolonged pressure or pressure in combinations with shear. The tolerance of soft tissue for pressure and shear may also be affected by microclimate, nutrition, perfusion, comorbidities, and conditions of the soft tissue (NPUAP, 2016).

- • Identify clients at risk for impaired skin integrity as a result of immobility, chronological age, malnutrition, incontinence, compromised perfusion, immunocompromised status, or chronic medical condition, such as diabetes mellitus, spinal cord injury, or renal failure.
- • Inspect and monitor skin condition at least once a day for color or texture changes, redness, localized heat, edema or induration, pressure damage, dermatological conditions, or lesions and any incontinence-associated dermatitis. Determine whether the client is experiencing loss of sensation or pain.
- • Monitor the client's skin care practices, noting type of soap or other cleansing agents used, temperature of water, and frequency of skin cleansing.
- • Keep skin clean and dry. Cleanse the skin gently with pH-balanced cleansers. Consider use of skin moisturizers to hydrate skin to reduce risk of skin damage. Protect skin from exposure to excessive moisture with a barrier product to reduce the risk of pressure-related damage (NPUAP/EPUAP, 2014).
- ▲ Develop and implement an individualized continence management plan. Cleanse the skin promptly after episodes of incontinence. Use incontinence skin barriers including creams, ointments, pastes, or film-forming skin protectants as needed to protect skin and maintain intact skin (Ratliff et al., 2017).
- • For clients with limited mobility, inspect and monitor condition of skin covering bony prominences.
- • Implement and communicate a client-specific prevention plan.
- • At-risk clients should be frequently repositioned. Frequency of repositioning will be influenced by variables concerning the individual's independent mobility and the support surface in use. Frequency of repositioning should be determined by the individual's tissue tolerance and medical condition (NPUAP/EPUAP, 2014). Use of heel suspension devices can remove pressure from the heels and support the lower extremity of individuals who are unable to keep pressure off the heels, without placing pressure on the Achilles tendon (Ratliff et al., 2017).
- • Evaluate for use of specialty mattresses, beds, or devices as appropriate (Lippoldt et al., 2014; Brienza et al., 2016).

- • Avoid massaging or vigorously rubbing over bony prominences.
- ▲ Assess the client's nutritional status; refer for a nutritional consult, and/or institute dietary supplements.

Geriatric

- • Limit the number of complete baths to two or three per week, and alternate them with partial baths. Use a tepid water temperature (between 90° F and 105° F) for bathing or use a no-rinse alternative product.
- • Use lotions and moisturizers to prevent skin from drying out, especially in the winter.
- • Increase fluid intake within cardiac and renal limits to a minimum of 1500 mL/day.
- • Increase humidity in the environment, especially during the winter, by using a humidifier or placing a container of water on a warm object.

Home Care

- • Assess client and caregiver ability to recognize potential risk for skin breakdown. Provide resources for client/caregiver to contact healthcare provider with questions/concerns related to skin and incontinence care as needed (Vrtis, 2013). Engage family, caregivers, or legal guardian when establishing goals of care and validate their understanding of these goals. Educate the individual and his or her caregiver regarding skin changes in aging and at end of life (NPUAP/EPUAP, 2014).
- ▲ Initiate a consultation in a case assignment with a wound care specialist or wound, ostomy, and continence nurse to establish a comprehensive plan as soon as possible (Vrtis, 2013).
- • See the care plan for Impaired **Skin** integrity.

Client/Family Teaching and Discharge Planning

- • Teach the client skin assessment and ways to monitor for impending skin breakdown. Early assessment and intervention help prevent the development of serious problems.
- • If consistent with overall client management goals, teach how to turn and reposition the client.
- • Teach the client and/or caregivers to use pillows, foam wedges, and pressure-reducing devices to prevent pressure injury (NPUAP/EPUAP, 2014).

Sleep Deprivation

NANDA-I Definition

Prolonged periods of time without sustained natural, periodic suspension of relative consciousness that provides rest

Defining Characteristics

Agitation; alteration in concentration; anxiety; apathy; combativeness; confusion; decrease in functional ability; decrease in reaction time; drowsiness; fatigue; fleeting nystagmus; hallucinations; hand tremors; heightened sensitivity to pain; irritability; lethargy; malaise; perceptual disorders; restlessness; transient paranoia

Related Factors

Age-related sleep stage shifts; average daily physical activity less than recommended for gender and age; environmental barrier; late day confusion; nonrestorative sleep pattern; overstimulating environment; prolonged discomfort; sleep terror; sleep walking; sustained circadian asynchrony; sustained inadequate sleep hygiene

At-Risk Population

Familial sleep paralysis

Associated Condition

Conditions with periodic limb movement; dementia; idiopathic central nervous system hypersomnolence; narcolepsy; nightmares; sleep apnea; sleep-related enuresis; sleep-related painful erections; treatment regimen

Client Outcomes

Client Will (Specify Time Frame)

- Verbalize plan that provides adequate time for sleep
- Identify actions that can be taken to ensure adequate sleep time
- Awaken refreshed once adequate time is spent sleeping
- Be less sleepy during the day once adequate time is spent sleeping

Nursing Interventions

- Assess the amount of sleep obtained each night compared with the amount of sleep needed.
- Assess the extent to which patients can be provided three to four consecutive hours of sleep time that is free from disturbance.
  - ❍ Minimize environmental factors that deprive clients of sleep. See Nursing Interventions and *Rationales* for Disturbed **Sleep** pattern.
  - ❍ Minimize personal factors that deprive clients of sleep. See Nursing Interventions and *Rationales* for **Insomnia.**
- When required nighttime care leaves patients sleep deprived, schedule a specific time for rest and sleep during the day.

- Assess for hypersensitivity to pain.
- When daytime drowsiness occurs despite adequate periods of undisturbed nighttime sleep, consider sleep apnea as a possible cause.
- Monitor caffeine intake (amounts and time of day) in sleep-deprived clients who may overuse caffeinated drinks to ward off daytime drowsiness.
- If evidence-based interventions are inadequate, consider and carefully evaluate unstudied but commonly used countermeasures for fighting drowsiness.

Pediatric

- Assess the amount of sleep obtained each night compared with the amount of sleep needed to avoid daytime drowsiness.
- Encourage daily schedules that allow for late awakening times for adolescents.
- See the Pediatric section of Nursing Interventions and *Rationales* for: Disturbed **Sleep** pattern.

Geriatric

▲ If an older client has daytime symptoms of sleep deprivation despite long nighttime sleep, refer to a sleep laboratory to evaluate the client for sleep apnea.
- Assess the amount of sleep obtained each night compared with the amount of sleep needed to function well during the day.
- Assess how much time the client spends in bed unable to sleep and client's comfort with low sleep efficiency.
- If a client is obtaining less sleep than required for optimal daytime function, explore if daytime napping will supplement, rather than replace, nighttime sleep.
- See the Geriatric section of Nursing Interventions and *Rationales* for disturbed **Sleep** pattern and **Insomnia.**

Multicultural

- Be aware of racial and ethnic disparities in sleep deprivation.

Home Care

- Teach family members about the short-term and long-term consequences of inadequate amounts of sleep for both clients and family caregivers.
- Teach client/family caregivers about the need for those with medical conditions to avoid schedules and commitments that interfere with obtaining adequate amounts of sleep.

- Promote adoption of behaviors that ensure adequate amounts of sleep for all family members. See Nursing Interventions and *Rationales* for Readiness for enhanced **Sleep.**
- Teach family members ways to avoid chronic sleep loss. See Nursing Interventions and *Rationales* for Disturbed **Sleep** pattern.
- Advise against chronic use of caffeinated drinks to overcome daytime fatigue and drowsiness while focusing on elimination of factors that lead to chronic sleep loss

Readiness for Enhanced Sleep

NANDA-I Definition

A pattern of natural, periodic suspension of relative consciousness to provide rest and sustain a desired lifestyle, which can be strengthened

Defining Characteristics

Expresses desire to enhance sleep

Client Outcomes

Client Will (Specify Time Frame)

- Verbalize a current interest in what constitutes normal sleep
- Reflect on own experiences and beliefs about sleep
- Verbalize an interest in nonpharmacological approaches to sleep promotion
- Take concrete steps to establish an environment conducive to sleep initiation and maintenance

S

Nursing Interventions

- Assess client's current knowledge and beliefs about sleep need and factors affecting sleep quantity and quality.
- Whenever there is a lack of knowledge or false beliefs about sleep requirements, provide information regarding sleep need and encourage clients to identify their personal sleep requirements.
- Based on assessment, focus on one or more of the following sleep hygiene strategies, choosing the most relevant.
  - Regular scheduling of the nighttime sleep period, daytime exposure to light, exercise, napping, and mealtimes characterized by (1) vigorous exercise during the day, (2) avoidance of long periods of daytime sleep (unless a night-shift worker), (3) avoidance of large meals before bed, and (4) arising at the same time each day even if sleep was poor during the previous night.

- Relaxing bedtime routine that includes (1) activities that calm the mind (e.g., mindfulness or other types of meditation, listening to music, prayer) and (2) activities that relax the body (e.g., warm baths, massage, progressive muscle relaxation).
- Creation of an environment conducive to sleep including (1) comfortable sleepwear, sleep surface, and room temperature; (2) low or masked levels of light and noise; and (3) a sleep space as free as possible from interruptions from others including pets.
- Management of any sources of pain as needed prior to sleep.
- Avoidance of late-day electronic device use.
- Monitoring of late-day intake of caffeine from all sources including energy drinks, coffee, colas, teas, and chocolate.
- Avoidance of alcoholic beverages to induce sleep.
- Avoidance of nicotine.
- Avoidance of a sedentary lifestyle.

Geriatric

- Interventions discussed previously can all be adapted for use with geriatric clients.
- Counsel the older client regarding normal age-related sleep changes.
- Elicit the older client's beliefs about sleep and correct any misconceptions, which may manifest as undue concern for some but too little concern for others.
- Review older client's prescription medications; use of over-the-counter (OTC) medications; and use of caffeine, tobacco, and alcohol.
- Assess and refer as appropriate if coexisting conditions may be affecting older client's sleep.
- Expand older client's awareness of sleep hygiene behaviors for improving sleep.
- Encourage the older client to walk and engage in other exercise outside unless contraindicated.

Home Care

- All interventions discussed previously can be adapted for home care use.
- Assess family caregivers' readiness for enhancing sleep.
- Assess the conduciveness of the home environment for promoting both caregiver and client sleep and the resources needed to improve the sleep environment.

Disturbed Sleep Pattern

NANDA-I Definition

Time-limited awakenings due to external factors

Defining Characteristics

Difficulty in daily functioning; difficulty initiating sleep; difficulty maintaining sleep state; dissatisfaction with sleep; feeling unrested; unintentional awakening

Related Factors

Disruption caused by sleep partner; environmental barrier; immobilization; insufficient privacy; nonrestorative sleep pattern

Client Outcomes

Client Will (Specify Time Frame)

- Verbalize plan to implement sleep promotion routines
- Maintain a regular schedule of sleep and waking
- Fall asleep without difficulty
- Remain asleep throughout the night
- Awaken naturally, feeling refreshed and is not fatigued during day

Nursing Interventions

- Obtain a sleep history to identify (1) noise, temperature, and light levels in the sleep environment; (2) activities occurring in the sleep environment during hours of sleep including use of handheld technology; (3) number of times awakened during the sleep period; and (4) when during the sleep period, time is available for undisturbed sleep.
- Negotiate use of handheld technology whenever clients have access to electronic devices in the care setting.
- Keep environment quiet during sleep periods.
- Consider masking hospital noise that cannot be eliminated.
- Offer earplugs when feasible.
- Dim the lights during sleep periods.
- Offer eye covers when lighting cannot be dimmed.
- Be aware that use of eye covers in intubated clients may lead to sensory deprivation and anxiety.
- Consolidate essential care to provide the opportunity for uninterrupted sleep the first 3 to 4 hours of the sleep period. Follow with periods of 90 to 110 minutes between interruptions.
- If the client must be disturbed the first 3 to 4 hours of the sleep period, attempt to protect 90- to 110-minute blocks of time between awakenings.
- Assess for medications and other stimulants that fragment sleep. Use caution when administering sleep medications. See Nursing Interventions and *Rationales* for **Insomnia.**

S

- Schedule newly ordered medications to avoid the need to wake the client the first few hours of the night.
- Combine the previously mentioned interventions as feasible to create a sleep promotion care bundle.

Pediatric

- Assess use of nighttime texting and consider limiting as needed to protect sleep.
- Adapt interventions for pediatric clients with caution because of limited empirical evidence regarding the effects of their use.

Geriatric

- Most interventions discussed previously can all be adapted for use with geriatric clients.
- Use of earplugs and eye covers with ataxic clients and clients with dementia may contribute to disorientation.

Multicultural

- Be aware that cultural sleep practices may alter the kinds of environmental sleep disruptors that require management.

Home Care

- Consider the unique characteristics of each home sleep environment when addressing sleep disruption.
- In addition, see the Home Care section of Nursing Interventions and *Rationales* for **Readiness for enhanced Sleep.**

Impaired Social Interaction

NANDA-I Definition

Insufficient or excessive quantity or ineffective quality of social exchange

Defining Characteristics

Anxiety during social interaction; dysfunctional interaction with others; expresses difficulty establishing satisfactory reciprocal interpersonal relations; expresses difficulty functioning socially; expresses difficulty performing social roles; expresses discomfort in social situations; expresses dissatisfaction with social connection; family reports altered interaction; inadequate psychosocial support system; inadequate use of social status toward others; low levels of social activities; minimal interaction with others; reports unsatisfactory social engagement; unhealthy competitive focus; unwillingness to cooperate with others

Related Factors

Altered self-concept; depressive symptoms; disturbed thought processes; environmental constraints; impaired physical mobility; inadequate communication skills; inadequate knowledge about how to enhance mutuality; inadequate personal hygiene; inadequate social skills; inadequate social support; maladaptive grieving; neurobehavioral manifestations; sociocultural dissonance

At-Risk Population

Individuals without a significant other

Associated Condition

Halitosis; mental diseases; neurodevelopmental disorders; therapeutic isolation

Client Outcomes

Client Will (Specify Time Frame)

- Identify barriers that cause impaired social interactions
- Discuss feelings that accompany impaired and successful social interactions
- Use available opportunities to practice interactions
- Use successful social interaction behaviors
- Report increased comfort in social situations
- Communicate, state feelings of belonging, demonstrate caring and interest in others
- Report effective interactions with others

Nursing Interventions

- • Monitor the client's use of defense mechanisms and support healthy defenses (e.g., the client focuses on the present and avoids placing blame on others for personal behavior).
- • Encourage the client to keep a gratitude journal.
- • Encourage dancing with Parkinson's programs for individuals with Parkinson's disease.
- • Model appropriate social interactions and use focused imitation interventions. Give positive verbal and nonverbal feedback for appropriate behavior (e.g., make statements such as, "I'm proud that you made it to work on time and did all the tasks assigned to you"; make eye contact). If not contraindicated, touch the client's arm or hand when speaking.
- • Consider use of social cognition and interaction training (SCIT) combined with social mentoring to improve social functioning.
- • Consider use of animal-assisted therapy (AAT).
- ▲ Refer client for social cognition training to increase social skills.
- ▲ Refer rehabilitation clients for assistive technologies to increase therapeutic engagement and promote social engagement.

S

- Refer to care plans for Risk for **Loneliness** and **Social** isolation for additional interventions.

Pediatric

- Provide supervised interaction opportunities for children of chronically ill parents.
- Encourage family style dining (FSD) for preschool children to promote social interactions during mealtimes.
- Use peer-mediated interaction (PMI) to increase social interactions of children on the autistic spectrum.
- Provide computers and Internet access to children with chronic disabilities that limit socialization.
- ▲ Refer children with autism for family-centered music therapy (FCMT).
- Consider the use of animal-assisted activities for children on the autistic spectrum.

Geriatric

- Assess for depression in clients with impaired social functioning.
- Assess older clients for hearing loss and refer for hearing aids as needed.
- Assess the communication patterns of clients with verbal domain problems for enactment strategies, paralinguistic features, and nonvocal communication.
- Encourage socialization through physical activity and meaningful activities incorporated into normal daily care practices.
- Provide live concert music for clients with dementia.
- ▲ Refer depressed clients to services for cognitive-behavioral therapy (CBT).
- Refer to care plans for **Frail Elderly** syndrome, Risk for **Loneliness,** and **Social** isolation for additional interventions.

Multicultural

- Approach individuals of color with respect, warmth, and professional courtesy.
- Use interpreters as needed.
- Refer to care plan for **Social** isolation for additional interventions.

Home Care

- Previously discussed interventions may be adapted for home care use.

Client/Family Teaching and Discharge Planning

- Previously discussed interventions may be adapted for client/family teaching and discharge planning.

S

Social Isolation

NANDA-I Definition

A state in which the individual lacks a sense of relatedness connected to positive, lasting, and significant interpersonal relationships.

Defining Characteristics

Expresses dissatisfaction with respect from others; expresses dissatisfaction with social connection; expresses dissatisfaction with social support; expresses loneliness; flat affect; hostility; impaired ability to meet expectations of others; low levels of social activities; minimal interaction with others; preoccupation with own thoughts; purposelessness; reduced eye contact; reports feeling different from others; reports feeling insecure in public; sad affect; seclusion imposed by others; sense of alienation; social behavior incongruent with cultural norms, social withdrawal

Related Factors

Difficulty establishing satisfactory reciprocal interpersonal relations; difficulty performing activities of daily living; difficulty sharing personal life expectations; fear of crime; fear of traffic; impaired physical mobility; inadequate psychosocial support system; inadequate social skills; inadequate social support; inadequate transportation; low self-esteem; negative perception of support system; neurobehavioral manifestations; values incongruent with cultural norms

S

At Risk Population

Economically disadvantaged individuals; immigrants; individuals experiencing altered social role; individuals experiencing loss of significant other; individuals living alone; individuals living far from significant others; individuals moving to unfamiliar locations; individuals with history of rejection; individuals with history of traumatic event; individuals with ill family member; individuals with no children; institutionalized individuals; older adults; widowed individuals

Associated Condition

Altered physical appearance; chronic disease; cognitive disorders

Client Outcomes

Client Will (Specify Time Frame)

- Identify feelings of isolation
- Practice social and communication skills needed to interact with others
- Initiate interactions with others; set and meet goals
- Participate in activities and programs at level of ability and desire
- Describe feelings of self-worth

Nursing Interventions

- Establish a therapeutic relationship with the client.
- Observe for barriers to social interaction.
- Discuss/assess causes of perceived or actual isolation.
- Allow the client opportunities to describe his or her daily life and to introduce any issues that may be of concern.
- Promote social interactions.
- Assist the client in identifying specific health and social problems and involve him or her in their resolution.
- Assist the client in identifying activities that encourage socialization.
- Identify available support systems and involve those individuals in the client's care.

▲ Refer clients and caregivers to support groups as necessary.

- Encourage interactions with others with similar interests.
- See the care plan for Risk for **Loneliness.**

Pediatric

▲ Refer obese adolescents for diet, exercise, and psychosocial support.

▲ Assess socially isolated adolescents. Refer to appropriate rehabilitation programs as needed.

Geriatric

▲ Assess physical and mental status to establish an early baseline for referring at-risk individuals to community resources.

S

- Assess for hearing.
- Involve client in planning activities.
- Involve nonprofessionals in activities and projects with the client.
- Suggest varied social activities that would decrease isolation and encourage participation.

▲ Consider the use of simulated presence therapy (see the care plan for **Hopelessness**).

- Consider using computers and the Internet to alleviate or reduce loneliness and social isolation.

Multicultural

- Acknowledge racial/ethnic differences at the onset of care.
- Assess for the influence of cultural beliefs, norms, values, and the client's personal cultural needs.
- Use a culturally competent, professional approach when working with clients of various ethnic groups.
- Promote a sense of ethnic attachment.
- Assess the client's feelings regarding social isolation.

- Assist those ethnic minorities who are underserved to access essential healthcare.

Home Care

- The interventions described previously may be adapted for home care use.
- Confirm that the home setting has health-safety systems in place.
- Consider the use of the computer and Internet to decrease isolation social interaction.
- Assess options for living that allow the client privacy but not isolation.
- Assist clients to interact with neighbors in the community when they move to supported housing.

Client/Family Teaching and Discharge Planning

- Assist the client in initiating contacts with self-help groups, counselors, and therapists.
- Provide information to the client about senior citizen services and community resources.
- Refer socially isolated caregivers to appropriate support groups.
- See the care plan for **Caregiver Role Strain**.

Chronic Sorrow

NANDA-I Definition

Cyclical, recurring, and potentially progressive pattern of pervasive sadness experienced (by parent, caregiver, individual with chronic illness or disability) in response to continual loss, throughout the trajectory of an illness or disability

Defining Characteristics

Feeling that interferes with well-being; overwhelming negative feelings; sadness

Related Factors

Crisis in disability management; crisis in illness management; missed milestones; missed opportunities

At-Risk Population

Death of significant other; developmental crisis; length of time as a caregiver

Associated Condition

Chronic disability; chronic illness

Client Outcomes

Client Will (Specify Time Frame)

- Express appropriate feelings of guilt, fear, anger, or sadness

- Identify problems associated with sorrow (e.g., changes in appetite, insomnia, nightmares, loss of libido, decreased energy, alteration in activity levels)
- Seek help in dealing with grief-associated problems
- Plan for the future one day at a time
- Function at normal developmental level

Nursing Interventions

- • Determine the client's degree of sorrow.
- • Assess for the four discrete stages of grieving in chronic obstructive pulmonary disease (COPD) clients.
- • Provide coping strategies for caregivers who may experience chronic sorrow.
- • Assess clients for chronic sorrow and provide them with coping strategies.
- • Develop a trusting relationship to care for clients with chronic sorrow.
- • Help the client understand that sorrow may be ongoing.
- • Urge the client to use positive coping techniques.
- ▲ Refer the client for mental health services if needed.
  - ❍ Refer clients for financial assistance if needed.

Pediatric

- • Encourage the parents of children with uncommon diseases to use online resources to manage their chronic sorrow.
- • Educate parents that an increase in chronic sorrow can occur after stressful events.
- • Nurses should assess for chronic sorrow and discuss coping strategies for parents of children who have been in the neonatal intensive care unit (NICU).
- • Allow children the opportunity to talk about the impending death of a parent or loved one.
- • Encourage parents to listen to their child's expression of grief.
- • Educate parents that children may grieve differently than adults.
- ▲ Refer grieving children to peer support groups.
- • Encourage children experiencing grief to participate in bereavement activities and camps.
- • Encourage children who are grieving to participate in other forms of therapy, in addition to individual counseling and psychotherapy.
- • Help the adolescent with chronic sorrow determine sources of support and refer for counseling if needed.
- • Provide family-centered care to parents of children with disabilities, and encourage parents to attend support groups.

S

- Encourage parents with chronic sorrow to participate in an online support group and learn coping strategies.
- Recognize that mothers who have a miscarriage or lose an infant often grieve and experience sorrow.

Geriatric

- Identify previous losses and assess the client for depression.
- Evaluate the social support system of the older client and refer for bereavement counseling if needed.

Home Care

- In-home bereavement follow-up by nurses should be considered if available.
- Assess the client for depression and refer for mental health services if appropriate.
- Encourage the client to participate in activities that are diversionary and uplifting as tolerated (e.g., outdoor activities, hobby groups, church-related activities, pet care).
- Encourage the client to participate in support groups appropriate to the area of loss or illness.
- Provide empathetic communication for family/caregivers.
- The interventions described previously may be adapted for home care use.
- See the care plans for Chronic low **Self-Esteem**, Risk for **Loneliness,** and **Hopelessness.**

S

Spiritual Distress

NANDA-I Definition

A state of suffering related to the impaired ability to integrate meaning and purpose in life through connections with self, others, the world, or a superior being

Defining Characteristics

Anger behaviors; crying; decreased expression of creativity; disinterested in nature; dysomnias; excessive guilt; expresses alienation; expresses anger; expresses anger toward power greater than self; expresses concern about beliefs; expresses concern about the future; expresses concern about values system; expresses concerns about family; expresses feeling abandoned by power greater than self; expresses feeling of emptiness; expresses feeling unloved; expresses feeling worthless; expresses insufficient courage; expresses loss of confidence; expresses loss of control; expresses loss of hope; expresses loss of serenity; expresses need for forgiveness; expresses regret; expresses suffering; fatigue; fear; impaired ability for introspection; inability to experience transcendence; maladaptive grieving; perceived loss of meaning in life; questions identity; questions meaning of life; questions meaning of suffering; questions own dignity; refuses to interact with others

Related Factors

Altered religious ritual; altered spiritual practice; anxiety; barrier to experiencing love; cultural conflict; depressive symptoms; difficulty accepting the aging process; inadequate environmental control; inadequate interpersonal relations; loneliness; loss of independence; low self-esteem; pain; perception of having unfinished business; self-alienation; separation from support system; social alienation; sociocultural deprivation; stressors; substance misuse

At-Risk Population

Individuals experiencing birth of a child; individuals experiencing death of a significant other; individuals experiencing infertility; individuals experiencing life transition; individuals experiencing racial conflict; individuals experiencing unexpected life event; individuals exposed to death; individuals exposed to natural disaster; individuals exposed to traumatic events; individuals receiving bad news; individuals receiving terminal care; individuals with low educational level

Associated Condition

Chronic disease; depression; loss of body part; loss of function of a body part; treatment regimen

Client Outcomes

Client Will (Specify Time Frame)

- Express meaning and purpose in life
- Express sense of hope in the future
- Express sense of connectedness with self
- Express sense of connectedness with family/friends
- Express ability to forgive
- Express acceptance of health status
- Find meaning in relationships with others
- Find meaning in relationship with Higher Power
- Find meaning in personal and healthcare treatment choices

Nursing Interventions

- Observe clients for cues indicating difficulties in finding meaning, purpose, or hope in life.
- Observe clients with chronic illness, poor prognosis, or life-changing conditions for loss of meaning, purpose, and hope in life.

- Promote a sense of love, caring, and compassion in nursing encounters.
- Be physically present and actively listen to the client.
- Help the client find a reason for living, be available for support, and promote hope.
- Respect the client's beliefs; avoid imposing your own spiritual beliefs on the client. Be aware of your own belief systems and accept the client's spirituality.
- Monitor and promote supportive social contacts.
- Integrate and assist family in searching for meaning in the client's healthcare situation.
- Offer spiritual support to family and caregivers.
- Screen for spiritual needs and, if a need arises, offer chaplain referral.
- Support mind–body interventions (e.g., meditation, guided imagery, relaxation, massage). Support outdoor activities.
- Encourage journaling.
- Provide privacy or a "sacred space."
- Integrate spiritual care in interprofessional palliative care teams.
- Encourage life review at end of life, including recalling, evaluating, and integrating life experiences.

Geriatric

- Identify client's past spiritual practices that have been helpful. Help the client explore his or her life and identify those experiences that are noteworthy.
- Offer opportunities to practice one's religion.

Pediatric

- ❍ Offer adolescents opportunities for reflection and storytelling to express their spirituality.
- ❍ Foster spiritual activities among adolescents.

Multicultural

- Recognize the importance of spirituality and provide culturally competent spiritual care to specific populations:
  - ❍ Muslims
  - ❍ Hispanic
  - ❍ African Americans (AAs)
  - ❍ Veterans of Armed Services. Recognize the unique spiritual needs of veterans and provide spiritual support or appropriate referrals.

Home Care

- All of the nursing interventions described previously apply in the home setting.

S

Risk for Spiritual Distress

NANDA-I Definition

Susceptible to an impaired ability to experience and integrate meaning and purpose in life through connectedness within self, literature, nature, and/or a power greater than oneself, which may compromise health

Risk Factors

Altered religious ritual; altered spiritual practice; anxiety; barrier to experiencing love; culture conflict; depressive symptoms; difficulty accepting the aging process; inadequate environmental control; inadequate interpersonal relations; loneliness; low self-esteem; pain; perception of having unfinished business; self-alienation; separation from support system; social alienation; sociocultural deprivation; stressors; substance misuse

At-Risk Population

Individuals experiencing birth of a child; individuals experiencing death of a significant other; individuals experiencing infertility; individuals experiencing life transition; individuals experiencing racial conflict; individuals experiencing unexpected life event; individuals exposed to death; individuals exposed to natural disaster; individuals exposed to traumatic events; individuals receiving bad news; individuals receiving terminal care; individuals with low educational level

Associated Condition

Chronic disease; depression; loss of a body part; loss of function of a body part; treatment regimen

Client Outcomes, Nursing Interventions

Refer to care plan for **Spiritual Distress**

Readiness for Enhanced Spiritual Well-Being

NANDA-I Definition

A pattern of experiencing and integrating meaning and purpose in life through connectedness with self, others, art, music, literature, nature, and/or a power greater than oneself, which can be strengthened

Defining Characteristics

Expresses desire to enhance acceptance; expresses desire to enhance capacity to self-comfort; expresses desire to enhance comfort in one's faith; expresses desire to enhance connection with nature; expresses desire to enhance connection with power greater than self; expresses desire to enhance coping; expresses desire to enhance courage; expresses desire to enhance creative energy; expresses desire to enhance forgiveness from others; expresses desire to enhance harmony in the environment; expresses desire to enhance hope;

expresses desire to enhance inner peace; expresses desire to enhance interaction with significant other; expresses desire to enhance joy; expresses desire to enhance love; expresses desire to enhance love of others; expresses desire to enhance meditative practice; expresses desire to enhance mystical experiences; expresses desire to enhance oneness with nature; expresses desire to enhance oneness with power greater than self; expresses desire to enhance participation in religious practices; expresses desire to enhance peace with power greater than self; expresses desire to enhance prayerfulness; expresses desire to enhance reverence; expresses desire to enhance satisfaction with life; expresses desire to enhance self-awareness; expresses desire to enhance self-forgiveness; expresses desire to enhance sense of awe; expresses desire to enhance sense of harmony within oneself; expresses desire to enhance sense of identity; expresses desire to enhance sense of magic in the environment; expresses desire to enhance serenity; expresses desire to enhance service to others; expresses desire to enhance strength in one's faith; expresses desire to enhance surrender

Client Outcomes

Client Will (Specify Time Frame)

- Express hope
- Express sense of meaning and purpose in life
- Express peace and serenity
- Express love
- Express acceptance
- Express surrender
- Express forgiveness of self and others
- Express satisfaction with philosophy of life
- Express joy
- Express courage
- Describe being able to cope
- Describe use of spiritual practices
- Describe providing service to others
- Describe interaction with spiritual leaders, friends, and family
- Describe appreciation for art, music, literature, and nature

Nursing Interventions

- Perform a spiritual assessment that includes the client's relationship with God, meaning and purpose in life, religious affiliation, and any other significant beliefs.
- Be present and actively listen to the client.
- Encourage the client to engage in other spiritual meditative or mind–body practices.

S

- Coordinate or encourage nurses to attend spiritual retreats or courses.
- Promote hope.
- Encourage clients to reflect on what is meaningful to them in life.
- Offer spiritual support to family and caregivers.
- Assist the client in identifying religious or spiritual beliefs that encourage integration of meaning and purpose in the client's life.
- Support spiritual practices, including meditation, guided imagery, journaling, relaxation, and involvement in art, music, or poetry.
- Encourage expressions of spirituality.
- Encourage integration of spirituality in healthy lifestyle choices.
- Encourage forgiveness.

Geriatric

- Offer opportunities to practice one's religion.
- For those with chronic disease, encourage individual spiritual practices that promote meaning and peace.
- For those with chronic illness, encourage patients to attend meaning-centered meditation programs, therapy, or counseling.
- Promote spiritual activities for those receiving palliative care.
- During bereavement, encourage bereavement life review to promote spiritual well-being and alleviate depression.

Pediatric

- ❍ Offer adolescents opportunities for reflection and storytelling to express their spirituality.
- ❍ Foster spiritual activities among adolescents.

Multicultural

- Recognize the importance of spirituality and provide culturally competent spiritual care to specific populations:
    - ❍ Muslims
    - ❍ Thai
    - ❍ Latinos
    - ❍ African Americans (AAs)
    - ❍ Sheltered Homeless
    - ❍ Chinese
    - ❍ Armed Forces
- Integrate spiritual practices in health-promoting programs, particularly within the AA community.

Home Care

- All of the nursing interventions described previously apply in the home setting.

Impaired Standing

NANDA-I Definition

Limitation of ability to independently and purposefully attain and/or maintain the body in an upright position from feet to head

Defining Characteristics

Impaired ability to adjust position of one or both lower limbs on uneven surface; impaired ability to attain a balanced position of the torso; impaired ability to extend one or both hips; impaired ability to extend one or both knees; impaired ability to flex one or both hips; impaired ability to flex one or both knees; impaired ability to maintain the torso in balanced position; impaired ability to stress torso with body weight

Related Factors

Emotional disturbance; insufficient endurance; insufficient energy; insufficient muscle strength; malnutrition; obesity; pain; self-imposed relief posture

Associated Condition

Circulatory perfusion disorder; impaired metabolic functioning; injury to lower extremity; neurological disorder; prescribed posture; sarcopenia; surgical procedure

Client Outcomes

Client Will (Specify Time Frame)

- Demonstrate optimal independence and safety when standing
- Demonstrate the proper use of assistive devices
- State benefits of standing

Nursing Interventions

- Encourage clients to stand at intervals throughout the day.
- Educate patients about the health risks of sitting.

Geriatric

- Advise older clients who have difficulty standing to use assistive devices.
- Encourage trunk exercises after clients have had strokes.
- Encourage clients who are unable to stand to consider chair exercises.
- Encourage clients poststroke to participate in rehabilitation interventions that promote standing.
- Raise the height of the bed and encourage the use of the client's hands when an older adult is rising from a sitting to standing position.
- Educate older adults who have fallen about the need for balance and muscle training of the ankle joint.
- Educate adults older than age 80 years on the need for vitamin D.

S

- Advise older clients who are at risk for falls to avoid doing multiple tasks at one time while standing.

Client/Family Teaching and Discharge Planning

- Educate clients that standing can be beneficial for their health.
- Teach clients about the need to take frequent breaks when standing for long periods.
- Instruct clients about the use of yoga for individuals who have difficulty with standing balance.

Stress Overload

NANDA-I Definition

Excessive amounts and types of demands that require action

Defining Characteristics

Excessive stress; feeling of pressure; impaired decision-making; impaired functioning; increase in anger; increase in anger behavior; increase in impatience; negative impact from stress; tension

Related Factors

Insufficient resources; repeated stressors; stressors

Client Outcomes

Client Will (Specify Time Frame)

- Review the amounts and types of stressors in daily living
- Identify stressors that can be modified or eliminated
- Mobilize social supports to facilitate lower stress levels
- Reduce stress levels through use of health promoting behaviors and other strategies

S

Nursing Interventions

- Assist client in identification of stress overload during vulnerable life events.
- Listen actively to descriptions of stressors and the stress response.
- In younger adult women, assess interpersonal stressors.
- Categorize stressors as modifiable or nonmodifiable.
- Help clients modify or mitigate stressors identified as modifiable.
- Help clients distinguish among short-term, chronic, and secondary stressors.
- Provide information as needed to reduce stress responses to acute and chronic illnesses.

▲ Explore possible therapeutic approaches such as cognitive-behavioral therapy, biofeedback, neurofeedback, acupuncture, pharmacological agents, and complementary and alternative therapies.

- Help the client reframe his or her perceptions of some of the stressors.
- Assist the client to mobilize social supports for dealing with recent stressors.

Pediatric

- With children, nurses should work with parents to help them reduce children's stressors.
- Help children manage their feelings related to self-concept.
- Help children deal with bullies and other sources of violence in schools and neighborhoods.
- Help children manage the complexities of chronic illnesses.

Geriatric

- Assess for chronic stress with older adults and provide a variety of stress relief techniques.
- ▲ Encourage older adults to seek appropriate counseling.

Multicultural

- Review cultural beliefs and acculturation level in relation to perceived stressors.

Home Care

- The preceding interventions may be adapted for home care use.
- Develop community-based programs for stress management as needed for groups with increased risk of stress overload (e.g., firefighters, policemen, military personnel, nurses).
- Support and encourage neighborhood stability.

Client/Family Teaching and Discharge Planning

- Diagnose the possibility of stress overload before teaching.
- Establish readiness for learning.
- Provide manageable amounts of information at the appropriate educational level.
- Evaluate the need for additional teaching and learning experiences.

Acute Substance Abuse Withdrawal Syndrome

NANDA-I Definition

Serious, multifactorial sequelae following abrupt cessation of an addictive compound

Defining Characteristics

Acute confusion (00128); anxiety (00146); disturbed sleep pattern (00198); nausea (00134); risk for electrolyte imbalance (00195); risk for injury (00035)

Related Factors

Developed dependence to alcohol or other addictive substance; heavy use of an addictive substance over time; malnutrition; sudden cessation of an addictive substance

At-Risk Population

History of previous withdrawal symptoms; older adults

Associated Condition

Comorbid mental disorder; comorbid serious physical illness

Client Outcomes

Client Will (Specify Time Frame)

- Will stabilize and remain free from physical injury
- Verbalizes effects of substances on body
- Maintain vital signs and lab values within normal range
- Verbalizes importance of adequate nutrition

Nursing Interventions

Alcohol-Induced Withdrawal Syndrome

- Assess for client's pattern of alcohol use, last drink, and current blood alcohol levels.
- Implement seizure precautions.
- Rule out other causes of symptoms.
- Monitor vital signs.
- Assess for progression of withdrawal symptoms such as insomnia, anxiety, nausea/vomiting, tremulousness, headache, diaphoresis, palpitations, increased body temperature, tachycardia, and hypertension.
- Monitor severity of withdrawal symptoms with the Clinical Institute Withdrawal Assessment (CIWA-Ar).
- Evaluate the client for progression to the delirium tremens (DTs).
- Assess nutritional status for risk of malnutrition. Assess for thiamine (B_1) deficiency, which is associated with chronic alcohol abuse, folate deficiency, and vitamin D deficiency associated with a history of inadequate exposure to sunlight. Consult with healthcare provider as needed for supplement order.
- Address hydration needs.
- Determine hepatic and renal functioning prior to administration of medications.

Opioid-Induced Withdrawal Syndrome

- Assess for client's opioid of choice, last use, and current withdrawal symptoms.

S

- Monitor severity of withdrawal symptoms with the Clinical Opiate Withdrawal Scale (COWS).
- Nurses should wait to administer the first dose of buprenorphine to opioid-dependent patients until clients are experiencing mild to moderate opioid withdrawal symptoms.
- Assess and manage early opioid withdrawal symptoms (agitation, anxiety, insomnia, muscle aches, increased lacrimation, rhinorrhea, sweating, and yawning) and late opioid withdrawal symptoms (abdominal cramping, diarrhea, pupillary dilation, nausea, vomiting, and piloerection).
- Monitor vital signs.
- Teach the client about the anticipated withdrawal symptoms and opioid cravings while offering support and encouragement.

▲ Monitor laboratory reports and report to healthcare provider.

Benzodiazepine-Induced Withdrawal Syndrome

- Assess for client's last benzodiazepine use and current withdrawal symptoms.
- Implement seizure precautions.
- Rule out delirium from other causes or other withdrawal syndromes.

▲ Anticipate use of the same treatment protocols as for alcohol withdrawal and use of a long-acting benzodiazepine in tapering doses over time.

Cocaine/Methamphetamine-Induced Withdrawal Syndrome

- Assess for client's last stimulant use and current withdrawal symptoms.

Cannabis-Induced Withdrawal Syndrome

- Assess for client's last cannabis use and current withdrawal symptoms.
- Direct nursing actions to address anxiety, irritability, sleep disturbances, and decreased appetite.

Nicotine-Induced Withdrawal Syndrome

- Assess for client's last nicotine use and current withdrawal symptoms.
- Rule out nicotine withdrawal as the cause of delirium in critically ill clients.

All Withdrawal Syndromes

- Obtain a drug and/or alcohol history using a tool such as the AUDIT-C or the DAST-10.
- Implement and follow institutional withdrawal protocols.
- Assess for signs of recent trauma or head injury.
- Assess client's level of consciousness, monitor for changes in behavior, and orient to reality as needed.

S

- Assess vital signs and monitor for existing medical conditions and current medications.
- Assess and monitor for expression of psychological distress.
- Collect urine/serum samples for laboratory tests.
- Address craving for substances with mindfulness-based techniques.
- Respond to agitated behavior with deescalation techniques.
- Administer as needed (prn) medications for agitation and symptom control as ordered.
- Provide a quiet room without dark shadows, noises, or other excessive stimuli.
- Provide suicide precautions and 1:1 staffing for clients that are delirious or who may present a danger to themselves or others.

Client/Family Teaching and Discharge Planning

▲ After withdrawal symptoms have subsided, refer client to substance use treatment.

▲ Refer for smoking cessation services that target nicotine craving.

Risk for Acute Substance Abuse Withdrawal Syndrome

S

NANDA-I Definition

Susceptible to serious, multifactorial sequelae following abrupt cessation of an addictive compound, which may compromise health

Risk Factors

Developed dependence to alcohol or other addictive substance; heavy use of an addictive substance over time; malnutrition; sudden cessation of an addictive substance

At-Risk Population

History of previous withdrawal symptoms; older adults

Associated Condition

Comorbid mental disorder; comorbid serious physical illness

Client Outcomes

Client Will (Specify Time Frame)

- Stabilize and remain free from physical injury
- Verbalize effects of substances on body
- Maintain vital signs and lab values within normal range
- Verbalize importance of adequate nutrition

Nursing Interventions

Risk for Alcohol-Induced Withdrawal Syndrome

- Assess for client's pattern of alcohol use, last drink, and current blood alcohol levels.
- Implement seizure precautions.
- Rule out other causes of symptoms.
- Monitor vital signs.
- Assess for progression of withdrawal symptoms such as insomnia, anxiety, nausea/vomiting, tremulousness, headache, diaphoresis, palpitations, increased body temperature, tachycardia, and hypertension.
- Monitor severity of withdrawal symptoms with the Clinical Institute Withdrawal Assessment (CIWA-Ar).
- Evaluate the client for progression to the delirium tremens (DTs).
- Assess nutritional status for risk of malnutrition, thiamine (B_1) deficiency associated with chronic alcohol abuse, folate deficiency, and vitamin D deficiency–associated history of inadequate exposure to sunlight. Consult with healthcare provider as needed for supplement order.
- Address hydration needs.
- Determine hepatic and renal functioning prior to administration of medications.

Risk for Opioid-Induced Withdrawal Syndrome

- Assess for client's opioid of choice, last use, and current withdrawal symptoms.
- Monitor severity of withdrawal symptoms with the Clinical Opiate Withdrawal Scale (COWS).
- Assess and manage early opioid withdrawal symptoms (agitation, anxiety, insomnia, muscle aches, increased lacrimation, rhinorrhea, sweating, and yawning) and late opioid withdrawal symptoms (abdominal cramping, diarrhea, pupillary dilation, nausea, vomiting, and piloerection).
- Monitor vital signs.
- Clients should be taught about risk of relapse and other safety concerns from using opioid withdrawal management as stand-alone treatment for opioid use disorder.
- Teach the client about the anticipated withdrawal symptoms and opioid cravings, while offering support and encouragement.

▲ Monitor laboratory reports and report to healthcare provider.

▲ Refer patient for buprenorphine or methadone treatment.

S

Risk for Benzodiazepine-Induced Withdrawal Syndrome

- • Assess for client's last benzodiazepine use, and current withdrawal symptoms.
- • Implement seizure precautions.
- • Rule out delirium from other causes or other withdrawal syndromes.
- ▲ Anticipate use of the same treatment protocols as for alcohol withdrawal and use of a long-acting benzodiazepine in tapering doses over time.

Risk for Cocaine/Methamphetamine-Induced Withdrawal Syndrome

- • Assess for client's last stimulant use and current withdrawal symptoms.

Risk for Cannabis-Induced Withdrawal Syndrome

- • Assess for client's last cannabis use and current withdrawal symptoms.
- • Direct nursing actions to address anxiety, irritability, sleep disturbances, and decreased appetite.

Risk for Nicotine-Induced Withdrawal Syndrome

- • Assess for client's last nicotine use and current withdrawal symptoms.
- • Rule out nicotine withdrawal as the cause of delirium in critically ill clients.

All Withdrawal Syndromes

S

- • Obtain a drug and/or alcohol history using a tool such as the AUDIT-C or the DAST-10.
- • Implement and follow institutional withdrawal protocols.
- • Assess for signs of recent trauma or head injury.
- • Assess client's level of consciousness, monitor for changes in behavior, and orient to reality as needed.
- • Assess vital signs and monitor for existing medical conditions and current medications.
- • Assess and monitor for expression of psychological distress.
- • Collect urine/serum samples for laboratory tests.
- • Address craving for substances with mindfulness-based techniques.
- • Respond to agitated behavior with deescalation techniques.
- • Administer as needed (PRN) medications for agitation and symptom control as ordered.
- • Provide a quiet room without dark shadows, noises, or other excessive stimuli.
- • Provide suicide precautions and 1:1 staffing for clients that are delirious or who may present a danger to themselves or others.

Client/Family Teaching and Discharge Planning

- ▲ After withdrawal symptoms have subsided, refer client to substance use treatment.
- ▲ Refer for smoking cessation services that target nicotine craving.

Risk for Sudden Infant Death

NANDA-I Definition

Susceptible to unpredicted death of an infant

Risk Factors

Delay in prenatal care; exposure to secondhand smoke; infant overheating; infant overwrapping; infant placed in prone position to sleep; infant placed in side-lying position to sleep; insufficient prenatal care; soft sleep surface; soft; loose objects placed near infant; infant less than 4 months; placed in sitting devices for routine sleep

At-Risk Population

African American ethnicity; age 2 to 4 months; infant not breastfed exclusively or fed with expressed breast milk; low birth weight; male gender; maternal smoking during pregnancy; Native American ethnicity; postnatal exposure to alcohol; postnatal exposure to elicit drug; prematurity; prenatal exposure to alcohol; prenatal exposure to elicit drug; young parental age

Associated Condition

Cold weather

Client Outcomes

Client Will (Specify Time Frame)

- Explain appropriate measures to prevent sudden infant death syndrome (SIDS)
- Demonstrate correct techniques for positioning and blanketing the infant, protecting the infant from harm

Nursing Interventions

- Position the infant supine to sleep during naps and night; do not position in the prone position or side-lying position (American Academy of Pediatrics [AAP], 2014a).
- Avoid use of bedding, such as blankets and loose sheets, for sleeping. Also keep quilts, pillows, bumpers, sheepskins, and soft toys out of the infant's bed. Dress the child in one-piece sleepers or wearable blankets (AAP, 2014b).
- Avoid over bundling, overheating, and swaddling the infant. The infant should not feel hot to touch.

- Provide the infant a certain amount of time in the prone position while the infant is awake and observed. Change the direction that the baby lies in the crib from one week to the next; avoid too much time in car seats and carriers.

Home Care

- Most of the interventions and client teaching information are relevant to home care.
- Evaluate home for potential safety hazards, such as inappropriate cribs, cradles, or strollers.
- Determine where and how the child sleeps, and provide instructions on safe sleeping positions and environments as needed.

Multicultural

- Encourage pregnant American Indian mothers and native Alaskan Indian mothers to avoid drinking alcohol and to avoid wrapping infants in excessive blankets or clothing.
- Encourage Hispanic and black mothers to find alternatives to bed sharing or placing infants for sleep on adult beds, sofas, or cots, and to avoid placing pillows, soft toys, and soft bedding in the sleep environment.

Client/Family Teaching and Discharge Planning

- Teach the safety guidelines for infant care in the previous interventions.
- Provide parents of both term and preterm infants with verbal and written education about SIDS and ways to reduce the risk of SIDS before discharge to home.
- Recommend breastfeeding.
- Teach parents the need to obtain a crib that conforms to the safety standards of the Consumer Product Safety Commission (CPSC).
- Teach the need to stop smoking during pregnancy and to not smoke around the infant. Do not allow the infant to be exposed to any secondhand smoke.
- Teach parents, especially mothers, not to use alcohol, medications, or illicit drugs while caring for or bed sharing with an infant.
- Teach parents not to sleep in the same bed with the infant, regardless of alcohol, medications, smoking, or illicit drug use.
- Teach parents not to place the infant on a cushion to sleep, or a sofa chair or other soft surface. Infants should sleep in a crib (AAP, 2014a).
- Recommend an alternative to sleeping with an infant of placing the infant's crib near their bed to allow for more convenient

breastfeeding and parent contact. *Parents should be advised to place the baby in his or her own crib next to the parent's bed* (AAP, 2014a).

- Recommend that parents with infants in child care make it very clear to the employees that the infant must always be placed in the supine position to sleep, not prone or in a side-lying position (AAP, 2014a).

Risk for Suffocation

NANDA-I Definition

Susceptable to inadequate air availability for inhalation, which may compromise health

Risk Factor

Access to empty refrigerator/freezer; eating large mouthfuls of food; emotional disturbance; gas leak; insufficient knowledge of safety precautions; low-strung clothesline; pacifier around infant's neck; playing with plastic bag; propped bottle placed in infant's crib; small object in airway; smoking in bed; soft underlayment; unattended in water; unvented fuel-burning heater; vehicle running in closed garage

Associated Condition

Alteration in cognitive functioning; alteration in olfactory function; face/neck disease; face/neck injury; impaired motor functioning

Client Outcomes

Client Will (Specify Time Frame)

- Undertake appropriate measures to prevent suffocation
- Demonstrate correct techniques for emergency rescue maneuvers (e.g., Heimlich maneuver, rescue breathing, cardiopulmonary resuscitation [CPR]) and describe situations that require them

Nursing Interventions

- Identify hospitalized clients at particular risk for suffocation, including the following:
  - Clients with altered levels of consciousness
  - Infants or young children
  - Clients with developmental delays
  - Clients with mental illness, especially schizophrenia
  - Clients who have been physically or chemically restrained

Pediatric

- Counsel families on the following for care of an infant:
  - Position infants on their back to sleep; do not position them on their side or prone.

S

- Position infants on their back to sleep; do not position them on their side or prone. Obtain a new crib that conforms to the safety standards of the Federal Safety Commission.
- Avoid use of loose bedding, such as blankets and sheets, for sleeping. If blankets are used, they should be tucked in around the crib mattress so the infant's face is less likely to become covered by bedding. The blanket should end at the level of the infant's chest.

- Assess for signs and symptoms of abuse such as Munchausen syndrome by proxy (MSBP).
- Conduct risk factor identification, noting special circumstances in which preventive or protective measures are indicated. Note the presence of environmental hazards, including plastic bags; cribs with slats wider than 2 inches; ill-fitting crib mattresses that can allow the infant to become wedged between the mattress and crib; pillows/loose bedding in cribs; placement of crib near windows with blinds or cords; co-sleeping; abandoned large appliances such as refrigerators, dishwashers, or freezers; clothing with cords or hoods that can become entangled; bibs; pacifiers on a string; necklaces in infants and children; drapery cords; and pull-toy strings.
- Counsel families to evaluate household furniture for safety, including large dressers, televisions, book shelves, and appliances, which may need to be anchored to the wall to prevent the child from climbing on the furniture and it falling forward and suffocating the child.
- Counsel families not to serve these foods to the child younger than 5 years of age: nuts, seeds, hot dogs, popcorn, pretzels, chips, chunks of meat, hard pieces of fruit or vegetables, raisins, whole grapes, hard candies, gum, chewable vitamins, fish with bones, snacks on toothpicks, and marshmallows.
- Counsel families to keep the following items away from the sight and reach of infants and toddlers: buttons, beads, jewelry, pins, nails, marbles, coins, stones, magnets, and balloons. Choose age-appropriate toys and games for children and check for any small parts that may be a choking hazard because children have the need to put everyday objects in their mouths (safekids.org, 2015).
- Stress water and pool safety precautions, including vigilant, uninterrupted parental supervision.
- Underscore the necessity of not allowing children to play with or near electric garage doors and of keeping garage door openers out of the reach of young children.

S

- For adolescents, watch for signs of depression that could result in suicide by suffocation.
- For geriatric clients, assess the status of the swallow reflex. Offer appropriate foods and beverages accordingly. Older adults, especially those receiving antipsychotic medications, have an increased incidence of choking. Refer to Impaired **Swallowing.**
- A swallowing assessment by a speech-language pathologist is recommended in patients with suspected or confirmed dysphagia to ensure the appropriate type and consistency of diet to mitigate choking and aspiration risk.
- Ensure proper positioning during and after feeding to decrease the risk of aspiration.
- Use care in pillow placement when positioning frail older clients who are on bed rest.
- Recognize that older adults in depression may use hanging, strangulation, and suffocation as a means of suicide.

Home Care

- Assess the home for potential safety hazards in systems that are not likely to be fixed (e.g., faulty pilot lights or gas leaks in gas stoves, carbon monoxide release from heating systems, kerosene fumes from portable heaters).
- Assist the family in having these areas assessed and making appropriate safety arrangements (e.g., installing detectors, making repairs, home safety inspections).
- Advise the family to have a safety plan for potential escape routes from the home in the event of detectors going off, fire, or other emergencies.

Client/Family Teaching and Discharge Planning

- Recommend that families who are seeking day care or in-home care for children, geriatric family members, or at-risk family members with developmental or functional disabilities inspect the environment for hazards and examine the first aid preparation and vigilance of providers.
- Recommend to families that they advise any caregivers of specific food consistency, types, and any feeding precautions and strategies required to decrease risk of choking and aspiration in high-risk children or adults.
- Ensure family members learn and practice rescue techniques, including treatment of choking and lack of breathing, as well as CPR.

S

Risk for Suicidal Behavior

NANDA-I Definition

Susceptible to self-injurious acts associated with some intent to die.

Related Factors

Behavioral

Apathy; difficulty asking for help; difficulty coping with unsatisfactory performance; difficulty expressing feelings; ineffective chronic pain self-management; self-injurious behavior; self-negligence; stockpiling of medication; substance misuse

Psychological

Anxiety; depressive symptoms; hostility; expresses deep sadness; expresses frustration; expresses loneliness; low self-esteem; maladaptive grieving; perceived dishonor; perceived failure; reports excessive guilt; reports helplessness; reports hopelessness; reports unhappiness; suicidal ideation

Situational

Easy access to weapon; loss of independence; loss of personal autonomy

Social

Dysfunctional family processes; inadequate social support; inappropriate peer pressure; legal difficulty; social deprivation; social devaluation; social isolation; unaddressed violence by others

At-Risk Population

S

Adolescents; adolescents living in foster care; economically disadvantaged individuals; individuals changing a will; individuals experiencing situational crisis; individuals facing discrimination; individuals giving away possessions; individuals living alone; individuals obtaining potentially lethal materials; individuals preparing a will; individuals who frequently seek care for vague symptomatology; individuals with disciplinary problems; individuals with family history of suicide; individuals with history of suicide attempt; individuals with history of violence; individuals with sudden euphoric recovery from major depression; institutionalized individuals; men; native American individuals; older adults

Associated Conditions

Depression; mental disorders; physical illness; terminal illness

Client Outcomes

Client Will (Specify Time Frame)

- Not harm self
- Maintain connectedness in relationships
- Disclose and discuss suicidal ideas if present; seek help
- Express decreased anxiety and control of impulses

- Talk about feelings; express anger appropriately
- Refrain from using mood-altering substances
- Obtain no access to harmful objects
- Yield access to harmful objects
- Maintain self-control without supervision

Nursing Interventions

The American Psychiatric Nurses Association (APNA, 2015) has adapted a set of essential competencies for psychiatric nurses, all of which can be useful for generalist nurses. These competencies have been incorporated in the following sections.

- Before implementing interventions in the face of suicidal behavior, nurses should examine their own emotional responses to incidents of suicide to ensure that interventions will not be based on countertransference reactions.
- Pursue an understanding of suicide as a phenomenon at all levels of nursing practice. Elements to be considered include the terminology used with suicidality and self-harm phenomena, the epidemiology of suicide, the risk and protective influences on suicide, and the evidence-based best practices in preventing and responding to suicidality (APNA, 2015).
- Assess for suicidal ideation when the history reveals the following: depression, substance abuse; bipolar disorder, schizophrenia, anxiety disorders, post-traumatic stress disorder, dissociative disorder, eating disorders, substance use disorders, antisocial or other personality disorders; attempted suicide, current or past; recent stressful life events (divorce and/or separation, relocation, problems with children); recent unemployment; recent bereavement; adult or childhood physical or sexual abuse; gay, lesbian, or bisexual gender orientation; family history of suicide; and history of chronic trauma. Assess all medical clients and clients with chronic illnesses, traumatic injuries, or pain for their perception of health status and suicidal ideation.
- Assess the client's ability to enter into a no-suicide contract. Contract (verbally or in writing) with the client for no self-harm if the client is appropriate for a contract; recontract at appropriate intervals.
- Be alert for the following warning signs of suicide: making statements such as, "I can't go on," "Nothing matters anymore," "I wish I were dead"; becoming depressed or withdrawn; behaving recklessly; getting affairs in order and giving away valued possessions;

S

showing a marked change in behavior, attitudes, or appearance; abusing drugs or alcohol; and suffering a major loss or life change.

- Take suicide notes seriously and ask if a note was left in any previous suicide attempts. Consider themes of notes in determining appropriate interventions.
- Question family members regarding the preparatory actions mentioned.
- Determine the presence and degree of suicidal risk. A number of questions will elicit the necessary information: Have you been thinking about hurting or killing yourself? How often do you have these thoughts and how long do they last? Do you have a plan? What is it? Do you have access to the means to carry out that plan? How likely is it that you could carry out the plan? Are there people or things that could prevent you from hurting yourself? What do you see in your future a year from now? Five years from now? What do you expect would happen if you died? What has kept you alive up to now?
- Observe, record, and report any changes in mood or behavior that may signify increasing suicide risk and document results of regular surveillance checks.
- Develop a positive therapeutic relationship with the client; do not make promises that may not be kept.
- Express desire to help client. Provide education about suicide and the effectiveness of intervention. Validate the client's experience of psychological pain while maintaining a safe environment for the client.
- ▲ Refer for mental health counseling and possible hospitalization if evidence of suicidal intent exists, which may include evidence of preparatory actions (e.g., obtaining a weapon, making a plan, putting affairs in order, giving away prized possessions, preparing a suicide note).
- Perform risk assessment for possible suicidality on admission to the hospital and thereafter during hospitalization. Alert treatment team to level of risk.
- Determine client's need for supervision and assign a hospitalized client to a room located near the nursing station.
- Search the newly hospitalized client and the client's personal belongings for weapons or potential weapons and hoarded medications during the inpatient admission procedure, as appropriate. Remove dangerous items.

- Limit access to windows and exits unless locked and shatterproof, as appropriate.
- Monitor the client during the use of potential weapons (e.g., razor, scissors).
- Increase surveillance of a hospitalized client at times when staffing is predictably low (e.g., staff meetings, change of shift report, periods of unit disruption).
- Ensure that all oncoming staff members have adequate information to assist the client, using the acronym SBARR: situation (current status, observations), background (relevant client history), assessment (including nurse's current risk assessment and relevant lab findings), recommendations (what the nurse believes is necessary going forward), and response feedback (verification of oncoming staff members' understanding) (APNA, 2015).

▲ If imminent suicide is suspected or an attempt has occurred, call for assistance and do not leave the client alone. Client and staff safety will be served by assistance in the response. The client may attempt additional self-harm if left alone.

- Place the client in the least restrictive, safe, and monitored environment that allows for the necessary level of observation. Assess suicidal risk at least daily and more frequently as warranted.
- Consider strategies to decrease isolation and opportunity to act on harmful thoughts (e.g., use of a sitter).
- Explain suicide precautions and relevant safety issues to the client and family (e.g., purpose, duration, behavioral expectations, and behavioral consequences).

▲ Refer for treatment and participate in the management of any psychiatric illness or symptoms that may be contributing to the client's suicidal ideation or behavior.

▲ Verify that the client has taken medications as ordered (e.g., conduct mouth checks after medication administration).

▲ Maintain increased surveillance of the client whenever use of an antidepressant has been initiated or the dose increased. Antidepressant medications take anywhere from 2 to 6 weeks to achieve full efficacy.

- Involve the client in treatment planning and self-care management of psychiatric disorders.

S

- • Explore with the client all circumstances and motivations related to the suicidality. Listen to the client's own views on his or her problems.
- • Explore with the client all perceived consequences that could act as a barrier to suicide (e.g., effect on family, religious beliefs).
- • Keep discussion oriented to the present and future.
- • Discuss plans for dealing with suicidal ideation in the future (e.g., how to identify precipitating factors, who to contact, where to go for help, and how to respond to desire for self-harm).
- • Assist the client in identifying a network of supportive persons and resources (e.g., clergy, family, care providers).
- ▲ Refer family members and friends to local mental health agencies and crisis intervention centers if the client has suicidal ideation or a suspicion of suicidal thoughts exists.
- ▲ Document client behavior in detail to support outpatient commitment or an overnight psychiatric observation program for an actively suicidal client.
- • Use cognitive-behavioral techniques that help the client modify thinking styles that promote depression, hopelessness, and a belief that suicide is a valid means of escaping the current situation.
- • Engage the client in group interventions that can be useful to address recurrent suicide attempts.
- • With the client's consent, facilitate family-oriented crisis intervention. Family-oriented crisis intervention can clarify stresses and allow assessment of family dynamics.
- • Involve the family in discharge planning (e.g., illness/medication teaching, recognition of increasing suicidal risk, client's plan for dealing with recurring suicidal thoughts, community resources).
- ▲ Before discharge from the hospital, ensure that the client has a supply of ordered medications, has a plan for outpatient follow-up, understands the plan or has a caregiver able and willing to follow the plan, and has the ability to access outpatient treatment.
- ▲ In the event of successful suicide, refer the family to a therapy group for survivors of suicide. Recommended clinical interventions include addressing psychological distress, normalizing denial as an effective coping strategy, working with concerns about family disintegration, and helping families deal with stigmatization.
- • See the care plans for Risk for self-directed **Violence, Hopelessness,** and Risk for **Self-Mutilation.**

S

Pediatric

- The previously mentioned interventions may be appropriate for pediatric clients.
- Use brief self-report measures to improve clinical management of at-risk cases.
- Recognize that the developmental issues of childhood and adolescence may heighten suicide risks and involve different issues from those with adults. Assess specific stressors for the pediatric client, including bullying.
- Assess for exposure to suicide of a significant other.
- Be alert to the presence of school victimization around lesbian, gay, bisexual, and transgender (LGBT) issues and be prepared to advocate for the client.
- Evaluate for the presence of self-mutilation and related risk factors. Refer to care plan for Risk for **Self-Mutilation** for additional information.
- Be aware that complete overlap does not exist between suicidal behavior and self-mutilation. The motivation may be different (ending life rather than coping with difficult feelings), and the method is usually different.
- Involve the adolescent in multimodal treatment programs.
- Before discharge from the hospital, ensure that the client's parent has a supply of ordered medications, has a plan for outpatient follow-up, has a caregiver who understands the plan or is able and willing to follow the plan, and has the ability to access outpatient treatment.
- Parental education groups can influence suicide risk factors.
- Support the implementation of school-based suicide prevention programs.

Geriatric

- Evaluate the older client's mental and physical health status and financial stressors.
- Explore with the client any concerns or pressures (physical and financial) regarding the ability to secure support of medical care, especially perceived pressures about being a burden on family.
- Conduct a thorough assessment of clients' medications.
- When assessing suicide risk factors, incorporate a higher degree of risk for older men and for some older adults who have lost a loved one in the previous year.

S

- Explore triggers of and barriers to suicidal behavior, with particular attention to real and perceived losses (e.g., professional role, health).
- An older adult who shows self-destructive behaviors should be evaluated for dementia.
- ▲ Advocate for the older client with other professionals in securing treatment for suicidal states. Primary care providers have been noted to under recognize and undertreat older adult clients with depression.
- Encourage physical activity in older adults.
- ▲ Refer older adults in primary care settings for care management.
- Consider telephone contacts as an effective intervention for suicidal older adults.

Multicultural

- Assess for the influence of cultural beliefs, norms, and values on the client's perceptions of suicide and on the nurse's perception and approach to suicide.
- Identify and acknowledge the stresses unique to culturally diverse individuals.
- Identify and acknowledge unique cultural responses to stressors in determining sensitive interventions to prevent suicide. Encourage family members to demonstrate and offer caring and support to each other.
- Validate the individual's feelings regarding concerns about the current crisis and family functioning.

Home Care

- Communicate the degree of risk to family and caregivers; assess the family and caregiving situation for the ability to protect the client and to understand the client's suicidal behavior. Provide the family and caregivers with guidelines on how to manage self-harm behaviors in the home environment.
- Assess risk factors in the home.
- If the client's suicidal ideation intensifies, or if a suicide plan with access to means becomes evident, institute an emergency plan for mental health intervention.
- Identify the client's concerns and implement interventions to address the consequences of disability in a client with medical illness. Refer to the care plans for **Hopelessness** and **Powerlessness.**

S

- ▲ Refer for homemaker or psychiatric home healthcare services for respite, client reassurance, and implementation of a therapeutic regimen.
- ▲ If the client is on psychotropic medications, assess the client's and family's knowledge of medication administration and side effects. Teach as necessary.
- ▲ Evaluate the effectiveness and side effects of medications and adherence to the medication regimen. Review with the client and family all medications kept in the home; encourage discarding of old prescriptions. Monitor the amount of medications ordered/provided by the healthcare provider; limiting the amount of medications to which the client has access may be necessary.

Client/Family Teaching and Discharge Planning

- • Establish a supportive relationship with family members.
- • Explain all relevant symptoms, procedures, treatments, and expected outcomes for suicidal ideation that is illness based (e.g., depression, bipolar disorder).
- • Teach the family how to recognize that the client is at increased risk for suicidal behavior (changes in behavior and verbal and nonverbal communication, withdrawal, depression, or sudden lifting of depression).
- • Provide written instructions for treatments and procedures for which the client will be responsible.
- • Instruct the client in coping strategies (assertiveness training, impulse control training, deep breathing, progressive muscle relaxation).
- • Teach cognitive-behavioral activities, such as active problem-solving, reframing (reappraising the situation from a different perspective), or thought stopping (in response to a negative thought, picturing a large stop sign and replacing the image with a prearranged positive alternative). Teach the client to confront his or her own negative thought patterns (or cognitive distortions), such as catastrophizing (expecting the very worst), dichotomous thinking (perceiving events in only one of two opposite categories), or magnification (placing distorted emphasis on a single event).
- • Provide the client and family with phone numbers of appropriate community agencies for therapy and counseling. The National Alliance on Mental Illness (NAMI) is an excellent resource for client and family support.

S

Delayed Surgical Recovery

NANDA-I Definition

Extension of the number of postoperative days required to initiate and perform activities that maintain life, health, and well-being

Defining Characteristics

Anorexia; difficulty in moving about; difficulty resuming employment; excessive time required for recuperation; expresses discomfort; fatigue; interrupted surgical area healing; perceives need for more time to recover postpones resumption of work; requires assistance for self-care

Related Factors

Delirium; impaired physical mobility; increased blood glucose level; malnutrition; negative emotional response to surgical outcome; obesity; persistent nausea; persistent pain; persistent vomiting; smoking

At-Risk Population

Individuals aged ≥ 80 years; individuals experiencing intraoperative hypothermia; individuals requiring emergency surgery; individuals requiring perioperative blood transfusion; individuals with American Society of Anesthesiolgists (ASA) Physical Status Classification score ≥ 3; individuals with history of myocardial infarction; individuals with low functional capacity; individuals with preoperative weight loss > 5%

Associated Condition

S

Anemia; diabetes mellitus; extensive surgical procedures; pharmaceutical preparations; prolonged duration of perioperative surgical wound infection; psychological disorder in postoperative period; surgical wound infection postoperative period; surgical site contamination; trauma at surgical site

Client Outcomes

Client Will (Specify Time Frame)

- Have surgical area that shows evidence of healing: no redness, induration, draining, or immobility
- State that appetite is regained
- State that no nausea is present
- Demonstrate ability to move about
- Demonstrate ability to complete self-care activities
- State that no fatigue is present
- State that pain is controlled or relieved after nursing interventions
- Resume employment activities/ADLs
- State no depression or anxiety related to surgical procedure

Nursing Interventions

- Encourage smoking cessation prior to surgery.
- Preoperatively, perform a thorough assessment of the client, including risk factors. Allow time to be with the client, and actively listen to client's concerns and questions about care, functional status, and recovery.
- Assess for the presence of medical conditions and treat appropriately before surgery. If the client is diabetic, maintain normal blood glucose levels before surgery.
- Carefully assess client's use of dietary supplements such as feverfew, fish oil, ginkgo biloba, garlic, ginseng, ginger, valerian, kava, St. John's wort, ephedra (Ma huang or metabolite), and Echinacea. It is recommended that all clients be advised to stop all dietary supplements at least 1 week before major surgical or diagnostic procedures.
- Assess and treat for depression and anxiety in a client before surgery and postoperatively.
- Play music of the client's choice preoperatively, intraoperatively, and postoperatively.
- Consider using healing touch and other mind-body-spirit interventions such as stress control, therapeutic massage, and imagery in the perianesthesia setting.
- Use reflective blankets to reduce heat loss during surgery.
- Postoperatively, discuss with the surgeon vital sign parameters, signs, and symptoms that could indicate early postoperative infection.
- Use careful aseptic technique when caring for wounds.
- Clients should be allowed to shower after surgery to maintain cleanliness if not contraindicated because of the presence of pacemaker wires.
- Promote early ambulation and deep breathing.
- The client should be provided with a complete, balanced therapeutic diet after the immediately postoperative period (24–48 hours).
- Encourage the client to use prayer as a form of spiritual coping if this is comfortable for the client.
- Carefully assess functional status of client postoperatively using a fall-risk stratification tool, such as the Morse Fall Scale, to identify clients at high risk for fall.
- See the care plans for **Anxiety,** Acute **Pain, Fatigue,** Risk for deficient **Fluid** volume, Risk for **Perioperative Positioning** injury, Impaired physical **Mobility,** and **Nausea.**

S

Pediatric

- Encourage children to ask questions about their procedures and postoperative expectations regarding pain, function, and long-term social and emotional care needs.
- Teach imagery and encourage distraction for children for postsurgical pain relief.

Geriatric

- Perform a thorough preoperative assessment, including a cardiac, social support, and skin assessment.
- Older clients are at increased risk of delayed surgical recovery associated with physical and psychological postsurgical stress, nutritional deficits, aging immune system, and comorbid disease states.
- Routinely assess pain in postoperative clients using a pain scale that is appropriate for clients with impaired cognition or inability to verbalize.
- Serially evaluate the client's vital signs, including temperature. Know what is normal and abnormal for each client. Check baseline vital signs and monitor trends.
- Ongoing evaluation of the older client for signs and symptoms of delirium should be incorporated into each assessment. Provide tools such as clocks, calendars, and other orientation tools to help reduce the risk of delirium in the postoperative area. Ensure that hearing aids and glasses are also available as needed.
- Offer spiritual support.

Home Care

- The preceding interventions may be adapted for the home setting.
- Provide supportive telephone calls from nurse to client as a means of decreasing anxiety and providing the psychosocial support necessary for recovery from surgery.

Client/Family Teaching and Discharge Planning

- Provide discharge planning and teaching in a language that is appropriate to the client and caregiver's education and literacy level.
- Meet with client and caregivers to create a discharge plan that includes measurable goals for functional ADLs and pain levels, discuss expectations for recovery, and address signs and symptoms of postoperative complications.
- Provide individualized teaching plans for the client with an ostomy. Assess client's ability to manage basic needs such as (1) maintenance of a pouching seal for a consistent, predictable wear time; (2) maintenance of peristomal skin integrity; and (3) social and

professional support. Referrals for home wound care or nursing visits may be necessary to help client maintain hygiene and prevent readmission for complications.

Risk for Delayed Surgical Recovery

NANDA-I Definition

Susceptible to an extension of the number of postoperative days required to initiate and perform activities that maintain life, health, and well-being, which may compromise health

Risk Factors

Delirium; impaired physical mobility; increased blood glucose level; malnutrition; negative emotional response to surgical outcome; obesity; persistent nausea; persistent pain; persistent vomiting; smoking

At-Risk Population

Individuals aged ≥ 80 years; individuals experiencing intraoperative hypothermia; individuals requiring emergency surgery; individuals requiring perioperative blood transfusion; individuals with American Society of Anesthesiolgists (ASA) Physical Status Classification score ≥ 3; individuals with history of myocardial infarction; individuals with low functional capacity; individuals with preoperative weight loss > 5%

Associated Condition

Anemia; diabetes mellitus; extensive surgical procedures; pharmaceutical preparations; prolonged duration of perioperative surgical wound infection; psychological disorder in postoperative period; surgical wound infection

Client Outcomes, Nursing Interventions, Client/Family Teaching and Discharge Planning

See the care plan for Delayed **Surgical** recovery

Impaired Swallowing

NANDA-I Definition

Abnormal functioning of the swallowing mechanism associated with deficits in oral, pharyngeal, or esophageal structure or function

Defining Characteristics

First Stage: Oral

Abnormal oral phase of swallow study; bruxism; choking prior to swallowing; choking when swallowing cold water; coughing prior to swallowing; drooling; food falls from mouth; food pushed out of mouth; gagging prior to swallowing; impaired ability to clear oral cavity; inadequate consumption during prolonged mealtime; inadequate lip closure; inadequate mastication; incidence of wet hoarseness twice within 30 seconds; inefficient nippling; inefficient suck; nasal reflux; piecemeal deglutition; pooling of bolus in lateral sulci; premature entry of bolus; prolonged bolus formation; tongue action ineffective in forming bolus

Second Stage: Pharyngeal

Abnormal pharyngeal phase of swallow study; altered head position; choking; coughing; delayed swallowing; fevers of unknown etiology; food refusal; gagging sensation; gurgly voice quality; inadequate laryngeal elevation; nasal reflux; recurrent pulmonary infection; repetitive swallowing

Third Stage: Esophageal

Abnormal esophageal phase of swallow study; acidic-smelling breath; difficulty swallowing; epigastric pain; food refusal; heartburn; hematemesis; hyperextension of head; nighttime awakening; nighttime coughing; odynophagia; regurgitation; repetitive swallowing; reports "something stuck"; unexplained irritability surrounding mealtimes; volume limiting; vomiting; vomitus on pillow

Related Factors

Behavioral feeding problem; altered attention; protein-energy malnutrition; self-injurious behavior

At-Risk Population

Individuals with history of enteral nutrition; older adults; premature infants

Associated Conditions

S

Acquired autonomic defects; brain injury; cerebral palsy; conditions with significant muscle hypotonia; congenital heart disease; cranial nerve involvement; developmental disabilities; esophageal achalasia; gastroesophageal reflux disease; gastroesophageal reflux disease; laryngeal diseases; mechanical obstruction; nasal defect; nasopharyngeal cavity defect; neurological problems; neuromuscular diseases; oropharynx abnormality; pharmaceutical preparations; prolonged intubation; respiratory condition; tracheal defect; trauma; upper airway anomaly; vocal cord dysfunction

Client Outcomes

Client Will (Specify Time Frame)

- Demonstrate effective swallowing without signs of aspiration (see the section Defining Characteristics)
- Remain free from aspiration (e.g., lungs clear, temperature within normal range)

Nursing Interventions

- Complete swallow screen per facility protocol.
- ▲ Do not feed clients with impaired swallowing orally until an appropriate diagnostic workup is completed.

- ▲ Ensure proper nutrition by consulting with a healthcare provider regarding alternative nutrition and hydration when oral nutrition is not safe/adequate.
- ▲ Refer to a speech-language pathologist for evaluation and diagnostic evaluation of swallowing to determine swallowing problems and solutions as soon as oral and/or pharyngeal dysphagia is suspected.
- ▲ To manage impaired swallowing, use a multidisciplinary dysphagia team composed of a speech pathologist, dietitian, nursing, healthcare provider, and medical staff. A comprehensive assessment from a multidisciplinary dysphagia team can lead to personalized therapeutic interventions that can help the client learn to swallow safely and maintain a good nutritional status.
- ▲ Observe the following feeding guidelines:
  - ❍ Before giving oral feedings, determine the client's readiness to eat (e.g., alert, able to hold head erect, follow instructions, move tongue in mouth, and manage oral secretions).
  - ❍ Monitor client during oral feedings and provide cueing as needed to ensure client follows swallowing guidelines/aspiration precautions recommended by speech-language pathologist or dysphagia specialist. Note: General aspiration precautions include the following: sit at 90 degrees for all oral feedings, take small bites/sips, eat at a slow rate, and no straws. However, client-specific strategies will be determined via bedside and/or instrumental swallowing evaluation performed by dysphagia specialist.
  - ❍ Keep bolus size to 5 mL or smaller.
- • During meals and all oral intake, observe for signs associated with swallowing problems such as coughing, choking, spitting of food, drooling, difficulty handling oral secretions, double swallowing or delay in swallowing, watering eyes, nasal discharge, wet or gurgling voice, decreased ability to move the tongue and lips, decreased mastication of food, decreased ability to move food to the back of the pharynx, and slow or scanning speech.
- ▲ Watch for uncoordinated chewing or swallowing; coughing immediately after eating or delayed coughing; pocketing of food; wet-sounding voice; sneezing when eating; delay of more than 1 second in swallowing; or a change in respiratory patterns. If any of these signs of dysphagia and/or aspiration is present, remove all food from the oral cavity, stop feedings, and consult with speech-language pathologist and dysphagia team.

S

- ▲ If signs of aspiration or pneumonia are present, auscultate lung sounds after feeding. Note new onset of crackles or wheezing, or elevated temperature.
- ▲ Assess for signs of malnutrition and dehydration and keep a record of food intake.
- ▲ Evaluate nutritional status daily. Weigh the client weekly to help evaluate nutritional status. If the client is not adequately nourished, work with the dysphagia team to determine whether the client needs therapeutic feeding only or needs enteral feedings until the client can swallow adequately.
- ▲ Assist client in following dysphagia specialist's recommendations and provide open, accurate, and effective communication with dysphagia team regarding client's diet tolerance.
- ▲ Document and notify the healthcare provider and dysphagia team of changes in medical, nutritional, or swallowing status.
- ▲ Work with the client on swallowing exercises prescribed by the dysphagia team.
- ▲ If needed, provide meals in a quiet environment away from excessive stimuli, such as a community dining room, for some clients who are easily distracted.
- ▲ For many adult clients, avoid the use of straws if recommended by the speech pathologist.
- ▲ Recognize that the client can aspirate oral feedings, even if there are no symptoms of coughing or distress. This phenomenon is called silent aspiration and is common.
- ▲ Ensure oral hygiene is maintained.
- ▲ Check the oral cavity for proper emptying after the client swallows and after the client finishes the meal. Provide oral care at the end of the meal. It may be necessary to manually remove food from the client's mouth. If this is the case, use gloves and keep the client's teeth apart with a padded tongue blade.
- ▲ Praise the client for successfully following directions and swallowing appropriately.
- ▲ Keep the client in an upright position for 45 minutes to an hour after a meal.
- ▲ Recognize that impaired swallowing may be caused by the medications the client is taking. Side effects of medications include xerostomia (antidepressants, anticholinergics, antihistamines, bronchodilators, antineoplastic, and anti-Parkinson), central nervous system depression

(anticonvulsants, benzodiazepines, antispasmodics, antidepressants, and antipsychotics), myopathy (corticosteroids, lipid-lowering agents, and colchicines), and decreased esophageal sphincter tone (antihistamines, diuretics, opiates, antipsychotics, antihypertensives, and anticholinergics).

▲ For clients receiving mechanical ventilation with a tracheostomy tube or after postextubation, request a referral to a speech-language pathologist or dysphagia specialist for an instrumental swallowing evaluation before beginning oral diet.

Pediatric

▲ Refer a child who has difficulty swallowing and symptoms such as difficulty manipulating food, delayed swallow response, and pocketing of a bolus of food to a speech-language pathologist (or dysphagia specialist) and a dietitian.

▲ Consult with a speech-language pathologist or dysphagia specialist regarding modifications to nipple, appropriate positioning and feeding strategies, and other therapeutic activities deemed most appropriate based on bedside and instrumental swallowing evaluation.

▲ The following are general feeding guidelines. Specific strategies to eliminate aspiration and maximize intake should be individualized and determined by a swallowing specialist through bedside and instrumental swallowing evaluation.

- Attempt feedings when infant is in an optimal behavioral feeding state (e.g., awake, alert, not agitated) and halt feedings if infant is not able to maintain or regain a proper feeding state.
- In a preterm infant, provide opportunities for patterned nonnutritive sucking (NNS).
- In a preterm infant, alter nipple flow rate to one that is easily managed by infant to facilitate intake while achieving physiological stability.
- Watch for indicators of aspiration and physiological instability during feeding: coughing, a change in vocal quality or wet vocal quality, perspiration and color changes, sneezing, apnea, and/or increased heart rate and breathing. Infants and children with silent aspiration may only have indicators of increased respiratory mucous, congestion and chronic wheeze or rhonchi, recurrent bronchitis, or recurrent pneumonia (Tutor & Gosa, 2012).
- Watch for warning signs of reflux such as sour-smelling breath after eating, sneezing, lack of interest in feeding, crying and fussing extraordinarily when feeding, pained expressions when feeding, and excessive chewing and swallowing after eating.

S

- Observe infant's behavior and cues and adjust feeding to promote a safe pleasurable feeding experience while eliminating aspiration and maximizing intake.

Geriatric

- ▲ Recognize that age-related changes can affect swallowing and these changes have a more pronounced effect when superimposed on disease such as neurological and other chronic medical problems.
- ▲ Evaluate medications the client is presently taking and consult with the pharmacist for assistance in monitoring for incorrect doses and drug interactions that could result in dysphagia.
- ▲ Ensure all nursing home residents are screened for swallowing problems.
- ▲ Encourage and provide good oral hygiene when indicated.
- ▲ Consult with occupational therapist for adaptive equipment when appropriate.
- ▲ Recognize that the older client with dementia may need a longer time to eat and is often easily distracted. Help optimize hydration and nutrition using the following techniques:
  - Encourage six small meals and hydration breaks per day.
  - Offer foods that are sweet, spicy, or sour to increase sensory input.
  - Allow clients to touch food and self-feed, if necessary (Tanner, 2013).
  - Eliminate from the tray or table nonfoods such as salt and pepper, or anything that can be distracting.
  - Keep desserts out of sight until the end of the meal.
  - Offer finger foods to the client who has trouble holding still to eat.
  - Allow clients to eat immediately when they come for the meal.
  - Recognize that the client with advanced dementia, who is unable to swallow, may or may not benefit from enteral tube feedings.

Home Care

- ▲ Refer to speech therapy. Speech-language pathologists can work with clients to enhance swallowing ability and teach compensatory strategies.

Client/Family Teaching and Discharge Planning

- ▲ Teach the client and family exercises prescribed by the dysphagia team.
- ▲ Teach the client a systematic method of swallowing effectively as prescribed by the dysphagia team.
- Educate the client, family, and all caregivers about rationales for food consistency and choices.
- Teach the family how to monitor the client to prevent and detect aspiration during eating.

Risk for Thermal Injury

NANDA-I Definition

Susceptible to extreme temperature damage to skin and mucous membranes, which may compromise health

Risk Factors

Fatigue; inadequate protective clothing; inadequate supervision; inattentiveness; insufficient caregiver knowledge of safety precautions; insufficient knowledge of safety precautions; smoking; unsafe environment

At-Risk Population

Extremes of age; extremes of environmental temperature

Associated Condition

Alcohol intoxication; alteration in cognitive functioning; drug intoxication; neuromuscular impairment; neuropathy; treatment regimen

Client Outcomes

Client Will (Specify Time Frame)

- Be free of thermal injury to skin or tissue
- Explain actions can take to protect self and others from thermal injury
- Explain actions can take to protect self and others in the work environment

Nursing Interventions

- Teach the following interventions to prevent fires in the home, to handle any possible fire, and to have a readily available exit from the home:
  - Avoid plugging several appliance cords into the same electrical socket.
  - Do not use open candles or allow smoking in the home.
  - Keep a fire extinguisher within reach in case a fire should occur.
  - Install smoke alarms on every level of the home and in every sleeping area.
  - Keep furniture and other heavy objects out of the way of doors and windows.
  - Develop a fire escape plan that includes two ways out of every room and an outside meeting place. Practice the escape plan at least twice a year.
- Teach clients about home grill safety to prevent thermal injury (propane and charcoal grills).
- Apply sunscreen as directed on the container when out in the sun. Also use sun-blocking clothing, and stay in the shade if possible.

- Teach clients safety measures to prevent fires in the home in which medical oxygen is in use:
  - **Never smoke** in a home in which medical oxygen is in use. "No smoking" signs should be posted inside and outside the home.
  - Do not wear oxygen near an ignition source (e.g., open flame, gas stove, fireplace, candles, cigarettes, matches, lighters, etc.). Note that petroleum jelly, lip balm, skin lotion, or the like will not spontaneously combust in the presence of supplemental oxygen without an ignition source, e.g., flame or spark, and are safe to use on the face and in bed in the presence of oxygen (Winslow & Jacobsen, 1998; Hadjiliadis, 2016).
  - Homes with medical oxygen must have working smoke alarms that are tested monthly.
  - Test fire extinguishers every 3 to 6 months. Keep a fire extinguisher within reach. If a fire occurs, turn off the oxygen, leave the home, and summon the fire department.
  - Develop a fire escape plan that includes two ways out of every room and an outside meeting place. Practice the escape plan at least twice a year.
- Be aware that thermal injury also includes injury from cold materials and environmental conditions, including freezing injury, nonfreezing injury, and hypothermia.
- Provide adequate environmental temperatures. Older clients and others at risk for temperature dysregulation can easily become hypothermic in air-conditioned environments (e.g., a surgical suite), with inadequate clothing, inhaling cold gases, or when exposed to room temperature or chilled fluids (e.g., intravenous, gastric lavage, bowel prep, continuous renal replacement therapy (CRRT), dialysis).
- Monitor temperature in vulnerable clients. Core temperature is the best measure to assess for hypothermia. If a pulmonary artery catheter is not available, use a thermometer calibrated for lower body temperature such as a distal esophageal probe or rectal or bladder temperature probe (Leon & Bouchama, 2015).
- Use active warming measures to help clients maintain body temperature (e.g., warming blankets, warmed fluids, forced warm air warming devices, foil wraps, radiant warmers) as indicated. Be aware that passive devices (e.g., socks or blankets) do not add heat to body tissues.

- Ensure that exposed skin is protected from cold with adequate clothing.
- Monitor for developing cold thermal injury by checking peripheral circulation, temperature, and sensation. Be aware that fine motor coordination decreases as a very early sign of hypothermia.
- Check the temperature of all equipment and other materials before allowing them to contact client skin, especially if client has increased risk factors for thermal injury.

Pediatric

- Teach the following activities to homes with small children:
  - Lock up matches and lighters out of sight and reach.
  - Never leave a hot stove unattended.
  - Do not allow small children to use the microwave until they are at least 7 or 8 years of age.
  - Keep all portable heaters out of children's reach and at least 3 feet away from anything that can burn.
  - Teach fire prevention and safety to older children.
- Install thermostatic mixer valves in a hot water system to prevent extreme hot water causing scalding burns.

Ineffective Thermoregulation

T

NANDA-I Definition

Temperature fluctuation between hypothermia and hyperthermia

Defining Characteristics

Cyanotic nail beds; flushed skin; hypertension; increase in body temperature above normal range; increase in respiratory rate; mild shivering; moderate pallor; piloerection; reduction in body temperature below normal range; seizure; skin cool to touch; skin warm to touch; slow capillary refill; tachycardia

Related Factors

Dehydration; fluctuating environmental temperature; inactivity; inappropriate clothing for environmental temperature; increase in oxygen demand; vigorous activity

At-Risk Population

Extremes of age; extremes of weight; extremes of environmental temperature; increased body surface area to weight ratio; insufficient supply of subcutaneous fat

Associated Condition

Alteration in metabolic rate; brain injury; condition affecting temperature regulation; decrease in sweat response; illness; inefficient nonshivering thermogenesis; pharmaceutical agent; sedation; sepsis; trauma

Client Outcomes

Client Will (Specify Time Frame)

- Maintain temperature within normal range
- Explain measures needed to maintain normal temperature
- Describe two to four symptoms of hypothermia or hyperthermia
- List two or three self-care measures to treat hypothermia or hyperthermia

Nursing Interventions

Temperature Measurement

- Measure and record the client's temperature using a consistent method of temperature measurement every 1 to 4 hours depending on the severity of the situation or whenever a change in condition occurs (e.g., chills, change in mental status).
- Select core, near core, or peripheral temperature monitoring mode based on ability to obtain an accurate temperature from that site and clinical situation dictating the need for mode of temperature monitoring required for clinical treatment decisions.
- Caution should be taken in interpreting extreme values of temperature (less than 35°C or greater than 39°C) from a near core temperature site device.
- Evaluate the significance of a decreased or increased temperature.

▲ Notify the healthcare provider of temperature according to institutional standards or written orders, or when temperature reaches 100.5°F (38.3°C) and above; use a lower threshold for immunocompromised clients who will be less likely to exhibit a fever when seriously ill (Niven et al., 2016). Also notify the healthcare provider of the presence of a change in mental status and temperature greater than 100.5°F (38.3°C) or less than 36°C.

Fever (Pyrexia)

- Recognize that fever is characterized as a temporary elevation in internal body temperature 1°C to 2°C higher than the client's normal body temperature.
- Recognize that fever is a normal physiological response to a perceived threat by the body, frequently in response to an infection.

▲ Review client history to include current medical diagnosis, medications, recent procedures/interventions, recent travel, environmental exposure to infectious agents, recent blood product administration, and review of laboratory analysis for cause of ineffective thermoregulation.

- Recognize that fever may be low grade (36°C–38°C) in response to an inflammatory process such as infection, allergy, trauma, illness, or surgery; moderate to high-grade fever (38°C–40°C) indicates a more concerted inflammatory response from a systemic infection; hyperpyrexia (40°C and higher) occurs as a result of damage of the hypothalamus, bacteremia, or an extremely overheated room (Munro, 2014; Niven et al., 2016).
- Recognize that fever has a predictable physiological pattern.
- Monitor and intervene to provide comfort during a fever by:
  - Obtaining vital signs and accurate intake and output
  - Checking laboratory analysis trends of white blood cell counts and other markers of infection
  - Providing blankets when the client complains of being cold, but removing surplus of blankets when the client is too warm
  - Encouraging fluid and nutrition
  - Limiting activity to conserve energy
  - Providing frequent oral care
  - Adjust room temperature for client comfort

Hypothermia

- Take vital signs frequently, noting changes associated with hypothermia, such as increased blood pressure, pulse, and respirations, that then advance to decreased values as hypothermia progresses.
- Monitor the client for signs of hypothermia (e.g., shivering, cool skin, piloerection, pallor, slow capillary refill, cyanotic nailbeds, decreased mentation, dysrhythmias) (Paal et al., 2016; Zafren, 2017).
- See the care plan for **Hypothermia** as appropriate.

Hyperthermia

- Recognize that hyperthermia is a different etiology than fever so the cause of the elevated body temperature should be explored for definitive treatment.
- Note changes in vital signs associated with hyperthermia, such as rapid, bounding pulse; increased respiratory rate; and decreased blood pressure, accompanied by orthostatic hypotension; and signs and symptoms of dehydration (Gaudio & Grissom, 2016; Niven, 2016).

- Monitor the client for signs of hyperthermia (e.g., headache, nausea and vomiting, weakness, extreme fatigue, delirium, coma).
- Adjust clothing to facilitate passive warming or cooling as appropriate.
- See the care plan for **Hyperthermia** as appropriate.

Pediatric

- For routine measurement of temperature, use an electronic thermometer in the axilla in infants younger than 4 weeks; for a child up to 5 years of age, use an electronic thermometer in the axilla or an infrared temporal artery thermometer.
- Recognize that pediatric clients have a decreased ability to adapt to temperature extremes. Take the following actions to maintain body temperature in the infant/child:
  - Keep the head covered.
  - Use blankets to keep the client warm.
  - Keep the client covered during procedures, transport, and diagnostic testing.
  - Keep the room temperature at 72°F (22.2°C).
- Recognize that the infant and small child are both vulnerable to develop heat stroke in hot weather; ensure that they receive sufficient fluids and are protected from hot environments.
- Antipyretic treatments typically are not indicated unless the child's temperature is higher than 38.3°C and may be given to provide comfort.

T

Geriatric

- Do not allow an older client to become chilled; keep the client covered when giving a bath and offer socks to wear in bed; be aware of factors such as room temperature (heating/air conditioning), clothing (layered/loose), and fluid intake.
- Recognize that the older client may have an infection without a significant rise in body temperature.
- Fever does not put the older adult at risk for long-term complications; thus fever should not be treated with antipyretic agents or other external methods of cooling, unless there is serious heart disease present.
- Ensure that older clients receive sufficient fluids during hot days and stay out of the sun.
- Assess the medication profile for the potential risk of drug-related altered body temperature.

Home Care

Treating Fever

- Instruct client/parents on the physiological benefits of fever and provide interventions to treat fever symptoms, avoiding antipyretic agents, and external cooling interventions.
- Ensure that client/parents know when to contact a healthcare provider for fever-related concerns.
- **Prevention of Hypothermia in Cold Weather**
  See the care plan **Hypothermia.**
- **Prevention of Hyperthermia in Hot Weather**
  See the care plan **Hyperthermia.**

Client/Family Teaching and Discharge Planning

- Teach the client and family the signs of fever, hypothermia, and hyperthermia and appropriate actions to take if either condition develops.
- Teach the client and family an age-appropriate method for taking the temperature.
- Teach the client to avoid alcohol and medications that depress cerebral function.

Risk for Ineffective Thermoregulation

NANDA-I Definition

Susceptible to temperature fluctuation between hypothermia and hyperthermia, which may compromise health

Risk Factors

Dehydration; fluctuating environmental temperature; inactivity; inappropriate clothing for environmental temperature; increase in oxygen demand; vigorous activity

At-Risk Population

Extremes of age; extremes of weight; extremes of environmental temperatures; increase body surface area to weight ratio; insufficient supply of subcutaneous fat

Associated Condition

Alteration in metabolic rate; brain injury; condition affecting temperature regulation; decrease in sweat response; illness; inefficient nonshivering thermogenesis; pharmaceutical agent; sedation; sepsis; trauma

Client Outcomes, Nursing Interventions

Refer to care plans for Ineffective **Thermoregulation** (fever), **Hyperthermia,** or **Hypothermia**

Impaired Tissue Integrity

NANDA-I Definition

Damage to the mucous membrane, cornea, integumentary system, muscular fascia, muscle, tendon, bone, cartilage, joint capsule, and/or ligament

Defining Characteristics

Abscess; acute pain; bleeding; decreased muscle strength; decreased range of motion; difficulty bearing weight; dry eye; hematoma; impaired skin integrity; localized area hot to touch; localized deformity; localized loss of hair; localized numbness; localized swelling; muscle spasm; reports lack of balance; reports tingling sensation; stiffness; tissue exposure below the epidermis

Related Factors

External Factors

Excretions; humidity; hyperthermia; hypothermia; inadequate caregiver knowledge about maintaining tissue integrity; inadequate caregiver knowledge about protecting tissue integrity; inadequate use of chemical agent; pressure over bony prominence; psychomotor agitation; secretions; shearing forces; surface friction; use of linen with insufficient moisture wicking property

Internal Factors

Body mass index above normal range for age and gender; body mass index below normal range for age and gender; decreased blinking frequency; decreased physical activity; fluid imbalance; impaired physical mobility; impaired postural balance; inadequate adherence to incontinence treatment regimen; inadequate blood glucose level management; inadequate knowledge about maintaining tissue integrity; inadequate knowledge about restoring tissue integrity; inadequate ostomy care; malnutrition; psychogenic factor; self mutilation; smoking; substance misuse

At-Risk Population

Homeless individuals; individuals at extremes of age; individuals exposed to environmental temperature extremes; individuals exposed to high-voltage power supply; individuals participating in contact sports; individuals participating in winter sports; individuals with family history of bone fracture; individuals with history of bone fracture

Associated Condition

Anemia; autism spectrum disorder; cardiovascular diseases; chronic neurological conditions; critical illness; decreased level of consciousness; decreased serum albumin level; decreased tissue oxygenation; decreased tissue perfusion; hemodynamic instability; immobilization; intellectual disability; medical devices; metabolic diseases; peripheral neuropathy; pharmaceutical preparations; sensation disorders; surgical procedures

Client Outcomes

Client Will (Specify Time Frame)

- Report any altered sensation or pain at site of tissue impairment
- Demonstrate understanding of plan to heal tissue and prevent reinjury
- Describe measures to protect and heal the tissue, including wound care
- Experience a wound that decreases in size and has increased granulation tissue

Nursing Interventions

- The National Pressure Ulcer Advisory Panel (NPUAP) redefined the definition of a pressure ulcer, which is now referred to as a pressure injury, during the NPUAP 2016 Staging Consensus Conference. The new definitions more accurately define alterations in tissue integrity from pressure as follows: A pressure injury is localized damage to the skin and underlying soft tissue usually over a bony prominence or related to a medical device or other device. The injury can present as intact skin or an open ulcer and may be painful. The injury occurs as a result of intense and/or prolonged pressure or pressure in combination with shear. The tolerance of soft tissue for pressure and shear may also be affected by microclimate, nutrition, perfusion, comorbidities, and condition of the soft tissue (NPUAP/European Pressure Ulcer Advisory Panel [EPUAP], 2016).
- The first step is to identify etiological factors or what is causing the impairment. A thorough assessment of the individual, not only the impairment, is crucial. This includes a comprehensive medical history, current medical status, medications, and family history (Murphree, 2017). Differentiate pressure injuries form other types of wounds such as moisture-associated skin damage (MASD) (Ratliff et al., 2017). A comprehensive assessment helps identify specific risk factors and systemic factors, which aids the clinician in a more successful wound management approach (Murphree, 2017).
- Determine the size (length, width) and depth of the wound. Select a uniform, consistent method for measuring wound length, width, or wound area, and depth to facilitate meaningful comparisons of wound measurements over time. A careful assessment should be performed to avoid causing injury when probing the depth of a wound bed or determining the extent of undermining or tunneling (NPUAP/EPUAP, 2014).

▲ Classify pressure injuries (NPUAP, 2016) using national guidelines and definitions (see http://www.npuap.org/resources/educational-and-clinical-resources/npuap-pressure-injury-stages/)
  - **Pressure Injury:** A pressure injury is localized damage to the skin and underlying soft tissue usually over a bony prominence or related to a medical or other device. The injury can present as intact skin or an open ulcer and may be painful. The injury occurs as a result of intense and/or prolonged pressure or pressure in combination with shear. The tolerance of soft tissue for pressure and shear may also be affected by microclimate, nutrition, perfusion, comorbidities, and condition of the soft tissue (NPUAP, 2016).
  - **Stage 1 Pressure Injury:** Nonblanchable erythema of intact skin
    Area of localized non-blanchable erythema that may appear differently in darkly pigmented skin, and changes in sensation, temperature, or firmness may precede visual changes. Color changes do not include purple or maroon discoloration, which is more likely to indicate deep tissue pressure injury (NPUAP, 2016).
  - **Stage 2 Pressure Injury:** Partial-thickness skin loss with exposed dermis
    Partial-thickness skin loss with exposed dermis in which the wound bed is pink/red and moist and adipose (fat) and deeper tissues are not visible. Granulation tissue, slough, and eschar are not present. A stage 2 pressure injury may also present as an intact or ruptured blister. These injuries commonly result from adverse microclimate and shear in the skin over the pelvis and shear in the heel. This stage should not be used to describe MASD including incontinence-associated dermatitis (IAD), intertriginous dermatitis (ITD), medical adhesive–related skin injury (MARSI), or traumatic wounds (skin tears, burns, and abrasions) (NPUAP, 2016).
  - **Stage 3 Pressure Injury:** Full-thickness skin loss
    Full-thickness loss of skin, in which adipose is visible and granulation tissue and epibole (rolled wound edges) are often present, and undermining/tunneling may occur. Slough and/or eschar may also be visible. Fascia, muscle, tendon, ligament, cartilage, and/or bone are not exposed. The depth of tissue damage varies by anatomical location, and areas of significant adiposity can develop deep wounds. If slough or eschar obscures the extent of tissue loss, this is an unstageable pressure injury (NPUAP, 2016).

- **Stage 4 Pressure Injury:** Full-thickness skin and tissue loss
  Full-thickness skin and tissue loss with exposed or directly palpable fascia, muscle, tendon, ligament, cartilage, or bone, and slough and/or eschar may be visible. Epibole, undermining, and/or tunneling often occur and depth varies by anatomical location. If slough or eschar obscures the extent of tissue loss, this is an unstageable pressure injury (NPUAP, 2016).
- **Deep Tissue Pressure Injury:** Persistent nonblanchable deep red, maroon, or purple discoloration
  Intact or nonintact skin with localized area of persistent nonblanchable deep red, maroon, or purple discoloration or epidermal separation revealing a dark wound bed or blood-filled blister. Pain and temperature change often precede skin color changes. Discoloration may appear differently in darkly pigmented skin. This injury results from intense and/or prolonged pressure and shear forces at the bone–muscle interface. The wound may evolve rapidly to reveal the actual extent of tissue injury, or it may resolve without tissue loss. If necrotic tissue, subcutaneous tissue, granulation tissue, fascia, muscle, or other underlying structures are visible, this indicates a full-thickness pressure injury (unstageable, stage 3, or stage 4). Do not use deep tissue pressure injury to describe vascular, traumatic, neuropathic, or dermatological conditions (NPUAP, 2016).
- **Unstageable Pressure Injury:** Obscured full-thickness skin and tissue loss
  Full-thickness skin and tissue loss in which the extent of tissue damage within the ulcer cannot be confirmed because it is obscured by slough or eschar. If slough or eschar is removed, a stage 3 or stage 4 pressure injury will be revealed. Stable eschar (i.e., dry, adherent, intact without erythema or fluctuance) on the heel or ischemic limb should not be softened or removed (NPUAP, 2016).

- Inspect and monitor the site of impaired tissue integrity at least once daily for color changes, redness, swelling, warmth, pain, or other signs of infection or per facility/agency policy. Monitor the status of the skin around the wound. Pay special attention to all high-risk areas such as bony prominences, skinfolds, sacrum, and heels. There is evidence that stage 1 pressure injuries are under detected in individuals with darkly pigmented skin because areas of redness are not easily identified.
- Assess for incontinence and implement an individualized plan for management. Differentiate wounds caused by incontinence from other

T

types of wounds. Cleanse the skin promptly after episodes of incontinence and use pH-balanced cleansers (NPUAP/EPUAP, 2014). Use incontinence skin barriers including creams, ointments, pastes, or film-forming skin protectants as needed to protect and maintain skin integrity with incontinent individuals (Ratliff et al., 2017).

- • Monitor for correct placement of tubes, catheters, and other devices. Assess the skin and tissue affected by the pressure of the devices and tape used to secure these devices.
- • Medical device–related pressure injury describes an etiology. Medical device–related pressure injuries result from the use of devices designed and applied for diagnostic or therapeutic purposes. The resultant pressure injury generally conforms to the pattern or shape of the device. The injury should be staged using the previously discussed staging system (NPUAP, 2016).
- • Assess frequently for correct placement of foot boards, restraints, traction, casts, or other devices, and assess skin and tissue integrity. Frequently assess for signs and symptoms of compartment syndrome (refer to the care plan for Risk for **Peripheral Neurovascular** dysfunction). Reposition the individual and/or the medical device to redistribute pressure and decrease shear force (NPUAP/EPUAP, 2014).
- • Implement and communicate a comprehensive treatment plan for the topical treatment of the skin impairment site.
- ▲ Identify a plan for debridement if necrotic tissue (eschar or slough) is present and if consistent with overall client management goals (i.e., curative versus palliative care).
- • Select a topical treatment that maintains a moist, wound-healing environment and also allows absorption of exudate and filling of dead space.
- • Avoid positioning the client on the site of impaired tissue integrity.
- • Evaluate for the use of support surfaces (specialty mattresses, beds) chair cushion, or devices as appropriate (Lippoldt, Pernicka, & Staudinger et al., 2014). Before replacing the existing mattress evaluate the effectiveness of previous and current prevention and treatment plans and set treatment goals consistent with the individual's goals and lifestyle (NPUAP/EPUAP, 2014). Continued repositioning of individuals placed on a pressure redistribution support surface is paramount (NPUAP/EPUAP, 2014).
- • If the goal of care is to keep the client comfortable (e.g., for a terminally ill client), repositioning may not be appropriate.

▲ Assess the client's nutritional status. Refer for a nutritional consult and/or institute dietary supplements as necessary. Review client nutrition plan evaluating for the intake of 1.25 to 1.5 g of protein per kilogram body weight daily, unless medically contraindicated, for adults at risk of a pressure injury or with existing pressure injuries. Offer 1 mL of fluid intake per kilocalorie per day, unless medically contraindicated (Ratliff et al., 2017). Reassess as condition changes (NPUAP/EPUAP, 2014).

▲ Develop a comprehensive plan of care that includes a thorough wound assessment, treatment interventions, support surfaces, nutritional products, adjunctive therapies, and evaluation of the outcome of care.

Home Care

- Some of the interventions previously described may be adapted for home care use.

▲ Assess the client's current phase of wound healing (inflammation, proliferation, or maturation) and stage of injury; initiate appropriate wound management.

- Instruct and assist the client and caregivers in understanding how to change dressings and in the importance of maintaining a clean environment. Provide written instructions and observe them completing the dressing change.

▲ Initiate a consultation in a case assignment with a wound specialist or wound, ostomy, and continence nurse to establish a comprehensive plan as soon as possible. Plan case conferencing to promote optimal wound care.

▲ Consult with other healthcare disciplines to provide a thorough, comprehensive assessment.

Client/Family Teaching and Discharge Planning

- Teach skin and wound assessment and ways to monitor for signs and symptoms of infection, complications, and healing.
- Teach the client why a topical treatment has been selected. Explain wound bed changes that the caregiver can expect to see. Instruct on when the dressing needs to be changed. Assess pressure injuries with each wound dressing change and confirm the appropriateness of the current dressing regimen (NPUAP/EPUAP, 2014).

▲ Teach the use of pillows, foam wedges, and pressure-reducing devices, on beds and chairs to prevent pressure injury. Pressure-redistributing surfaces serve as adjuncts and not replacements to regular repositioning (Ratliff et al., 2017).

Risk for Impaired Tissue Integrity

NANDA-I Definition

Susceptible to damage to the mucous membrane, cornea, integumentary system, muscular fascia, muscle, tendon, bone, cartilage, joint capsule, and/or ligament, which may compromise health

Risk Factors

External Factors

Excretions; humidity; hyperthermia; hypothermia; inadequate caregiver knowledge about maintaining tissue integrity; inadequate caregiver knowledge about protecting tissue integrity; inadequate use of chemical agent; pressure over bony prominence; psychomotor agitation; secretions; shearing forces; surface friction; use of linen with insufficient moisture wicking property

Internal Factors

Body mass index above normal range for age and gender; body mass index below normal range for age and gender; decreased blinking frequency; decreased physical activity; fluid imbalance; impaired physical mobility; impaired postural balance; inadequate adherence to incontinence treatment regimen; inadequate blood glucose level management; inadequate knowledge about maintaining tissue integrity; inadequate knowledge about restoring tissue integrity; inadequate ostomy care; malnutrition; psychogenic factor; self mutilation; smoking; substance misuse

At-Risk Population

Homeless individuals; individuals at extremes of age; individuals exposed to environmental temperature extremes; individuals exposed to high-voltage power supply; individuals participating in contact sports; individuals participating in winter sports; individuals with family history of bone fracture; individuals with history of bone fracture

Associated Condition

Anemia; autism spectrum disorder; cardiovascular diseases; chronic neurological conditions; critical illness; decreased level of consciousness; decreased serum albumin level; decreased tissue oxygenation; decreased tissue perfusion; hemodynamic instability; immobilization; intellectual disability; medical devices; metabolic diseases; peripheral neuropathy; pharmaceutical preparations; sensation disorders; surgical procedures

Client Outcomes, Nursing Interventions, Client/Family Teaching and Discharge Planning

Refer to care plan for Impaired **Tissue** integrity

Ineffective Peripheral Tissue Perfusion

NANDA-I Definition

Decrease in blood circulation to the periphery, which may compromise health

Defining Characteristics

Absence of peripheral pulses; alteration in motor function; alteration skin characteristic; ankle-brachial index < 0.90; capillary refill time >3 seconds; color does not return to lowered limb after 1 minute of leg elevation; decrease in blood pressure in extremities; decrease in pain-free distances during a 6-minute walk test; decrease in peripheral pulses; delay in peripheral wound healing; distance in the 6-minute walk test below normal range; edema; extremity pain; femoral bruit; intermittent claudication; paresthesia; skin color pales with limb elevation

Related Factors

Excessive sodium intake; insufficient knowledge of disease process; insufficient knowledge of modifiable factors; sedentary lifestyle; smoking

Associated Condition

Diabetes mellitus; endovascular procedure; hypertension; trauma

Client Outcomes

Client Will (Specify Time Frame)

- Demonstrate adequate tissue perfusion as evidenced by palpable peripheral pulses, warm and dry skin, adequate urine output, and absence of respiratory distress
- Verbalize knowledge of treatment regimen, including appropriate exercise and medications and their actions and possible side effects
- Identify changes in lifestyle needed to increase tissue perfusion

Nursing Interventions

▲ Check the brachial, radial, dorsalis pedis, posterior tibial, and popliteal pulses bilaterally. If unable to find them, use a Doppler stethoscope and notify the healthcare provider immediately if new onset of absence of pulses along with a cold extremity.

- Note skin color and feel the temperature of the skin. Check capillary refill.
- Assess for pain in the extremities, noting severity, quality, timing, and exacerbating and alleviating factors. Differentiate venous from arterial disease.
- Note skin texture and the presence of hair, ulcers, or gangrenous areas on the legs or feet.

- • Note the presence of edema in the extremities and rate severity on a four-point scale. Measure the circumference of the ankle and calf at the same time each day in the early morning (Busti, 2016).
- ▲ Prepare for vascular lab.

Arterial Insufficiency

- ▲ Monitor peripheral pulses. If there is new onset of loss of pulses with bluish, purple, or black areas and extreme pain, notify the healthcare provider immediately.
- ▲ Measure ABI via Doppler imaging.
- • Avoid elevating the legs above the level of the heart. With arterial insufficiency, leg elevation decreases arterial blood supply to the legs.
- ▲ For early arterial insufficiency, encourage exercise such as walking or riding an exercise bicycle from 30 to 60 minutes per day as ordered by the healthcare provider.
- • Keep the client warm and have the client wear socks and shoes or sheepskin-lined slippers when mobile. Do not apply heat. Clients with arterial insufficiency report being constantly cold; keep extremities warm to maintain vasodilation and blood supply. Heat application can easily damage ischemic tissues.
- ▲ Pay meticulous attention to foot care. Refer to a podiatrist if the client has a foot or nail abnormality. Ischemic feet are vulnerable to injury; meticulous foot care can prevent further injury.
- • If the client has ischemic arterial ulcers, refer to the care plan for Impaired **Tissue** integrity.
- ▲ If the client smokes, aggressively counsel the client to stop smoking and refer to the healthcare provider for medications to support nicotine withdrawal and a smoking withdrawal program.
- ▲ Educate on use and safety of antiplatelet medications.

Venous Insufficiency

- ▲ Elevate edematous legs as ordered and ensure no pressure under the knee and heels to prevent pressure ulcers.
- ▲ Apply graduated compression stockings as ordered. Ensure proper fit by measuring accurately. Remove the stockings at least twice a day, in the morning with the bath and in the evening, to assess the condition of the extremity, then reapply. Knee length is preferred rather than thigh length.
- • Encourage the client to walk with compression stockings on and perform toe-up and point-flex exercises.
- • If the client is overweight, encourage weight loss to decrease venous disease.

• If the client has venous leg ulcers, encourage the client to avoid prolonged sitting, standing, and elevation of the involved leg. Encourage proper use of compression stockings. Pain may prevent compliance.

▲ If the client is mostly immobile, consult with the healthcare provider regarding use of a calf-high pneumatic compression device for prevention of deep venous thrombosis (DVT).

• Observe for signs of DVT, including pain, tenderness, swelling in the calf and thigh, and redness in the involved extremity. Take serial leg measurements of the thigh and calf circumferences. In some clients a tender venous cord can be felt in the popliteal fossa. Do not rely on Homan's sign.

▲ Note the results of a D-dimer test and ultrasounds.

• If DVT is present, observe for symptoms of a PE.

▲ Educate on use and safety of anticoagulant medications.

Geriatric

• Complete a thorough lower extremity assessment, documenting the smallest change from previous assessment, and implement a plan immediately.

• Recognize that older adults have an increased risk for development of PE.

Home Care

• The interventions previously described may be adapted for home care use.

• If arterial disease is present and the client smokes, aggressively encourage smoking cessation.

• Examine the feet carefully at frequent intervals for changes and new ulcerations. Encourage the client to perform regular assessment of the feet.

▲ Assess the client's nutritional status, paying special attention to obesity, hyperlipidemia, and malnutrition. Refer to a dietitian if appropriate.

• Monitor for development of gangrene, venous ulceration, and symptoms of cellulitis (redness, pain, and increased swelling in an extremity).

Client/Family Teaching and Discharge Planning

• Explain the importance of good foot care. Teach the client and family to wash and inspect the feet daily. Recommend that the diabetic client wear comfortable shoes and break them in slowly, watching for blisters (Armstrong, 2017).

▲ Teach the diabetic client that he or she should have a comprehensive foot examination at least annually (which includes an analysis for predicting foot ulceration risk), which includes assessment of sensation using the Semmes–Weinstein monofilaments. If good sensation is not present, refer to a footwear professional for fitting of therapeutic shoes and inserts, the cost of which is covered by Medicare.

- For arterial disease, stress the importance of not smoking, following a weight loss program (if the client is obese), carefully controlling a diabetic condition, controlling hyperlipidemia and hypertension, maintaining intake of antiplatelet therapy, and reducing stress.
- Teach the client to avoid exposure to cold; limit exposure to brief periods if going out in cold weather and wear warm clothing.
- For venous disease, teach the importance of wearing compression stockings as ordered, elevating the legs at intervals, and watching for skin breakdown on the legs.
- Teach the client to recognize the signs and symptoms that should be reported to a healthcare provider (e.g., change in skin temperature, color, or sensation, or the presence of a new lesion on the foot).
- Provide clear, simple instructions about plan of care.
- Instruct and provide emotional support for client undergoing hyperoxygenation treatment.

Risk for Ineffective Peripheral Tissue Perfusion

NANDA-I Definition

Susceptible to a decrease in blood circulation to the periphery, which may compromise health

Risk Factors

Excessive sodium intake; insufficient knowledge of disease process; insufficient knowledge of modifiable factors; sedentary lifestyle; smoking

Associated Condition

Diabetes mellitus; endovascular procedure; hypertension; trauma

Client Outcomes, Nursing Interventions, Client/Family Teaching and Discharge Planning

Refer to care plan for Ineffective peripheral **Tissue Perfusion**

Impaired Transfer Ability

NANDA-I Definition

Limitation of independent movement between two nearby surfaces

Defining Characteristics

Impaired ability to transfer between bed and chair; impaired ability to transfer between bed and standing position; impaired ability to transfer between car and chair; impaired ability to transfer between chair and floor; impaired ability to transfer between chair and standing position; impaired ability to transfer between floor and standing position; impaired ability to transfer between uneven levels; impaired ability to transfer in or out of bath tub; impaired ability to transfer in or out of shower; impaired ability to transfer on or off a commode; impaired ability to transfer on or off a toilet

Related Factors

Environmental barrier; impaired balance; insufficient knowledge of transfer techniques; insufficient muscle strength; obesity; physical deconditioning; pain

Associated Condition

Alteration in cognitive functioning; impaired vision; musculoskeletal impairment; neuromuscular impairment

Client Outcomes

Client Will (Specify Time Frame)

- Transfer from bed to chair and back successfully
- Transfer from chair to chair successfully
- Transfer from wheelchair to toilet and back successfully
- Transfer from wheelchair to car and back successfully

Nursing Interventions

- Specify level of independence using a standardized functional scale.
- Assess level of patient ability to perform specific tasks prior to transfer of patient.
- ▲ Complications associated with immobility and resultant muscle loss begins within 48 hours of onset or injury and is greatest during the first 2 to 3 weeks (Cameron et al., 2015). Request consult for a physical and/or occupational therapist (PT and OT) to develop plan of care for safe patient handling and mobility.
- Assess client's dependence, weight, strength, balance, tolerance to position change, cooperation, fatigue level, and cognition plus available equipment and staff ratio/experience to decide whether to do a manual or device-assisted transfer (Cohen et al., 2010; American Nurses Association [ANA] 2013).
- ▲ Obtain a consult for a PT, OT, or orthotist to evaluate and fit clients with proper orthoses, braces, collars, and walking aids before helping them stand.
- ▲ Help client put on/take off collars, braces, prostheses in bed, and put on/take off antiembolism stockings and abdominal binders. If applying antiembolism stockings is prescribed to reduce the risk of deep vein thrombosis (DVT), apply while the client is in bed for ease of application.

▲ Collaborate with PT and OT to use algorithms to identify technological aids to handle and transfer dependent and obese clients. Use assistive mobility devices such as gait belts, lifts, and transport devices to move obese clients to avoid harm to both client and healthcare professional (Choi & Brings, 2015).
• Implement and document type of transfer (e.g., slide board, pivot), weight-bearing status (non–weight-bearing, partial), equipment (walker, sling lift), and level of assistance (standby, moderate) on care plan, white board in room, and/or electronic medical record.
• Apply a gait belt with handles before transferring clients with partial weight-bearing abilities; keep the belt and client close to provider during the transfer.
• Help clients when wearing shoes with nonskid soles and socks/hose.
• Remove or swivel wheelchair armrests, leg rests, and footplates to the side, especially with squat or slide board transfers.
• Adjust transfer surfaces so they are similar in height. For example, lower a hospital bed to about an inch higher than commode height.
• Place wheelchair and commode at a slight angle toward the surface onto which client will transfer.
• Teach client to consistently lock brakes on wheelchair/commode/shower chair before transferring.
• Give clear, simple instructions, allow client time to process information, and let him or her do as much of the transfer as possible.
▲ Remind clients to comply with weight-bearing restrictions ordered by their healthcare provider.
• Place client in set position before standing him or her, for example, sitting on edge of surface with bilateral weight-bearing on buttocks and hips, with knees flexed, balls of feet aligned under knees, and head in midline.
• Support and stabilize client's weak knees by placing one or both of your knees next to or encircling client's knees, rather than blocking them.
  ○ Squat transfer: client leans well forward, slightly raises flexed hips off the surface, pivots, and sits down on new surface.
  ○ Standing pivot transfer: client leans forward with hips flexed and pushes up with hands from seat surface (or arms of chair), then stands erect, pivots, and sits down on new surface.
  ○ Slide board transfer: client should have on pants or have a pillowcase over the board. Remove arm and leg rest from wheelchair on one side, then slightly angle chair toward new

surface. Help client lean sideways, shifting his or her weight so the transfer board can be placed well under the upper thigh of the leg next to new surface. Make sure the board is safely angled across both surfaces. Help client sit upright and place one hand on the board and the other hand on the surface. Remind and help client perform a series of pushups with arms while leaning slightly forward and lifting (not sliding) hips in small increments across the board with each pushup.

- Position walking aids appropriately so a standing client can grasp and use them once he or she is upright. These aids help provide support, balance, and stability to help client stand and step safely (Kalisch, Dabney, & Lee, 2013; Mayeda-Letourneau, 2014).
- Reinforce to clients who use walkers to place one hand on walker and push with opposite hand against chair arm or surface from which they are arising to stand up.
- Use ceiling-mounted or bedside mechanical bariatric lifts to transfer dependent bariatric (extremely obese) clients.
- Use bariatric devices and use available safe client handling equipment for lifting, transferring, positioning, and sliding client (Cohen et al., 2010; ANA 2013; Choi & Brings, 2015).
- Place a mechanical lift sling in the wheelchair preventively. Place two transfer sheets or a slide board under the bariatric client.
- Perform initial and subsequent fall risk assessment.

▲ Collaborate with PT, OT, and pharmacist for individualized preventive/postfall plans, for example, scheduled toileting, balance and strength training, removal of hazards, chair alarms, call system/ phone in reach, and review of medications.

- Coordinate a follow-up encounter within 30 days of discharge from any inpatient facility with a licensed provider to perform a medication reconciliation to include all medications the client has been taking or receiving prior to the outpatient visit to provide quality care and improve quality of communication related to medications (Agency for Healthcare Research and Quality [AHRQ], 2015).
- Encourage an exercise component such as Tai chi, physical therapy, or other exercise for balance, gait, and strength training in group programs or at home.
- Integrate structured and progressive exercise protocols into a client's plan of care and innovative partnerships with other providers to create longer duration interventions for clients at risk of falling.

T

- • Modify environment for safety; recommend vision assessment and consideration for cataract removal.
- • To reduce the risk of falling, assess the physical environment (e.g., poor lighting, high bed position, improper equipment).
- • Recommend polypharmacy assessment with special consideration to sedatives, antidepressants, and drugs affecting the central nervous system; recommend evaluation for orthostatic hypotension and irregular heartbeats; and recommend vitamin D supplementation 800 IU per day (AHRQ, 2015).

Home Care

- ▲ Obtain referral for OT and PT to teach home exercises and balance and fall prevention and recovery. They also evaluate for potential modifications such as an entry ramp, elevated toilet seat/toilevator (raised base under toilet), tub seat or shower chair, need for shower stall with built-in seat or wheel-in shower stall without a curb/threshold, handheld flexible shower head, lever-type facets, pull-out drawers with loop handles versus cupboards, standing lift, and so on.
- • Develop a multifactorial/multicomponent interventions risk strategy to reduce the risk for falls that include adaptation or modification of the home environment; withdrawal or minimization of psychoactive medications; withdrawal of minimization of other medications; management of postural hypotension; management of foot problems and footwear; and exercise, particularly balance, strength, and gait training (AHRQ, 2013; Skelton et al., 2013).
- • Assess for adequate lighting and hazards such as throw/area rugs, clutter, cords, and unfitted bedspreads. Suggest safe floor surfaces, such as use of adhesive nonslip strips in tubs/thresholds/areas in which floor height changes; removal of wax from slippery floors; and installing low-pile carpet/nonglazed or nonglossy tiles/wood/linoleum coverings. Stress relocating commonly used items to shelves/drawers in reach; applying remote controls to appliances; and optimizing furniture placement for function, maneuverability, and stability.
- • Assess clients for impairment of vision because this can result in a loss of function in activities of daily living and, consequently, in impaired functional capacity and is an important risk factor for falls.

T

- Nurses can provide further safety assessments by suggesting installing hand rails in bathrooms and by stairs, ensuring client's slippers and clothes fit properly, and recommending repairing or discarding broken equipment in the home (Taylor et al., 2011).
- ▲ Involve social worker or case manager to educate clients about potential assistive technology, financial cost and benefits, regulations of payers, and local resources.
- ▲ Implement approaches for home care staff and family to safely handle and transfer clients.
- For further information, refer to care plans for Impaired physical **Mobility** and Impaired **Walking.**

Client/Family Teaching and Discharge Planning

- Assess for readiness to learn and use teaching modalities conducive to personal learning styles, including written instructions for home use.
- Supervise practice sessions in which client and family apply items such as gait belts, braces, and orthoses. Check skin once aids are removed.
- Teach and monitor client/family for consistent use of safety precautions for transfers (e.g., nonskid shoes, correctly placed equipment/chairs, locked brakes, leg rests swiveled away) and for correct performance of transfer or use of lifts/slings.
- Teach client/family how to check brakes on chairs to ensure they engage and how to check tires for adequate air pressure; advise routine inspection and annual tune-up of devices.
- Offer information on safe use of shower and commode chairs to prevent discomfort, pressure, and falls during transfer, transport, care, and hygiene.
- For further information, refer to the care plans for Impaired physical **Mobility,** Impaired **Walking,** and Impaired wheelchair **Mobility.**

T

Risk for Physical Trauma

NANDA-I Definition

Susceptible to physical injury of sudden onset and severity which require immediate attention.

Risk Factors

External

Absence of call-for-aid device; absence of stairway gate; absence of window guard; access to weapon; bathing in very hot water; bed in high position; children riding in front seat of car; defective appliance; delay in ignition of gas appliance; dysfunctional call-for-aid device; electrical hazard; exposure to corrosive product; exposure to dangerous machinery; exposure to radiation; exposure to toxic chemical; flammable object; grease on stove; icicles hanging from roof; inadequate stair rails; inadequately stored combustible; inadequately stored corrosive; insufficient anti-slip material in bathroom; insufficient lighting; insufficient protection from heat source; misuse of headgear; misuse of seat restraint; nonuse of seat restraints; obstructed passageway; playing with dangerous object; playing with explosive; pot handle facing front of stove; proximity to vehicle pathway; slippery floor; smoking in bed; smoking near oxygen; struggling with restraints; unanchored electric wires; unsafe operation of heavy equipment; unsafe road; unsafe walkway; use of cracked dishware; use of throw rugs; use of unstable chair; use of unstable ladder; wearing loose clothing around open flame

Internal

Emotional disturbance; Impaired Balance; insufficient knowledge of safety precautions; Insufficient vision; weakness

At-Risk Population

Economically disadvantaged; extremes of environmental temperature; gas leak; high crime neighborhood; history of trauma

Associated Condition

Alteration in cognitive functioning; alteration in sensation; decrease in eye-hand coordination; decrease in muscle coordination;

Client Outcomes

Client Will (Specify Time Frame)

- Remain free from trauma
- Explain actions that can be taken to prevent trauma

Nursing Interventions

- Provide vision aids for visually impaired clients.
- Assist the client with ambulation. Encourage the client to use assistive devices in activities of daily living (ADLs) as needed.
- Evaluate client's risk for burn injury.
- Assess the client for causes of impaired cognition.
- Provide assistive devices in the home.
- ▲ Question the client concerning his/her sense of safety.

- ▲ Assess for a substance abuse problem and refer to appropriate resources for drug and alcohol education.
- • Review drug profile for potential side effects that may inhibit performance of ADLs.
- • See care plans for Risk for **Aspiration,** Risk for Adult **Falls,** Ineffective **Home** Maintenance Behaviors, Risk for **Injury,** Risk for **Poisoning,** and Risk for **Suffocation.**

Pediatric

- • Assess the client's socioeconomic status.
- • Never leave young children unsupervised.
- • Keep flammable and potentially flammable articles out of reach of young children.
- • Lock up harmful objects such as guns.

Geriatric

- • Assess the geriatric client's cognitive level of functioning.
- • Assess for routine eye examinations.
- • Perform a home safety assessment and recommend the following preventive measures: keep electrical cords out of the flow of traffic; remove small rugs or make sure they are slip resistant; increase lighting in hallways and other dark areas; place a light in the bathroom; keep towels, curtains, and other items that might catch fire away from the stove; store harmful products away from food products; provide at least one grab bar in tubs and showers; check prescribed medications for appropriate labels; store medications in original containers or in a dispenser of some type (e.g., egg carton, 7-day plastic dispenser). If the client cannot administer medications according to directions, secure someone to administer medications. Mark stove knobs with bright colors (yellow or red) and outline the borders of steps.
- • Discourage driving at night.
- • Encourage the client to participate in resistance and impact exercise programs as tolerated.

Client/Family Teaching and Discharge Planning

- • Educate the family regarding age-appropriate child safety precautions, environmental safety precautions, and intervention in an emergency.
- • Teach the family to assess the child care provider's knowledge regarding child safety.
- • Educate the client and family regarding helmet use during recreation and sports activities.
- • Encourage the proper use of car seats and safety belts.

- Teach parents to restrict driving for teens.
- Teach parents the importance of monitoring children after school.
- Teach firearm safety.
- For further information, refer to care plans for Risk for **Aspiration,** Risk for Adult **Falls,** Ineffective **Home** Maintenance Behaviors, Risk for **Injury,** Risk for **Poisoning,** and Risk for **Suffocation.**

Unilateral Neglect

NANDA-I Definition

Impairment in sensory and motor response, mental representation, and spatial attention of the body, and the corresponding environment, characterized by inattention to one side and overattention to the opposite side. Left-side neglect is more severe and persistent than right-side neglect

Defining Characteristics

Alteration in safety behavior on neglected side; disturbance of sound lateralization; failure to dress neglected side; failure to eat food from portion of plate on neglected side; failure to groom neglected side; failure to move eyes in the neglected hemisphere; failure to move head in the neglected hemisphere; failure to move limbs in the neglected hemisphere; failure to move trunk in the neglected hemisphere; failure to notice people approaching from the neglected side; hemianopsia; impaired performance on line cancellation; line bisection; and target cancellation tests; left hemiplegia from cerebrovascular accident; marked deviation of the eyes to stimuli on the non-neglected side; marked deviation of the trunk to stimuli on the non-neglected side; omission of drawing on the neglected side; perseveration; representational neglect; substitution of letters to form alternative words when reading; transfer of pain sensation to the non-neglected side; unaware of positioning of neglected limb; unilateral visuospatial neglect; use of vertical half of page only when writing

Related Factors

To be developed

Associated Condition

Brain injury

Client Outcomes

Client Will (Specify Time Frame)

- Use techniques that can be used to minimize unilateral neglect (UN)
- Care for both sides of the body appropriately and keep affected side free from harm

- Return to the highest functioning level possible based on personal goals and abilities
- Remain free from injury

Nursing Interventions

▲ Assess the client for signs of UN (e.g., not washing, shaving, or dressing one side of the body; sitting or lying inappropriately on affected arm or leg; failing to respond to environmental stimuli contralateral to the side of lesion; eating food on only one side of plate; or failing to look to one side of the body).

▲ Collaborate with healthcare provider for referral to a rehabilitation team (including, but not limited to, rehabilitation clinical nurse specialist, physical medicine and rehabilitation healthcare provider, neuropsychologist, occupational therapist, physical therapist, and speech and language pathologist) for continued help in dealing with UN.

- Use the principles of rehabilitation to progressively increase the client's ability to compensate for UN by using assistive devices, feedback, and support.
- Teach the client to be aware of the problem and modify behavior and environment.
- Set up the environment so that essential activity is on the unaffected side:
  - Place the client's personal items within view and on the unaffected side.
  - Position the bed so that client is approached from the unaffected side.
  - Monitor and assist the client to achieve adequate food and fluid intake.
- Implement fall prevention interventions.
- Position affected extremity in a safe and functional manner.

▲ Collaborate closely with rehabilitation professionals to identify and reinforce therapies aimed at reducing neglect symptoms.

Home Care

- Many of the previously listed interventions may be adapted for use in the home care setting.
- Position bed at home so that client gets out of bed on unaffected side.

Client/Family Teaching and Discharge Planning

- Engage discharge planning specialists for comprehensive assessment and planning early in the client's stay.
- Encourage family participation in care.
- Explain pathology and symptoms of UN to both the client and family.

• = Independent ▲ = Collaborative

U

- Teach the client how to scan regularly to check the position of body parts and to regularly turn head from side to side for safety when ambulating, using a wheelchair, or doing self-care tasks.
- Teach caregivers to cue the client to the environment.

Impaired Urinary Elimination

NANDA-I Definition

Dysfunction in urine elimination

Defining Characteristics

Dysuria; frequent voiding; nocturia; urinary hesitancy; urinary incontinence; urinary retention; urinary urgency

Related Factors

Alcohol consumption; altered environmental factor; caffeine consumption; environmental constraints; fecal impaction; improper toileting posture; ineffective toileting habits; insufficient privacy; involuntary sphincter relaxation; obesity; pelvic organ prolapse; smoking; use of aspartame; weakened bladder muscle; weakened supportive pelvic structure

At Risk Population

Older adults; women

Associated Conditions

Anatomic obstruction; diabetes mellitus; sensory motor impairment; urinary tract infection

Client Outcomes

Client Will (Specify Time Frame)

- State absence of pain or excessive urgency during urination
- Demonstrate voiding frequency no more than every 2 hours

Nursing Interventions

- Ask the client about urinary elimination patterns and concerns. Urinary elimination problems have many presenting signs and symptoms. Asking the client questions may help understand the subtle signs and symptoms associated with urinary elimination (Mayo Clinic, 2017).
- Question the client regarding the following:
  - Presence of symptoms such as incontinence, dribbling, frequency, urgency, dysuria, and nocturia
  - Presence of pain in the area of the bladder
  - Pattern of urination and approximate amount
  - Possible aggravating and alleviating factors for urinary problems

- • Ask the client to keep a bladder diary/bladder log.
- • For interventions on urinary incontinence, refer to the following nursing diagnosis care plans as appropriate: Stress urinary **Incontinence,** Urge urinary **Incontinence,** or Disability-associated urinary **Incontinence.**
- ▲ Perform a focused physical assessment including inspecting the perineal skin integrity, percussion, and palpation of the lower abdomen looking for obvious bladder distention or an enlarged kidney.
- ▲ Check for costovertebral tenderness.
- ▲ Review results of urinalysis for the presence of urinary infection such as white blood cells, red blood cells, bacteria, and positive nitrites. If urinalysis results are not available, request a midstream specimen of urine (urine obtained during voiding, discarding the first and last portions) for a urinalysis (Pietrucha-Dilanchian & Hooton, 2016).
- ▲ If blood or protein is present in the urine, recognize that both hematuria and proteinuria are serious symptoms, and the client should be referred to a urologist to receive a workup to rule out pathology.
- • Inquire about the client's history of smoking.

Urinary Tract Infection

- ▲ Consult the provider for a culture and sensitivity testing and antibiotic treatment in the individual with evidence of a symptomatic UTI.
- ▲ Teach the client to recognize symptoms of UTI, such as dysuria that crescendos as the bladder nears complete evacuation; urgency to urinate followed by micturition of only a few drops; suprapubic aching discomfort; malaise; voiding frequency; sudden exacerbation of urinary incontinence with or without fever, chills, and flank pain. Recognize that a cloudy or malodorous urine, in the absence of other lower urinary tract symptoms, may not indicate the presence of a UTI and that asymptomatic bacteriuria in the older adult does not justify a course of antibiotics.
- ▲ Refer the individual with chronic lower urinary tract pain to a urologist or specialist in the management of pelvic pain.

Geriatric

- • Evidence for behavioral interventions include the following: (1) prompted voiding is effective in the treatment of daytime symptoms when patients and caregivers comply; (2) prompted voiding is ineffective and should not be used for people who need the assistance of more than one person to transfer, instead manage with "check and change"; (3) promoted voiding should not be continued in people who have less than

U

20% reduction in wet checks or toilet successfully less than two-thirds of the time after a 3-day trial; and (4) interventions combining toileting, exercise, food, and fluids are effective (Wagg et al., 2014).

- • Encourage older women to consume one to two servings of fresh blueberries and consider drinking at least 10 ounces of cranberry juice daily or supplement the diet with cranberry concentrate capsules as ordered.
- ▲ Refer the older woman with recurrent UTIs to her healthcare provider for possible use of topical estrogen creams for treatment of atrophic vaginal mucosa from decreased hormonal stimulation, which can predispose to UTIs (Aydin et al., 2014; Nicolle & Norrby, 2016).
- • Postresidual volumes (PRVs) should be assessed in older women with overactive bladder (OAB). A volume of greater than 200 mL is significant. A history of back or pelvic injury or surgery increases the risk of greater PRV (Park and Palmer, 2015).
- ▲ Recognize that UTIs in older men are typically associated with prostatic hyperplasia or strictures of the urethra. Refer the client to a urologist (Nicolle & Norrby, 2016).
- • Analysis of urinary elimination patterns of clients could help in clinical follow-up of elderly postoperative patients and in the selection of best nursing interventions.
- • Practice recommendations when caring for older clients include: (1) frailty, not age should guide urinary elimination treatment decisions; (2) caring for individuals with urinary incontinence and cognitive impairment needs to be tailored to the individuals abilities; and (3) be cautious of anticholinergic medications and weigh the risk and benefits for antimuscarinics (Wagg et al., 2014).

U

Client/Family Teaching and Discharge Planning

- • Teach the client/family methods to keep the urinary tract healthy. Refer to Client/Family Teaching in the care plan for Readiness for enhanced **Urinary** elimination.
- • Teach the following measures to women to decrease the incidence of UTIs:
  - ❍ Urinate at appropriate intervals. Do not ignore need to void, which can result in stasis of urine.
  - ❍ Drink plenty of liquids, especially water.
  - ❍ Wipe from front to back.
  - ❍ Wear underpants that have a cotton crotch.
  - ❍ Avoid potentially irritating feminine products.

- Teach the sexually active woman with recurrent UTIs prevention measures including:
  - Void after intercourse to flush bacteria out of the urethra and bladder.
  - Use a lubricating agent as needed during intercourse to protect the vagina from trauma and decrease the incidence of vaginitis.
  - Watch for signs of vaginitis and seek treatment as needed.
  - Avoid use of diaphragms with spermicide.
- Teach clients with spinal cord injury and neurogenic bladder dysfunction to consider adding cranberry extract tablets or cranberry juice, or fruits containing D-mannose (e.g., apples, oranges, peaches, blueberries) on a daily basis, monitor fluid intake. The client is encouraged to discuss the use of probiotics and antibiotic therapy with the provider for frequent recurrent symptomatic UTIs.
- Teach all persons to recognize hematuria and to promptly seek care if this symptom occurs.

Urinary Retention

NANDA-I Definition

Incomplete emptying of the bladder.

Defining Characteristics

Absence of urinary output; bladder distention; dysuria; increased daytime urinary frequency; minimal void volume; overflow incontinence; reports sensation of bladder fullness; reports sensation of residual urine; weak urine stream

Related Factors

Environmental constraints; fecal impaction; improper toileting posture; inadequate relaxation of pelvic floor muscles; insufficient privacy; pelvic organ prolapse; weakened bladder muscle

At Risk Population

Puerperal women

Associated Conditions

Benign prostatic hyperplasia; diabetes mellitus; nervous system diseases; pharmaceutical preparations; urinary tract obstruction

Client Outcomes

Client Will (Specify Time Frame)

- Demonstrate consistent ability to urinate when desire to void is perceived
- Have measured urinary residual volume of less than 300 mL

- Experience correction or relief from dysuria, nocturia, postvoid dribbling, and voiding frequently
- Be free of a urinary tract infection

Nursing Interventions

- Obtain a focused urinary history including questioning the client about episodes of acute urinary retention (UR; complete inability to void) or chronic retention (documented elevated postvoid residual volumes), as well as symptoms such as dysuria, nocturia, postvoid dribbling, and voiding frequently.
- Question the client concerning specific risk factors for UR including:
  - Spinal cord injuries
  - Ischemic stroke
  - Metabolic disorders such as diabetes mellitus, chronic alcoholism, and related conditions associated with polyuria and peripheral polyneuropathies
  - Herpetic infection
  - Heavy-metal poisoning (lead, mercury) causing peripheral polyneuropathies
  - Advanced-stage HIV infection
  - Medications including antispasmodics/parasympatholytics, alpha-adrenergic agonists, antidepressants, sedatives, narcotics, psychotropic medications, illicit drugs
  - Recent surgery requiring general or spinal anesthesia
  - Vaginal delivery within the past 48 hours
  - Bowel elimination patterns, history of fecal impaction, encopresis
  - Recent surgical procedures
  - Recent prostatic biopsy
- Complete a pain assessment including pain intensity using a self-report pain tool, such as the 0 to 10 numerical pain rating scale. Also determine location, quality, onset/duration, intensity, aggravating/alleviating factors, and effects of pain on function and quality of life.
- Perform a focused physical assessment including perineal skin integrity and inspection, percussion, and palpation of the lower abdomen, looking for obvious bladder distention or an enlarged kidney.
- Recognize that unrelieved obstruction of urine can result in kidney damage and, if severe, kidney failure. UR can be a medical

emergency and should be reported to the primary provider as soon as possible.

- Review laboratory test results including serum electrolytes, blood urea nitrogen (BUN) and creatinine, along with calcium, phosphate, magnesium, uric acid, and albumin.
- Monitor for signs of dehydration, peripheral edema, elevating blood pressure, and heart failure.

Ask the client to complete a bladder diary including patterns of urine elimination, urine loss (if present), nocturia, and volume and type of fluids consumed for a period of 3 to 7 days.

- Consult with the provider concerning eliminating or altering medications suspected of producing or exacerbating UR.
- Both men and women may develop UR from obstruction of the bladder outlet and abnormalities in detrusor contractility.
- In clients treated with an indwelling urethral catheter (IUC), complications such as catheter-associated urinary tract infections are common, whereas underuse of IUC may cause harmful UR.
- Advise the male client with UR related to benign prostatic hyperplasia (BPH) to avoid risk factors associated with acute UR:
  - Avoid over-the-counter (OTC) cold remedies containing a decongestant (alpha-adrenergic agonist) or antihistamine such as diphenhydramine, which has anticholinergic effects.
  - Avoid taking OTC dietary medications (frequently contain alpha-adrenergic agonists).
  - Discuss voiding problems with a healthcare provider before beginning new prescription medications.
  - After prolonged exposure to cool weather, warm the body before attempting to urinate.
  - Avoid overfilling the bladder by regular urination patterns and refrain from excessive intake of alcohol.
- Advise the client who is unable to void of specific strategies to manage this potential medical emergency as follows:
  - Attempt urination in complete privacy.
  - Place the feet solidly on the floor.
  - If unable to void using these strategies, take a warm sitz bath or shower and void (if possible) while still in the tub or shower.
  - Drink a warm cup of caffeinated coffee or tea to stimulate the bladder, which may promote voiding.

U

- • If unable to void within 6 hours or if bladder distention is producing significant pain, seek urgent or emergency care.
- • Perform sterile (in acute care) or clean intermittent catheterization at home as ordered for clients with UR.
- ▲ Insert an indwelling catheter only as ordered by a healthcare provider. Understand the indication for the urinary catheter to be placed as part of client management. Catheter-associated urinary tract infections (CAUTIs) are among the most common healthcare–associated infections. Each CAUTI episode is estimated to cost $600, rising to $2800 per episode when a CAUTI leads to a bloodstream infection. Although certain conditions among hospitalized clients may require the use of a urinary catheter, limiting their use and decreasing the length of use are the most effective methods of reducing clients' exposure to CAUTIs (Choosing Wisely and the American Academy of Nursing, 2014).
- • Nurse-led and computer-based reminders are both successful in reducing how long urinary catheters remain in place (Bernard, Hunter, & Moore, 2012).
- • Nurse-driven practice recommendations to reduce CAUTI risk include securing catheters; maintaining drainage bags lower than level of bladder; emptying drainage bags every 8 hours, when two-thirds full, and before any transfer; daily evaluation of catheter indication/need to promote removal; and use of bladder scanner to prevent reinsertion.
- • Current practice recommendations support aseptic catheter insertions, whereas the use of hydrophilic-coated catheters for clean intermittent catheters can reduce the rate of CAUTIs. Suprapubic catheterization is not more effective than urethral catheterization in reducing the incidence of catheter-related bacteremia.
- • For the individual with UR who is not a suitable candidate for intermittent catheterization, recognize that the catheter can be a significant cause of harm to the client through development of a CAUTI or through genitourinary trauma when the catheter is pulled.
- • Advise clients with indwelling catheters that bacteria in the urine is an almost universal finding after the catheter has remained in place

for more than 1 week and that only symptomatic infections warrant treatment.

- Use the following strategies to reduce the risk for CAUTI whenever feasible:
  - Insert the indwelling catheter with sterile technique, only when insertion is indicated.
  - Remove the indwelling catheter as soon as possible; acute care facilities should institute a policy for regular review of the necessity of an indwelling catheter.
  - Maintain a closed drainage system whenever feasible.
  - Maintain unobstructed urine flow, avoiding kinks in the tubing and keeping the collecting bag below the level of the bladder at all times.
  - Regularly cleanse the urethral meatus with a gentle cleanser to remove apparent soiling.
  - Change the long-term catheter every 4 weeks; more frequent catheter changes should be reserved for clients who experience catheter encrustation and blockage.
- Educate staff about the risks for CAUTI development and specific strategies to reduce these risks.

Postoperative Urinary Retention

- UR is a common complication of surgery, anesthesia, and advancing age. If conservative measures do not help the client pass urine, then the bladder needs to be drained using either an intermittent catheter or IUC, which places the client at risk for development of CAUTI (Steggall, Treacy, & Jones, 2013).
- Remove the IUC at midnight in the hospitalized postoperative client to reduce the risk for acute UR.
- Perform a bladder scan before considering inserting a catheter to determine PVR volume after surgery.
- The overall incidence of postoperative urinary catheterization is 40% for total hip and knee arthroplasties.

Geriatric

- Aggressively assess older clients, particularly those with dribbling urinary incontinence, urinary tract infection, and related conditions for UR.
- Assess older clients for impaction when UR is documented or suspected: Monitor older male clients for retention related to BPH or prostate cancer.

Home Care

- Encourage the client to report any inability to void.
- Maintain an up-to-date medication list; evaluate side effect profiles for risk of UR.
- Refer the client for healthcare provider evaluation if UR occurs.

Client/Family Teaching and Discharge Planning

- Teach the client with mild to moderate obstructive symptoms to double void by urinating, resting in the bathroom for 3 to 5 minutes, and then trying again to urinate.
- Teach the client with UR and infrequent voiding to urinate by the clock.
- Teach the client with an indwelling catheter to assess the tube for patency, maintain the drainage system below the level of the symphysis pubis, and routinely cleanse the bedside bag as directed.
- Teach the client with an indwelling catheter or undergoing intermittent catheterization the symptoms of a significant urinary infection, including hematuria, acute-onset incontinence, dysuria, flank pain, fever, or acute confusion.

Risk for Vascular Trauma

NANDA-I Definition

V

Susceptible to damage to vein and its surrounding tissues related to the presence of a catheter and/or infusion solutions, which may compromise health

Risk Factors

Inadequate available insertion site; prolonged period of time catheter is in place

Associated Condition

Irritating solution; rapid infusion rate

Client Outcomes

Client Will (Specify Time Frame)

- Remain free from vascular trauma
- Remain free from signs and symptoms that indicate vascular trauma
- Remain free of signs and symptoms of vascular inflammation or infection
- Remain free from impaired tissue and/or skin

- Maintain skin integrity, tissue perfusion, usual tissue temperature, color, and pigment
- Report any altered sensation or pain
- State site is comfortable

Nursing Interventions

Client Preparation

- ▲ Verify objective and estimate duration of treatment. Check healthcare provider's order.
- • Assess client's clinical situation when venous infusion is indicated.
- • Assess if client is prepared for an IV procedure. Explain the procedure if necessary to decrease stress.
- • Provide privacy and make the client comfortable during the IV insertion.
- • Teach the client what symptoms of possible vascular trauma he or she should be alert to and to immediately inform staff if any of these symptoms are noticed.

Insertion

- • Wash hands before and after touching the client, as well as when inserting, replacing, accessing, repairing, or dressing an intravascular catheter (Infusion Nurses Society [INS], 2016).
- • Maintain aseptic technique for the insertion and care of intravascular catheters.
- • In preparation, assess the patient's medical history for disease processes such as diabetes and hypertension, frequent venipuncture, variations in skin color, skin alteration, age, obesity, fluid volume deficit, and IV drug use.
- • When vascular visualization is difficult, consider the use of visible light devices that provide transillumination of the peripheral veins or ultrasonography (INS, 2016).
- • Avoid areas of joint flexion or bony prominences.
- • Avoid the use of the antecubital area.
- ▲ Avoid the dorsal hand, radial wrist, and the volar (inner) wrist, if possible.
- ▲ Consider topical anesthetic prior to IV cannula insertion.
- • Choose an appropriate vascular access device (VAD) based on the types and characteristics of the devices and insertion site. Consider the following:
    - ○ Peripheral cannulae: these are short devices that are placed into a peripheral vein. They can be straight, winged, or ported and winged.

- ❍ Midline catheters or peripherally inserted central catheters (PICCs) that range from 7.5 to 20 cm.
- ❍ Central venous access devices (CVADs) are terminated in the central venous circulation and are available in a range of gauge sizes; they can be nontunneled catheters, skin-tunneled catheters, implantable injection ports, or PICCs.
- ❍ Polyurethane venous devices and silicone rubber may cause less friction and, consequently, may reduce the risk of mechanical phlebitis (Phillips, 2014).

▲ Choose a device with consideration of the nature, volume, and flow of prescribed solution.

- If possible, choose the venous access site considering the client's preference.
- Select the gauge of the venous device according to the duration of treatment, purpose of the procedure, and size of the vein.
- Verify whether the client is allergic to fixation or device material.
- Disinfect the venipuncture site. Assess that skin is dry before puncturing.
- Provide a comfortable, safe, hypoallergenic, easily removable stabilization dressing, allowing for visualization of the access site.
- Use sterile, transparent, semipermeable dressing to cover catheter site.
- Document insertion date, site, type of VAD, number of punctures performed, other occurrences, and measures/arrangements.
- Always decontaminate the device before infusing medication or manipulating IV equipment (Xue, 2014; Helm et al., 2015).

▲ Verify the sequence of drugs to be administrated. Vesicants should always be administered first in a sequence of drugs (Loubani & Green, 2015).

Monitoring Infusion

- Monitor permeability and flow rate at regular intervals.
- Monitor catheter–skin junction and surrounding tissues at regular intervals, observing possible appearance of burning, pain, erythema, altered local temperature, infiltration, extravasation, edema, secretion, tenderness, or induration. Remove promptly.

▲ Replace device according to institution protocol.

▲ Flush vascular access according to organizational policies and procedures, and as recommended by the manufacturer. When locking a catheter, use enough fluid to fill the entire catheter and use a positive pressure technique when disconnecting the syringe (Porritt, 2016).

- Remove catheter on suspected contamination, if the client develops signs of phlebitis or infection, the catheter is malfunctioning, or when the catheter no longer required.
- Encourage clients to report any discomfort such as pain, burning, swelling, or bleeding (Xue, 2014).

Pediatric

- The preceding interventions may be adapted for the pediatric client.
- Inform the client and family about the IV procedure; obtain permissions, maintain client's comfort, and perform appropriate assessment prior to venipuncture. Assess the client for any allergies or sensitivities to tape, antiseptics, or latex.
- Consider using a two-dimensional ultrasound for venous cannulation.
- The use of an appropriate device to obtain blood samples reduces discomfort in the pediatric client.
- Avoid areas of joint flexion or bony prominences.
- ▲ Consider whether sedation or the use of local anesthetic is suitable for insertion of a catheter, taking into consideration the age of the pediatric client.
- ▲ Use diversion while performing the procedure.

Geriatric

- The preceding interventions may be adapted for the geriatric client.
- Consider the physical, emotional, and cognitive changes related to older adults.
- Use strict aseptic technique for venipuncture of older clients.

Home Care

- Some devices may remain after discharge. Provide device-specific education to the client and family members about care of the selected device.
- Help in the choice of actions that support self-care. The nurse can provide valuable information that can be used to guide decision-making to maximize the self-care abilities of clients receiving home infusion therapy.
- Select, with the client, the insertion site most compatible with the development of activities of daily living (ADLs) (McGowan, 2014; Xue, 2014).
- Minimize the use of continuous IV therapy whenever possible.

V

Impaired Spontaneous Ventilation

NANDA-I Definition

Inability to initiate and/or maintain independent breathing that is adequate to support life

Defining Characteristics

Apprehensiveness; decrease in arterial oxygen saturation (SaO_2); decrease in cooperation; decrease in partial pressure of oxygen (PO_2); decrease in tidal volume; dyspnea; increase in accessory muscle use; increase in heart rate; increase in metabolic rate; increase in partial pressure of carbon dioxide (PCO_2); restlessness

Related Factors

Respiratory muscle fatigue

Associated Condition

Alteration in metabolism

Client Outcomes

Client Will (Specify Time Frame)

- Maintain arterial blood gases within safe parameters
- Remain free of dyspnea or restlessness
- Effectively maintain airway
- Effectively mobilize secretions

Nursing Interventions

▲ Collaborate with the client, family, and healthcare provider regarding possible intubation and ventilation. Ask whether the client has advanced directives and, if so, integrate them into the plan of care with clinical data regarding overall health and reversibility of the medical condition.

V

- Assess and respond to changes in the client's respiratory status. Monitor the client for dyspnea, increase in respiratory rate, use of accessory muscles, retraction of intercostal muscles, flaring of nostrils, decrease in O_2 saturation, cyanosis, and subjective complaints (Kjellström & van der Wal, 2013; Gallagher, 2017).
- Have the client use a numerical scale (0–10) or visual analog scale to self-report dyspnea before and after interventions.
- Assess for history of chronic respiratory disorders when administering oxygen.

▲ Collaborate with the healthcare provider and respiratory therapists in determining the appropriateness of noninvasive positive pressure ventilation (NPPV) and noninvasive ventilation (NIV) for the decompensated client with COPD. Ventilatory support in a COPD exacerbation can be provided by either noninvasive or invasive ventilation (GOLD, 2017). NIV improves respiratory acidosis and decreases respiratory rate, severity of breathlessness, incidence of ventilator-associated pneumonia (VAP), and hospital length of stay (Mas & Masip, 2014; American Association of Critical Care Nurses [AACN], 2017a; GOLD, 2017).

- ▲ Assist with implementation, client support, and monitoring if NPPV/NIV is used.
- • If the client has apnea, respiratory muscle fatigue, somnolence, hypoxemia, and/or acute respiratory acidosis, then prepare the client for possible intubation and mechanical ventilation.

Ventilator Support

- ▲ Explain the endotracheal intubation and mechanical ventilation process to the client and family as appropriate, and during intubation administer sedation for client comfort according to the healthcare provider's orders.
- • Secure the endotracheal tube in place using either tape or a commercial available device, auscultate bilateral breath sounds, use a CO_2 detector, and obtain a chest radiograph to confirm endotracheal tube placement.
- • Review ventilator settings with the healthcare provider and respiratory therapy to ensure support is appropriate to meet the client's minute ventilation requirements (Chacko et al., 2015; Stacy, 2018).
- ▲ Suction as needed and hyperoxygenate according to facility policy. Refer to the care plan for Ineffective **Airway** clearance for further information on suctioning.
- • Check that monitor alarms are set appropriately at the start of each shift.
- • Respond to ventilator alarms promptly. If unable to immediately locate the source/cause of an alarm, use a manual self-inflating resuscitation bag to ventilate the client while waiting for assistance.
- • Prevent unplanned extubation by maintaining stability of the endotracheal tube (Goodrich, 2017b).
- • Drain collected fluid from condensation out of ventilator tubing as needed.

- Note ventilator settings of flow of inspired oxygen, peak inspiratory pressure, tidal volume, and alarm activation at intervals and when removing the client from the ventilator for any reason (Gallagher, 2017).
- ▲ Administer analgesics and sedatives as needed to facilitate client comfort and rest. Use behavioral and sedation scales for nonverbal clients to provide a consistent way of monitoring pain and sedation levels and ensuring that therapeutic outcomes are being met (Barr et al., 2013; Dale et al., 2014; Reade & Finfer, 2014). Clients receiving mechanical ventilation frequently require sedation to help attenuate the anxiety, pain, and agitation associated with this intervention (Barr et al., 2013). The overall goal of sedation during mechanical ventilation is to provide physiological stability, ventilator synchrony, and comfort for clients (Makic et al., 2015).
- Tools such as the Riker Sedation-Agitation Scale, the Motor Activity Assessment Scale, the Ramsey Scale, or the Richmond Agitation-Sedation Scale may be useful in monitoring levels of sedation.
- Alternatives to medications for decreasing anxiety should be attempted, such as music therapy with selections of the client's choice played on headphones at intervals.
- Analyze and respond to arterial blood gas results, end-tidal CO_2 levels, and pulse oximetry values.
- Use an effective means of verbal and nonverbal communication with the client. Barriers to communication include endotracheal tubes, sedation, and general weakness associated with a critical illness. Basic technologies should be readily available to the client, including eyeglasses and hearing aids. A variety of communication devices are available, including electronic voice output communication aids, alphabet boards, picture boards, computers, and writing slate. Ask the client for input into their care as appropriate (ten Hoorn et al., 2016).
- Move the endotracheal tube from side to side at least every 24 hours, and tape it or secure it with a commercially available device. Assess and document client's skin condition, and ensure correct tube placement at lip line (National Pressure Ulcer Advisory Panel, 2013; Vollman, Sole, & Quinn, 2017).

V

- Implement steps to prevent ventilator-associated events (VAE), such as VAP, including continuous removal of subglottic secretions, elevation of the head of bed to 30 to 45 degrees (AACN, 2017b) unless medically contraindicated, change of the ventilator circuit no more than every 48 hours, and handwashing before and after contact with each client.
- Use endotracheal tubes that allow for the continuous aspiration of subglottic secretions (Frost et al., 2013; Vollman, Sole, & Quinn, 2017).
- Position the client in a semirecumbent position with the head of the bed at a 30 to 45 degree angle to decrease the aspiration of gastric, oral, and nasal secretions (AACN, 2017b; Vollman, Sole, & Quinn, 2017). Consider use of kinetic therapy, using a kinetic bed that slowly moves the client with 40 degree turns.
- Perform handwashing using both soap and water and alcohol-based solution before and after all mechanically ventilated client contact to prevent spread of infections (Makic et al., 2013; Centers for Disease Control and Prevention, 2014).
- Provide routine oral care using toothbrushing and oral rinsing with an antimicrobial agent if needed (Joanna Briggs Institute, 2014; AACN, 2017a, 2017b; Vollman, Sole, & Quinn et al., 2017).
- Maintain proper cuff inflation for both endotracheal tubes and cuffed tracheostomy tubes with minimal leak volume or minimal occlusion volume to decrease risk of aspiration and reduce incidence of VAP (AACN, 2016, Johnson, 2017; Stacy, 2018).
- Reposition the client as needed. Use rotational bed or kinetic bed therapy in clients for whom side-to-side turning is contraindicated or difficult.

▲ Patients mechanically ventilated for more than 24 hours can benefit from protocolized rehabilitation directed toward early mobilization (Schmidt et al., 2017).

- Assess bilateral anterior and posterior breath sounds every 2 to 4 hours and as needed; respond to any relevant changes (Gallagher, 2017).
- Assess responsiveness to ventilator support; monitor for subjective complaints and sensation of dyspnea (Gallagher, 2017).

▲ Collaborate with the interdisciplinary team in treating clients with ARF to meet the client's ventilator care needs and avoid complications (Karthika et al., 2016).

Geriatric

- Recognize that critically ill older adults have a high rate of morbidity when mechanically ventilated.
- ▲ NPPV may be used during acute treatment of older clients with impaired ventilation.

Home Care

- ▲ Some of the interventions listed previously may be adapted for home care use. Begin discharge planning as soon as possible with the case manager or social worker to assess the need for home support systems, assistive devices, and community or home health services.
- ▲ With help from a medical social worker, assist the client and family to determine the fiscal effect of care in the home versus an extended care facility.
- Assess the home setting during the discharge process to ensure the home can safely accommodate ventilator support (e.g., adequate space and electricity).
- Have the family contact the electric company and place the client residence on a high-risk list in case of a power outage.
- Assess the caregivers for commitment to supporting a ventilator-dependent client in the home.
- Be sure that the client and family or caregivers are familiar with operation of all ventilation devices, know how to suction secretions if needed, are competent in doing tracheostomy care, and know schedules for cleaning equipment. Have the designated caregiver or caregivers demonstrate care before discharge.
- Assess client and caregiver knowledge of the disease, client needs, and medications to be administered via ventilation-assistive devices. Avoid analgesics. Assess knowledge of how to use equipment. Teach as necessary.
- Establish an emergency plan and criteria for use. Identify emergency procedures to be used until medical assistance arrives. Teach and role-play emergency care.

Client/Family Teaching and Discharge Planning

- Explain to the client the potential sensations that will be experienced, including relief of dyspnea, the feeling of lung inflations, the noise of the ventilator, and the reality of alarms.
- Explain to the client and family about being unable to speak, and work out an alternative system of communication. See previously mentioned interventions (Gallagher, 2017).

- Demonstrate to the family how to perform simple procedures, such as suctioning secretions in the mouth with a tonsil-tip catheter, providing range-of-motion exercises, and reconnecting the ventilator immediately if it becomes disconnected.
- Offer both the client and family explanations about how the ventilator works and answer any questions.

Dysfunctional Ventilatory Weaning Response

NANDA-I Definition

Inability to adjust to lowered levels of mechanical ventilator support that interrupts and prolongs the weaning process

Defining Characteristics

Mild

Breathing discomfort; fatigue; fear of machine malfunction; feeling warm; increase in focus on breathing; mild increase in respiratory rate over baseline; perceived need for increase in oxygen; restlessness

Moderate

Abnormal skin color; apprehensiveness; decrease in air entry on auscultation; diaphoresis; facial expression of fear; hyperfocused on activities; impaired ability to cooperate; impaired ability to respond to coaching; increase in blood pressure from baseline (<20 mmHg); increase in heart rate from baseline (<20 beats/min); minimal use of respiratory accessory muscles; moderate increase in respiratory rate over baseline

Severe

Abnormal skin color; adventitious breath sounds; agitation; asynchronized breathing with the ventilator; decrease in level of consciousness; deterioration in arterial blood gases from baseline; gasping breaths; increase in blood pressure from baseline (≥20 mmHg); increase in heart rate from baseline (≥20 beats/minute); paradoxical abdominal breathing; profuse diaphoresis; shallow breathing; significant increase in respiratory rate above baseline; use of significant respiratory accessory muscles

Related Factors

Physiological

Alteration in sleep pattern; inadequate nutrition; ineffective airway clearance; pain

Psychological

Anxiety; decrease in motivation; fear; hopelessness; insufficient knowledge of weaning process; insufficient trust in healthcare professional; low self-esteem; powerlessness; uncertainty about ability to wean

Situational

Environmental barrier; inappropriate pace of weaning process; insufficient social support; uncontrolled episodic energy demands

Associated Condition

History of unsuccessful weaning attempt; history of ventilator dependence >4 days

Client Outcomes

Client Will (Specify Time Frame)

- Wean from ventilator with adequate arterial blood gases
- Remain free of unresolved dyspnea or restlessness
- Effectively clear secretions

Nursing Interventions

- Assess client's readiness for weaning as evidenced by the following:
  - Physiological and psychological readiness; there has been little research devoted to the study of psychological readiness to wean.
  - Resolution of initial medical problem that led to ventilator dependence.
  - Hemodynamic stability.
  - Normal hemoglobin levels.
  - Absence of fever.
  - Normal state of consciousness.
  - Metabolic, fluid, and electrolyte balance.
  - Adequate nutritional status with serum albumin levels >2.5 g/dL.
  - Adequate sleep.
  - Adequate pain management and minimal sedation.

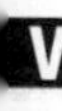

- ▲ Noninvasive weaning may be used in place of invasive mechanical support in adults with respiratory failure.
- ▲ A spontaneous awakening trial (SAT) in conjunction with a daily weaning assessment has a great effect on ventilator liberation outcomes (Haas & Loik, 2012; Jones et al., 2014, Klompas et al., 2015; Penuelas, Thille, & Esteban, 2015).
- Provide adequate nutrition to ventilated clients, using enteral feeding when possible.
- Use evidence-based weaning and extubation protocols as appropriate.

- • Identify reasons for previous unsuccessful weaning attempts, and include that information in the development of the weaning plan.
- • Reducing the size of artificial airways can increase airway resistance and overly increase energy expenditures of the diaphragm (Penuelas, Thille, & Esteban, 2015).
- ▲ Collaborate with an interdisciplinary team (healthcare provider, nurse, respiratory therapist, physical therapist, and dietitian) to develop a weaning plan with a time line and goals; revise this plan throughout the weaning period.
- • In clients with COPD who fail extubation, NIV facilitates weaning, prevents reintubation, and reduces mortality. Early NIV after extubation reduces the risk for respiratory failure and lowers 90-day mortality in clients with hypercapnia during an SBT (Mas & Masip, 2014; Ward & Fulbrook, 2016).
- • Assist client to identify personal strategies that result in relaxation and comfort (e.g., music, visualization, relaxation techniques, reading, television, family visits). Support implementation of these strategies. Music intervention can be used to allay anxiety and can be a powerful distractor from distressful sounds and thoughts in the ICU (Tracy & Chlan, 2011; Bradt & Dileo, 2014).
- • Provide a safe and comfortable environment.
- • If unable to stay, make the call light button readily available and assure the client that needs will be met responsively.
- ▲ Coordinate pain and sedation medications to minimize sedative effects. Appropriate levels of sedation may be key to successful weaning (Reade & Finfer, 2014).
- • Administer analgesics and sedatives as needed to facilitate client comfort and rest. Use behavioral and sedation scales for nonverbal clients to provide a consistent way of monitoring pain and sedation levels and ensuring that therapeutic outcomes are being met (Barr et al., 2013; Dale et al., 2014; Reade & Finfer, 2014).
- • Tools such as the Riker Sedation-Agitation Scale, the Motor Activity Assessment Scale, the Ramsey Scale, or the Richmond Agitation-Sedation Scale may be useful in monitoring levels of sedation (Balas et al., 2012; Barr et al., 2013; Dale et al., 2014).
- • Schedule weaning periods for the time of day when the client is most rested. Cluster care activities to promote successful weaning. Avoid other procedures during weaning: keep the environment quiet and promote restful activities between weaning periods.

V

- • Promote a normal sleep-wake cycle, allowing uninterrupted periods of nighttime sleep.
- • During weaning, monitor the client's physiological and psychological responses; acknowledge and respond to fears and subjective complaints. Validate the client's efforts during the weaning process.
- • Involve the client and family in the weaning plan. Inform them of the weaning plan and possible client responses to the weaning process (e.g., potential feelings of dyspnea). Foster a partnership between clients and nurses in care planning for weaning.
- • Coach the client through episodes of increased anxiety. Remain with the client or place a supportive and calm significant other in this role. Give positive reinforcement and, with permission, use touch to communicate support and concern.
- • Terminate weaning when the client demonstrates predetermined criteria or when the following signs of weaning intolerance occur:
  - Tachypnea, dyspnea, or chest and abdominal asynchrony
  - Agitation or mental status changes
  - Decreased oxygen saturation: $Sao_2 < 90\%$
  - Increased $Paco_2$ or $EtCO_2$
  - Change in pulse rate or blood pressure or onset of new dysrhythmias
- ▲ If the dysfunctional weaning response is severe, consider slowing weaning to brief periods (e.g., 5 minutes). Continue to collaborate with the team to determine whether an untreated physiological cause for the dysfunctional weaning pattern remains. Consult with healthcare provider regarding use of NIV immediately after discontinuing ventilation. Consider an alternative care setting (subacute, rehabilitation facility, or home) for clients with prolonged ventilator dependence as a strategy that can positively affect outcomes.

Geriatric

- • Recognize that older clients may require longer periods to wean.
- • Frequently assess the older client for hypodelirium and hyperdelirium states.

Home Care

- • Weaning from a ventilator at home should be based on client stability and comfort of the client and caregivers under an intermittent care plan.

Risk for Other-Directed Violence

NANDA-I Definition

Susceptible to behaviors in which an individual demonstrates that he or she can be physically, emotionally, and/or sexually harmful to others

Risk Factors

Access to weapon; impulsiveness; negative body language; pattern of indirect violence; pattern of other-directed violence; pattern of threatening violence; pattern of violent anti-social behavior; suicidal behavior

At-Risk Population

History of childhood abuse; history of cruelty to animals; history of fire-setting; history of motor vehicle offense; history of substance misuse; history of witnessing family violence

Associated Condition

Alteration in cognitive functioning; neurological impairment; pathological intoxication; perinatal complications; prenatal complications; psychotic disorder

Client Outcomes

Client Will (Specify Time Frame)

- Stop all forms of abuse (physical, emotional, sexual; neglect; financial exploitation)
- Have cessation of abuse reported by victim
- Display no aggressive activity
- Refrain from verbal outbursts
- Refrain from violating others' personal space
- Refrain from antisocial behaviors
- Maintain relaxed body language and decreased motor activity
- Identify factors contributing to abusive/aggressive behavior
- Demonstrate impulse control or state feelings of control
- Identify impulsive behaviors
- Identify feelings/behaviors that lead to impulsive actions
- Identify consequences of impulsive actions to self or others
- Avoid high-risk environments and situations
- Identify and talk about feelings; express anger appropriately
- Express decreased anxiety and control of hallucinations as applicable
- Displace anger to meaningful activities
- Communicate needs appropriately
- Identify responsibility to maintain control
- Express empathy for victim

- Obtain no access or yield access to harmful objects
- Use alternative coping mechanisms for stress
- Obtain and follow through with counseling
- Demonstrate knowledge of correct role behaviors

Victim (and Children if Applicable) Will (Specify Time Frame)

- Have safe plan for leaving situation or avoiding abuse
- Resolve depression or traumatic response

Parent Will (Specify Time Frame)

- Monitor social/play contacts
- Provide supervision and nurturing environment
- Intervene to prevent high-risk social behaviors

Nursing Interventions

Client Violence

- Aggressive/violent behavior may be impulsive, but more commonly it evolves in reaction to the environment (internal or external). In either case, nursing staff must go through specialized training to be prepared for a quick response.
- Monitor the environment, evaluate situations that could become violent, and intervene early to deescalate the situation. Know and follow institutional policies and procedures concerning violence. Consider that family members or other staff may initiate violence in all settings. Enlist support from other staff rather than attempting to handle situations alone.
- Assess causes of aggression, such as social versus biological.
- Assess the client for risk factors of violence, including those in the following categories: personal history (e.g., past violent behavior, especially violent behavior in the community within 2 weeks of admission); psychiatric disorders (particularly psychoses, paranoid or bipolar disorders, substance abuse, post-traumatic stress disorder [PTSD], antisocial personality, borderline personality disorder); neurological disorders (e.g., head injury, temporal lobe epilepsy, cardiovascular accident, dementia or senility), medical disorders (e.g., hypoxia, hypoglycemia, hyperglycemia), psychological precursors (e.g., low tolerance for stress, impulsivity, hostility), coping difficulties (e.g., inability to plan solutions or see long-term consequences of behavior), younger age, risk of suicide, and childhood or adolescent disorders (e.g., conduct disorders, hyperactivity, autism, learning disability).

V

- Measures of violence may be useful in predicting or tracking behavior and serving as outcome measures.
- Assess the client with a history of previous assaults, especially violent behavior in the community within 2 weeks of admission. Listen to and acknowledge feelings of anger, observe for increased motor activity, and prepare to intervene if the client becomes aggressive.
- Assess the client for physiological signs and external signs of anger. Internal signs of anger include increased pulse rate, respiration rate, and blood pressure; chills; prickly sensations; numbness; choking sensation; nausea; and vertigo. External signs include increased muscle tone, changes in body posture (clenched fists, set jaw), eye changes (eyebrows lower and drawn together, eyelids tense, eyes assuming a "hard" appearance), lips pressed together, flushing or pallor, goose bumps, twitching, and sweating.
- Assess for the presence of hallucinations.
- Apply STAMPEDAR as an acronym for assessing the immediate potential for violence.
- Determine the presence and degree of homicidal or suicidal risk. A number of questions will elicit the necessary information: Have you been thinking about harming someone? If yes, who? How often do you have these thoughts, and how long do they last? Do you have a plan? What is it? Do you have access to the means to carry out that plan? What has kept you from hurting the person until now? Refer to the care plan for Risk for **Suicidal Behavior.** Mental health providers are required to report harm or threats of harm to another person, referred to as the "duty to warn." State laws and mental health codes should be checked to determine local mandates for threat reporting by specific healthcare professionals.
- Take action to minimize personal risk; use nonthreatening body language. Respect personal space and boundaries. Maintain at least an arm's length distance from the client; do not touch the client without permission (unless physical restraint is the goal). Do not allow the client to block access to an exit. If speaking with the client alone, keep the door to the room open. Be aware of where other staff is at all times. Notify other staff of where you are at all times. Take verbal threats seriously and notify other staff. Wear clothing and

V

accessories that are not restricting and that will not be dangerous (e.g., sandals or shoes with heels can lead to twisted ankles; necklaces or dangling earrings could be grabbed). Ensure staff training to deal with violence.

- Remove potential weapons from the environment. Be prepared to remove obstructions to staff response from the environment. Search the client and his or her belongings for weapons or potential weapons on admission to the hospital as appropriate.
- Inform the client of unit expectations for appropriate behavior and the consequences of not meeting these expectations. Emphasize that the client must comply with the rules of the unit. Give positive reinforcement for compliance. Increase surveillance of the hospitalized client at smoking, meal, and medication times.
- Assign a single room to the client with a potential for violence toward others. The client will be able to take time away from unit stimulation to calm self as needed. Another client will not be placed at risk as a roommate.
- Maintain a calm attitude in response to the client. Provide a low level of stimulation in the client's environment; place the client in a safe, quiet place, and speak slowly and quietly. Anxiety is contagious.
- Redirect possible violent behaviors into physical activities (e.g., walking, jogging) if the client is physically able. Using a punching bag or hitting a pillow is not indicated because these are not calming activities and they continue patterning violent behavior. However, activities that distract while draining excess energy help build a repertoire of alternative behaviors for stress reduction.
- Provide sufficient staff if a show of force is necessary to demonstrate control to the client.
- Deescalation is the first and most important action in response to anger and hostility. Close observation supervision may be implemented.
- Protect other clients in the environment from harm. Remove other individuals from the vicinity of a violent or potentially violent client. Follow safety protocols of the department. The risk of a violent client to others in the area (other clients, visitors) should be anticipated, even as efforts proceed to deescalate the situation with the client.

- • Maintain a secluded area for the client to be placed when violent. Ensure that staff is continuously present and available to client during seclusion.
- ▲ Recognize legal requirements that the least restrictive alternative of treatment should be used with aggressive clients. The hierarchy of intervention is as follows: promote a milieu that provides structure and calmness, with negotiation and collaboration taking precedence over control; maintain vigilance of the unit and respond to behavioral changes early; talk with client to calm and promote understanding of emotional state; use chemical restraints as ordered; increase to manual restraint if needed; increase to mechanical restraint and seclusion as a last resort.
- ▲ Use mechanical restraints if ordered and as necessary. Physical restraint can be therapeutic to keep the client and others safe.
- ▲ Follow the institutional protocol for releasing restraints. Observe the client closely, remain calm, and provide positive feedback as the client's behavior becomes controlled.
- ▲ After a violent event on a unit, debriefing and support of both staff and clients should be made available.
- • Form a therapeutic alliance with the client, remaining calm, identifying the source of anger as external to both nurse and client, and using the therapeutic relationship to prevent the need for seclusion or restraint. The development of a therapeutic relationship before aggressive behavior occurs provides an alternative for working through anger and frustration. Assisting the client to identify a source of anger or frustration that is external to both the nurse and client prevents the need for defensiveness by both and directs energy at solving an external problem.
- • Allow, encourage, and assist the client to verbalize feelings appropriately either one-on-one or in a group setting. Actively listen to the client; explore the source of the client's anger, and negotiate resolution when possible. Teach healthy ways to express feelings/anger, appropriate gender roles, and how to communicate needs appropriately.
- • Identify with client the stimuli that initiate violence and the means of dealing with the stimuli. Have the client keep an anger diary and discuss alternative responses together. Teach cognitive-behavioral techniques. Assisting the client to identify situations and people that upset him or her provides information needed for problem-solving.

V

The client may then identify alternative responses (e.g., leaving the stimulus; using relaxation techniques, such as deep breathing; initiating thought stopping; initiating a distracting activity; responding assertively rather than aggressively).

▲ Initiate and promote staff attendance at aggression management training programs.

Intimate Partner Violence/Domestic Violence

Note: Before implementation of interventions in the face of domestic violence, nurses should examine their own emotional responses to abuse, their knowledge base about abuse, and systemic elements within the emergency department (ED) to ensure that interventions will be compassionate and appropriate.

- Screen for possible abuse in women or children with a pattern of multiple injuries, particularly if any suspicion exists that the physical findings are inconsistent with the explanation of how the injuries were incurred.

▲ Report suspected child abuse to Child Protective Services. Refer women suspected of being in a spousal abuse situation to an area crisis center and provide phone number of area crisis hotline.

- Assess for physical and mental concerns of women, including risk of HIV.
- Assist the client in negotiating the healthcare system and overcoming barriers.
- With women who repeatedly experience injuries from domestic violence, maintain a nonjudgmental approach and continue to offer resources/referrals. If the woman voices a willingness to leave her situation, assist with developing an emergency plan that will consider all contingencies possible (e.g., safe location, financial resources, care of children, when to leave safely). A woman in a domestic violence situation may change her mind several times before actually leaving. Proactive organization of an emergency plan helps increase the possibility that women will be able to leave safely. The most dangerous time of a domestic violence situation is when the spouse tries to leave.
- Maintain a nonjudgmental response when clients return to husbands or refuse to leave them. Women have many reasons for remaining in an abusive relationship, including economic concerns (especially with children), socialization about the woman's role,

V

political or legal obstacles, powerlessness, and a realistic fear of retaliation or death. Refer to the care plan for **Powerlessness.** Experienced nurses working with abused women define success as client personal growth over time, rather than the woman leaving the relationship.

- • Focus on providing support, ensuring safety, and promoting self-efficacy while encouraging disclosure about IPV events.
- • Pregnancy is a particular risk period for interpersonal violence. Screen pregnant women for the potential for domestic violence during pregnancy, especially in teenage pregnancies.
- • Women with physical or mental disabilities require extended assessment, including a comprehensive functional assessment, with attention to cultural issues, the nature of the disability, and needed resources. Women with disabilities may experience abuse from multiple sources, and particular attention should be paid to the additional emotional stressors present. Difficulties leaving home, physical needs that a shelter may not be able to accommodate, and the undesirability of nursing home placement are just a few stressors. Personal assistance providers may be abusive or take advantage financially.
- ▲ Referral for spiritual counseling may be considered, but be aware that clergy vary in their helpfulness.
- • Evaluate medical and mental illness as precursors to elder abuse.
- • Consider risk versus benefit when deciding if, when, and in how great a depth to explore client responses to abuse or violence.
- ▲ When spouse or child abuse accompanies substance abuse, refer the abusive client to a substance abuse treatment program. Refer the spouse receiving abuse to Al-Anon and the children to Alateen.
- ▲ When an adult reveals a history of unresolved/untreated sexual abuse as a child, referral to a local Adults Molested as Children (AMAC) group may be helpful. Refer to the care plans for Risk for **Suicidal Behavior, Self-Mutilation,** and Risk for **Self-Mutilation.**
- ▲ Referral of women for psychiatric/psychological treatment or parenting classes should be considered as an appropriate intervention.
- ▲ Referral of children for psychiatric/psychological treatment should be considered as an appropriate intervention.
- ▲ Refer to batterer intervention programs that are often available and may be court mandated.

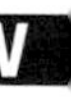

Social Violence

- • Assess for acute stress disorder (ASD) and PTSD among victims of violence.
- ▲ Assess the support network of women who become victims of violent crime and refer for appropriate levels of assistance. Of particular concern would be women who do not have family or friends to provide support or who have difficulty accessing other types of assistance.
- • Be aware that hate crime is increasing, particularly toward gay and transgendered individuals, and it requires support and advocacy for victims.
- ▲ Victims of violence seen in the ED should receive an assessment for needed services and assignment to case management.

Rape-Trauma Syndrome

- • Brief relationship abuse instruction with counseling in a student health center can be effective in preventing and responding to episodes of sexual coercion.
- • Assist client to cope with potential stalking activity.
- • Approach client with sensitivity.
- ▲ Monitor for paradoxical drug reactions and report any to the healthcare provider. Violent behavior can be stimulated by a medication intended to calm the client.
- • Assess for brain insults, such as recent falls or injuries, strokes, or transient ischemic attacks. Clients with brain injuries may respond to stimulus control, problem-solving, social skills training, relaxation training, and anger management to reduce aggressive behaviors. Brain injuries, lowered impulse control, and reduced coping can cause violent reactions to self or others. Brain injury symptoms may be mistaken for mental illness.
- • Decrease environmental stimuli if violence is directed at others. Removal of the client to a quiet area can reduce violent impulses. Use a calm voice to "talk down" the client.
- • Assess holistic needs of the client.
- • Discuss with client her wishes regarding use of an emergency contraceptive.
- ▲ If abuse or neglect of an older client is suspected, report the suspicion to an adult protective services agency with jurisdiction over the geographical area in which the client lives.

Pediatric
- Assess for predictors of anger that can lead to violent behavior.
- Be alert for both shaken baby syndrome and exposure of children to violence.
- Pregnant teens should be assessed for abuse, particularly if they are with an older partner.

▲ In the case of child abuse or neglect, refer for early childhood home visitation.

Geriatric
- Be alert to the potential for elder abuse in clients, including the possibility of psychological abuse.
- Assess for presence or client history of mental illness or treatment.
- Assess and observe for aggressive behavior in older clients at long-term care facilities.
- Observe clients for dementia and delirium.
- For clients with dementia, provide music therapy.
- Be aware of laws and regulations in the appropriate jurisdiction in which the client is located.
- Document and record suspected elder abuse according to mandatory regulations.
- Apart from mandated requirements, abide by the older client's wishes regarding action to be taken in response to abuse. Avoid interventions that increase the risk of abuse.
- Develop a safety plan and provide referrals to all relevant agencies or services.

Multicultural
- Exercise cultural competence when dealing with domestic violence.
- Identify and respond to unique needs of immigrant women who experience IPV.
- Assist with acculturation and activating social support.

Home Care
- Be alert to the potential for violent behavior in the home setting. Respond to verbal aggression with interventions to deescalate negative emotional states. Violence is a process that can be recognized early. Deescalation involves reducing client stressors, responding to the client with respect, acknowledging the client's feeling state, and assisting the client to regain control. If deescalation does not work, the nurse should leave the home.

- • Assess family members or caregivers for their ability to protect the client and themselves. The safety of the client between home visits is a nursing priority. Caregivers often need assistance with recognizing or admitting fear of or danger from a loved one.
- • Include an initial and ongoing assessment and evaluation of potential abuse and neglect. Photograph evidence of abuse or neglect when possible. Refer to the care plan for **Powerlessness.**
- ▲ If neglect or abuse is suspected, identify an emergency plan that addresses the problem immediately, ensures client safety, and includes a report to the appropriate authorities. Discuss when to use hotlines and 911. Role-play access to emergency resources with the client and caregivers.
- • Encourage appropriate safety behaviors in abused women; call the client at intervals during a 6-month period to determine whether safety behaviors are being performed.
- • Assess the home environment for harmful objects. Have the family remove or lock objects as able.
- ▲ Refer for homemaker or psychiatric home healthcare services for respite, client reassurance, and implementation of a therapeutic regimen. Responsibility for a person who may become violent provides high caregiver stress. Respite decreases caregiver stress. The presence of caring individuals is reassuring to both the client and caregivers, especially during periods of client anxiety. Individuals exhibiting violent behaviors can respond to the interventions described previously, modified for the home setting.
- ▲ If the client is taking psychotropic medications, assess client and family knowledge of medication and its administration and side effects. Teach as necessary. Knowledge of the medical regimen supports compliance.
- ▲ Evaluate effectiveness and side effects of medications. Accurate clinical feedback improves the healthcare provider's ability to prescribe an effective medical regimen specific to a client's needs.
- • If client displays mildly intensifying aggressive behavior, attempt to diffuse anger or violence (e.g., ask for a glass of water to distract client). Later in the visit, explain that aggressive behavior is not acceptable and present consequences of continued aggressive behavior (i.e., right of agency to discontinue services).

- • Document all acts or verbalizations of aggression. Safety of the staff is a primary responsibility of home health agencies. Law enforcement intervention may be necessary.
- ▲ If client verbalizes or displays threatening behavior, notify your supervisor and plan to make joint visits with another staff person or a security escort.
- • If the client's behavior is not overtly threatening but makes the nurse uncomfortable, a meeting may be held outside the home in sight of others (e.g., front porch).
- • Never enter a home or remain in a home if aggression threatens your well-being.
- ▲ Never challenge a show of force, such as a gun threat. Leave and notify your supervisor and the appropriate authorities. Document the incident.
- ▲ If client behaviors intensify, refer for immediate mental health intervention. The degree of disturbance and ability to manage care safely at home determines the level of services needed to protect the client.

Client/Family Teaching and Discharge Planning

- • Instruct victims of IPV in the dynamics and prognosis of domestic violence behavior, as well as the effect on children who witness or are victims of domestic violence.
- • Teach relaxation and exercise as ways to release anger and deal with stress.
- • Teach cognitive-behavioral activities, such as active problem-solving, reframing (reappraising the situation from a different perspective), or thought stopping (in response to a negative thought, picture a large stop sign and replace the image with a prearranged positive alternative). Teach the client to confront his or her own negative thought patterns (or cognitive distortions), such as catastrophizing (expecting the very worst), dichotomous thinking (perceiving events in only one of two opposite categories), magnification (placing distorted emphasis on a single event), or unrealistic expectations (e.g., "should get what I want when I want it").
- ▲ Refer to individual or group therapy.
- • Teach the adolescent client violence prevention, and encourage him or her to become involved in community service activities. School programs that couple community service with classroom health

instruction can have a measurable effect on violent behaviors of young adolescents at high risk for being both the perpetrators and victims of peer violence. Community service programs may be a valuable part of multicomponent violence prevention programs.

- Teach the use of appropriate community resources in emergency situations (e.g., hotline, community mental health agency, ED, 911 in most places in the US, the toll-free National Domestic Violence Hotline [1-800-799-SAFE]). Internet resources are increasing and should be made available to clients. It is necessary to get immediate help when violence occurs.
- Encourage the use of self-help groups in nonemergency situations.
- Inform the client and family about any applicable medication actions, side effects, target symptoms, and toxic reactions.

Risk for Self-Directed Violence

NANDA-I Definition

Susceptible to behaviors in which an individual demonstrates that he or she can be physically, emotionally, and/or sexually harmful to self

Risk Factors

Behavioral cues of suicidal intent; conflict about sexual orientation; conflict in interpersonal relationship(s); employment concern; engagement in autoerotic sexual acts; insufficient personal resources; social isolation; suicidal ideation; suicidal plan; verbal cues of suicidal intent

At-Risk Population

Age ≥45 years; age 15–19 years; history of multiple suicide attempts; marital status; occupation; pattern of difficulties in family background

Associated Condition

Mental health issue; physical health issue; psychological disorder

Client Outcomes, Nursing Interventions, Client/Family Teaching and Discharge Planning

Refer to care plans for Risk for **Suicidal Behavior, Self-Mutilation,** and Risk for **Self-Mutilation**

Impaired Walking

NANDA-I Definition

Limitation of independent movement within the environment on foot

Defining Characteristics

Impaired ability to climb stairs; impaired ability to navigate curbs; impaired ability to walk on decline; impaired ability to walk on incline; impaired ability to walk on uneven surface; impaired ability to walk required distance

Related Factors

Alteration in mood; decrease in endurance; environmental barrier; fear of falling; insufficient knowledge of mobility strategies; insufficient muscle strength; obesity; pain; physical deconditioning

Associated Condition

Alteration in cognitive functioning; impaired balance; impaired vision; musculoskeletal impairment; neuromuscular impairment

Client Outcomes/Goals

Client Will (Specify Time Frame)

- Demonstrate optimal independence and safety in walking
- Demonstrate the ability to direct others on how to assist with walking
- Demonstrate the ability to use and care for assistive walking devices properly and safely

Nursing Interventions

- • Progressive mobilization as tolerated (gradually raising head of bed [HOB], sitting in reclined chair, standing, with assistance). Progressing mobility gradually from bedrest to increased sit to stand times to short distance walking and timed testing can provide goals for the client and staged mobility successes (Ellison et al., 2016). See also **Impaired Physical Mobility.**
- • Consider and monitor for side effects of prescribed hydration and medications; physical condition; length of immobility contributing to orthostatic hypotension; and/or if lightheadedness, dizziness, syncope, or unexplained falls occur.
- ▲ Assess for orthostatic hypotension if systolic pressure falls 15 mm Hg or diastolic pressure falls 7 mm Hg from sitting to standing within 3 minutes. If this occurs, then replace client in bed and notify prescriber (Arnold & Raj, 2017).
- • Apply thromboembolic deterrent (TED) stockings and/or elastic leg wraps and abdominal binders as prescribed; raise HOB slowly in

W

small increments to sitting, have client move feet/legs up and down, and then stand slowly; avoid prolonged standing.

- Assess for cognitive, neuromuscular, and sensory deficits that will affect safety when walking (e.g., stroke, diabetic neuropathy, history of falls).
- ▲ Take pulse rate/rhythm, respiratory rate, and pulse oximetry before walking clients, and reassess within 5 minutes of walking, then ongoing as needed. If abnormal, have the client sit 5 minutes, then remeasure. If still abnormal, walk clients more slowly and with more help or for a shorter time, or notify physician. If uncontrolled diabetes/angina/arrhythmias/tachycardia (100 beats per minute or more) or resting systolic blood pressure (SBP) at or above 200 mm Hg or diastolic blood pressure (DBP) at or above 110 mm Hg occurs, do not initiate walking exercise. Refer to the care plan **Decreased Activity Tolerance.**
- Assist clients to apply orthosis, immobilizers, splints, braces, and compression stockings as prescribed before walking.
- Eat frequent small, low-carbohydrate meals.
- Reinforce correct use of prescribed mobility devices, and remind clients of weight-bearing restrictions.
- Emphasize the importance of wearing properly fitting, low-heeled shoes with nonskid soles and socks/hose, and of seeking medical care for foot pain or problems with abnormal toenails, corns, calluses, or diabetes. Refer to podiatric consult if indicated.
- ▲ Use a snug gait belt with handles and assistive devices while walking clients, as recommended by the physical therapist (PT).
- Walk clients frequently with an appropriate number of people; have one team member state short, simple motor instructions.
- Cue and manually guide clients with neglect as they walk.
- Document the number of helpers, level of assistance (maximum, standby, etc.), type of assistance, and devices needed in communication tools (e.g., plan of care, client room signage, verbal report).

Special Considerations: Lower Extremity Amputation

- Teach clients to don stump socks, liner, immediate postoperative prostheses (IPOP), or traditional prosthesis correctly before standing/walking.
- Teach clients the importance of avoiding prolonged hip and knee flexion. If contractures occur, they will affect prosthesis fit and function.

W

Geriatric

- ▲ Assess for swaying, poor balance, weakness, and fear of falling while elders stand/walk. If present, implement fall protection precautions and refer for PT evaluation and recommendations.
- ▲ Review medications for polypharmacy (more than five drugs) and medications that increase the risk of falls, including sedatives, antidepressants, and drugs affecting the central nervous system (CNS).
- • Encourage Tai chi, PT, or other exercise for balance, gait, and strength training in group programs or at home.
- • Recommend vision assessment and consideration for cataract removal if needed.

Home Care

- • Establish a support system for emergency and contingency care (e.g., wearable medical alert alarm; notify local emergency medicine services [EMS] of potential need).
- • Assess for and modify any barriers to walking in the home environment.
- ▲ Refer to occupational therapist (OT)/PT for home assessment and evaluation for home assessment for barriers, individualized strength, balance retraining, an exercise plan, and environmental modifications for safety (Peterson et al., 2016).
- ▲ Make referrals for home health services for support and assistance with activities of daily living (ADLs). An activity program pairing trained healthcare assistants with frail elders resulted in significant improvements in health outcomes and functional activity (Muramatsu et al., 2017).

Client/Family Teaching and Discharge Planning

- • Teach clients to check ambulation devices weekly for cracks, loose nuts, or worn tips and to clean dust and dirt on tips.
- • Teach diabetics that they are at risk for foot ulcers and teach them preventive interventions. See care plan **Risk for Ineffective Peripheral Tissue Perfusion.**
- ▲ Instruct clients at risk for osteoporosis or hip fracture to bear weight, walk, engage in resistance exercise (with appropriate adjustments for conditions), ensure good nutrition (especially adequate intake of calcium and vitamin D), drink milk, stop smoking, monitor alcohol intake, and consult a physician for appropriate medications.

Wandering

NANDA-I Definition

Meandering, aimless, or repetitive locomotion that exposes the individual to harm; frequently incongruent with boundaries, limits, or obstacles

Defining Characteristics

Continuous movement from place to place; eloping behavior; frequent movement from place to place; fretful locomotion; haphazard locomotion; hyperactivity; impaired ability to locate landmarks in a familiar setting; locomotion into unauthorized spaces; locomotion resulting in getting lost; locomotion that cannot be easily dissuaded; long periods of locomotion without an apparent destination; pacing; periods of locomotion interspersed with periods of nonlocomotion; persistent locomotion in search of something; scanning behavior; searching behavior; shadowing a caregiver's locomotion; trespassing

Related Factors

Alteration in sleep-wake cycle; desire to go home; overstimulating environment; physiological stage; separation from familiar environment

At-Risk Population

Premorbid behavior

Associated Condition

Alteration in cognitive functioning; cortical atrophy; psychological disorder; sedation

Client Outcomes

Client Will (Specify Time Frame)

- Maintain psychological well-being and reduce need to wander
- Reduce episodes of wandering in restricted areas/getting lost/elopement
- Maintain appropriate body weight
- Remain safe and free from falls
- Maintain physical activity and remain comfortable and free of pain

Caregiver Will (Specify Time Frame)

- Be able to explain interventions he or she can use to provide a safe environment for a care receiver who displays wandering behavior
- Develop strategies to reduce caregiver stress levels

Nursing Interventions

- Assess for physical distress or unmet needs (e.g., hunger, thirst, pain/discomfort, elimination needs).
- Assess for emotional or psychological distress, such as anxiety, fear, or feeling lost, considering the situated experience of the client.

- Assess and document the pattern, rhythm, and frequency of wandering over time.
- Obtain a psychosocial history including stress-coping behaviors.
- Observe the location and environmental conditions in which wandering is occurring and modify those that appear to induce wandering.
- Assess the client's environment and advocate for appropriate modifications using a survey such as the Wayfinding Evidence-Based Checklist and Rating (WEBCAR) instrument (Benbow, 2013).
- Use a full-length mirror in front of exit doors to deter elopement.
- Use camouflage (a cloth panel or wall hanging) to cover door knobs or locks to prevent elopement (check fire safety code/policy first).
- Change floor pattern to create subjective barrier (illusion of a step, hole, or pit) at exit door.
- Increase social interaction and offer structured activity and stress-reducing approaches, such as walking and exercise, music, massage, or a rocking chair.
- Create a familiar, low-stress or home-like environment with familiar belongings and regular daily activities.
- Provide safe and secure surroundings that deter and detect accidental elopements, using perimeter control devices or electronic tracking systems (including radiofrequency identification [RFID] tags, *global positioning system* [GPS] locator, smart watch, or cell phone application).
- When using electronic tracking technologies, an approach emphasizing relationships, respect, and the individual needs of patients and caretakers is best suited to finding solutions that both protect and empower.
- Develop and update unit and facility procedures and staff education related to wandering.
- Role-model person-centered care and provide appropriate supervision, support, and education of direct-care staff.
  - Establish a caring, calm, friendly and inviting climate in which relationships are valued.
  - Develop a culture of team spirit in which staff feel valued.
  - Support the development and maintenance of staff competencies in dementia care.
  - Encourage discussion of ethical issues and conflicts that arise during care.

W

- Help residents find their room by placing a sign with their name and a portrait of themselves at a younger age next to the doorway.
- Provide a regularly scheduled and supervised exercise or walking program, particularly if wandering occurs excessively during the night or at times that are inconvenient in the setting (Jensen & Padilla, 2017).
- Keep a current client photograph on file to help with identification (see **Client/Family Teaching and Discharge Planning** section regarding community safe return programs including AMBER and Silver alerts).
- Refer to the care plan for **Caregiver Role Strain.**
- For clients with dementia, also see care plan for **Chronic Confusion**.

Multicultural

- Assess for cultural assets, beliefs, life experiences, and values on the family's understanding of wandering behavior and caregiving.
- Assess client preferences for use of social services and family caregivers' availability and willingness to provide care.

Client/Family Teaching and Discharge Planning

- Use a broad range of descriptions for the term "wandering" to enhance caregivers' understanding.
- Teach caregivers about AMBER and Silver alert, Safe Return/Safely Home, and/or Project Lifesaver programs.
- Refer to supportive community and social services such as a psychiatric home health nurse and companion or respite care to assist with the impact of caregiving for the wandering client.

Home Care

W

- The previously mentioned interventions may be adapted for home care use.
- Help the caregiver set up a plan to reduce and manage wandering behavior including a plan of action to use if the client elopes:
  - Assess the home environment for modifications that will protect the client and prevent elopement.
  - Provide information about therapy dog/assistance dog resources.

APPENDIX

Nursing Care Plans for Hearing Loss and Vision Loss

Hearing Loss

Definition

A condition where there is the inability to detect some or all frequencies of sound and may involve complete or partial impairment of the ability to hear

Note: **Hearing Loss** is not a NANDA-I accepted diagnosis, but it is included here because of the frequency of occurrence of hearing loss, especially in the geriatric population.

Defining Characteristics

Inability to hear in noisy environments; difficulty following conversations with more than one person; change in speech; change in usual response to stimuli; disorientation; impaired communication; irritability; poor concentration; restlessness; sensory distortions

Related Factors

Altered sensory integration; altered sensory reception; altered sensory transmission; biochemical imbalance; electrolyte imbalance; excessive noise exposure; psychological stress

Client Outcomes

Client Will (Specify Time Frame)

- Demonstrate understanding by a verbal, written, or signed response
- Demonstrate relaxed body movements and facial expressions
- Explain plan to modify lifestyle to accommodate hearing impairment
- Demonstrate familiarity with hearing assistive devices

Nursing Interventions

- Observe for signs of hearing loss, especially in people exposed to loud noise and people older than 60 years of age.
- Use the National Institutes of Health (NIH) Toolbox to test hearing as available.
- Recognize that certain populations are especially vulnerable to noise-induced hearing loss, including farmers, industrial workers,

firefighters, construction workers, musicians, and music lovers using personal listening devices.

- ▲ Refer client to otolaryngologist and/or audiologist.
- • Keep background noise to a minimum. Turn off the television and radio when communicating with the client. If in a noisy environment, take the client to a private room and shut the door.
- • Stand or sit directly in front of the client when communicating. Make sure adequate light is on the nurse's face, avoid chewing gum or covering mouth or face with hands while speaking, establish eye contact, and use nonverbal gestures.
- • Speak clearly in lower voice tones if possible. Do not over-enunciate or shout at the client.
- • Verify that the client understands critical information by asking the client to repeat the information.
- • If necessary, provide a communication board, personnel who know sign language, or any method helpful to increase understanding for the hearing-impaired client.
- • Prepare pictures or diagrams depicting tests or procedures; have books with relevant pictures available for more detailed discussions.
- • Watch for signs of depression such as withdrawal, impaired sleep, and flat affect, and refer for treatment if needed.
- • Encourage the client to wear a hearing aid if available.
- • Recognize that clients with a hearing aid may choose to wear a hearing aid intermittently because hearing aids can create distortion of speech and extraneous noise that is bothersome (Shah & Lotke, 2017).
- • Review the client's nutritional status and suggest a diet diary to evaluate nutritional habits.
- • Ask the client about smoking. Refer the client to a smoking cessation program if indicated.
- • Review the client's environmental risk factors for hearing loss to include occupational noise.

Critical Care

- • Develop a communication cart to foster communication with hearing-impaired clients. Contents can include spiral notebooks, felt-tip markers, clipboards, communication boards (picture, word, entire phrases, and alphabet), hearing aid batteries, and electronic speech generators.

- • Develop good communication skills to interact with hearing impaired clients. It is unfair to expect critically ill older adults to understand what is being said to them only through auditory means.

Pediatric

- ▲ Refer infants or children for hearing tests as indicated so that treatment/therapy begins early as needed.
- • In the child, recommend that parents watch for signs of hearing loss including worsening speech or school performance, withdrawal from social activities, playing alone, and playing the television and music increasingly more loudly (Shah & Lotke, 2017).
- • Refer the child to an audiologist to explore the use of computer-based auditory training programs.
- • Recognize that children who are deaf or hard of hearing are particularly vulnerable to abuse, both by parents/caregivers and by sexual predators.
- • Recommend that teenagers avoid use of personal listening devices, or try to keep the volume down. Use culturally appropriate teaching materials. *There is an increased rate of hearing loss in teenagers 12 to 19 years of age* (Shah & Lokte, 2017).

Geriatric

- ▲ Routinely screen geriatric clients for presence of hearing loss because up to two-thirds of all people age 70 or older have hearing loss (Bainbridge & Wallhagen, 2014).
- ▲ Inspect the ear canal for wax buildup.
- • Work with the client to ensure contact with others and maintenance of meaningful activities to strengthen the social network and maintain cognitive abilities.

Home Care

- • The previously listed interventions are applicable in the home care setting.
- • Recommend that the client change the home environment if needed for better acoustics. Avoid glossy walls, high and reflective ceilings, reflective glass counters, and tiled floors. Use acoustic paneling if needed.
- • Suggest installation of devices such as strobe lights for the telephone, alarm clock, fire alarms, and doorbell; sensors that detect an infant's cry; alarm clocks that vibrate the bed; and closed caption decoders for television sets. Other helpful devices include telephone amplifiers,

speakerphones, cell phones with text messaging or instant messaging, pocket talker personal listening systems, and FM and infrared amplification systems that connect directly to a television or audio output jack. Also available is a telecommunication device, which is a typewriter keyboard with an alphanumeric display that allows the hearing-impaired person to send typed messages over the telephone line. Use of hearing ear dogs (dogs specially trained to alert their owners to specific sounds) may also be helpful.

Client/Family Teaching and Discharge Planning

- Teach the client to avoid excessive noise at work or at home and to wear hearing protection when necessary.
- Teach the client to avoid inserting objects such as cotton-tipped swabs or bobby pins into the ears.

Vision Loss

Definition

Decreased or absence of vision when it existed previously; vision loss can be either acute in onset or occur as a slow progressive chronic visual loss

Note: Vision Loss is not a NANDA-I nursing diagnosis. The authors have identified this health problem because vision loss is commonly seen in nursing practice.

Defining Characteristics

Change in behavior pattern; change in problem-solving abilities; disorientation; decreased visual acuity; loss of vision; visual hallucinations

Related Factors

Aging; diabetes mellitus; exposure to ultraviolet (UV) light; impaired visual function; impaired visual integration; impaired visual reception; impaired visual transmission; nutritional deficiency

(Adapted from the work of NANDA-I.)

Client Outcomes

Client Will (Specify Time Frame)

- Demonstrate relaxed body movements and facial expressions
- Remain as independent as possible
- Explain plan to modify lifestyle to accommodate visual impairment
- Incorporate use of lighting to maximize visual abilities
- Demonstrate familiarity with vision assistive devices
- Remain free of physical harm resulting from loss of vision

Nursing Interventions

- When providing sensitive care, post visual impairment signage for interprofessional team service support (Luckowski & Luckowski, 2015).
- Knock before entering and address client by name. Introduce yourself and title. If you want to shake hands, verbalize intent first, and in a normal natural tone of voice explain exactly what you are going to do. Check the call bell to ensure it is in place and usable. Place other items such as the phone and bedside table within reach and let the client know where they are located. Describe the bedrail controls and room layout, including the bathroom. Keep area clean and free from clutter. Indicate when a conversation is over and when you are leaving the room (Luckowski & Luckowski, 2015).
- When handing an item, place it directly in the client's hand or place the client's hand on top of the item. Use the sight-guided technique to assist ambulation. Offer the back of your arm just above the elbow and walk one step ahead. Inform the client of stairs or turns. When sitting, guide the client's hand to the back of the chair or place to sit on the bed (Luckowski & Luckowski, 2015).
- Use the clock's coordinates to describe the location of food on the plate. Open containers as requested. Encourage utilization of talking clocks and watches, books, radio, and service dogs. Read education and discharge information to the client and refer for social support services as required (Luckowski & Luckowski, 2015).
- Provide environmental predictability. Consistently remind staff, family members, and visitors to tell the client when something is added or removed from the environment.
- Make doorframes and light switches a contrasting color to the walls.
- Ensure access to eyeglasses or magnifying devices as needed. Vision aid devices include readers, microscopes, handheld magnifiers, and stand magnifiers (Ventocilla, 2013).
- Encourage expression of feelings and expect grieving behavior if onset of vision loss and/or blindness is new. People grieve the loss of vision and experience a loss of identity and control over their lives.
- Recommend that client have vision evaluated by an optometrist or ophthalmologist as appropriate to determine whether an improvement in visual acuity is possible.
- Question the client regarding the presence of visual hallucinations (Charles Bonnet syndrome).

- Take protective measures to prevent falls. Refer to the care plan for Risk for **Adult Falls.**
- Explore and enhance available support systems to ensure a safe discharge. Caregivers and/or family may not have the ability to assist the client after discharge. See care plan for Risk for **Injury** or Risk for **Adult Falls.**
- Assess the client's visual and other sensory loss using valid and reliable tools such as the Snellen eye chart (visual acuity) or Amsler grid (central vision loss with macular degeneration).
- Annual dilated eye examinations for diabetic clients are recommended.
- Encourage the client to implement lifestyle strategies that promote avoidance of cardiovascular disease and diabetes to prevent vision loss.
- Nursing actions that create a sense of good nursing care in clients with wet age-related macular degeneration identified two main areas of focus. The first theme was related to being perceived as an individual, specifically being respected, and answering questions politely and focusing on them as individuals and being engaged. The second theme was client empowerment through encouragement of participation to create confidence. Creating trust by building partnerships and shared decision-making is best (Emsfors, Christensson, & Elgand, 2017).

Multicultural

- Consider race/ethnicity as a possible related factor to vision loss.

Geriatric

- Low vision is defined as central acuity of 20/70 or worse corrected. Legal blindness is defined as 20/200 or worse. Determination of legal blindness may qualify people for Social Security and Disability benefits. Driving contraindications must be heeded for safety (Pelletier, Rojas-Roldan, & Coffin, 2016).
- Sight loss is linked to increasing age and can have a profound effect on quality of life.

▲ Three important implications for practice include: (1) untreatable vision loss is not an inevitable consequence of aging, and any vision loss should be investigated; (2) cataract extraction is a common procedure and results in visual rehabilitation; and (3) eye drops are often prescribed medications. Missed doses can cause untreatable vision loss (Marsden, 2017).

- Older people with sight loss are more prone to falls and the risk of injury, including hip fractures, which double in older clients.
- Evidence supports daily age-related eye disease study (AREDS) vitamin supplementation to delay vision loss with age-related macular degeneration. Intravitreal injections of vascular endothelial growth factor stabilize vision in clients with neovascular macular degeneration or diabetic edema (Pelletier, Rojas-Roldan, & Coffin, 2016).
- Low vision rehabilitation to promote independence while reducing risk for injury must incorporate aging adults' perspective on risk and analysis of environmental factors (Laliberte Rudman et al., 2016).
- Keep the environment quiet, soothing, and familiar. Use consistent caregivers. These measures are comforting to older adults with a sensory loss and help decrease confusion (Lawrence, 2011).

▲ The leading causes of sight loss in older people are uncorrected refractive error (treatable with prescriptions), cataracts (treatable with surgery), glaucoma (preventable), diabetic retinopathy (preventable with good glycemic control), and age-related macular degeneration (sometimes treatable) (Marsden, 2017).

- Cataracts are the leading cause of reversible vision impairment and may increase the risk for falls in older adults.
- Hearing and vision rehabilitation services need to screen for dual sensory impairment.

▲ Refer to a comprehensive vision rehabilitation center early in the disease process of macular degeneration to prevent some of the negative consequences of vision loss (Maturi, 2011).

- Teach the client methods to preserve remaining vision as much as possible, including avoiding smoking or breathing secondhand smoke, protecting the eyes from sunlight, and including fish and leafy green vegetables in the diet (Maturi, 2011; Young, 2015).
- Vision impairment is independently associated with malnutrition.
- Monitor for signs of new onset of increased vision loss, such as not recognizing familiar people, difficulty seeing in bright light or low light, new problems with reading, and complaints of tired eyes and/or vision problems with current glasses facilitating effective vision (Ventocilla, 2013).
- Age-related visual problems can also occur with stroke.

- Watch for signs of depression such as decreased appetite, withdrawal from usual life activities, flat affect, excessive time in bed, and somatization.
- For the client with both vision loss and dementia, provide the following nursing care:
    - Recognize that vision loss can increase problems for the client with dementia, including decreased orientation, decreased recognition of others, less recall, impaired judgment, and possibly aggression (Young, 2015).
    - Use one-to-one conversations to maintain socialization.
    - Obtain and use visual aids to help maintain orientation and contact with the environment, including such things as talking clocks, speaking Freeview digital boxes to give an auditory version of what is on the television, and use of memory photo dial pads so that clients can use the telephone to maintain contact with others (Barrand, 2013; Young, 2015).

Home Care

- Most of the listed interventions are applicable in the home care setting.
- Monitor home care clients for recent visual loss and resulting decrease in social activity.
- Enable the visually impaired client to do things for himself or herself to maintain independence as long as possible (Cattan, 2011).

Client/Family Teaching and Discharge Planning

Low Vision

- Use contrast to increase visibility of items; for example, place a dark background around the light switch so that it can be located more easily.
- Place red, yellow, or orange identifiers on important items that need to be seen, such as a red strip at the edge of steps, a red marker behind a light switch, or a red dot on a stove or washing machine to indicate how far to turn the knob, or use a dial marker that will offer a tactile cue to the client to turn on ovens, stoves, and washing machines.
- Use a watch or clock that verbally tells time and a phone with large numerals and emergency numbers programmed into it (Ventocilla et al., 2013).
- Teach blind clients how to feed themselves; associate food on the plate with hours on a clock so that the client can identify the location of food.

- Use low vision aids including magnifying devices for near vision and telescopes for seeing objects at a distance, a closed-circuit television that magnifies print, and guides for writing checks and envelopes.
- Teach the client with vision loss to do the following:
  - Use a magnifying mirror to shave or apply makeup; use an electric razor only.
  - Put personal care products in brightly colored pump containers (red, yellow, or orange) for identification.
  - Use tactile clues such as safety pins or buttons placed in hems to help client match clothing, or place matching outfits of clothing in separate plastic bags.
  - Use a prefilled medication organizer with large lettering or three-dimensional (3D) markers.
- ▲ Increase lighting in the home to help vision in the following ways:
  - Ensure adequate illumination of the entire home, adding light fixtures and increasing wattage of existing bulbs as needed.
  - Decrease glare; where light reflects on shiny surfaces, move or cover objects.
  - Use nonglare wax on the floor.
  - Use motion lights that turn on automatically when a person enters the room for nighttime use.
  - Add indoor strip or "runway"-type lighting to baseboards.
- ▲ Refer the client to an occupational therapist for assistance in dealing with vision loss and learning how to meet personal needs to maintain maximum independence.
- Encourage the client to wear a hat and sunglasses when out in the sun.
- Work with the client to find rewarding recreational pursuits.
- Arrange transportation sources because driving is contraindicated.

BIBLIOGRAPHY

Aalbers, S., Fusar-Poli, L., Freeman, R. E., Spreen, M., Ket, J. C. F., Vink, A. C., et al. (2017). Music therapy for depression. *Cochrane Library*, *11*, doi:10.1002/14651858.CD004517.pub3.

Abrams, P., et al. (2010). The standardization of terminology of lower urinary tract function: Report from the standardization sub-committee of the international continence society. *American Journal of Obstetrics and Gynecology*, *187*(1), 116–126.

Agency for Healthcare Research and Quality, U.S. Department of Health and Human Services. (2015). *Geriatrics: percentage of patients aged 65 and older discharged from any inpatient facility (e.g., hospital, skilled nursing facility, or rehabilitation facility) and seen within 30 days of discharge in the office by the physician, prescribing practitioner, registered nurse, or clinical pharmacist who had reconciliation of the discharge medications with the current medication list in the outpatient medical record documented.* https://www.qualitymeasures.ahrq.gov/summaries/summary/49756/fall-risk-management-the-percentage-of-medicare-members-75-years-of-age-and-older-or-65-to-74-years-of-age-with-balance-or-walking-problems-or-a-fall-in-the-past-12-months-who-were-seen-by-a-practitioner-in-the-past-12-months-and-who-discussed-falls-or-problem?q=medications+and+older+adults+and+falls. Retrieved January 2, 2018.

Agency for Toxic Substances and Disease Registry (ATSDR). (2014). *Medical management guideline for parathion.* Retrieved from http://www.atsdr.cdc.gov/MMG/MMG.asp?id=1140&tid=246.

Allen, L. A., Stevenson, L. W., Grady, K. L., et al. (2012). Decision making in advanced heart failure: A scientific statement from the American Heart Association. *Circulation*, *125*, 1928–1952.

Allison, J., & George, M. (2014). Using preoperative assessment and patient instruction to improve patient safety. *Association of Operating Room Nurses*, *99*(3), 364–375.

American Academy of Audiology. (2017). *Facts about hearing loss*. Retrieved October 31, 2017, from https://www.audiology.org/publications-resources/consumer-information/fact-sheets.

American Academy of Ophthalmology (AAO). (2015). *Four ways to fight dry eyes. The Ophthalmic News and Education Network.* Retrieved from https://www.aao.org/eye-health/tips-prevention/four-ways-to-fight-dry-eye. Retrieved February 10, 2018.

American Academy of Ophthalmology (AAO). (2018). *Seven tips for battling dry eye.* The Ophthalmic News and Education Network. Retrieved from https://www.aao.org/eye-health/tips-prevention/dry-eye-tips. Retrieved February 10, 2018.

American Academy of Oral Medicine. (2016). AAOM Clinical Practice Statement. Subject: Clinical management of cancer therapy-induced salivary gland hypofunction and xerostomia. *Oral Surgery, Oral Medicine, Oral Pathology and Oral Radiology*, *122*(3), 310–312. http://dx/doi/10.1016/j.oooo.2016.04.015.

American Academy of Pediatrics (AAP). (2014a). *Preventing SIDS*. Retrieved from http://www.healthychildren.org/English/ages-stages/baby/sleep/Pages/Preventing-SIDS.aspx.

American Academy of Pediatrics (AAP). (2014b). *Winter safety tips*. Retrieved from http://www.aap.org/en-us/about-the-aap/aap-press-room/news-features-and-safety-tips/Pages/Winter-Safety-Tips.aspx.

American Association of Critical Care Nurses. (2016). *AACN Practice Alert–Prevention of aspiration in adults. American Association of Critical Care Nurses.* Retrieved from https://www.aacn.org/~/media/aacn-website/clincial-resources/practice-alerts/preventionaspirationpracticealert.pdf. Retrieved February 20, 2018.

American Association of Critical Care Nurses. (2016a). *AACN Practice Alert-Prevention of Aspiration in Adults*. American Association of Critical Care Nurses. Retrieved from: https://www.aacn.org/~/media/aacn-website/clincial-resources/practice-alerts/preventionaspirationpracticealert.pdf.

American Association of Critical Care Nurses. (2017). *AACN Practice Alert-Prevention of ventilator-associated pneumonia in adults. American Association of Critical Care Nurses.* Retrieved February 20, 2018, from https://www.aacn.org/~/media/aacn-website/clincial-resources/practice-alerts/preventingvapinadults2017.pdf.

American Association of Critical Care Nurses. (2017a). *AACN Practice Alert-Prevention of Ventilator-Associated Pneumonia in Adults*. American Association of Critical Care Nurses. Retrieved February 10, 2018, from https://www.aacn.org/~/media/aacn-website/clincial-resources/practice-alerts/preventingvapinadults2017.pdf.

American Association of Critical Care Nurses. (2017b). *AACN Practice Alert-Oral Care for Acutely and Critically Ill Patients*. American Association of Critical Care Nurses. Retrived February 10, 2018, from https://www.aacn.org/~/media/aacn-website/clincial-resources/practice-alerts/oralcarepractalert2017.pdf.

American College of Nurse-Midwives. (2010). Position Statement: Nitrous oxide for labor analgesia. *Journal of Midwifery and Women's Health*, 55(3).

American Dental Association. (2015). *Managing xerostomia and salivary gland hypofunction. A Report on the ADA Council of Scientific Affairs*. Retrieved from http://jada.ada.org/content/145/8/867.abstract.

American Dental Association. (2017). *Home oral care*. Retrieved February 26, 2018, from http://www.ada.org/en/member-center/oral-health-topics/home-care.

American Dental Association (ADA). (2017a). *Oral health topics:* Home oral care. http://www.ada.org/en/member-center/oral-health-topics/home-care. Retrieved February 3, 2018.

American Dental Association (ADA). (2017b). *Mouth Healthy:* Halitosis. http://www.mouthhealthy.org/en/az-topics/h/Halitosis. Retrieved February 3, 2018.

American Dental Association (ADA). (2017c). *MouthHealthy: Brushing your teeth.* http://www.mouthhealthy.org/en/az-topics/b/brushing-your-teeth. Retrieved February 3, 2018.

American Dental Association (ADA). (2017d). *Mouth Healthy: Mouthwash.* http://www.mouthhealthy.org/en/az-topics/m/mouthwash. Retrieved February 3, 2018.

American Geriatrics Society. (2015). Updated Beers criteria for potentially inappropriate medication use in older adults. *Journal of the American Geriatrics Society*, *63*(11), 2227–2246. doi:10.1111/jgs.13702.

American Nurses Association. (2013). *Safe Patient Handling and Mobility: Interprofessional National Standards*. Spring Field, MD. Nursebooks. http://www.nursesbooks.org/ebooks/download/SPHM-Standards.pdf. Retrieved January 1, 2018.

American Psychiatric Association (APA). (2015). *Practice guidelines for the treatment of psychiatric disorders: Compendium*, http://psychiatryonline.org/guidelines.

American Psychiatric Nurses Association. (2015). *Psychiatric-mental health nurse essential competencies for assessment and management of individuals at risk for suicide*. Retrieved from http://www.apna.org/i4a/pages/index.cfm?pageid=5684.

American Society of PeriAnesthesia Nurses (ASPAN). (2015). *Normothermia clinical guideline*. http://www.aspan.org/Clinical-Practice/Clinical-Guidelines/Normothermia. Retrieved January 9, 2018.

Amsterdam, E. A., Wenger, N. K., Brindis, R. G., et al. (2014). AHA/ACC guideline for the management of patients with non-ST elevation acute coronary syndromes: A report of the American College of Cardiology/American Heart Association Task Force on Practice Guidelines. *Circulation*, *23*(30), e344–e426.

Andersen, L. S., Magidson, J. F., O'Cleirigh, C., Remmert, J. E., Kagee, A., Leaver, M., et al. (2018). A pilot study of a nurse-delivered cognitive behavioral therapy intervention (Ziphamandla) for adherence and depression in HIV in South Africa. *Journal of Health Psychology*, *23*(6), 776–787. doi: 10.1177/1359105316643375. Epub 2016 Apr 26.

Anderson, D. J., Podgorny, K., Berrios-Torres, S. I., et al. (2014). Strategies to prevent surgical site infections in acute care hospitals: 2014 Update. *Infection Control and Hospital Epidemiology*, *35*(6), 605–627.

Anderson, E. T., & McFarlane, J. (2011). *Community as partner: Theory and practice in nursing* (6th ed.). Philadelphia: Lippincott Williams & Wilkins.

Anderson, K., Ewen, H., Miles, E., et al. (2010). The grief support in healthcare scale: Development and testing. *Nursing Research*, *59*(6), 372–379.

Andrews, A., & Morgan, G. (2013). Constipation in palliative care: Treatment options and considerations for individual patient management. *International Journal of Palliative Nursing*, *19*(6), 226–273.

Apold, J., & Rydrych, D. (2012). Preventing device-related pressure ulcers: Using data to guide statewide change. *Journal of Nursing Care Quality*, *27*(1), 28–34.

Appleton, R., Kinsella, J., & Quasim, T. (2015). The incidence of intensive care unit-acquired weakness syndromes: A systematic review. *Journal of the Intensive Care Society*, *16*(2), 126–136.

Arnold, A., & Raj, S. (2017). Orthostatic hypotension: A practical approach to investigation and management. *The Canadian Journal of Cardiology*, *33*(12), 1725–1728.

Arockisamy, V., Holsti, L., & Albersheim, S. (2008). Fathers' experience in the neonatal intensive care unit: A search for control. *Pediatrics*, *121*(2), e215–e222.

Aronson, J. (2017). Medication reconciliation. *BMJ: British Medical Journal (Online)*, 356. http://dx.doi.org.proxy.lib.umich.edu/10.1136/bmj.i5336.

Assaad, S., Popescu, W., & Perrino, A. (2013). Fluid management in thoracic surgery. *Current Opinion in Anaesthesiology*, *26*, 31–39.

Attaluri, A., et al. (2011). Randomized clinical trial: Dried plums (prunes) vs psyllium for constipation. *Alimentary Pharmacology and Therapeutics*, *33*, 822–828.

Austin, P., Jenkins, S., & Hines, A. (2017). Thromboembolic events in PICU: A descriptive study. *Pediatric Nursing*, *43*(3), 132–137.

Avery, G. (2013). *Law and ethics in nursing and healthcare: An introduction* London: Sage Publications Inc.

Aydin, A., Ahmed, K., Zaman, I., et al. (2014). Recurrent urinary tract infections in women. *International Urogynecology Journal*, *26*(6), 795–804.

Babaee, S., Shafiei, Z., Sadeghi, M. M., Nik, A. Y., & Valiani, M. (2012). Effectiveness of massage therapy on the mood of patients after open heart surgery. *Iranian Journal Nursing Midwifery Research*, *17*(2 Suppl 1), S120

Baer, A. N. (2017). *Treatment of dry mouth and other non-ocular sicca symptoms in Sjögren's syndrome*. Retrieved from https://www-uptodate-com.proxy.hsl.ucdenver.edu/contents/treatment-of-dry-mouth-and-other-non-ocular-sicca-symptoms-in-sjogrens-syndrome/print?source=search_result&search=xerostomia%20treatment&selectedTitle=1~150.

Bainbridge, K. E., & Wallhagen, M. I. (2014). Hearing loss in an aging American population: Extent, impact and management. *Annual Review of Public Health*, *35*, 139–152.

Balas, M. C., Vasilevskis, E. E., Burke, W. J., et al. (2012). Critical care nurses' role in implementing the "ABCDE Bundle" into practice. *Critical Care Nurse*, *32*(2), 35–38, 40–48.

Ban, K. A., Minei, J. P., Laronga, C., et al. (2016). American College of Surgeons and Surgical Infection Society: Surgical site infection guidelines, 2016 update. *Journal of the American College of Surgeons*, *22*(1), 59–74.

Baranoski, S., & Ayello, E. A. (Eds.). (2016). *Wound care essentials: Practice principles* (4th ed.). Ambler, PA: Lippincott Williams & Wilkins.

Barr, J., Fraser, G. L., Puntillo, K., et al. (2013). Clinical practice guidelines for the management of pain, agitation, and delirium in adult patients in the intensive care unit. *Critical Care Medicine*, *41*(1), 263–306.

Barrand, J. (2013). *Supporting sight loss and dementia*. Retrieved October 31, 2017, from http://www.magonlinelibrary.com/doi/abs/10.12968/nrec.2011.13.9.448.

Barton, G., Vanderspank-Wright, B., & Shea, J. (2016). Optimizing oxygenation in the mechanically ventilated patient nursing practice implications. *Critical Care Nursing Clinics of North America*, *28*, 425–435.

Beeckman, D. (2017). A decade of research on Incontinence-Associated Dermatitis (IAD): Evidence, knowledge gaps and next steps. *Journal of Tissue Viability*, *26*(1), 47–56. doi:10.1016/j.jtv.2016.02.004.

Benbow, W. (2013). Evidence-based checklist for wayfinding design in dementia care facilities. *Canadian Nursing Home*, *24*(1), 4–10.

Benfield, R., et al. (2010). The effects of hydrotherapy on anxiety, pain, neuroendocrine response, and contractions dynamics during labor. *Biological Research for Nursing*, *12*(1), 18–36.

Berger, A. M., Mitchell, S. A., Jacobsen, P. B., & Pirl, W. F. (2015). Screening, evaluation, and management of cancer-related fatigue: Ready for implementation to practice? *CA: A Cancer Journal for Clinicians*, *65*(3), 190–211. doi:10.3322/caac.21268.

Berríos-Torres, S. I., Umscheid, C. A., Bratzler, D. W., et al. (2017). Healthcare infection control practices advisory committee. Centers for Disease Control and Prevention guideline for prevention of surgical site infection, 2017. *JAMA Surgery*, *152*(8), 784–791.

Bickley, L. S., & Szilagyi, P. (2016). *Bate's guide to physical examination* (12th ed.). Philadelphia: Lippincott.

Billeter, A. T., Hohmann, S. F., Dren, D., et al. (2014). Unintentional perioperative hypothermia is associated with severe complications and high mortality in elective operations. *Surgery*, *156*, 1245–1252.

Black, D. S., O'Reilly, G. A., Olmstead, R., Breen, E. C., & Irwin, M. R. (2015). Mindfulness meditation and improvement in sleep quality and daytime impairment among older adults with sleep disturbances: A randomized clinical trial. *JAMA Internal Medicine*, *175*(4), 494–501. doi:10.1001/jamainternmed.2014.8081.

Blakeman, T. (2013). Evidence for oxygen use in the hospitalized patient: Is more really the enemy of good? *Respiratory Care*, *58*(10), 1679–1693.

Bliss, D. Z., Funk, T., Jacobson, M., & Savik, K. (2015). Incidence and characteristics of incontinence-associated dermatitis in community-dwelling persons with fecal incontinence. *Journal of Wound Ostomy Continence Nursing*, *42*(5), 525–530. doi:10.1097/WON.0000000000000159.

Bolen, B. B. (2017). *What not to eat with diarrhea*. Retrieved from http://ibs.about.com/od/ibsfood/qt/EatforDiarrhea.htm. https://www.verywell.com/what-to-eat-for-diarrhea-1944822. Retrieved January 26, 2018.

Bossola, M. (2015). Nutritional interventions in head and neck cancer patients undergoing chemoradiotherapy: A narrative review. *Nutrients*, 265–276.

Boynton, T., Kelly, L., Perez, A., et al. (2014). Banner mobility assessment tool for nurses: Instrument validation. *American Journal of Safe Patient Handling & Mobility*, *493*, 86–92.

Bozkurt, B., Aguilar, D., Deswal, A., et al. (2016). Contributory risk and management of comorbidities of hypertension, obesity, diabetes mellitus, hyperlipidemia, and metabolic syndrome in chronic heart failure: A scientific statement from the American Heart Association. *Circulation*, *134*, e535–e578.

Bradt, J., & Dileo, C. (2014). Music interventions for mechanically ventilated patients. *The Cochrane Database of Systematic Reviews*, (12), CD006902, doi:10.1002/14651858.CD006902.pub3.

Bratzler, D. W., Dellinger, E. P., Olsen, M. K., et al. (2013). Clinical practice guidelines for antimicrobial prophylaxis in surgery. *American Journal Health-System Pharmacists*, *70*, 195–283.

Brett, L., Traynor, V., & Stapley, P. (2016). Effects of physical exercise on health and well-being of individuals living with a dementia in nursing homes: A systematic review. *Journal of the American Medical Directors Association*, *17*(2), 104–116.

Brienza, D. M., et al. (2016). Pressure redistribution: Seating, positioning, and support surfaces. In S. Baranoski & E. A. Ayello (Eds.), *Wound care essentials: Practice principles* (4th ed.). Ambler, PA: Lippincott Williams & Wilkins.

Bruderer, U., Fisler, A., Steurer, P., & Steurer, M. (2017). Post-discharge nausea and vomiting after total intravenous anaesthesia and standardized PONV prophylaxis for ambulatory surgery. *Acta Anaesthesiologica Scandinavica*, *61*, 758–766.

Burkett, K., Morris, E., Anthony, J., Shambley-Ebron, D., & Manning-Courtney, P. (2017). Parenting African American children with autism: The influence of respect and faith in mother, father, single-, and two-parent care. *Journal of Transcultural Nursing*, *28*(5), 496–504.

Burns, K., Lellouche, F., Nisenbaum, R., et al. (2014). Automated weaning and SBT systems versus non-automated weaning strategies for weaning time in invasively ventilated critically ill adults. *The Cochrane Database of Systematic Reviews*, (9), CD008638.

Busti, A. (2016). *Pitting Edema Assessment*. https://www.ebmconsult.com/articles/pitting-edema-assessment. Retrieved September 2016.

Cagir, B. (2016). *Ileus: Drugs and diseases*. Medscape. Retrieved from https://emedicine.medscape.com/article/2242141-overview on November 4, 2017.

Cajanding, R. J. M. (2016). The effectiveness of a nurse-led cognitive-behavioral therapy on the quality of life, self-esteem and mood among Filipino patients living with heart failure: A randomized controlled trial. *Applied Nursing Research*, *31*, 86–93. doi: 10.1016/j.apnr.2016.01.002. Epub 2016 Jan 20.

Cameron, S., Ball, I., Cepinskas, G., et al. (2015). Early mobilization in the critical care unit: A review of adult and pediatric literature. *Journal of Critical Care*, *30*, 664–672.

Campbell, G., Alderson, P., Smith, A. F., et al. (2015). Warming of intravenous and irrigation fluids for preventing inadvertent perioperative hypothermia (review). *The Cochrane Collaboration*, (4), CD009891.

Campbell, M. L. (2017). Dyspnea. *Critical Care Clinics of North America*, *29*(4), 461–470.

Carrière, K., et al. (2018). Mindfulness-based interventions for weight loss: A systematic review and meta-analysis. *Obesity Reviews: An Official Journal of the International Association for the Study of Obesity*, *19*(2), 164–177. doi:10.1111/obr.12623.

Carter, T., Morres, I., Repper, J., & Callaghan, P. (2016). Exercise for adolescents with depression: Valued aspects and perceived change. *Journal of Psychiatric and Mental Health Nursing*, *23*, 37–44. doi:10.1111/jpm.12261.

Caruso, D., Gater, D., Harnish, C., & Clin Auton Res. (2015). *Prevention of recurrent autonomic dysreflexia: A Survey of current practice*. 25: 293. https://doi-org.auraria library.idm.oclc.org/10.1007/s10286-015-0303-0.

Cattan, M. (2011). How to assist residents with sight loss in your home. *Nursing and Residential Care*, *13*(2), 91–93.

Centers for Disease Control and Prevention (CDC). (2007). *Healthcare Infection Control Practices Advisory Committee: guideline for isolation precautions: preventing transmission of infectious agents in healthcare settings*. From http://www

.cdc.gov/ncidad/dh9p/pdf/guidelines/isolation2007.pdf. Updated 2014, accessed September 6, 2017.

Centers for Disease Control and Prevention (CDC). (2011). *Guideline for the prevention of intravascular catheter related infections*. Retrieved from http://www.cdc.gov/hicpac. Accessed May 8, 2017.

Centers for Disease Control and Prevention (CDC). (2014). *Hand hygiene basics*. Retrieved February 10, 2018 http://www.cdc.gov/handhygiene/Basics.html.

Centers for Disease Control and Prevention (CDC). (2014b). *International adoption and prevention of lead poisoning*. Retrieved from http://www.cdc.gov/nceh/lead/tips/adoption.htm.

Centers for Disease Control and Prevention (CDC). (2014c). *Vaccine information Statement (VIS) Influenza*. Accessed July 2017.

Centers for Disease Control and Prevention (CDC). (2015). *Healthy Weight—it's not a diet, it's a lifestyle!* http://www.cdc.gov/healthyweight/assessing/bmi/index.html. Retrieved 25 March 2018.

Centers for Disease Control and Prevention (CDC). (2016). *National Center for Health Statistics*. Atlanta, GA: Author.

Centers for Disease Control and Prevention (CDC). (2016). *The ABCs of hepatitis*. Retrieved January 21, 2018, from https://www.cdc.gov/hepatitis/resources/professionals/pdfs/abctable.pdf.

Centers for Disease Control and Prevention (CDC). (2017). *Health Effects of Cigarette Smoking*. https://www.cdc.gov/tobacco/data_statistics/fact_sheets/health_effects/effects_cig_smoking/index.htm.

Centers for Disease Control and Prevention (CDC). (2017). *Heat stress. NIOSH workplace safety and health tips*. From https://www.cdc.gov/niosh/topics/heatstress/. Retrieved August 24, 2017.

Centers for Disease Control and Prevention (CDC). (2017). *Guidelines for prevention of catheter-associated urinary tract infections*. Retrieved October 30, 2017, from https://www.cdc.gov/infectioncontrol/pdf/guidelines/cauti-guidelines.pdf.

Centers for Disease Control and Prevention (CDC). (2017). *Clostridium Difficile*. https://www.cdc.gov/hai/organisms/cdiff/cdiff_clinicians.html. Retrieved November 12, 2017.

Centers for Disease Control and Prevention (CDC). (2017). *Adult immunization schedules*. Retrieved from http://www.cdc.gov/vaccines/schedules/hcp/adult.html.

Centers for Disease Control and Prevention (CDC). (2018). *Surgical Site Infection Event*. https://www.cdc.gov/nhsn/PDFs/pscManual/9pscSSIcurrent.pdf. Retrieved January 9, 2018.

Centers for Disease Control and Prevention (CDC). (2018). *Workplace safety and health*. https://www.cdc.gov/niosh/injury/data.html. Retrieved May, 1, 2018.

Chacko, B., Peter, J. V., Tharyan, P. I., et al. (2015). Pressure-controlled versus volume-controlled ventilation for acute respiratory failure due to acute lung injury (ALI) or acute respiratory distress syndrome (ARDS). *The Cochrane Database of Systematic Reviews*, (1), Art. No.: CD008807.

Chang, S. J., & Huang, H. H. (2013). Diarrhea in enterally fed patients: Blame the diet? *Current Opinion in Clinical Nutrition and Metabolic Care, 2013*(16), 588–594.

Chassiakos, L. R., et al. (2016). Children and adolescents and digital media. *Pediatrics*, *138*(5), e1–e18. doi:10.1542/peds.2016-2593.

Clarke, K., Tong, D., Pan, Y., et al. (2013). Reduction in catheter-associated urinary tract infections by bundling interventions. *International Journal for Quality Health Care*, *25*(1), 43–49.

Choi, S. D., & Brings, K. (2015). Work-related musculoskeletal risks associated with nurses and nursing assistants handling overweight and obese patients: A literature review. *Work (Reading, Mass.)*, *53*(2), 439–448.

Cohen, M. H., et al. (2010). *Patient handling and movement assessments: A white paper, The Facility Guideline Institute*, http://www.wsha.org/wp-content/uploads/Worker-Safety_4-Equipment-needs-FGI_PHAMA_whitepaper_042810.pdf. (Retrieved 2 January 2018).

College of Nurses of Ontario. (2014). *Practice standard: Medication*. Retrieved from http://www.cno.org/Global/docs/prac/41007_Medication.pdf.

Contou, D., & de Prost, N. (2016). Skin mottling. *The New England Journal of Medicine*, *375*, 2187. doi:10.1056/NEJMicm1602055.

Corbett, K., & Hannison, E. (2016). Non-pharmacological interventions for the prevention of venous thromboembolism: A literature review. *Nursing Standard*, *31*(8), 48–57.

Costa, D. K., White, M. R., Ginier, E., et al. (2017). Identifying barriers to delivering the awakening and breathing coordination, delirium, and early exercise/mobility bundle to minimize adverse outcomes for mechanically ventilated patients: A systemic review. *Chest*, *152*(2), 304–311.

Coyer, F., Gardner, A., & Doubrovsky, A. (2017). An interventional skin care protocol (InSPiRE) to reduce incontinence-associated dermatitis in critically ill patients in the intensive care unit: A before and after study. *Intensive and Critical Care Nursing*, 40(X), doi.org/10.1016/j.iccn.2016.12.001.

Croucher, B. (2014). The challenge of diagnosing dyspnea. *AACN Advanced Critical Care*, *25*(3), 284–290.

Crowe, M., Beaglehole, B., & Inder, M. (2016). Social rhythm interventions for bipolar disorder: A systematic review and rationale for practice. *Journal of Psychiatric and Mental Health Nursing*, *23*, 3–11. 10.1111/jpm.12271.

Da Fonseca, M. A., & Avenetti, D. (2017). Social determinants of pediatric oral health. *Dental Clinics of North America*, *61*(3), 519–532. doi:10.1016/j.cden.2017.02.002.

Dale, C., Kannas, D., Fan, V., et al. (2014). Improved analgesia, sedation, and delirium protocol associated with decreased duration of delirium and mechanical ventilation. *Annals of the American Thoracic Society*, *11*(3), 367–374.

Danzl, D. F. (2012). Hypothermia and frostbite. In A. S. Fauci (Ed.), *Harrison's principles of internal medicine* (18th ed.). New York: McGraw-Hill.

David Armstrong. (2017) *Diabetes and Foot Problems. National Institute of Diabetes and Digestive and Kidney Diseases.* https://www.niddk.nih.gov/health-information/diabetes/overview/preventing-problems/foot-problems.

De Almeida, L. M., & Braga, C. G. (2006). Construction and validation of an instrument to assess powerlessness. *International Journal of Nursing Terminologies and Classifications*, *17*, 67.

deAraujo, T., Maeve, V., Gomes, P. C., & Caporossi, C. (2014). Enteral nutrition in critical patients; should the administration be continuous or intermittent? *Nutra hosp*, *29*(5), 563–567.

Dirks, J. (2017). Continuous venous oxygen monitoring. In D. L. Wiegand (Ed.), *AACN procedure manual for high acuity, progressive, and critical care* (7th ed.). Philadelphia: Saunders Elsevier.

Ditah, I., Devaki, P., Luma, H. N., Ditah, C., Njei, B., et al. (2014). Prevalence, trends, and risk factors for fecal incontinence in United States adults, 2005–2010. *Clinical Gastroenterology and Hepatology*, *12*(4), 636–643 .e2.

Doenges, M. E., Moorhouse, M. F., & Murr, A. C. (2016). *A nurse's pocket guide: Diagnoses, prioritized interventions and rationales* (14th ed.). Philadelphia: Davis Company.

Douglas, M. K., Rosenkoetter, M., Pacquiao, D. F., et al. (2014). Guidelines for implementing culturally competent nursing care. *Journal of Transcultural Nursing*, *25*(2), 109–121.

Downing, L. J., Caprio, T. V., & Lyness, J. M. (2013). Geriatric psychiatry review: Differential diagnosis and treatment of the 3 D's—delirium, dementia, and depression. *Current Psychiatry Reports*, *15*(6), 365.

Drennan, V. M., Greenwood, N., & Cole, L. (2014). Continence care for people with dementia at home. *Nursing Times*.

Dumoulin, C., Hay-Smith, J., & Mac Habbe-Seguin, G. (2014). *Pelvic floor muscle training versus no treatment, or interactive control treatments, for urinary incontinence in women. The Cochrane Library*. doi:10.1002/14651858.CD005654.pub3.

Dunn, N., & Ramos, R. (2017). Preventing venous thromboembolism: The role of nursing with intermittent pneumatic compression. *American Journal of Critical Care*, *26*(2), 164–167. https://doi.org/10.4037/ajcc2017504.

Dupuis, L. L., Sung, L., Molassiotis, A., Orsey, A. D., Tissing, W., & van de Wetering, M. (2017). 2016 updated MASCC/ESMO consensus recommendations: Prevention of acute chemotherapy-induced nausea and vomiting in children. *Supportive Care in Cancer*, *25*, 323–331.

Eckel, R. H., Jakicic, J. M., Ard, J. D., et al. (2013). 2013 AHA/ACC guideline on lifestyle management to reduce cardiovascular risk: A report of the American College of Cardiology/American Heart Association Task Force on Practice Guidelines. *Circulation*, *129*(Suppl. 2), S76–S99.

Eilers, J., Harris, D., Henry, K., et al. (2014). Evidence-based interventions for cancer treatment-related mucositis: Putting evidence into practice. *Clinical Journal of Oncology Nursing*, *18*(6), 80–96.

Eisenstadt, E. S. (2010). Dysphagia and aspiration pneumonia in older adults. *Journal of American Academy Nursing Practitioners*, *22*(1), 17–22.

Eksterowicz, N., & Dimaggio, T. J. (2018). Acute pain management. In M. L. Czarnecki & H. N. Turner (Eds.), *Core curriculum*. St. Louis, MO: Mosby Elsevier.

Ellison, J., Drummond, M., Dickinson, J., McGaugh, J., Paddon-Jones, D., & Volpi, E. (2016). Short-term intensive rehabilitation induces recovery of physical function after 7 days of bed rest in older adults. *Journal of Acute Care Physical Therapy*, 7(4), 156–163.

Eman, S. M., & Lohrmann, C. (2015). Prevalence of fecal and double fecal and urinary incontinence in hospitalized patients. *Journal of Wound, Ostomy & Continence Nursing*, *42*(1), 89–93. doi:10.1097/WON.0000000000000082.

Emerson, J. A., Hurley, K. M., Caulfield, L. E., & Black, M. M. (2017). Maternal mental health symptoms are positively related to emotional and restrained eating attitudes in a statewide sample of mothers participating in a supplemental nutrition program for women, infants and young children. *Maternal & Child Nutrition*, *13*(1), doi:10.1111/mcn.12247.

Emsfors, A., Christensson, L., & Elgand, C. (2017). Nursing actions that create a sense of good nursing care in patients with wet age-related macular degeneration. *Journal of Clinical Nursing*, *26*, 2680–2688.

Environmental Protection Agency (EPA). (2017). *Protect your family from lead in your home*. Retrieved from http://www.epa.gov/lead/protect-your-family-lead-your-home.

Ersan, T., & Schwer, W. A. (2015). *Perioperative Management of the Geriatric Patient*. https://emedicine.medscape.com/article/285433-overview#a2. Accessed February 17, 2018.

Fabrellas, N. (2017). Research about nursing care for persons with liver disease: A step in the right direction. *Nursing Research*, *66*(6), 419–420.

Faigenbaum, A. D., et al. (2018). Pediatric inactivity triad: A risky PIT. *Current Sports Medicine Reports*, *17*(2), 45–47. doi:10.1249/JSR.0000000000000450.

Fielding, F., & Long, C. O. (2014). The death rattle dilemma. *Journal of Hospice & Palliative Nursing*, *16*(8). Retrieved http://www.medscape.com/viewarticle/834898. February 22, 2018.

Flaherman, V. J., Gay, B., Scott, C., et al. (2012). Randomised trial comparing hand expression with breast pumping for mothers of term newborns feeding poorly. *Archives of Disease in Childhood. Fetal and Neonatal Edition*, *97*(1), F18–F23.

Fowler, J. (1981). *Stages of faith: The psychology of human development and quest for meaning*. San Francisco: Harper & Row.

Fowler, J. (1987). *Faith development and pastoral care*. Philadelphia: Fortress Press.

Fox, J., Gutierrez, D., Haas, J., & Durnford, S. (2016). Centering prayer's effects on psycho-spiritual outcomes: A pilot outcome study. *Mental Health, Religion & Culture*, *19*(4), 379–392. doi:10.1080/13674676.2016.1203299.

Frost, S. A., Azeem, A., Alexandrou, E., et al. (2013). Subglottic secretion drainage for preventing ventilator associated pneumonia: A meta-analysis. *Australian Critical Care : Official Journal of the Confederation of Australian Critical Care Nurses*, *26*(4), 180–188.

Fulkerson, J. A., et al. (2018). Family home food environment and nutrition-related parent and child personal and behavioral outcomes of the healthy home offerings via the mealtime environment (HOME) plus program: A randomized controlled trial. *Journal of the Academy of Nutrition and Dietetics*, *118*(2), 240–251. doi-org.proxy.lib.umich.edu/10.1016/j.jand.2017.04.006.

Gallagher, J. (2017). Invasive mechanical ventilation (through an artificial airway): Volume and pressure modes. In D. L. Wiegand (Ed.), *AACN procedure manual for high acuity, progressive, and critical care* (7th ed.). Philadelphia: Saunders Elsevier.

Gaudio, F. G., & Grissom, C. K. (2016). Cooling methods in heat stroke. *The Journal of Emergency Medicine*, *50*, 607–616. doi:10.1016/j.jemermed.2015.09.014.

Gillibrand, W. (2012). Faecal incontinence in the elderly: Issues and interventions in the home. *British Journal of Community Nursing*, *17*(8), 364–368.

Gleason, L. J., Benton, E. A., Alvarez-Nebreda, M. L., Weaver, M. J., Harris, M. B., & Javedan, H. (2017). FRAIL questionnaire screening tool and short-term outcomes in geriatric fracture patients. *Journal of the American Medical Directors Association*, doi:10.1016/j.jamda.2017.07.005. [Epub ahead of print]; Aug 30. pii: S1525-8610(17)30403-6.

GOLD Global strategy for the diagnosis, management, and prevention of COPD (revised 2017), Global Initiative for Chronic Obstructive Lung Disease. Retrieved February 10, 2018. http://goldcopd.org/wp-content/uploads/2016/12/wms-GOLD-2017-Pocket-Guide.pdf.

Gold, K. (2013). But does it do any good? Measuring the impact of music therapy on people with advanced dementia. *Dementia (Basel, Switzerland)*, *13*(2), 258–264. doi:10.1177/1471301213494512.

GOLD. *Global strategy for the diagnosis, management, and prevention of COPD (revised 2017),* Global Initiative for Chronic Obstructive Lung Disease. http://www.goldcopd.org. Accessed February 20, 2018.

Goldberg, J. L. (2017). Guideline Implementation; hand hygiene. *AORN Journal*, *105*(2), *203–212*.

Goodrich, C. (2017b). Endotracheal intubation (perform). In D. L. Wiegand (Ed.), *AACN procedure manual for high acuity, progressive, and critical care* (7th ed.). Philadelphia: Saunders Elsevier.

Gosselink, R., Bott, J., Johnson, M., et al. (2008). Physiotherapy for adult patients with critical illness: Recommendations of the European Respiratory Society and European Society of Critical Care Medicine Task Force on Physiotherapy for Critically Ill Patients. *Intensive Care Medicine*, *34*(7), 1188–1199.

Grabiner, M. D. (2013). Exercise-based fall prevention programmes decrease fall-related injuries. *Evidence-Based Nursing*, *17*(4), 125.

Grap, M. (2009). Not-so-trivial pursuit: Mechanical ventilation risk reduction. *American Journal of Critical Care*, *18*(4), 299–309.

Graves, N. S. (2013). Acute gastroenteritis. *Primary Care*, *40*(3), 727–741.

Gray-Miceli, D. (2016). Preventing falls in acute care. In M. Boltz, E. Capezuti, T. Fulmer, & D. Zwicker (Eds.), *Evidence-based geriatric nursing protocols for best practice* (5th ed.). New York: Springer Publishing Company.

Greenberg, S. A. (2011). Try this:® *Best practices in nursing care to older adults. Fall risk assessment for older adults: Falls Efficacy Scale-International (FES-I)*. New York: Hartford Institute for Geriatric Nursing. https://consultgeri.org/try-this/general-assessment/issue-29. (Accessed 29 October 2017).

Greenberg, S. A. (2012). Analysis of measurement tools of fear of falling among high-risk, community-dwelling older adults. *Clinical Nursing Research*, *21*(1), 113–130. doi:10.1177/1054773811433824.

Greenberg, S. A. (2016). Try this:® *Issue 16: The 2015 American geriatrics society updated beers criteria for potentially inappropriate medication use in older adults.*

New York: Hartford Institute for Geriatric Nursing and The American Geriatrics Society. https://consultgeri.org/try-this/general-assessment/16beers2016-r2.pdf. (Accessed 29 October 2017).

Grossman, E., & Messerli, F. H. (2012). Drug-induced hypertension: An unappreciated cause of secondary hypertension. *The American Journal of Medicine*, *125*, 14–22.

Guandalini, S., Frye, R. E., Tamer, M. A., et al. (2017). *Diarrhea. Medscape Reference*. https://emedicine.medscape.com/article/928598-overview. Retrieved December 6, 2017.

Guenter, P. (2010). Safe practices for enteral nutrition in critically ill patients. *Critical Care Nurse Clinics of North America*, *22*(2), 197–208.

Gupta, K., & Trautner, B. (2011). Urinary tract infections, pyelonephritis and prostatitis. In D. L. Longo, et al. (Eds.), *Harrison's principles of internal medicine* (18th ed.). New York: McGraw-Hill.

Gupta, R. (2016). Diarrhea. In R. Wyllie, J. S. Hyams, & M. Kay (Eds.), *Pediatric gastrointestinal and liver disease* (5th ed., pp. 104–114). Philadelphia: Elsevier.

Haas, C. F., Eakin, R. M., Konkle, M. A., et al. (2014). Endotracheal tubes: Old and new. *Respiratory Care*, *59*(6), 933–955.

Haas, C. F., & Loik, P. S. (2012). Ventilator discontinuation protocols. *Respiratory Care*, *57*(10), 1649–1662.

Hamilton, L. A., Collins-Yoder, A., & Collins, R. E. (2016). Drug-induced liver injury. *AACN Critical Care*, *27*(4), 430–440.

Hansson, L., & Bjorkman, T. (2005). Empowerment in people with a mental illness: Reliability and validity of the Swedish version of an empowerment scale. *Scandinavian Journal of Caring Sciences*, *19*, 32.

Headley, J., & Giuliano, K. (2011). Continuous venous oxygen saturation monitoring. In D. J. Lynn-McHale (Ed.), *AACN procedure manual for critical care* (6th ed.). Philadelphia: Saunders Elsevier.

Healthy People 2020. *Hearing and other sensory or communication disorders*. Retrieved September 12, 2014, from www.healthypeople.gov/2020/topicsobjectives2020/overviewaspx?topicid=20.

Heeringa, J., Deirdre, A. M., van der Kuip, A., et al. (2006). Prevalence, incidence and lifetime risk of atrial fibrillation: The Rotterdam study. *European Heart Journal*, *27*(8), 949–953. https://doi.org/10.1093/eurheartj/ehi825.

Helm, R. E., Klausner, J. D., Klemperer, J. D., et al. (2015). Accepted but unacceptable: Peripheral IV catheter failure. *Journal of Infusion Nursing*, *38*(3), 189–201.

Hendrich, A. (2016). Try this:® *Best practices in nursing care to older adults. Fall risk assessment for older adults: The hendrich II fall risk model™*. New York: Hartford Institute for Geriatric Nursing. https://consultgeri.org/try-this/general-assessment/issue-8.pdf. (Accessed 29 October 2017).

Heo, S., McSweeney, J., Ounpraseuth, S., Shaw-Devine, A., Fier, A., & Moser, D. K. (2017). Testing a holistic meditation intervention to address psychosocial distress in patients with heart failure: A pilot study. *Journal of Cardiovascular Nursing*, Jun 28, [Epub ahead of print]. doi:10.1097/JCN.0000000000000435.

Herr, K., Coyne, P. J., McCaffrey, M., Manworren, R., & Merkel, S. (2011). Pain assessment in the patient unable to self-report: Position statement with clinical practice recommendations. *Pain Management Nursing*, *12*(4), 230–250.

Hill, E., & Fauerbach, L. A. (2014). Falls and fall prevention in older adults. *Journal of Legal Nurse Consulting*, *25*(2), 24–29.

Ho, K. M., & Harahsheh, Y. (2016). Intermittent pneumatic compression is effective in reducing proximal DVT. *Evidence-Based Nursing*, *19*(2), 47.

Ho, S. S. M., Kwong, A. N. L., Wan, K. W. S., Ho, R. M. L., & Chow, K. M. (2017). Esperiences of aromatherapy massage among adult female cancer patients: A qualitative study. *Journal of Clinical Nursing*, *1-8*, doi:10.1111/jocn.13784.

Hoffman, A. J., Brintnall, R. A., Given, B. A., von Eye, A., Jones, L. W., & Brown, J. K. (2017). Using perceived self-efficacy to improve fatigue and fatigability in postsurgical lung cancer patients: A pilot randomized controlled trial. *Cancer Nursing*, *40*(1), 1–12.

Hogan, N. S., Worden, J. W., & Schmidt, L. A. (2004). An empirical study of the proposed complicated grief disorder criteria. *Omega*, *48*(3), 263–277.

Howatson-Jones, L., Standing, M., & Roberts, S. (Eds.). (2012). *Patient assessment and care planning in nursing*. London: Sage Publications.

Huffman, M. (2016). Advancing the practice of health coaching—differentiation from wellness coaching. *Workplace Health & Safety*, *64*(9), 400–403.

Husebo, B. S., Ballard, C., Fritze, F., Sandvik, K., & Aarsland, D. (2014). Efficacy of pain treatment on mood syndrome in patients with dementia: A randomized clinical trial. *Geriatric Psychiatry*, *29*, 828–836.

Hutzler, L., & Williams, J. (2017). Decreasing the incidence of surgical site infections following joint replacement surgery. *Bulletin of the Hospital for Joint Diseases*, *75*(4), 268–273.

Infusion Nurses Society (INS). (2013). *Recommendations for improving safety practices with short peripheral catheters*. Retrieved from http://www.ins1.org/i4a/pages/index.cfm?pageid=3412.

Infusion Nurses Society (INS). (2016). *Infusion therapy standards of practice*. Available at http://ins.tizrapublisher.com/hai13r/.

Institute for Healthcare Improvement. (2012a). *How-to-Guide: Prevent Surgical Site Infections*. Cambridge, MA: Institute for Healthcare Improvement. Available at www.ihi.org. Retrieved January 9, 2018.

International Foundation for Functional Gastrointestinal Disorders. (2017). *Nutritional strategies for managing diarrhea*. https://www.iffgd.org/gi-disorders/motility-disorders.html#incontinence.

Irwin, M., & Johnson, L. A. (2014). *Putting evidence into practice: A pocket guide to cancer symptom management*. Pittsburgh, PA: Oncology Nursing Society.

Islam, S. (2015). Gastroparesis in children. *Current Opinion in Pediatrics*, *27*(3), 377–382.

Jackson, R. (2017). ADA case review. *Journal of Legal Nurse Consulting*, *28*(4), 22–25.

Jacobs, D. S. (2017). *Corneal Abrasions and Injury*. http://www.uptodate.com/contents/corneal-abrasions-and-corneal-foreign-bodies-management?source=see_link. Retrieved October 31, 2017.

Jauch, E. C., Saver, J. L., Adams, H. P., et al. (2013). Guidelines for the early management of patients with acute ischemic stroke: A guideline for healthcare professionals from the AHA/ASA. *Stroke; a Journal of Cerebral Circulation*, *44*, 870–947.

Jelovsek, J. E., Chen, Z., Markland, A. D., Brubaker, L., Keisha, Y., Meikle, S., et al. (2014). Minimum important differences for scales assessing symptom severity and quality of life in patients with fecal incontinence. *Female Pelvic Medical Reconstructive Surgery*, *20*(6), 342–348. doi:10.1097/SPV.0000000000000078.

Jensen, L., & Padilla, R. (2017). Effectiveness of environment-based interventions that address behavior, perception, and falls in people with Alzheimer's disease and related major neurocognitive disorders: A systematic review. *The American Journal of Occupational Therapy*, *71*(5), 7105180030p7105180031-7105180030p7105180010. doi:10.5014/ajot.2017.027409.

Joanna Briggs Institute. (2014). *Ventilator-associated pneumonia prevention*.

Johnson, R. (2017). Tracheostomy cuff and tube care. In D. L. Wiegand (Ed.), *AACN procedure manual for high acuity, progressive, and critical care* (7th ed.). Philadelphia: Saunders Elsevier.

Johnson, D. M., Worell, J., & Chandler, R. K. (2005). Assessing psychological health and empowerment in women: The personal progress scale revised. *Women and Health*, *41*(1), 109.

Joling, K. J., Windle, G., Dröes, R. M., Huisman, M., Hertogh, C. M. P. M., & Woods, R. T. (2017). What are the essential features of resilience for informal caregivers of people living with dementia? A Delphi consensus examination. *Aging & Mental Health*, *21*(5), 509–517. doi:10.1080/13607863.2015.1124836.

Jones, K., Newhouse, R., Johnson, K., et al. (2014). Achieving quality health outcomes through the implementation of a spontaneous awakening and spontaneous breathing trial protocol. *AACN Advanced Critical Care*, *25*(1), 33–42.

Jordan, A. H., & Litz, B. T. (2014). Prolonged grief disorder: Diagnostic, assessment, and treatment considerations. *Professional Psychology, Research and Practice*, *45*(3), 180–187.

Jorgensen, A. L. (2013). Contrast-induced nephropathy: Pathophysiology and preventive strategies. *Critical Care Nurse*, *33*(1), 37–47. doi http://dx.doi.org/10.4037/ccn2013680.

Judd, S. R. (2017). Uncovering common sleep disorders and their impacts on occupational performance. *Workplace Health and Safety*, *65*(5), 232.

Kahn, S., et al. (2012). *Antithrombotic therapy and prevention of thrombosis*, ed 9, American College of Chest Physician Evidence-Based clinical practice guidelines online only articles. *Chest*, *141*(Suppl. 2), e195S–e226S.

Kaiser, A. M., Orangio, G. R., Zutshi, M., et al. (2014). Current status: New technologies for the treatment of patients with fecal incontinence. *Surgical Endoscopy*, *28*, 2277–2301.

Kalisch, B. J., Dabney, B. W., & Lee, S. (2013). Safety of mobilizing hospitalized adults: Review of the literature. *Journal of Nursing Care Quality*, *28*(2), 162–168.

Karthika, M., Al Enezi, F. A., Pillai, L. V., & Arabi, Y. M. (2016). Rapid shallow breathing index. *Annals of Thoracic Medicine*, *11*(3), 167–176. http://doi.org/10.4103/1817-1737.176876.

Kaya, S., Turkan, A., Ceren, G., et al. (2015). Short-term effect of adding pelvic floor muscle training to bladder training for female urinary incontinence: A randomized controlled trial. *The International Urogynacological Journal*, *26*(2), 285–293.

Keles, E., Bayraktar, D., Alpaydin, A. O., & Ozalevli, S. (2016). Comparison of physical activity levels and fatigue severity in young and elderly males with COPD. *European Respiratory Journal, 48*, PA1898.

Kentson, M., Tödt, K., Skargren, E., Jakobsson, P., Ernerudh, J., Unosson, M., et al. (2016). Factors associated with experience of fatigue, and functional limitations due to fatigue in patients with stable COPD. *Therapeutic Advances in Respiratory Disease, 10*(5), 410–424. doi:10.1177/1753465816661930.

Khan, M. H., Kunselman, A. R., et al. (2002). Attenuated sympathetic nerve responses after 24 hours of bed rest. *American Journal of Physiology, Heart and Circulatory Physiology, 282*(6), H2210–H2215.

Kim, J., et al. (2017). Overweight or obesity in children aged 0 to 6 and the risk of adult metabolic syndrome: A systematic review and meta-analysis. *Journal of Clinical Nursing, 26*(23–24), 3869–3880. doi-org.proxy.lib.umich.edu/10.1111/jocn.13802.

Kim, Y. H., Choi, K. S., Han, K., & Kim, H. W. (2017). A psychological intervention programme for patients with breast cancer under chemotherapy and at a high risk of depression: A randomised clinical trial. *Journal of Clinical Nursing*, 1–10, doi:10.1111/jocn.13910.

Kjellstrom, B., & van der Wal, M. H. L. (2013). Old and new tools to assess dyspnea in the hospitalized patient. *Current Heart Failure Reports, 10*, 204–211.

Klompas, M., Anderson, D., & Trick, W. (2015). The preventability of ventilator-associated events. The CDC Prevention Epicenters Wake Up and Breathe Collaborative. *American Journal of Respiratory and Critical Care Medicine, 191*, 292–301.

Kolanowski, A., Boltz, M., Galik, E., Gitlin, L. N., Kales, H. C., Resnick, B., et al. (2017). Determinants of behavioral and psychological symptoms of dementia: A scoping review of the evidence. *Nursing Outlook, 65*(5), 515–529. doi:10.1016/j.outlook.2017.06.006.

Kolcaba, K. (2003). *Comfort theory and practice*. New York: Springer.

Koren, P. E., DeChillo, N., & Friesen, B. J. (1992). Measuring empowerment in families whose children have emotional disabilities: A brief questionnaire. *Rehabilitation Psychology, 37*, 305–321. doi:10.1037/h0079106.

Kuo, Y. W., Yen, M., Fetzer, S., & Lee, J. D. (2013). Toothbrushing versus toothbrushing plus tongue cleaning in reducing halitosis and tongue coating: A systematic review and meta-analysis. *Nursing Research, 62*(6), 422–429.

Kwekkeboom, K. L., & Bratzke, L. C. (2016). A systematic review of relaxation, meditation, and guided imagery strategies for symptom management in heart failure. *Journal of Cardiovascular Nursing, 31*(5), 457–468. doi:10.1097/JCN.0000000000000274.

Laliberte Rudman, D., Egan, M., McGrath, E., Kessler, D., Gardner, P., King, J., et al. (2016). Low vision rehabilitation, age-related vision loss and risk: A critical interpretive synthesis. *The Gerontologist, 58*(3), e32–e45.

Lareau, S., Meek, P., & ZuWallack, R. (2014). Effect of pulmonary rehabilitation on dyspnea. In D. A. Mahler & D. E. O'Donnell (Eds.), *Dyspnea mechanisms, measurement and management*. Boca Raton, FL: CRC Press Taylor & Francis Group.

Larson, J., et al. (2005). Spouse's life situation after partner's stroke: Psychometric testing of a questionnaire. *Journal of Advanced Nursing, 52*, 300.

Lawrence, V. (2011). Caring for older people with dementia and sight loss. *Nursing and Residential Care, 13*(4), 186–188.

Leaver, R. (2017). Assessing patients with urinary incontinence: The basics. *Journal of Community Nursing, 31*(1), 40–46.

Lee, D. (2017). Oxygen saturation monitoring with pulse oximetry. In D. Wiegand (Ed.), *AACN procedure manual for critical care* (7th ed.). Phildelphia: Saunders Elsevier.

Lee, D. (2017). Oxygen saturation monitoring with pulse oximetry. In D. L. Wiegand (Ed.), *AACN procedure manual for high acuity, progressive, and critical care* (7th ed.). Philadelphia: Saunders Elsevier.

Leon, L. R., & Bouchama, A. (2015). Heat stroke. *Comprehensive Physiology, 5*, 611–647. doi:10.1002/cphy.c140017.

Lippoldt, J., Pernicka, E., & Staudinger, T. (2014). Interface pressure at different degrees of backrest elevation with various types of pressure redistribution surfaces. *American Journal of Critical Care, 23*(2), 119–126.

Lippoldt, J., & Staudinger, T. (2014). Interface pressure at different degrees of backrest elevation with various types of pressure redistribution surfaces. *American Journal of Critical Care, 23*(2), 119–126.

Lin, Y. B., & Gardiner, M. F. (2014). Fingernail-induced corneal abrasions: Case series from an ophthalmology emergency department. *Cornea, 33*(7), 691–695.

Lipman, G. S., Eifling, K. P., Ellis, M. A., Gaudio, F. G., Otten, E. M., & Grissom, C. K. (2013). Wilderness Medical Society Practice Guidelines for the prevention and treatment of heat-related illness. *Wilderness & Environmental Medicine, 24*, 351–361. doi:10.1016/j.wem.2014.07.017.

Lo, E., Nicolle, L. E., Coffin, S. E., Gould, C., Maragakis, L. L., Meddings, J., et al. (2014). Strategies to prevent catheter-associated urinary tract infections in acute care hospitals: 2014 update. *Infection Control and Hospital Epidemiology, 35*(Suppl. 2), S32–S47. doi:10.1086/675718.

Loscalzo, J. (2016). Hypoxia and cyanosis. In J. Loscalzo (Ed.), *Harrison's pulmonary and critical care medicine* (3rd ed.). New York: McGraw Hill Education Medical.

Loubani, O. M., & Green, R. S. (2015). A systematic review of extravasation and local tissue injury from administration of vasopressors through peripheral intravenous catheters and central venous catheters. *Journal of Critical Care, 30*(3), 653–659.

Lough, M. (2018). Cardiovacular diagnostic procedures. In L. Urden, K. Stacy, & M. Lough (Eds.), *Critical care nursing diagnosis and management* (8th ed.). Maryland Heights, MO: Elsevier.

Luckowski, A., & Luckowski, M. (2015). Caring for a patient with vision loss. *Nursing, 2015*(11), 55–58.

Magidson, P. D., & Martinez, J. P. (2016). Abdominal pain in the geriatric patient. *Emergency Medical Clinics of North America, 34*, 559–574.

Mahler, D. (2014). Other treatments for dyspnea. In D. A. Mahler & D. E. O'Donnell (Eds.), *Dyspnea mechanisms, measurement and management*. Boca Raton, FL: CRC Press Taylor & Francis Group.

Makic, M. B. F., Martin, S. A., Burns, S., et al. (2013). Putting evidence into nursing practice: Four traditional practices not supported by the evidence. *Critical Care Nurse, 33*(2), 28–42.

Makic, M., Rauen, C., Jones, K., et al. (2015). Continuing to challenge practice to be evidence based. *Critical Care Nurse*, *35*(2), 39–50.

Makris, M., Van Veen, J. J., Tait, C. R., et al. (2013). Guideline on the management of bleeding in patients on antithrombotic agents. *British Journal of Haematology*, *160*, 35–46.

Malafa, M., Coleman, E., Bowman, R., & Rohrich, R. (2016). Perioperative corneal abrasion: Updated guidelines for prevention and management. *American Society of Plastic Surgeons*, *137*, 790e.

Maria, O. M., Eliopoulos, N., & Muanza, T. (2017). Radiation-induced oral mucositis. *Frontiers in Oncology*, *7*, 89. doi:10.3389/fonc.2017.00089.

Marsden, J. (2017). Preserving vision and promoting visual health in older people. *Nursing Older People*, *29*(6), 22–26.

Martin-Plank, L. (2014). *Chest Disorders*. In L. Kennedy-Malone, K. R. Fletcher, & L. Martin-Plank (Eds.).

Marzuillo, P., del Guidice, E. M., & Santoro, N. (2014). Pediatric fatty liver disease: Role of ethnicity and genetics. *World Journal of Gastroenterology*, *20*(23), 7347–7355.

Maturi, R. K. (2011). *Nonexudative ARMD. Medscape Review*. Retrieved October 31, 2017, from http://emedicine.medscape.com/article/1223154-overview.

Mas, A., & Masip, J. (2014). Noninvasive ventilation in acute respiratory failure. *International Journal of Chronic Obstructive Pulmonary Disease*, *9*, 837–852.

Mayeda-Letourneau, J. (2014). Safe patient handling and movement: A literature review. *Rehabilitation Nursing*, *39*, 123–129.

Mayo Clinic. (2017). *Prevention of urinary tract infections*. From http://www.mayoclinic.com/health/urinary-tract-infection/DS00286/DSECTION=prevention. Retrieved October 31, 2017.

McClurg, D., & Norton, C. (2016). What is the best way to manage neurogenic bowel dysfunction? *British Medical Journal*, *354*, i3931. doi:10.1136/bmj.i3931.

McFadden, B. (2013). Is there a safe coital position after a total hip arthroplasty? *Orthopaedic Nursing*, *32*(4), 223–226. doi:10.1097/NOR.0b013e31829b0349.

McGowan, D. (2014). Peripheral intravenous cannulation: What is considered best practice? *The British Journal of Nursing*, *23*(14), S26–S28.

McNeil, A. (2016). Using evidence to structure discharge planning. *Nursing Management*, *47*(5), 22–23.

Meddings, J., Rogers, M. A. M., Krein, S. L., Fakih, M. G., Olmsted, R. N., & Saint, S. (2014). Reducing unnecessary urinary catheter use and other strategies to prevent catheter-associated urinary tract infection: An integrative review. *BMJ Quality & Safety*, *23*(4), 277–289.

Medline Plus. (2017). *Indwelling catheter care*. Retrieved October 31, 2017, from https://medlineplus.gov/ency/patientinstructions/000140.htm.

Miller, J., Sabol, V., & Pastva, A. (2017). Promoting older adult physical activity throughout care transitions using and interprofessional approach. *The Journal for Nurse Practitioners*, *13*(1), 64–71.

Momani, T. G., & Berry, D. L. (2017). Integrative therapeutic approaches for the management and control of nausea in children undergoing cancer treatment: A systematic review. *Journal of Pediatric Oncology Nursing*, *34*(3), 173–184.

Morse, J. M., Tylko, S. J., & Dixon, H. A. (1987). Characteristics of the fall-prone patient. *The Gerontologist*, *27*(4), 516–522.

Munro, N. (2014). Fever in acute and critical care: A diagnostic approach. *AACN Advanced Critical Care*, *25*, 237–248. doi:10.1097/NCI.0000000000000041.

Muramatsu, N., Yin, L., Berbaum, M., et al. (2017). Promoting seniors' health with home care aides: A pilot. *The Gerontologist*, gnx101. https://doi.org/10.1093/geront/gnx101.

Murphree, R. W. (2017). Impairments in skin integrity. *Nursing Clinics of North America*, *52*(3), 405–417.

Nagarwala, J., Dev, S., & Markin, A. (2016). The vomiting patient: Small bowel obstruction, cyclic vomiting, and gastroparesis. *Emergency Medical Clinics of North America*, *34*, 271–291. http://dx.doi.org/10.1016/j.emc.2015.12.005.

Nasiri, M., Rahimian, B., Jahanshahi, M., Fotoukian, Z., & Chaboki, A. M. O. (2016). Study of fatigue and associated factors in patients with chronic heart failure. *Critical Care Nursing Journal*, *9*(3), e8124.

National Center for Public Policy Research. (2005). *Income of U.S. Workforce Projected to Decline if Education Doesn't Improve*. Retrieved April 12, 2018, from http://www.highereducation.org/reports/pa_decline/index.shtml.

National Consensus Project for Quality Palliative Care. (2013). *Clinical Practice Guidelines for Quality Palliative Care (3rd edition)*. Retrieved from https://www.nationalcoalitionhpc.org/ncp-guidelines-2013/.

National Council on Aging. (2015). *Falls Free®: 2015 National Falls Prevention Action Plan*. https://www.ncoa.org/resources/2015-falls-free-national-falls-prevention-action-plan/. Accessed October 29, 2017.

National Health Service (NHS) England. (2014). *Dry eye syndrome—self-help*. Retrieved from http://www.nhs.uk/Conditions/Dry-eye-syndrome/Pages/Prevention.aspx.

National Institute for Health and Care Excellence. (2015). *Constipation*. Clinical Knowledge summaries accessed at http://cks.nice.org.uk/constipation. Accessed October 18, 2017.

National Interagency Fire Center. (2014). *CISM Information Sheets*. From http://gacc.nifc.gov/wgbc/cism/effectsoftrauma.pdf. Retrieved October 23, 2014.

National Prescribing Service Limited (NPS). (2017). *Medicines that affect blood glucose levels*. Retrieved from https://www.nps.org.au/medical-info/consumer-info/medicines-and-type-2-diabetes.

National Pressure Ulcer Advisory Panel. (2013). *Best practices for prevention of medical device-related pressure ulcers in critical care*. Retrieved February 10, 2018, from http://www.npuap.org/wp-content/uploads/2013/04/BestPractices-CriticalCare1.pdf.

National Pressure Ulcer Advisory Panel (NPUAP). (2016). *Pressure Injury Stages*. http://www.npuap.org/resources/educational-and-clinical-resources/npuap-pressure-injury-stages/. Retrieved November 28, 2017.

National Pressure Ulcer Advisory Panel (NPUAP) and European Pressure Ulcer Advisory Panel (EPUAP). (2014). In E. Haesler (Ed.), *Prevention and treatment of pressure ulcers*. Perth, Australia: Cambridge Media.

National Pressure Ulcer Advisory Panel (NPUAP) and European Pressure Ulcer Advisory Panel (EPUAP). (2016). *Pressure Injury Stages*. http://www.npuap.

org/resources/educational-and-clinical-resources/npuap-pressure-injury-stages/. Retrieved December 5, 2017.

National Pressure Ulcer Advisory Panel, European Pressure Ulcer Advisory Panel and Pan Pacific Pressure Injury Alliance. (2014). *Prevention and Treatment of Pressure Ulcers: Clinical Practice Guideline*. Emily Haesler (Ed.). Cambridge Media: Osborne Park, Western Australia.

National Pressure Ulcer Advisory Panel, European Pressure Ulcer Advisory Panel and Pan Pacific Pressure Injury Alliance. (2014). *Prevention and Treatment of Pressure Ulcers: Quick Reference Guide*. Emily Haesler (Ed.). Cambridge Media: Osborne Park, Australia.

Neifert, M., & Bunik, M. (2013). Overcoming clinical barriers to exclusive breastfeeding. *Pediatric Clinics of North America*, *60*, 115–145.

Nicolle, L. E., & Norrby, S. R. (2016). Approach to the patient with urinary tract infection. In L. Goldman & A. Schafer (Eds.), *Goldman's Cecil medicine* (25th ed., pp. 1872–1876). St. Louis, MO: Saunders/Elsevier.

Nielsen, S., et al. (2011). Adequacy of milk intake during exclusive breastfeeding: A longitudinal study. *Pediatrics*, *128*(4), 907–914.

Niven, D. J., & Laupland, K. B. (2016). Pyrexia: Aetiology in the ICU. *Critical Care: The Official Journal of the Critical Care Forum*, *20*, 247. doi:10.1186/s13054-016-1406-2.

Oates, L. L., & Price, C. I. (2017). Clinical assessments and care interventions to promote oral hydration amongst older patients: A narrative systemic review. *BMC Nursing*, *16*, 4.

Odom-Forren, J., Hooper, V., Moser, D. K., et al. (2014). Postdischarge nausea and vomiting: Management strategies and outcomes over 7 days. *Journal of Perianesthesia Nursing*, *29*(4), 275–284.

Oerther, S. E. (2011). Plant poisonings: Common plants that contain cardiac glycosides. *Journal of Emergency Nursing*, *37*(1), 102–103.

Ortega, A., Sanchez-Manzanares, M., Gil, F., et al. (2013). Enhancing team learning in nursing teams through beliefs about interpersonal contexts. *The Journal of advanced Nursing*, *69*(1), 363–370.

Paal, P., Gordon, L., Strapazzon, G., Maeder, M. B., Putzer, G., Walpoth, B., et al. (2016). Accidental hypothermia—an update: The content of this review is endorsed by the International Commission for Mountain Emergency Medicine (ICAR MEDCOM). *Scandinavian Journal of Trauma, Resuscitation and Emergency Medicine*, *24*, 111. doi:10.1186/s13049-016-0303-7.

Paden, M. S., Franjic, L., & Halcomb, E. (2013). Hyperthermia caused by drug interactions and adverse reaction. *Emergency Medicine Clinics of North America*, *31*, 1035–1044. doi:10.1016/j.emc.2013.07.003.

Pan American Health Organization. (2012). *Mental health and psychosocial support in disaster situations in the Caribbean*. Washington, DC: PAHO.

Park, J., & Palmer, M. (2015). Factors associated with incomplete bladder emptying in older women with overactive bladder symptoms. *Journal of the American Geriatrics Society*, *63*, 1426–1431.

Parshall, M. B., Schwartzstein, R. M., Adams, L., et al. (2012). An official American Thoracic Society statement: Update on the mechanisms, assessment, and management of dyspnea. *American Journal of Respiratory and Critical Care Medicine*, *185*(4), 435–452.

Patel, P., Robinson, P. D., Thackray, J., Flank, J., Holdsworth, M. T., Gibson, P., et al. (2017). Guideline for the prevention of acute chemotherapy-induced nausea and vomiting in pediatric cancer patients: A focused update. *Pediatric Blood & Cancer*, *64*, e26542. https://doiorg/10.1002/pbc.26542.

Pelletier, A., Ledy, R., & Coffin, J. (2016). Vision loss in older adult. *American Family Physician*, *94*(3), 219–226.

Penuelas, O., Thille, A., & Esteban, A. (2015). Discontinuation of ventilatory support: New solutions to old dilemmas. *Current Opinion in Critical Care*, *21*(1), 74–81.

Perme, C., Nawa, R. K., Winkelman, C., & Masud, F. (2014). A tool to assess mobility status in critically ill patients: The perme intensive care unit mobility score. *Methodist DeBakey Cardiovascular Journal*, *10*(1), 41–49.

Peterson, M., Goodman, S., et al. (2016). Attitudes and plans for low-income elderly homeowners to age in place. *The American Journal of Occupational Therapy*, *70*, 7011500074p1. doi:10.5014/ajot.2016.70S1-PO7023.

Petrone, P. (2014). Management of accidental hypothermia and cold injury. *Current Problems in Surgery*, *51*(10), 417–431. doi:10.1067/j.cpsurg.2014.07.004.

Peyrani, P. (2014). Pneumonia. In *APIC test of infection control and epidemiology* (4th ed.). Washington, DC: Association for Professionals in Infection Control and Epidemiology. Last revised 6/6/14. (Accessed 14 September 2017).

Phillips, K. W., Rothbard, N. P., & Dumas, T. L. (2009). To disclose or not disclose: Status distance and self-disclosure in diverse environments. *Academy of Management Journal*, *2009*(34), 710–732.

Pietrucha-Dilanchian, P., & Hooton, T. M. (2016). Diagnosis, treatment and prevention of urinary track infection. *Microbiolspec*, *4*(6), doi:10.1128/microbiolspec.UTI-0021-2015.

Pileggi, D. J., & Cook, A. M. (2016). Neuroleptic malignant syndrome: Focus on treatment and rechallenge. *The Annals of Pharmacotherapy*, *50*, 973–981. doi:10.1177/1060028016657553.

Plemons, J. M., Al-Hashimi, I., & Marek, C. (2014). Managing xerostomia and salivary gland hypofunction. *The Journal of the American Dental Association*, *145*(8), 867–873. https://dx.doi.org/10.14219/jada.archive.2007.0358.

Podsiadlo, D., & Richardson, S. (1991). The timed "Up & Go": A test of basic functional mobility for frail elderly persons. *Journal of the American Geriatrics Society*, *39*(2), 142–148.

Porritt, K. (2015a). *Peripheral intravenous cannula: Insertion.* JoAnn Briggs Institute EBP Database. JBI14045.

Porritt, K. (2016). *Intravascular Therapy: Maintaining catheter lumen patency.* JoAnn Briggs Institute EBP Database. JBI14448.

Preas, M. A., O'Hara, L., & Thom, K. (2017). *2017 HICPAC-CDC Guideline for Prevention of Surgical Site Infection: What the infection preventionist needs to know. Fall 2017 APIC Prevention strategist.* https://apic.org/Resource_/TinyMceFileManager/Periodical_images/SSI_2017_Fall_PS.pdf. Retrieved January 23, 2018.

Prentiss, A. S. (2012). Early recognition of pediatric venous thromboembolism: A risk-assessment tool. *American Journal of Critical Care*, *21*(3), 178–183.

Puntillo, K. A., Max, A., Timsit, J.-F., et al. (2014). Determinants of procedural pain intensity in the intensive care unit. The European study. *American Journal of Respiratory and Critical Care Medicine*, *189*(1), 39–47.

Quinlan, N., Marcantonio, E. R., Inouye, S. K., et al. (2011). Vulnerability: The crossroads of frailty and delirium. *Journal of the American Geriatrics Society, 59*(Suppl. 2), S262–S268.

Radiology & Biomedical Imaging. (2017b). *Vascular access and use of central lines and ports in pediatrics. University of California San Francisco*. Retrieved from https://radiology.ucsf.edu/patient-care/patient-safety/contrast/iodinated/vascular-access-pediatrics.

Radiology and Biomedical Imaging. (2017a). *Vascular access and use of central lines and ports in adults. University of California San Francisco*. Retrieved from http://www.radiology.ucsf.edu/patient-care/patient-safety/contrast/iodinated/vascular-access-adults.

Radvansky, L. J., Pace, M. B., & Siddiqui, A. (2013). Prevention and management of radiation-induced dermatitis, mucositis, and xerostomia. *American Journal of Health-System Pharmacy, 70*, 1025–1032.

Ratliff, C. R., Droste, L. R., Bonham, P., Crestodina, L., Johnson, J. J., Kelechi, T., et al. (2017). WOCN 2016 guideline for prevention and management of pressure injuries (ulcers). An Executive Summary, Wound, Ostomy and Continence Nurses Society-Wound Guidelines Task Force. *Journal of Wound, Ostomy, and Continence Nursing, 44*(3), 241–246.

Ratwani, R. M., Trafton, J. G., & Myers, C. (2006). *Helpful or harmful? Examining the effects of interruptions on task performance.* Proceedings of the Human Factors and Ergonomics Society 50th Annual Meeting (pp. 372-375).

Raynor, H. A., & Champagne, C. M. (2016). Position of the academy of nutrition and dietetics: Interventions for the treatment of overweight and obesity in adults. *Journal of the Academy of Nutrition and Dietetics, 116*(1), 129–147.

Reade, M., & Finfer, S. (2014). Sedation and delirium in the intensive care unit. *The New England Journal of Medicine, 370*, 444–454.

Rees, H. C. (2013). Care of patients requiring oxygen therapy or tracheostomy. In D. Ignatavicius & M. L. Workman (Eds.), *Medical-surgical nursing: Patient-centered collaborative care* (7th ed., pp. 562–580). St. Louis, MO: W.B. Saunders Company.

Reid, J. (2014). Managing urinary incontinence: Guidelines for community nurses. *Journal of Christian Nursing, 28*(6), 20–26.

Requejo, P. S., Furumasu, J., & Mulroy, S. J. (2015). Evidence-based strategies for preserving mobility for elders and aging manual wheelchair users. *Topics in Geriatric Rehabilitation, 31*(1), 26–41.

Resnick, B., et al. (2011). Testing the effect of function-focused care in assisted living. *Journal of the American Geriatrics Society, 59*, 2233–2240.

Resnick, B., & D'Adamo, C. (2011). Factors associated with exercise among older adults in a continuing care retirement community. *Rehabilitation Nursing, 36*(2), 47–53, 82.

Resnick, B., & Jenkins, L. S. (2000). Testing the reliability and validity of the self-efficacy for exercise scale. *Nursing Research, 49*(3), 154–159.

Rhodes, A., Evans, L. E., Alhazzani, W., Levy, M. M., Antonelli, M., Ferrer, R., et al. (2017). Surviving sepsis campaign: International guidelines for management of sepsis and septic shock: 2016. *Critical Care Medicine, 45*(3), 486–552.

Rich, M. W., & Nienaber, W. J. (2014). Polypharmacy and adverse drug reactions in the aging population with heart failure. In B. I. Jugdutt (Ed.), *Aging and heart failure* (pp. 107–116). New York: Springer.

Riebe, D., Franklin, B., et al. (2015). Updating American College of Sports Medicine's recommendations for exercise preparticipation health screening. *Medicine & Science in Sports & Exercise*, *47*(11), 2473–2479. doi:10.1249/MSS.0000000000000664.

Rischall, M. L., & Rowland-Fisher, A. (2016). Evidence-based management of accidental hypothermia in the emergency department. *Emergency Medicine Practice*, *18*(1), 1–18.

Roberts, L., Gulliver, B., Fisher, J., & Cloyes, K. (2010). The coping with labor algorithm: An alternative pain assessment tool for the laboring woman. *Journal of Midwifery and Women's Health*, *55*(2), 107–116.

Rodgers, G. B., Franklin, R. L., & Midgett, J. D. (2012). Unintentional paediatric ingestion poisonings and the role of imitative behavior. *Injury Prevention*, *18*(2), 103–108.

Romo, L. K. (2018). An examination of how people who have lost weight communicatively negotiate interpersonal challenges to weight management, health communication. *Health Communication*, *33*(4), 469–477. doi:10.1080/10410236.2016.1278497.

Rosenberg, H., Pollock, N., Schiemann, A., Bulger, T., & Stowell, K. (2015). Orphanet. *Journal of Rare Diseases*, *10*, 93. doi:10.1186/s13023-015-0310-1.

Rubin, F. H., Neal, K., Fenlon, K., et al. (2011). Sustainability and scalability of the hospital elder life program at a community hospital. *Journal of the American Geriatrics Society*, *59*(2), 359–365.

Safekids.org. (2015). *Choking and Strangulation Prevention Tips*. Retrieved from https://www.safekids.org/safetytips/field_risks/choking_and_strangulation.

Sanders, M., et al. (2015). New formulation of sustained released naloxone can reverse opioid induced constipation without compromising the desired opioid effects. *Pain Medicine*, *16*, 1540–1550.

Schallom, M., Dykeman, B., Kirby, J., et al. (2015). Head-of-bed elevation and early outcomes of gastric reflux, aspiration, and pressure ulcers: A feasibility study. *American Journal of Critical Care*, *24*(1), 57–66.

Schattner, M. A., & Grossman, E. B. (2016). Nutritional management. In M. Feldman, L. Friedman, & L. J. Brandt (Eds.), *Sleisenger and Fordtran's gastrointestinal and liver disease* (10th ed., pp. 83–101). Philadelphia: Elsevier.

Schiller, L. R., & Sellin, J. H. (2016). Diarrhea. In M. Feldman, L. Friedman, & L. J. Brandt (Eds.), *Sleisenger and Fordtran's gastrointestinal and liver disease* (10th ed., pp. 221–241). Philadelphia: Elsevier.

Schmidt, C., Girard, T., Kress, J., et al. (2017). Official Exective Summary of an American Thoracic Society/American College of Chest Physicians Clinical Practice Guideline: Liberation from mechanical ventilation in critically ill adults. *American Journal of Respiratory and Critical Care Medicine*, *195*(1), 115–119.

Schnur, J., & John, R. M. (2014). Childhood lead poisoning and the new centers for disease control and prevention guidelines for lead exposure. *Journal of the American Association of Nurse Practitioners*, *26*, 238–247.

Scott, R. A., Oman, K. S., Makic, M. B. F., et al. (2014). Reducing indwelling urinary catheter use in the emergency department: A successful quality-improvement initiative. *Journal of Emergency Nursing*, *40*, 237–240.

Seckel, M. (2017). Suctioning: Endotracheal tube or tracheostomy tube. In D. Wiegland (Ed.), *AACN procedure manual for critical care* (7th ed.). Philadelphia: Saunders Elsevier.

Segal, K. L., Fleischut, P. M., Kim, C., et al. (2014). Evaluation and treatment of perioperative corneal abrasions. *Journal of Ophthalmology*, 320–326. http://dx.doi.org/10.1155/2014/901901. (Retrieved 31 October 2017).

Shah, R., & Lotke, M. (2017). Hearing impairment. *Medscape*. Retrieved February 10, 2018, from http://emedicine.medscape.com/article/994159-overview#a0199.

Shahoei, R., Shahghebi, S., Rezaei, M., & Naqshband, S. (2017). The effect of transcutaneous electrical nerve stimulation on the severity of labor pain among nulliparous women: A clinical trial. *Complementary Therapies in Clinical Practice*, *28*, 176–180.

Siela, D. (2010). Evaluation standards for management of artificial airways. *Critical Care Nurse*, *30*(4), 76–78.

Siela, D., & Kidd, M. (2017). Oxygen requirements for acutely and critically ill patients. *Critical Care Nurse*, *37*(4), 58–70.

Simkin, P., & Bolding, A. (2004). Update on nonpharmacologic approaches to relieve labor pain and prevent suffering. *Journal of Midwifery and Women's Health*, *49*(6), 489–504.

Simkin, P., & Klein, M. (2017) Nonpharmacological approaches to management of labor pain. *UpToDate*. Retrieved January 1, 2018, from https://www.uptodate.com/contents/nonpharmacologic-approaches-to-management-of-labor-pain?source=search_result&search=pharmacological%20managemet%20of%20pain%20during%20labor&selectedTitle=2~150.

Simons, S. R., & Abdallah, L. M. (2012). Bedside assessment of enteral tube placement aligning practice with evidence. *American Journal of Nursing*, *112*(2), 40–48.

Singer, M. (2016). The new sepsis consensus definitions (Sepsis-3): The good, the not-so-bad, and the actually-quite-pretty. *Intensive Care Medicine*, *42*(12), 2027–2029.

Singh, R., Singla, P., & Chaudhary, U. (2014). Surgical site infections: Classification, risk factors, pathogenesis and preventive management. *International Journal of Pharma Research and Health Sciences*, *2*(3), 203–214.

Skelton, D. A., et al. (2013). Environmental and behavioural interventions for reducing physical activity limitation in community-dwelling visually impaired older people. *The Cochrane Database of Systematic Reviews*, accessed online November 2017, doi:10.1002/14651858.CD009233.pub2.

Smith, M. A., & Dahlen, N. R. (2013). Clinical practice guideline surgical site infection prevention. *Journal of Orthopaedic Nursing*, *32*(5), 242–248.

Sofka, K. (2011). *Technology Corner: It's All Downhill-Ramps, Part 1, JNLCP XI.3:438 ff and Part 2, JNLCP XI.4: 476 ff.*

Soreide, K. (2014). Clinical and translational aspects of hypothermia in major trauma patients: From pathophysiology to prevention, prognosis and potential preservation. *Injury*, *45*, 647–654.

Sorrell, J. (2010). Use of feeding tubes in patients with advanced dementia. *Journal of Psychosocial Nursing and Mental Health Services*, *48*(5), 15–18.

Spiller, H. A., Beuhler, M. C., Ryan, M. L., et al. (2013). Evaluation of changes in poisoning in young children 2000-2010. *Pediatric Emergency Care*, *29*(5), 635–640.

Sprigle, S., & Sonenblum, S. (2011). Assessing evidence supporting redistribution of pressure for pressure ulcer prevention: A review. *Journal of Rehabilitation Research and Development*, *48*(3), 203–214.

Spruce, L., & Van Wicklin, S. A. (2014). Back to basics: Positioning the patient. *AORN Journal*, *100*(3), 299–302.

St Aubyn, B., & Andrews, A. (2015). If it's not written down; it didn't happen. *Journal of Community Nursing*, *29*(5), 20–22.

St. Clair, MacDermott, J. (2017). Continuous lateral rotation therapy. In D. L. Wiegand (Ed.), *AACN procedure manual for critical care* (7th ed.). Philadelphia: Saunders Elsevier.

Stacy, K. M. (2018). Pulmonary therapeutic management. In L. D. Urden, K. M. Stacy, & M. E. Lough (Eds.), *Critical care nursing: Diagnosis and management* (8th ed.). Maryland Heights, MO: Elsevier.

Steinke, E. E. (2013a). How can heart failure patients and their partners be counseled on sexual activity? *Current Heart Failure Reports*, *10*(3), 262–269. doi:10.1007/s11897-013-0138-8.

Steinke, E. E. (2013b). Sexuality and chronic illness. *Journal of Gerontological Nursing*, *39*(11), 18–27. doi:10.3928/00989134-20130916-01.

Steinke, E. E., Jaarsma, T., Barnason, S. A., Byrne, M., Doherty, S., Dougherty, C. M., et al. (2013). Sexual counseling for individuals with cardiovascular disease and their partners: A consensus document from the American Heart Association and the ESC Council on Cardiovascular Nursing and Allied Health Professionals (CCNAP). *Circulation*, *128*(18), 2075–2096. doi:10.1161/CIR.0b013e31829c2e53.

Strathearn, L., & Kim, S. (2013). Mothers' amygdala response to positive or negative infant affect is modulated by personal relevance. *Frontiers in Neuroscience*, *7*, 176.

Strothers, L., & Friedman, B. (2011). Risk factors for the development of stress urinary incontinence in women. *Current Urology Reports*, *12*, 363–369.

Suzumura, E. A., Figueiro, M., Normilio-Silva, K., et al. (2014). Effects of alveolar recruitment maneuvers on clinical outcomes in aptients with acute respiratory distress syndrome: A systematic review and meta-analysis. *Intensive Care Medicine*, *40*, 1227–1240.

Tadros, A., et al. (2016). Emergency department visits by pediatric patients for poisoning by prescription opioids. *The American Journal of Drug and Alcohol Abuse*, *42*(5), 550–555. doi-org.proxy.lib.umich.edu/10.1080/00952990.2016.1194851.

Tanasiewicz, M., & Hildebrandt, T. (2016). Xerostomia of various etiologies: A review of the literature. *Advances in Clinical and Experimental Medicine*, *25*(1), 199–206. doi:10.17219/acem/29375.

Tanner, D. (2013). CNA observations could save a resident: An interview. *Nursing Assistant. Cengage Learning*, *18*(8).

Taylor, B. E., McClave, S. A., Martindale, R. G., et al. (2016). Guidelines for the provision and assessment of nutrition support therapy in the adult critically ill patient: Society of Critical Care Medicine (SCCM) and American Society for Parenteral and Enteral Nutrition (A.S.P.E.N.). *Critical Care Medicine*, *44*(2), 390–438. doi:10.1097/CCM.0000000000001525.

Taylor, C. R., et al. (2011). Safety, security and emergency preparedness. In C. R. Taylor, et al. (Eds.), *Fundamentals of nursing, the art and science of nursing care* (7th ed.). Philadelphia: Lippincott Williams & Wilkins.

ten Hoorn, S., Elbers, P. W., Girbes, A. R., et al. (2016). Communicating with conscious and mechanically ventilated critically ill patients: A systematic review. *Critical Care: The Official Journal of the Critical Care Forum*, *20*, 333. doi:10.1186/s13054-016-1483-2. https://www.ncbi.nlm.nih.gov/pmc/articles/PMC5070186/pdf/13054_2016_Article_1483.pdf. Retrieved February 10, 2018.

The American Geriatrics Society (AGS). (2010). *AGS/BGS Clinical Practice Guideline (2011). Prevention of falls in older persons. Summary of recommendations.* https://hsctc.org/wp-content/uploads/2017/07/2010-American-Geriatrics-Society-Guideline_-Prevention-of-Falls-in-Older-Persons.pdf.

The Joint Commission. (2017). *Accreditation program: home care. 2017 national patient safety goals. Goal 9. Reduce the risk of falls.* https://www.jointcommission.org/assets/1/6/NPSG_Chapter_OME_Jan2017.pdf. Accessed October 8, 2009.

The Joint Commission. (2014). *National patient safety goals effective January 1, 2014.* Hospital accreditation program. Retrieved from http://www.jointcommission.org/assets/1/6HAP_NPSG_Chapter_2014.pdf.

Thompson, M. C., & Wachs, J. E. (2012). Occupational health nursing in the united states. *Workplace Health and Safety*, *60*(3), 127–133.

Tinetti, M. E. (2003). Preventing falls in elderly persons. *The New England Journal of Medicine*, *348*(1), 42–49.

Torossian, A., Bräuer, A., Höcker, J., Bein, B., Wulf, H., & Horn, E. P. (2015). Preventing inadvertent perioperative hypothermia. *Deutsches Ärzteblatt International*, *112*(10), 166–172.

Torossian, A., Van Gerven, E., Geertsen, K., Horn, B., Van de Velde, M., & Raeder, J. (2016). Active perioperative patient warming using a self-warming blanket (BARRIER EasyWarm) is superior to passive thermal insulation: A multinational, multicenter, randomized trial. *Journal of Clinical Anesthesia*, *34*, 547–554. doi:10.1016/j.jclinane.2016.06.030.

Tracy, M. F., & Chlan, L. (2011). Nonpharmacological interventions to manage common symptoms in patients receiving mechanical ventilation. *Critical Care Nurse*, *31*(3), 19–29.

Tutor, J. D., & Gosa, M. M. (2012). Dysphagia and aspiration in children. *Pediatric Pulmonology*, *47*(4), 321–337.

Twomey, S., & Dowling, M. (2013). Management of death rattle at end of life. *British Journal of Nursing (Mark Allen Publishing)*, *22*(2), 81–85.

U.S. Army Medical Research Institute of Infectious Diseases (2014). *USAMRIID's medical management of biological casualties handbook* (8th ed.). Fort Detrick, MD: Author.

Udoh, I. (2016). Understanding venous thromboembolism in patients with cancer. *The Journal for Nurse Practitioners*, *12*(1), 53–59.

United States Department of Labor. Occupational Safety and Health Administration (OSHA). (2011). *Access to Medical and Exposure Records.* September

2013. Retrieved December 10, 2017, from https://www.osha.gov/Publications/osha3110.pdf.

United States Department of Labor. Occupational Safety and Health Administration (OSHA). (2016). *Recommended Practices for Safety and Health Programs.* Retrieved January 4, 2018, from https://www.osha.gov/shpguidelines/docs/OSHA_SHP_Recommended_Practices.pdf.

US Department of Health and Human Services. (2008). *2008 Physical Activity.* Guidelines for Americans. https://health.gov/paguidelines/2008/pdf/paguide.pdf.

US Department of Health and Human Services. (2018). *Physical activity guidelines for Americans: Youth physical activity recommendations.* Washington, DC: U.S. Department of Health and Human Services.

US Food and Drug Administration. (2014). *Consumer updates > Have a baby or young child with a cold? Most don't need medicines.* Retrieved from http://www.fda.gov/ForConsumers/ConsumerUpdates/ucm422465.htm.

Van Bree, S. H. J., Bemelman, W. A., Hollman, M. W., et al. (2014). Identification of clinical outcome measures for recovery of gastrointestinal motility in postoperative ileus. *Annals of Surgery, 259*(4), 708–714.

Van der Gucht, N., & Lewis, K. (2015). Women's experience of coping with pain during childbirth: A critical review of qualitative research. *Midwifery, 31*, 349–358.

van der Lee, J., Bakker, T. J., Duivenvoorden, H. J., & Dröes, R. M. (2014). Multivariate models of subjective caregiver burden in dementia: A systematic review. *Ageing Research Reviews, 15*, 76–93. doi:10.1016/j.arr.2014.03.003.

Van Horn, L., Carson, J. S., Appel, L. J., et al. (2016). Recommended dietary pattern to achieve adherence to the American Heart Association/American College of Cardiology (AHA/ACC) guidelines: A scientific statement from the American Heart Association. *Circulation, 134*, e505–e529

Van Wicklin, S. A. (2017). Guideline for positioning the patient. In R. Conner (Ed.), *Guidelines for perioperative practice* (Vol. 1). Denver, CO. AORN.

Vardakas, K. Z., Trigkidis, K. K., & Boukouvala, E. (2016). Clostridium difficile infection following systemic antibiotic administration is randomized controlled trials: A systematic review and meta-analysis. *International Journal of Antimicrobial Agents, 48*, 1–10. http://www.ijaaonline.com/article/S0924-8579.(16)30055-3/fulltext.

Veenema, T. G. (2013). *Disaster nursing and emergency preparedness for chemical, biological and radiological terrorism and other hazards* (3rd ed.). New York: Springer.

Ventocilla, M. (2013). Low vision therapy. *Medscape*. Retrieved October 31, 2017, from http://emedicine.medscape.com/article/1832033-overview.

Verma, A., & Khan, H. R. (2014). *Corneal Abrasion*. Retrieved October 31, 2017, from http://emedicine.medscape.com/article/1195402-overview.

Villa, A., Wolff, A., Aframian, D., Vissink, A., Ekström, J., Proctor, G., et al. (2015). World Workshop on Oral Medicine VI: A systematic review of medication-induced salivary gland dysfunction: prevalence, diagnosis, and treatment. *Clinical Oral Investigations, 19*(7), 1563–1580. doi:10.1007/s00784-015-1488-2.

Volkert, D., et al. (2015). ESPEN guideline on nutrition in dementia. *Clinical Nutrition: Official Journal of the European Society of Parenteral and Enteral Nutrition*, *34*, 1052–1073.

Vollman, K., Dickinson, S., & Powers, J. (2017). Pronation therapy. In D. L. Wiegand (Ed.), *AACN procedure manual for high acuity, progressive, and critical care* (7th ed.). Philadelphia: Saunders Elsevier.

Vollman, K., Sole, M., & Quinn, B. (2017). Endotracheal tube care and oral care practices for ventilated and non-ventilated patients. In D. L. Wiegand (Ed.), *AACN procedure manual for high acuity, progressive, and critical care* (7th ed.). Philadelphia: Saunders Elsevier.

von Leupoldt, A., Van den Bergh, O., & Davenport, P. (2014). Anxiety, depression, and panic. In D. A. Mahler & D. E. O'Donnell (Eds.), *Dyspnea mechanisms, measurement and management*. Boca Raton, FL: CRC Press Taylor & Francis Group.

Vorvick, L. J. (2014). *Corneal Injury*. http://umm.edu/health/medical/ency/articles/corneal-injury. Retrieved October 31, 2017.

Vrtis, M. C. (2013). The economic impact of complex wound care on home health agencies. *Journal of Wound, Ostomy, and Continence Nursing*, *40*(4), 360–363.

Wachs, J. (2005). Building the occupational health team keys to successful interdisciplinary collaboration. *Workplace Health and Safety*, *53*(4), 166–171.

Wagg, A., Gibson, W., Ostaszkiewicz, J., Johnson, T., Markland, A., Palmer, M., et al. (2014). Urinary incontinence in frail elderly persons: Report from the 5th international consultation on incontinence. *Neurourology and Urodynamics*, *34*, 398–406.

Wagner, K. D., & Hardin-Pierce, M. G. (2014). *High acuity nursing* (6th ed.). Boston, MA: Prentice Hall.

Wakai, A., Lawrenson, J. G., Lawrenson, A. L., Wang, Y., Brown, M. D., Quirke, M., et al. (2017). Topical non-steroidal anti-inflammatory drugs for analgesia in traumatic corneal abrasion. *Cochrane Database of Systematic Reviews*, (5).

Wan, D., & Krassioukov, A. (2014). Life-threatening outcomes associated with autonomic dysreflexia: A clinical review. *The Journal of Spinal Cord Medicine*, *37*(1), 2–10.

Ward, D., & Fulbrook, P. (2016). Nursing strategies for effective weaning of the critically ill mechanically ventilated patient. *Critical Care Nursing Clinics of North America*, *28*(4), 499–512.

Watson, K. B., Carlson, S. A., Gunn, J. P., Galuska, D. A., O'Connor, A., Greenlund, K. J., et al. (2016). Physical activity among adults aged 50 years and older—United States, 2014. *MMWR. Morbidity & Mortality Weekly Report*, *65*(36), 954–958.

WebMD.com. (2017). *Smoking Cessation Health Center*. Retrieved April 12, 2018, from https://www.webmd.com/smoking-cessation/default.htm.

Westfal, M. L., & Goldstein, A. M. (2017). Pediatric enteric neuropathies: Diagnosis and current management. *Current Opinion in Pediatrics*, *29*(3), 347–353.

Whelton, P. K., Carey, R. M., Aronow, W. S., et al. (2017). ACC/AHA/AAPA/ABC/ACPM/AGS/APhA/ASH/ASPC/NMA/PCNA guidelines for the prevention, detection, evaluation, and management of high blood pressure in adults. A report of the American Collage of Cardiology/American Heart Association Task Forces on Clinical Practice Guidelines. *Journal of the American College of Cardiology*, *71*, e127–e248. http://www.onlinejacc.org/content/71/19/e127?_ga=2.66372653.2004839219.1542569578-506177100.1542569578.

White, J., Guenter, P., & Gordon, J. (2012). Consensus statement of the academy of nutrition and dietetics/American society for parenteral and enteral nutrition: Characteristics recommended for the identification and documentation of adult malnutrition. *Journal of the Academy of Nutrition and Dietetics*, *112*, 730–738.

Whitehead, W. E., Palsson, O. S., & Simren, M. (2016). Treating fecal incontinence: An unmet need in primary care medicine. *North Carolina Medical Journal*, *77*(3), 211–215.

Willson, M. M., Angyus, M., Beals, D., et al. (2014). Executive summary: A quick reference guide for managing fecal incontinence. *Journal of Wound, Ostomy, and Continence Nursing*, *41*(1), 61–69

Winslow, E. H., & Jacobson, A. F. (1998). Dispelling the petroleum jelly myth. *Asian Journal of Nursing*, *98*(11), 16.

Witt, D. M., Clark, N. P., Kaatz, S., et al. (2016). Guidance for the practical management of warfarin therapy in the treatment of venous thromboembolism. *Journal of Thrombosis and Thrombolysis*, *41*, 187–205.

Wolf, P. A., Abbott, R. D., & Kannel, W. B. (1991). Atrial fibrillation as an independent risk factor for stroke: The Framingham Study. *Stroke; a Journal of Cerebral Circulation*, *22p*, 983–988.

World Health Organization. (2016). *Global guidelines for the prevention of surgical site infection*. Geneva. Switzerland: WHO Press. http://www.who.int/gpsc/ssi-guidelines/en/.

Xue, Y. (2014). *Peripheral intravenous line: Insertion*. JoAnn Briggs Institute EBP Database. JB11841.

Yancy, C. W., Jessup, M., Bozkurt, B., et al. (2013). ACCF/AHA guideline for the management of heart failure: A report of the American College of Cardiology Foundation/American Heart Association Task Force on Practice Guidelines. *Circulation*, *128*, e240–e327.

Yancy, C. W., Jessup, M., Bozkurt, B., et al. (2017). ACCF/AHA/HFSA focused update of the 2013 ACCF/AHA guideline for the management of heart failure: A report of the American College of Cardiology Foundation/American Heart Association Task Force on Clinical Practice Guidelines and the Heart Failure Society of America. *Circulation*, 1–75.

Yardley, L., Beyer, N., Hauer, K., et al. (2005). Development and initial validation of the falls efficacy scale-international (FES-I). *Age and Ageing*, *34*(6), 614–619.

Yokoe, D. S., Anderson, D. J., Berenholtz, S. M., Calfee, D. P., Dubberke, E. R., Ellingson, K. D., et al. (2014). A compendium of strategies to prevent healthcare-associated infections in the acute care hospitals: 2014 updates. *Infection Control and Hospital Epidemiology*, *35*(8), 967–977.

Yorio, P. L., & Wachter, J. K. (2014). Safety-and-health-specific high-performance work practices & occupational injury and illness prevention: The mediating role of task & team safety proficiency behaviors. *ASSE Journal of Safety, Health & Environmental Research*, *10*(1), 123–134.

Young, J. S. (2015). Age-related eye disease and recommendations for low vision AIDS. *Home Healthcare Now*, *33*(1), 10–17.

Young, C. J., Zahid, A., Koh, C. E., & Young, J. M. (2017). Hypothesized summative anal physiology score correlates but poorly predicts incontinence severity. *World Journal of Gastroenterology*, *59*(2), 99–105.

Zafren, K. (2017). Out-of-hospital evaluation and treatment of accidental hypothermia. *Emergency Medicine Clinics of North America*, *35*, 261–279. doi:10.1016/j.emc.2017.01.003.

Zafren, K., & Griesbrecht, G. (2014). *State of Alaska: Cold injuries guidelines.* Retrieved from http://dhss.alaska.gov/dph/Emergency/Documents/ems/documents/Alaska%20DHSS%20EMS%20Cold%20Injuries%20Guidelines%20June%202014.pdf.

INDEX

E

M

N

O

Q

R

S

U